CDC Health Information for International Travel 2010

THE YELLOW BOOK

For Elsevier

Commissioning Editor: Sue Hodgson
Development Editor: Joanne Scott
Editorial Assistant: Rachael Harrison
Project Manager: Susan Stuart
Design: Stewart Larking
Marketing Managers (UK/USA): Clara Toombs, Courtney Ingram
Production: Helius

CDC Health Information for International Travel 2010

THE YELLOW BOOK

Managing Editor

Gary W. Brunette, MD, MS

Medical Editors

Phyllis E. Kozarsky, MD
Alan J. Magill, MD
David R. Shlim, MD

Associate Editor

Amanda D. Whatley, MPH

U.S. DEPARTMENT OF HEALTH AND HUMAN SERVICES
Public Health Service
Centers for Disease Control and Prevention
National Center for Preparedness, Detection, and Control of Infectious Diseases
Division of Global Migration and Quarantine
Atlanta, Georgia

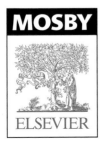

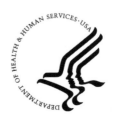

MOSBY

ELSEVIER

MOSBY is an imprint of Elsevier Inc.

© 2009, Elsevier Inc. All rights reserved.

ISBN: 978-0-7020-3481-7

Suggested Citation

Centers for Disease Control and Prevention. CDC Health Information for International Travel 2010. Atlanta: U.S. Department of Health and Human Services, Public Health Service, 2009.

Readers are invited to send comments and suggestions regarding this publication to Gary W. Brunette, Managing Editor, Centers for Disease Control and Prevention, Division of Global Migration and Quarantine (E-03), Geographic Medicine and Health Promotion Branch, 1600 Clifton Road NE, Atlanta, Georgia 30333, USA.

Disclaimers

Both generic and trade names are used in this text. In all cases, the decision to use one or the other was made based on recognition factors and was done for the convenience of the intended audience. Therefore, the use of trade names and commercial sources in this publication is for identification only and does not imply endorsement by the U.S. Department of Health and Human Services, the Public Health Service, or the Centers for Disease Control and Prevention.

References to non-CDC sites on the Internet are provided as a service to readers and do not constitute or imply endorsement of these organizations or their programs by the U.S. Department of Health and Human Services, the Public Health Service, or the Centers for Disease Control and Prevention. CDC is not responsible for the content of these sites. URL addresses were current as of the date of publication.

Notice

Medical knowledge is constantly changing. Standard safety precautions must be followed, but as new research and clinical experience broaden our knowledge, changes in treatment and drug therapy may become necessary or appropriate. Readers are advised to check the most current product information provided by the manufacturer of each drug to be administered to verify the recommended dose, the method and duration of administration, and contraindications. It is the responsibility of the practitioner, relying on experience and knowledge of the patient, to determine dosages and the best treatment for each individual patient. Neither the publisher nor the authors assume any liability for any injury and/or damage to persons or property arising from this publication.

The Publisher

For additional copies, please contact Elsevier Inc. Order online at www.elsevierhealth.com

British Library Cataloguing in Publication Data

CDC health information for international travel 2010.
1. Travel—Health aspects.
I. Health information for international travel 2010
II. Yellow book
III. Brunette, Gary W.
IV. Centers for Disease Control and Prevention
613.6′8-dc22
ISBN-13: 9780702034817

Library of Congress Cataloging in Publication Data

A catalog record for this book is available from the Library of Congress.

Printed in Spain

Last digit is the print number: 9 8 7 6 5 4 3 2 1

Contents

List of Tables

List of Maps

List of Figures

List of Boxes

CDC Contributors

Adjemian, Jennifer
Alexander, James P.
Alexander, Nicole T.
Anderson, Alicia
Ansari, Armin
Arguin, Paul M.
Ari, Mary D.
Atkinson, William
Bair-Brake, Heather
Balaban, Victor
Barskey, Albert E., IV
Barzilay, Ezra J.
Batts, Dahna
Beach, Michael
Benzekri, Noelle A.
Bern, Caryn
Boore, Amy L.
Brooks, John T.
Brown, Clive M.
Brunette, Gary W.
Cano, Maria V.
Chaves, Sandra S.
Chiller, Tom
Chosewood, L. Casey
Cohn, Amanda
Dasch, Gregory A.
Davis, Xiaohong Mao
De, Barun K.
Deming, Michael
Dorell, Christina
Dunne, Eileen F.
Dykewicz, Clare A.
Eremeeva, Marina E.
Fagan, Ryan P.
Farnon, Eileen C.
Fischer, Marc
Fox, LeAnne M.
Gallagher, Kathleen M.
Gallagher, Nancy M.
Galland, G. Gale
Gee, Jay E.
Gershman, Mark

Gould, L. Hannah
Green, Michael D.
Griggs, Anne
Guerra, Marta A.
Hall, Aron J.
Herwaldt, Barbara L.
Hicks, Lauri A.
Hlavsa, Michele C.
Holmberg, Scott
Illig, Petra A.
Jackson, Michael L.
Jentes, Emily S.
Johnston, Stephanie P.
Jones, Jeffrey L.
Joyce, M. Patricia
Kozarsky, Phyllis E.
Kroger, Andrew
Kutty, Preeta K.
Lawson, Carl
LoBue, Philip
Lynch, Michael
Mali, Sonja
Malilay, Josephine
Maloney, Susan
Marano, Nina
Marienau, Karen J.
McCarron, Margaret
McQuiston, Jennifer
Mead, Paul S.
Miller, Charles W.
Mintz, Eric
Mitruka, Kiren
Montgomery, Susan
Moore, Anne
Moro, Pedro L.
Mullan, Robert J.
Nasci, Roger S.
Naughton, Mary P.
Nuorti, J. Pekka
Ortega, Luis S.
Park, Benjamin
Parker, Amy A.

Powers, Ann M.
Reed, Christie M.
Reef, Susan E.
Reynolds, Mary G.
Rollin, Pierre E.
Roy, Sharon
Rupprecht, Charles E.
Schantz, Peter M.
Schilling, Katharine
Schroeder, Betsy
Shadomy, Sean V.
Shay, David K.
Shealy, Katherine
Skoff, Tami H.
Sleet, David A.
Smith, Theresa L.
Sommers, Theresa
Staples, J. Erin
Steele, Stefanie F.
Stoddard, Robyn
Sutton, Madeline
Tan, Kathrine R.
Teo, Chong-Gee
Thomas, Cynthia G.
Tiwari, Tejpratap S. P.
Tomashek, Kay M.
Uzicanin, Amra
Viray, Melissa
Wallace, L. J. David
Warnock, Eli W., III
Wassilak, Steven
Watson, John C.
Weber, Ingrid B.
Weinberg, Michelle
Weinberg, Nicholas
Whatley, Amanda D.
Widdowson, Marc-Alain
Wiersma, Steven T.
Wirtz, Robert A.
Workowski, Kimberly
Yanni, Emad
Zielinski-Gutierrez, Emily

External Contributors

Acosta, Rebecca W.   Traveler's Medical Service of New York, New York, NY
Ansdell, Vernon E.   University of Hawaii, Honolulu, HI
Backer, Howard D.   California Department of Public Health, Richmond, CA

Barbeau, Deborah Nicolls	Tulane University, New Orleans, LA
Barnett, Elizabeth D.	Boston University School of Medicine and Boston Medical Center, Boston, MA
Borwein, Sarah T.	TravelSafe, Hong Kong, China
Carroll, I. Dale	The Pregnant Traveler, Spring Lake, MI
Chavez, Gilberto F.	California Department of Public Health, Sacramento, CA
Connor, Bradley A.	Weill Medical College of Cornell University, New York, NY
Franco-Paredes, Carlos	Emory University, Atlanta, GA
Freedman, David O.	University of Alabama, Birmingham, AL
Guerrant, Richard L.	University of Virginia School of Medicine, Charlottesville, VA
Gushulak, Brian D.	Migration Health Consultants, Cheltenham, Canada
Hackett, Peter H.	Institute for Altitude Medicine, Telluride, CO
Harriman, Kathleen H.	California Department of Public Health, Richmond, CA
Hidron, Alicia I.	Emory University, Atlanta, GA
Howard, Cynthia R.	University of Minnesota, Minneapolis, MN
John, Chandy C.	University of Minnesota, Minneapolis, MN
Jong, Elaine C.	University of Washington, Seattle, WA
Kain, Kevin C.	University of Toronto, Toronto, Canada
Keystone, Jay S.	University of Toronto, Toronto, Canada
LaRocque, Regina C.	Massachusetts General Hospital and Harvard University, Boston, MA
Mackell, Sheila M.	Mountain View Pediatrics, Flagstaff, AZ
Magill, Alan J.	Walter Reed Army Institute of Research, Silver Spring, MD
McCarthy, Anne E.	University of Ottawa, Ottawa, Canada
Nord, Daniel A.	Divers Alert Network, Durham, NC
Ostroff, Stephen M.	Pennsylvania Department of Health, Harrisburg, PA
Pawlowski, Sean W.	University of Virginia School of Medicine, Charlottesville, VA
Ryan, Edward T.	Massachusetts General Hospital and Harvard University, Boston, MA
Shlim, David R.	Jackson Hole Travel and Tropical Medicine, Jackson Hole, WY
Stauffer, William M.	University of Minnesota, Minneapolis, MN and CDC Atlanta, GA
Walker, Patricia F.	HealthPartners, Center for International Health, St. Paul, MN
Wilson, Mary Elizabeth	Harvard Medical School and Harvard School of Public Health, Boston, MA

All contributors have signed a statement indicating that they have no conflicts of interest with the subject matter or materials discussed in the document(s) that they have written or reviewed for this book and that the information that they have written or reviewed for this book is objective and free from bias.

Acknowledgments

The *CDC Health Information for International Travel 2010* editorial team gratefully acknowledges all the authors and reviewers for their commitment to this new edition. We extend sincere thanks to the following individuals and groups for their contributions to the production of this book:

- Kevin Liske, Jeffery Henry, and Robert Neurath (Geospatial Research, Analysis and Services Program of the Agency for Toxic Substances and Disease Registry) for creating all the maps contained in this publication;
- Tiffany Bailey, Amanda Crowell, Linda Frank, Shannon Omisore, Jacqui Read, and Cathy Young in CDC's Writer–Editor Services Branch;
- Kelly Holton, Theresa Sommers, Heather Bair-Brake, Katherine Mues, Laurie Dieterich, and Tricia Schwartz for their additional assistance in preparing the text for publication; and
- Elise Beltrami, Clive Brown, Mark Gershman, Emily Jentes, Katherine Johnson, Nina Marano, and Ava Navin for their extensive review of the text.

Preface

The *CDC Health Information for International Travel 2010* has been extensively revised for this latest edition in an effort to stay on the cutting edge of travel health information. The book is meant to be a guide to the practice of travel medicine, as well as the authoritative source of U.S. government recommendations for immunizations and prophylaxis for foreign travel. International travel is becoming more and more commonplace, and thus having at least a basic understanding of the medical problems that travelers face has become a necessary aspect of practicing medicine. The goal of this book is to be a comprehensive resource for the practitioner and public to find the answers to their travel-related questions, whether before travel, during travel, or post-travel.

NATIONAL CENTER FOR PREPAREDNESS, DETECTION AND CONTROL
OF INFECTIOUS DISEASES
Rima Khabbaz, MD, Director

DIVISION OF GLOBAL MIGRATION AND QUARANTINE
Martin S. Cetron, MD, Director

Nina Marano, DVM, MPH, Chief, Geographic Medicine and Health Promotion Branch

Phyllis E. Kozarsky, MD, Expert Consultant, Travelers' Health

Gary W. Brunette, MD, MS, Medical Epidemiologist

Amanda D. Whatley, MPH, CHES, Health Communications Specialist

1

Introduction

INTRODUCTION TO TRAVEL HEALTH AND THE YELLOW BOOK

Amanda D. Whatley, Phyllis E. Kozarsky

Travel Health

International travel continues to grow substantially every year. Not only are more travelers moving about, but they are heading to areas that have rarely been visited in the past. The travelers range in age from very young infants and small children to centenarians; they may have pre-existing medical conditions, may be immunosuppressed, or may be pregnant or contemplating pregnancy. Additionally, people travel internationally for a variety of reasons other than tourism including: business, study abroad and research programs, visiting friends and relatives, ecotourism, adventure, medical tourism, mission work, or responding to an international disaster. The infectious disease risks that travelers face are a shifting target—some travel destinations have become safer, but in others, new diseases have emerged and old ones have re-emerged.

The risk of becoming ill or injured during international travel depends on many factors, such as the region of the world visited, a traveler's age and health status, the length of the trip, and the diversity of planned activities. The Centers for Disease Control and Prevention (CDC) provides travel health information to address the many different health risks a traveler may face, with the aim of assisting travelers and their health-care providers to better understand the measures necessary to prevent illness and injury during international travel. This publication and the CDC Travelers' Health website (www.cdc.gov/travel) are the two primary avenues of communication with these audiences.

The History and Roles of the Yellow Book and the International Health Regulations

CDC Health Information for International Travel ("The Yellow Book") has been a trusted resource since 1967. Originally, it was a small pamphlet published to satisfy the World

Health Organization (WHO) International Health Regulations' (IHR) requirements. As a member state, the United States is responsible for informing the public about health requirements for entering other countries, such as the necessity of being vaccinated against yellow fever. The purpose of the IHR is to ensure maximum security against the international spread of diseases, with minimum interference with world travel and commerce. Epidemics have always been catalysts for intensive multilateral collaboration in public health. A copy of the current IHR and its supporting information can be found on the WHO website at www.who.int/csr/ihr/en/.

The IHR were originally intended to help monitor and control six serious infectious diseases: cholera, plague, relapsing fever, smallpox, typhus, and yellow fever. Under the 2005 IHR, as part of the notification requirement, member states are required to assess whether events may constitute a public health emergency of international concern (PHEIC). The occurrence of smallpox, SARS, wild poliovirus, and novel influenza, irrespective of context, requires immediate notification to the WHO. A PHEIC is an event that constitutes a public health risk to other member states with international consequences, such as the spread of disease, and that potentially requires a coordinated international response, as in the case of smallpox, SARS, wild poliovirus, or novel influenza. The 2005 IHR revisions require that these events be assessed and notified to the WHO. This definition broadens the scope of the IHR to cover existing, new, and re-emerging diseases, including emergencies caused by chemical, biological, or radiological agents and the context surrounding these events. As a member state of the WHO, the United States adheres to the IHR and participated in their development.

Most immunizations are not required under the IHR but may be recommended to protect the health of the traveler. However, an International Certificate of Vaccination or Prophylaxis (ICVP) documenting yellow fever vaccine administration is required of all travelers by some countries as a condition for entry, while other countries require vaccination against yellow fever only if travelers arrive from a country where the disease is present. The Yellow Book and the CDC Travelers' Health website aim to define and communicate requirements under the IHR. Although this publication includes the most current available information regarding these requirements, requirements can change. Current information must be accessed to ensure that these requirements are met; the CDC Travelers' Health website may be checked for regularly updated information.

The Yellow Book is written primarily for health-care providers, including physicians, nurses, and pharmacists. Others, such as the travel industry, multinational corporations, missionary and volunteer organizations, and travelers themselves, can also find a wealth of information here.

This text is authored by subject-matter experts from within CDC and outside the agency. The guidelines presented in this book are evidence-based and supported by best practices. Internal text citations have not been included; however, references are included at the end of each section for those who would like to obtain more detailed information. *CDC Health Information for International Travel 2010* is produced by the Division of Global Migration and Quarantine, National Center for Preparedness, Detection, and Control of Infectious Diseases, Centers for Disease Control and Prevention. The 2010 edition is the third edition published by Elsevier Inc., publishers of numerous authoritative texts on infectious diseases and travel medicine.

In addition to the hard-copy text, a searchable online version of the Yellow Book can be found on the CDC Travelers' Health website at www.cdc.gov/yellowbook.

New in the 2010 Edition

Readers of previous versions will notice several differences in the 2010 edition of the Yellow Book. As with previous editions, the 2010 edition covers new and updated vaccine guidelines and new developments in the prevention and treatment of malaria and other health risks. The Yellow Book's scope has also been broadened to address emerging infectious diseases and travel health issues. To aid in quick scanning and utility, authors and editors have taken a more streamlined approach to presenting information, including more bullets separating concepts.

Chapter Notes

A few chapters contain important changes in the 2010 edition and are highlighted below.

Chapter 2: The Pre-Travel Consultation

Since the primary audience of the Yellow Book is clinicians who will be assisting individuals in their travel preparation, the layout of the book has been set up to match the inherent chronology of travel—the pre-travel planning and medical visit, issues that can occur during travel, and conditions that must be dealt with after travel. Topics and diseases most commonly discussed in a pre-travel consultation are found in Chapter 2. Just as in most pre-travel consultations, issues concerning both travel-related and routine vaccines are discussed first. The text continues with malaria information, self-treatable disease topics, and finally concludes with topics generally discussed when counseling travelers about healthy behaviors that may decrease risk of illness and injury. Yellow fever requirements and recommendations by country remain in chart format, identifiable by yellow edges for quick reference. Country-specific malaria risk information and recommendations, previously listed in the same chart as yellow fever risk, are now located in a separate chart, identifiable by red edges.

Chapter 3: Select Destinations and Travel Itineraries

In this entirely new chapter, some popular tourist destinations and routes are discussed by authors who have lived in or visited these areas. The purpose of this chapter is to better orient providers who may not have had the opportunity to travel to these destinations, frequented by many travelers and from which many questions are generated. Similar to a guide book, authors discuss the destination along with the reality of various health risks to aid clinicians in preparing travelers. These sections are editorial in nature, containing the author's expressed opinions and aim to present topics for consideration; they should not necessarily be taken as a prescription for pre-travel care.

Chapter 5: Other Infectious Diseases Related to Travel

This chapter highlights diseases related to travel that are not as commonly discussed during the pre-travel consultation. They are important diseases with which to become familiar, especially if one also sees patients after travel or wishes to triage quickly prior to referral. Readers may notice that these sections have taken on a new format to aid in quick reference in the clinical setting.

Chapter 9: Health Considerations for Newly Arrived Immigrants and Refugees

This chapter is also new and discusses health issues related to immigrants and refugees. Many clinicians giving pre-travel care may also give care to these populations. Additionally, these groups of people may be more likely to travel to their home country to visit friends and relatives in the future and are at very high risk of travel-related diseases.

Appendices

Be sure to note the new Appendices that have been added as reference material in travel medicine:

- Appendix A: Promotion of Quality in the Practice of Travel Medicine—including a discussion about the growing field of Travel Medicine
- Appendix B: Essential Electronic Resources for the Travel Medicine Practitioner—including links to many helpful online resources containing travel health information
- Appendix C: Travel Vaccine Summary Table—including information helpful in administering or prescribing travel-related vaccines

Editorial Sections—*Perspectives*

An exciting new feature in the 2010 edition is the incorporation of editorial sections, bordered in green and entitled *Perspectives*. Although there is an increasing body of evidence-based knowledge in this new and growing field of travel medicine, there is also recognition that the practice of this specialty is not only science, but art, as well. Thus, readers will notice a few sections that contain editorial discussions aiming to add depth and clinical perspective, as well as to discuss some controversies or differences in opinions and practice.

Contact Information for CDC

Questions, comments, and suggestions for CDC Travelers' Health, including comments about this publication, may be made through the CDC-INFO contact center (toll-free at 800-CDC-INFO or cdcinfo@cdc.gov). Travelers with specific health questions should call their health-care provider. Health-care providers with urgent health questions about their patients should contact their local or state health department.

Additionally, health-care providers needing assistance with the diagnosis or management of suspected cases of malaria can contact CDC's Malaria Branch Telephone Hotline at 770-488-7788 during business hours. After hours and on weekends, a Malaria Branch clinician may be reached by calling 770-488-7100.

PLANNING FOR HEALTHY TRAVEL: RESPONSIBILITIES OF THE TRAVELER, CLINICIAN, AND TRAVEL INDUSTRY

Amanda D. Whatley, Nina Marano, Phyllis E. Kozarsky

In 2007, approximately 14% of adult U.S. residents spent at least one night outside the United States. Additionally, there were over 64 million trips outside the country, a 21% increase since 1997. As international travel has increased dramatically over the past decades and as travelers choose more varied destinations and activities, the responsibilities of the traveler, clinician, and travel industry become more complex and interdependent. This section outlines how these groups can work together so that travel may be safer and healthier, and more enjoyable.

Responsibilities of the Traveler

Although studies have shown that the majority of travelers from the United States and other countries do not seek pre-travel health advice, travelers do need to understand the health risks that traveling internationally may pose and take an active part in health preparation. Whether a person is a frequent international traveler or on the trip of a lifetime, he or she can take steps to plan for healthy and safe travel.

- **Gather information about the travel destination(s) and possible activities.**
  - Regardless of whether travelers are planning their own trips or joining a tour group, travelers should find out as many details as possible about their travel destinations, modes of travel, lodging, food, and activities during the trip.
  - These details are important to tailoring the travel health advice individually for each person. For example, two travelers to the same country but who have different itineraries and planned activities may be provided different vaccines, medications, and detailed advice in preparation for their trips.
- **Visit the CDC Travelers' Health website for health information.**
  - The website (www.cdc.gov/travel) is kept current with latest recommendations concerning endemic diseases, as well as outbreaks around the world and other health-related situations, such as effects of natural disasters.

- o Of particular interest are the destination pages with country-specific health information.
  - o The information provided on the website, along with that from a health-care provider, will equip travelers with what they need to know to remain as healthy as possible.
- **Seek pre-travel health advice from a health-care provider familiar with travel.**
  - o Travelers should make certain that there is enough time (ideally 4–6 weeks) to see a health-care provider and obtain any necessary vaccinations before they travel. Those with imminent travel, such as business travelers, should still seek travel health advice from an expert.
  - o Even healthy young adults going to developed areas should be up-to-date on their routine vaccinations. Vaccination practices in other parts of the world vary. Travel anywhere outside the United States, even to industrialized regions, such as Western Europe, presents a risk for exposure to measles and other vaccine-preventable conditions, such as influenza and hepatitis A.
  - o One of the most important ways that travelers can prepare for their visit with a health-care provider is to come to the clinic with helpful details that will facilitate a pre-travel consultation (Box 1-1).
  - o The CDC Travelers' Health website provides help in locating a clinic for pre-travel consultation. The site provides links to directories of travel medicine clinicians who are members of the International Society of Travel Medicine and the American Society of Tropical Medicine and Hygiene. The site also provides links to state health departments and the Yellow Fever Vaccination Clinic Registry that lists facilities approved to provide yellow fever vaccinations (wwwn.cdc.gov/travel/contentTravelClinics.aspx).
- **Prevent illness during travel.**
  - o Even with travel advice, vaccines, and medications, a person is not 100% protected against all diseases or injuries. Healthy behaviors, such as being careful about food and water, protecting against insect and mosquito bites, and washing hands frequently, are important ways of preventing many common travel illnesses.
  - o Travelers should prepare and carry a travel health kit (see the Travel Health Kits section in Chapter 2), equipped with many items that can help prevent and treat common travel-related illnesses and injuries.
  - o Increased awareness of cough hygiene or respiratory etiquette (such as covering one's mouth when coughing) is not only a courtesy, but if generally practiced, would help reduce transmission of respiratory and influenza-like illnesses. Travelers should exercise appropriate precautions and try not to travel if they are ill with a communicable disease that is spread easily to other people (see the Obtaining Health Care Abroad for the Ill Traveler section in Chapter 2).

Responsibilities of the Clinician

Regardless of their specialty, most clinicians will encounter a traveling patient at some point in their practice. It is important for clinicians, especially those in primary care, to know some basic travel health information to determine the extent of health advice their patients should access prior to traveling and to recognize common post-travel health symptoms and syndromes.

- **Incorporate the subject of travel medicine into one's practice.**
  - o This might be as basic as asking patients if they are planning to travel internationally, particularly to a developing country destination, and referring them to a travel medicine clinic.
  - o Clinicians should emphasize the importance of a pre-travel consultation and the fact that international travel can pose special health risks that should be addressed.

Box 1-1. Questions for persons preparing to travel

The following questions are a starting point for planning the health aspects of one's travel. Travelers will be well prepared for their travel medicine encounter if they know most of the answers to these questions.

Details of your trip and travel history

- When are you traveling, and how long will you be at each location?
- Where are you traveling?
  - In what countries will you be traveling?
  - Where within the country or countries will you be traveling?
  - Are these destinations urban areas or rural areas?
  - What are the conditions of your lodging (such as hotel with air conditioning, screened cabin, or open-air tents)?
- What activities will you be doing while traveling (such as hiking, backpacking, or scuba diving, sightseeing)?
- Have you traveled internationally in the past?
  - Where did you go?
  - When did you travel?

Personal health-related questions

- How old are you?
- What vaccinations have you had previously?
  - When did you have these vaccinations?
  - How many doses did you have of a particular vaccine (for example, some vaccines, such as the hepatitis A and B vaccines or the measles–mumps–rubella (MMR) vaccine, require multiple doses for long-term protection)?
  - Did you have any allergies or reactions to any previous vaccines?
- Do you have any other allergies (for example, medications, foods, or environmental)?
  - In particular, do you have an allergy to eggs, latex, yeast, mercury, or thimerosal?
- What is your medical history and current health status (for example, past illnesses and surgeries, chronic health problems, or other underlying medical conditions)?
- What medications are you currently taking or have you taken in the past 3 months?
- Do you have a weakened immune system?
- If you are a woman,
  - Are you pregnant now?
  - Are you trying to become pregnant, or will you try to become pregnant in the next 3 months?
  - Are you breastfeeding?
- Do you plan to seek medical care during your trip?

- Health-care providers should be particularly aware of individuals who have migrated to the United States from another country or who may be visiting friends or relatives in developing countries. The goal of inquiring well in advance would either allow the time for the individual to access a specialist in travel medicine or allow the health-care provider the opportunity to convey risk information over time, provide vaccine immunity by administering needed vaccines well in advance, and provide the patient the opportunity to consider possible costs over several months rather than require the patient to make a decision based on a single interaction.
- **Determine one's own limitations in giving pre-travel advice.**
  - Before evaluating an individual for a pre-travel consultation, the clinician should determine what level of information he or she is comfortable in giving to the patient regarding their travel plans. Choices are—
    - Referring all travelers to a travel clinic or a travel medicine specialist.
    - Offering basic pre-travel advice for less complex situations, such as advising travelers who are going on a short vacation to a popular tourist destination, like Mexico or the Caribbean. In such cases, updating routine vaccinations, providing hepatitis A and B vaccines, and providing education about healthy behaviors to prevent diseases and injuries may be all that is necessary.
    - Providing complex pre-travel consultations and making a commitment to the practice of travel medicine.

- **Give a comprehensive pre-travel consultation.**
  - For more information, see The Pre-Travel Consultation in Chapter 2. Basic components of a pre-travel consultation will include a risk assessment, providing health counseling and advice, and selection and administration of appropriate vaccinations and medications. There are several ways clinicians can extend their knowledge to provide comprehensive pre-travel care and more complex consultations.
  - The International Society of Travel Medicine (ISTM) provides educational resources, including the Journal of Travel Medicine, an active listserv, and a Certificate of Knowledge in Travel Health (CTH), awarded upon completion of an exam.
  - Numerous conferences are held throughout the year, both nationally and internationally, on the subject of travel medicine.
  - The Body of Knowledge for the Practice of Travel Medicine, which is the scope of the specialty of travel medicine, has been published, recently updated, and is available on the ISTM website (www.istm.org).
  - As the subject matter of travel medicine is quite dynamic, clinicians who will be regularly advising travelers in pre-travel consultations need to maintain a current base of knowledge. Many different Internet resources and databases, although sometimes incomplete or in conflict with one another, are available for clinicians to use to keep abreast of the health issues in international travel (see Appendix B).
  - In addition to general pre-travel consultations, some clinicians may also wish to become registered yellow fever vaccine providers. This process is initiated with one's state health department.
- **Recognize common disease symptoms and syndromes of international travelers.**
  - When assessing a patient who is ill, simply asking about their recent travel history is the first step in providing post-travel medical care. This can be a major clue in determining the cause of the ailment. For example, a patient who returns from sub-Saharan Africa with a fever and flu-like symptoms needs emergency attention to rule out malaria.
  - The extent of the care given by each clinician is personally determined. Knowing when one will refer a patient to a specialist and who that specialist would be are important decisions to make before patients come into the office seeking medical care, or even pre-travel health advice.
  - Patients needing more extensive post-travel care can be referred to a clinician in infectious diseases or clinical tropical medicine. The American Society of Tropical Medicine and Hygiene provides a listing of such clinicians on its website (www.astmh.org).
  - Further information about post-travel medical care can be found in Chapter 4.

Responsibilities of the Travel Industry

The responsibilities of the travel industry, including travel agencies, tour operators, and air and cruise lines, do not culminate with the final booking of the tickets or hotel rooms. These members of the travel industry, too, should learn about the basics of travel medicine as it affects the areas of the world where their customers are traveling.

- **Learn about health risks around the world.**
  - Access the CDC Travelers' Health website for information about many travel destinations (www.cdc.gov/travel).
- **Acknowledge travel health risks and provide resources for education for travelers.**
  - Studies have shown that customers often look to their travel agents to advise them on all aspects of their trip, including health risks and preventive actions they should take.

    ○ Although the role of the travel industry is not to provide personal medical consultations, mentioning that health risks exist and referring travelers to a clinic or to the ISTM website are appropriate actions.

    ○ Most travelers will likely travel regardless of possible health risks if they know that they can take actions to help prevent getting sick. A healthy trip and a positive experience, as a result of proper preventive health behaviors, will be motivation to travel again in the future.

Resources for Travel Health Advice: CDC Website

Travelers' Health Website

Destination Pages

CDC's Travelers' Health website now features destination-specific pages with information on current CDC assessments of disease risk and recommendations for healthy travel (wwwn.cdc.gov/travel/destinationList.aspx).

Travel Notices

Prior to embarking on a trip, travelers and their health-care providers should consult sources such as the Travel Notice section of the website (wwwn.cdc.gov/travel/notices.aspx) for the latest information on outbreaks or other health-related issues.

CDC's Travel Notices are presented in the following four levels of increasing precautionary guidance to assist the traveler (Table 1-1). Most notices posted on the website appear under "In the News" or "Outbreak." In only one instance, during the outbreak of SARS in 2003, has postponement of nonessential travel to affected areas been recommended in a Travel Health Warning.

1. **In The News** provides information about sporadic cases of disease or an occurrence of a disease of public health significance affecting a traveler or travel destination. The risk for an individual traveler does not differ from the usual risk in that area.
2. **Outbreak Notice** provides information about a disease outbreak in a limited geographic area or setting. The risk to travelers is defined and limited, and the notice will remind travelers about standard or enhanced travel recommendations, such as vaccinations.
3. **Travel Health Precaution** provides specific information about a disease outbreak of greater scope and over a larger geographic area so travelers can take measures to reduce the risk of infection. CDC does not recommend against travel to a specific area but may recommend limiting exposure to a defined setting, such as poultry farms or health-care settings.
4. **Travel Health Warning** recommends against nonessential travel to an area because a disease of public health concern is expanding outside the areas or populations that were initially affected. The purpose of a travel warning is to reduce the volume of traffic to affected areas, thus limiting the risk of spreading the disease to unaffected areas.

Occasionally, travel notices may feature changes to existing recommendations, such as adding antimalarial prophylaxis for an area previously thought to be malaria free. If the outbreak resolves, the recommendation may be withdrawn. If the new recommendation becomes permanent, it will be highlighted and incorporated into the text of the online version of *CDC Health Information for International Travel 2010* at www.cdc.gov/yellowbook. A complete description of the definitions and criteria for issuing and removing travel notices can also be found in Table 1-1 and at wwwn.cdc.gov/travel/notices.aspx.

Malaria Website

CDC's Malaria website contains informational tools, educational materials, and cautionary tales of real people who acquired malaria after travel without adequate prophylactic measures (www.cdc.gov/malaria/travel/index.htm).

Table 1-1. Travel notice definitions

Type of Notice/ Level of Concern	Scope[1]	Risk for Travelers[2]	Preventive Measures	Example of Notice	Example of Recommended Measures
In the News	Reports of sporadic cases	No increased risk over baseline for travelers observing standard recommendations	Keeping travelers informed and reinforcing standard prevention recommendations	Report of dengue in Mexico in 2001	Reinforced standard recommendations for protection against insect bites
Outbreak Notice	Outbreak in limited geographic area or setting	Increased risk, but definable, and limited to specific settings	Reminders about standard and enhanced recommendations for the region	Outbreak of yellow fever in a state in Brazil in 2003	Reinforced enhanced recommendations, such as vaccination
Travel Health Precaution	Outbreak of greater scope affecting a larger geographic area	Increased risk in some settings along with risk for spread to other areas	Specific precautions to reduce risk during the stay, and what to do before and after travel[3]	Outbreak of avian influenza among poultry and humans in several countries in Southeast Asia in early 2004	Recommended specific precautions, including avoiding areas with live poultry, such as live animal markets and poultry farms; ensuring poultry and eggs are thoroughly cooked; monitoring health
Travel Health Warning	Evidence that outbreak is expanding outside the area or populations initially affected	Increased risk because evidence of transmission outside defined settings and/or inadequate containment measures	In addition to the specific precautions cited above, postpone nonessential travel[3]	SARS outbreak in Asia in 2003	Recommended travelers to postpone nonessential travel because of level of risk

1 The term "scope" incorporates the size, magnitude, and rapidity of spread of an outbreak.
2 Risk for travelers is dependent on patterns of transmission, as well as severity of illness.
3 Preventive measures other than the standard advice for the region may be recommended depending on the circumstances (i.e., travelers may be requested to monitor their health for a certain period after their return, or arriving passengers may be screened at ports of entry).

CDC's Malaria Risk Map is an interactive map that provides location-specific information on current CDC assessments of malaria risk and recommendations for preventive malaria treatment (www.cdc.gov/malaria/features/risk_map.htm).

References

1. Wolfe M, Acosta RW. Structure and organization of the pre-travel consultation and general advice for travelers. In: Keystone JS, Kozarsky PE, Freedman DO, Nothdurft HD, Connor BA, editors. Travel medicine. 2nd ed. Philadelphia: Mosby; 2008. p. 35–45.
2. CDC. Hepatitis Surveillance Report No. 61. Atlanta: US Department of Health and Human Services, Centers for Disease Control and Prevention; 2006.
3. Uyeki T, Zane SB, Bodnar UR, et al. Alaska/Yukon Territory respiratory outbreak investigation team: Large summertime influenza A outbreak among tourists in Alaska and the Yukon Territory. Clin Infect Dis. 2003;36(9):1095–102.
4. Kozarsky PE, Keystone JS. Body of knowledge for the practice of travel medicine. J Travel Med. 2002;9(2):112–5.
5. Keystone JS, Kozarsky PE, Freedman DO.

Internet- and computer-based resources for travel medicine practitioners. Clin Infect Dis. 2001;32(5):757–65.

6. Hamer DH, Connor BA. Travel health knowledge, attitudes and practices among United States travelers. J Travel Med. 2004;11(1):23–6.

7. Van Herck K, Van Damme P, Castelli F, et al. Knowledge, attitudes and practices in travel-related infectious diseases: The European Airport Survey. J Travel Med. 2004;11(1):3–8.

8. Toovey S, Jamieson A, Holloway M. Travelers' knowledge, attitudes and practices on the prevention of infectious diseases: Results

from a study at Johannesburg International Airport. J Travel Med 2004;11(1):16–22.

9. Provost S, Soto JC. Predictors of pretravel consultation in tourists from Québec (Canada). J Travel Med. 2001;8(2):66–75.

10. Provost S, Gaulin C, Piquet-Gauthier B, et al. Travel agents and the prevention of health problems among travelers in Québec. J Travel Med. 2002;9(1):3–9.

11. MacDougall LA, Gyorkos TW, Leffondré K, et al. Increasing referral of at-risk travelers to travel health clinics: evaluation of a health promotion intervention targeted to travel agents. J Travel Med. 2001;8(5):232–42.

TRAVEL EPIDEMIOLOGY

David O. Freedman

To prescribe optimal pre-travel advice, preventive measures, and education, travel health professionals must be aware of the absolute and relative magnitude of the many travel-related health risks. Such knowledge allows health-care providers to perform an epidemiologic and host-related risk assessment so that these measures can be appropriately prioritized for each traveler. Health problems are self-reported by 22%–64% of travelers to the developing world; most of these problems are mild, self-limited illnesses such as diarrhea, respiratory infections, and skin disorders. Approximately 8% of the more than 50 million travelers to developing regions, or 4 million persons, are ill enough to seek health care, either while abroad or upon returning home.

Limitations of Current Epidemiologic Knowledge

Knowledge of the precise risk for a specific disease in a specific location has proved elusive despite several decades of interest and investigation. (For additional discussion, see the Risks Travelers Face section later in this chapter.) A reasonably exact estimate of the number of cases of the disease or infection in all travelers over a time period at a location is difficult to determine, as many will have returned to their home countries by the time the disease manifests symptoms. Similarly difficult to obtain is an exact denominator reflecting the total numbers of travelers to that location, due to poor infrastructure in many destination countries. An accurate numerator must be divided by an accurate denominator to calculate a true incidence rate or risk. Even this standard population-based approach assumes that past experience predicts future risk. In addition, disease risks are not stable over time, and current or real-time data are rarely available. Much of the frequently quoted numerical data regarding the incidence of infection in travelers are based on extrapolations of limited data collected in limited samples of travelers anywhere from a few to more than 20 years ago. This knowledge base includes morbidity studies of various methodologic designs, each with its own set of strengths and weaknesses. These studies have mostly examined a few key individual diseases in all travelers regardless of destination; profiles of disease occurrence at a few specific high-risk destinations; and disease occurrence in certain types of travelers with certain behaviors. Many have been single-clinic or single-destination studies that can lead to conclusions that are not generalizable to groups of travelers with different local, national, or cultural backgrounds.

Incidence Rates and Estimates of Risk

A compilation of best available numerical incidence rate estimates, given the above limitations, is available and is frequently updated (Figure 1-1). With the notable exception of malaria, the major preventable travel-related diseases are associated with relatively low risks, ranging from 1 in 100 for influenza to less than 1 in 100,000 for several diseases that often concern travelers. Hepatitis A may be taken as an example of a prototypical vaccine-preventable disease, with an estimated overall uncorrected incidence of approximately 1 in 5,000 travelers to the developing world. Thus, the odds against acquiring hepatitis A on a single short trip are greatly in the traveler's favor, and many travelers are sophisticated enough to realize this. Any considered vaccination should be presented in context as insurance against a relatively uncommon event but one that may result in significant illness or consequences.

For diseases with poor or fatal outcomes, the context of less tolerance of even small risks needs to be communicated to travelers to help them make informed decisions about all available interventions. The incidence rates in Figure 1-1 are reflective of aggregate data and studies and do not consider variations in risk behaviors, destination, season, duration of travel, or general style of travel. For many diseases, research into

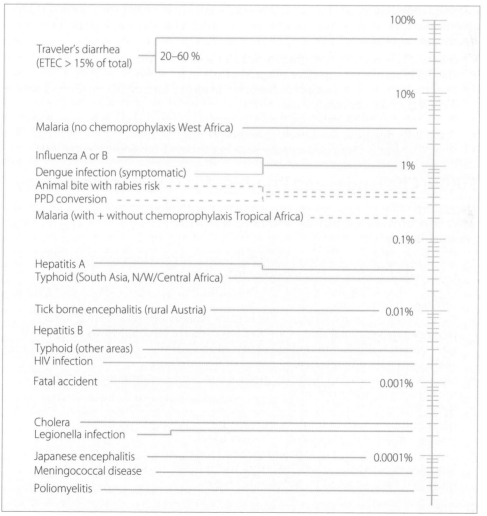

Figure 1-1. Incidence rate per month of health problems during a stay in developing countries—2008. (From Steffen R, Amitirigala I, Mutsch M. Health risks among travelers—need for regular updates. J Travel Med. 2008;15(3):145–6. Reprinted with permission from Wiley-Blackwell.)

increased or decreased risk according to these variables is still in its infancy due to difficulties in tracking outcomes at remote destinations.

Surveillance Networks and Tracking of Disease Profiles

A more recent and novel approach to defining disease epidemiology in travelers has involved the use of collaborative networks of specialized travel medicine clinics to collect and aggregate data on large samples of ill travelers who have been exposed in many countries and who are seen after their return home. One such network, GeoSentinel, a collaborative effort of the International Society of Travel Medicine and CDC has developed a profile of the relative likelihood of travel-related disease stratified by region of travel in the developing world (Figure 1-2).

Based on 17,353 ill returned travelers seen at 31 clinical sites on six continents, the destination-specific differences in relative frequencies are apparent for most diseases. Figure 1-2 shows destination-specific proportions of ill returned travelers with each diagnosis and not numerical incidence rates, which can be used to assist with risk-profiling of prospective travelers during the pre-travel medical consultation. When individual diagnoses were collected into syndrome groups and examined for all regions together, 226 of every 1,000 ill returned travelers seen by participating clinicians had a systemic febrile illness, 222 had acute diarrhea, 170 had a dermatologic disorder, 113 had chronic diarrhea, and 77 had a respiratory disorder. Important region-specific disease occurrence data indicated that—

- Febrile illness is most likely from Africa and Southeast Asia.
- Malaria is among the top three diagnoses from every region.
- Over the past decade dengue has become the most common febrile illness from every region outside sub-Saharan Africa.
- In sub-Saharan Africa, rickettsial disease is second only to malaria as a cause of fever.
- Respiratory disease is most likely in Southeast Asia.
- Acute diarrhea is disproportionately seen in travelers from South Central Asia.

Future Challenges and Priorities for Travel Epidemiology

Issues surrounding the relative merits of different methodologic approaches to defining travel-associated disease risk have recently been reviewed at length. Some epidemiologic priorities include:

- Travel-related data for many existing and potentially vaccine-preventable diseases. Current data are sparse, and incidence in local populations is often not reflective of travelers' risk due to different risk behaviors, previous infection, or pre-existing vaccination campaigns.
- Development of better surrogate markers for malaria exposure during travel to facilitate interventional studies for novel malaria chemoprophylaxis drugs. Such information is difficult to obtain because of the inability to perform placebo drug studies given the life-threatening nature of the infection.
- Studies of the impact of high-risk medical conditions or immunocompromising medications on travel outcome.
- Better understanding is needed of the impact of host behavior related to differing travel purposes, such as tourism, business travel, travel to visit friends and relatives, missionary travel, and volunteer travel.
- More insight is needed of exposure-related factors, such as urban vs. rural travel, long-stay vs. short-stay travel, luxury vs. rough travel, season of travel, and organized package travel vs. self-directed travel.

References

1. Steffen R, deBernardis C, Baños A. Travel epidemiology—a global perspective. Int J
Antimicrob Agents. 2003;21(2):89–95.
2. Steffen R, Rickenbach M, Wilhelm U, et al.

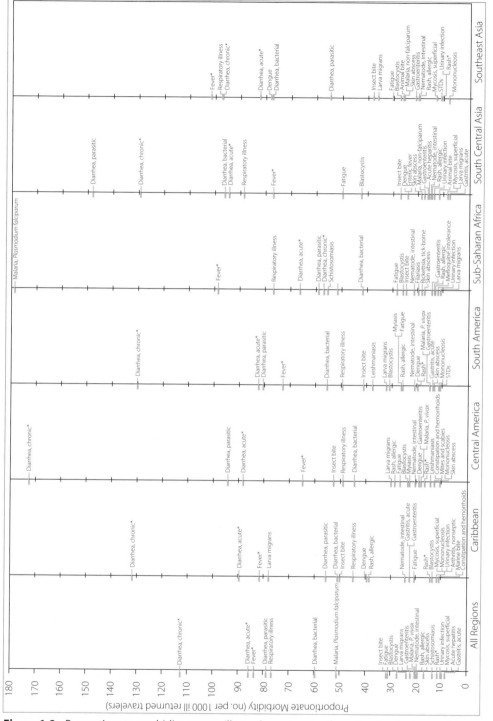

Figure 1-2. Proportionate morbidity among ill travelers returning from the developing world, according to region of travel.

The proportions are shown, not incidence rates, of each of the top 22 specific diagnoses for all ill returned travelers within each of the regions. STD denotes sexually transmitted disease. Asterisks indicated syndromic diagnoses for which specific etiologic diagnoses could not be assigned.

(From Freedman DO, Weld LH, Kozarsky PE, et al. GeoSentinel Surveillance Network. Spectrum of disease and relation to place of exposure among ill returned travelers. N Engl J Med. 2006;354(2): 119–30. Reprinted with permission from Massachusetts Medical Society.)

Health problems after travel to developing countries. J Infect Dis. 1987;156(1):84–91.

3. Hill DR. Health problems in a large cohort of Americans traveling to developing countries. J Travel Med. 2000;7(5):259–66.

4. Leder K, Wilson ME, Freedman DO, Torresi J. A comparative analysis of methodological approaches used for estimating risk in travel medicine. J Travel Med. 2008;15(4):263–72.

5. Caumes E, Ehya N, Nguyen J, Bricaire F. Typhoid and paratyphoid fever: A 10-year retrospective study of 41 cases in a Parisian hospital. J Travel Med. 2001;8(6):293–7.

6. Shah S, Filler S, Causer LM, et al. Malaria surveillance—United States, 2002. MMWR Surveill Summ. 2004;53(1):21–34.

7. Raoult D, Fournier PE, Fenollar F, et al. *Rickettsia africae*, a tick-borne pathogen in travelers to sub-Saharan Africa. N Engl J Med. 2001;344(20):1504–10.

8. Whitty CJ, Mabey DC, Armstrong M, et al. Presentation and outcome of 1107 cases of schistosomiasis from Africa diagnosed in a non-endemic country. Trans R Soc Trop Med Hyg. 2000;94(5):531–4.

9. Schwartz E, Weld LH, Wilder-Smith A, et al. GeoSentinel Surveillance Network. Seasonality, annual trends, and characteristics of dengue among ill returned travelers, 1997–2006.

Emerg Infect Dis. 2008;14(7):1081–8.

10. Taylor DN, Houston R, Shlim DR, et al. Etiology of diarrhea among travelers and foreign residents in Nepal. JAMA. 1988;260(9):1245–8.

11. Liese B, Mundt KA, Dell LD, et al. Medical insurance claims associated with international business travel. Occup Environ Med. 1997;54(7):499–503.

12. Herwaldt BL, de Arroyave KR, Roberts JM, Juranek DD. A multiyear prospective study of the risk factors for and incidence of diarrheal illness in a cohort of Peace Corps volunteers in Guatemala. Ann Intern Med. 2000;132(12):982–8.

13. Patel D, Easmon CJ, Dow C, et al. Medical repatriation of British diplomats resident overseas. J Travel Med. 2000;7(2):64–9.

14. Steffen R, Amitirigala I, Mutsch M. Health risks among travelers-need for regular updates. J Travel Med. 2008;15(3):145–6.

15. Mutsch M, Spicher VM, Gut C, Steffen R. Hepatitis A virus infections in travelers, 1988–2004. Clin Infect Dis. 2006;42(4):490–7.

16. Freedman DO, Weld LH, Kozarsky PE, et al. GeoSentinel Surveillance Network. Spectrum of disease and relation to place of exposure among ill returned travelers. N Engl J Med. 2006;354(2):119–30.

Perspectives: Risks Travelers Face

David R. Shlim

Travel medicine is based on the concept of the reduction of risk. In the context of travel medicine, "risk" refers to the possibility of harm during the course of a planned trip. Some risks may be avoidable, and others may not. Vaccine-preventable diseases may be mostly avoidable depending on the risk of the disease and the protective efficacy of the vaccine. The risk of malaria depends on the combination of the degree of local risk, behavior, efficacy of the prophylactic medication, and compliance by the traveler in taking the medication. Some risks are common but not life-threatening, such as travelers' diarrhea, or rare but severe, such as Japanese encephalitis. Nondisease risks, such as motor vehicle accidents or drowning, account for a much higher percentage of deaths among travelers than infectious diseases.

For most travelers, the perception of risk colors their choice of destinations, activities, and health concerns. Travel medicine practitioners may know statistics for a given risk, but whether the risk is considered high or low depends on the perception of the traveler. For example, the risk of dying while trekking in Nepal was shown to be 15 of every 100,000 trekkers. Although that was an accurate figure for the risk, there is no objective way to determine whether this is a high risk or a low risk. When the manuscript on trekking deaths was reviewed by two peer reviewers prior to acceptance by the journal, the first reviewer wrote, "You need to emphasize that these data show how dangerous trekking actually is." The second reviewer wrote, "You should make a point of stating that these data show how safe trekking is."

The subjective sense of risk is based on one's perception of risk ("15 per 100,000 means it's dangerous"), and one's tolerance for risk ("it may be 15 per 100,000, but it's worth it"). This subjective sense of risk suffuses the field of travel medicine, from the practitioner to the traveler, but it is rarely discussed. Some travelers canceled travel plans to Asia due to their fear of H5N1 avian influenza, even though the actual risk to travelers had been almost zero. Other travelers plan to ascend Mt. Everest, even though the risk of dying during an Everest climb is 1 in 40.

Regardless of the perception and tolerance of risk, the hazards associated with travel cannot be eliminated, just as the risks of staying home are not zero. Even the act of trying to prevent a risk—such as the risk of yellow fever—can lead to a fatal reaction to the vaccine. Therefore, the goal in travel and in travel medicine should be the skillful management of risk, rather than trying to eliminate risk. The pre-travel visit is an opportunity to discuss risks and develop plans that minimize the risks, based on evaluation of risks versus benefits. Each traveler may have individual concepts about the risks and benefits of vaccines, prophylaxis, and behavior modification. A traveler who is told that there is a low risk of typhoid fever at the destination may choose not to have the typhoid vaccine, while another traveler may say, "I'm the kind of person who doesn't like to take any risks, so I'd like the vaccine."

Travelers should consider the psychological and emotional aspects of foreign travel. Culture shock can occur on either end of a journey: on arrival when one encounters an entirely strange new world, and on return when one's own world may temporarily appear unfamiliar. Travelers with underlying psychiatric conditions should be cautious when heading out to a new environment that may prove stressful, particularly if they are traveling alone.

All travelers should contemplate the concept of commitment, which is a term to describe the fact that certain parts of a journey cannot easily be reversed. A person trekking into a remote area may have to realize that rescue, if available at all, may be delayed for days. A person who has a myocardial infarction in a country with no advanced cardiac services may have a difficult time getting to definitive medical care. If the traveler has already contemplated these concerns and accepted them, it is easier to deal with them in the remote chance that they actually come to pass.

Finally, travelers should be encouraged to travel with compassion. It is all too easy to fall into a pattern of blaming the destination country for frustrating inefficiency, shortages, delays, and corruption, without stopping to think that most of the local population have to live with these problems their whole lives.

The goal of travel medicine, apart from helping advise people with regard to travel-related risks should also be to help people match their interests, abilities, fitness, and sense of adventure with the right destination. Evaluating underlying illness and helping to guide a traveler to the right type of trip is also a key part of travel medicine. Travel is one of the main activities that helps break down the barriers between cultures and human beings around the world and enriches the lives of travelers. Despite the risks of travel, we should never lose sight of the benefits.

Perspectives: Why Guidelines Differ

Alan J. Magill, David R. Shlim

INTRODUCTION

Numerous international, national, and professional organizations publish guidelines and recommendations that assist travel medicine practitioners in providing the best possible advice to prospective travelers. The CDC Yellow Book is an example of one of these published guidelines. However, it is quickly apparent to both practitioners and patients that guidelines and recommendations differ, sometimes dramatically. Conflicting messages from "authoritative sources" may confuse the patient and the practitioner and thus undermine the credibility of the source. It can be unsettling for patients to receive travel medicine advice, vaccines, and malaria prescription from one provider, only to find that the recommendations conflict with what they have obtained from other sources or even heard from other advisors. The skillful travel medicine practitioner will be able to help the traveler run this gantlet of conflicting advice by knowing more about why guidelines differ.

HOW ARE GUIDELINES CREATED?

Most guidelines that concern travel medicine practitioners and travelers focus on recommendations for immunizations, prophylactic medications, and self-treatment regimens (such as those for travelers' diarrhea). Guidelines come from many sources. A regulatory agency in each country must approve the safety and efficacy of each vaccine or medication. International organizations such as the World Health Organization (WHO) promote their own sets of guidelines. At national levels, agencies such as the Centers for Disease Control and Prevention (CDC) in the United States make recommendations for the use of approved vaccines and medications for travelers. In addition, professional organizations may create consensus guidelines based on published medical literature and expert opinion. Travel medicine-specific subscription services use experts to organize and present travel medicine recommendations for practitioners. However, these services have greater flexibility in using information that may not be fully validated by national and international authorities. Finally, there are the vast, unregulated opinions published on the Internet. The person who is new to travel medicine may not be aware of the decision-making process or the source information that results in formal recommendations from these organizations.

Regulatory authorities

A national regulatory authority is the government body that approves vaccines and drugs. In the United States, this is the Food and Drug Administration (FDA). For the vaccines and medications commonly prescribed in a pre-travel consultation, providers are expected to use the products in accordance with the current product label as approved by the FDA. The product label is a valuable source of information that is as accurate as possible at the time it is published. Manufacturers submit a very detailed application that undergoes rigorous, multidisciplinary review. The approved product label reflects the information provided by the manufacturer in response to the requirements specified by a large body of regulatory law developed over many years. Since each country has different laws and requirements, it is easy to see why the approved products and their product labels may differ from country to country. This difference is then reflected in the national guidelines in relation to that product.

International organizations

Important travelers' health information is provided by the WHO's publication *International Travel and Health* (the "Green Book") and also in the WHO International Health Regulations 2005. Countries with less developed or nonexistent regulatory agencies often default to the WHO guidelines, while more developed countries with resources devoted to travelers' health may be aware of the WHO recommendations but may not be able to reconcile WHO recommendations with their own country's recommendations in every situation.

U.S. national organizations

CDC provides recommendations for travelers' health and publishes those recommendations in this book. Experts at CDC review information in their area of expertise and formulate recommendations. For vaccines, the Advisory Committee on Immunization Practices (ACIP) develops written recommendations for the administration of vaccines, including travelers' vaccines, to children and adults in the civilian population. Recommendations include age for vaccine administration, number of doses and dosing interval, and precautions and contraindications. The ACIP, which is the only entity in the federal government that makes such recommendations, consists of 15 experts in fields associated with immunization who have been selected to provide advice and guidance to CDC on the control of vaccine-preventable diseases.

Professional organizations

Professional organizations often develop, write, and publish practice guidelines using committees of experts from their membership. These practice guidelines typically follow an evidence-based medicine (EBM) approach that links recommendations to the strength and quality of the evidence as assessed by the committee members. The Infectious Disease Society of America (IDSA) has published a travel medicine practice guideline that many find useful. Practice guidelines by their nature are consensus documents.

Peer-reviewed medical literature and open sources

As experience with a vaccine or a drug is acquired over the years, these results are often published in the peer-reviewed medical literature. In addition, individuals who use these products gain experience over time and develop their own opinions ("experience-based medicine"). The actual data that would be most useful in deciding how to use a vaccine or medication may not be available in the published reports, so expert opinion attempts to interpret the available information or provide background perspective.

WHY DO GUIDELINES DIFFER?

Guidelines in different countries and organizations may differ in significant ways. Some of the reasons why guidelines differ include availability of products in different countries, a different cultural perception of risk, lack of evidence (or differing interpretations of the same evidence), and sometimes just honest differences in opinion among experts. Occasionally, public opinion may have an influence on recommendations (for example, the widespread adverse publicity about mefloquine that was reported in the media).

Availability of products

Travel medicine providers can only use the products that are available to them. Availability is determined by the regulatory approval status of the product and to a lesser extent the marketing and distribution plan of the manufacturer. Among the various vaccines and antimalarial drugs commercially available worldwide, the process for regulatory approvals varies greatly. For example, it is a very costly and rigorous process to register a new vaccine or antimalarial drug in the United States. If the market is insufficient to justify the expense of registration, then a commercial company may choose not to seek registration in a particular country. The standards for licensure vary, and what may be sufficient for one regulatory authority may not suffice for another. For example, primaquine, an option for antimalarial prophylaxis in the United States, is not registered or commercially available in Switzerland. Atovaquone–proguanil (Malarone, GlaxoSmithKline) was available for malaria chemoprophylaxis in the United States prior to its availability for this purpose in many other countries. On the other hand, Dukoral (Chiron Vaccines) is an oral vaccine against cholera that is approved for use and widely available in many other countries, but is not approved by the U.S. FDA. Therefore, CDC and ACIP guidelines do not include any recommendations for the use of Dukoral.

Even when the same products are available, the recommendations for their use may differ. The capsular polysaccharide typhoid vaccine (Typhim Vi) and the oral typhoid vaccine (Vivotif, or Ty21a) are examples. In the United States, a booster of Typhim Vi is recommended after 2 years, but in most European countries a booster is recommended after 3 years. In the United States, a packet of four oral typhoid capsules is dispensed, whereas in Europe, three doses are considered adequate. The regulatory agencies may have reviewed the same data and drawn different conclusions, or they may have reviewed different data at different times and reached different conclusions. It is unusual that regulatory submissions to different agencies are ready and occur at the same time; therefore, the data available for review by different agencies may be different for legitimate reasons.

Perception of risk

Groups from different backgrounds can view the same risk data and come to different conclusions as to the cost and benefit of preventing that risk. For example, national-level recommendations to prevent malaria while traveling to India vary widely. German recommendations are to not use standard prophylaxis for any travel to an Indian destination; stand-by emergency treatment (SBET or self-treatment) is the recommendation for identified risk destinations. The guidelines in the United Kingdom (U.K.) recommend only awareness and mosquito bite prevention for more than half the Indian subcontinent, including large cities and popular tourist destinations in the north and south, while recommending an individual risk assessment based on activities and types of travelers. Standard prophylaxis recommended in the U.K. guidelines is the combination of chloroquine plus proguanil (an option not available in the United States) for much of the middle of the subcontinent. However, CDC recommends malaria prophylaxis for any Indian destination except for some mountainous areas of northern states above 2,000 meters. Is one of these guidelines better than the others? Not necessarily, as the recommendations may be based on the national experience with different types of travelers, and the risk assessment approach of the organization formulating the national guidelines. For example, India (121 cases) was second only to Nigeria (278 cases) for total reported cases on the list of countries where malaria was acquired for cases reported in the US in 2006, yet was close to the median for estimated relative case rates. India does report active transmission in all provinces in the country. Based on the extremely large population of India, some of these provinces have high absolute numbers of cases but low case rates. Some countries chose to base their recommendations on these relatively low case rates while it is the assessment of others that the high absolute numbers of cases results in large numbers of infective mosquitoes that can in turn, infect travelers. In any case, travelers to India are likely to encounter a great diversity of recommendations for the prevention of malaria while searching the Internet or from speaking with fellow travelers after arriving at the destination.

The best available data should always be used to balance the risk of the intervention—and the costs—against the risk of the disease, so that the decision to recommend a vaccine or prophylactic medicine may be understood by the practitioner and the traveler.

Lack of evidence

In many cases limited or no data are available from which to make an evidence-based assessment. In this setting, travel medicine providers defer to expert opinion or an extrapolation from very limited data in conjunction with expert opinion. In travel medicine, it is rare to have actual prospective numerator and denominator data on the risk of any vaccine-preventable diseases in travelers. For example, any data that we currently obtain on the risk of hepatitis A in travelers would have to account for the immunization rate with hepatitis A vaccine. These data are rarely available, and therefore we often rely on historical data that captured very few actual cases.

CAN WE HARMONIZE GUIDELINES?

The complex nature of how we obtain, evaluate, and verify data, combined with the fundamental differences in risk perception, make it likely that multiple, overlapping, and at times conflicting guidelines will continue to exist. In addition, the marriage of the science and the art of medicine is often not an easy one. Nonetheless, the role of the travel medicine practitioner is to become more sophisticated in his or her understanding of the various differences in guidelines, in interpreting this information, and in conveying it in an assured and comforting manner to travelers.

REFERENCES

1. Chiodini P, Hill D, Lalloo D, et al. Guidelines for malaria prevention in travellers from the United Kingdom. London, Health Protection Agency; 2007 [Internet]. [cited 2008 Nov 25]. Available from: http://www.hpa.org.uk/web/HPAwebFile/HPAweb_C/1203496943523.

2. German Society for Tropical Medicine and International Health Association (DTG). Deutsche Gesellschaft für Tropenmedizin und Internationale Gesundheit. [cited 2008 Nov 25]. Available in German from: http://www.dtg.org.

3. Health Canada. Canadian recommendations for the prevention and treatment of malaria among international travelers. CCDR. 2004;30S1:1–62.

4. World Health Organization. International Health Regulations, 2005. [cited 2008 Nov 25]. Available from: http://www.who.int/csr/ihr/en/index.html.

5. WHO. International travel and health, 2008. Geneva: World Health Organization; 2008. [cited 2008 Nov 25]. Available from: http://www.who.int/ith/en/.

6. CDC. Advisory Committee on Immunization Practices (ACIP). [cited 2008 Nov 25]. Available from: http://www.cdc.gov/vaccines/recs/ACIP/default.htm.

7. Hill DR, Ericsson CD, Pearson RD, et al. Infectious Diseases Society of America. The practice of travel medicine: guidelines by the Infectious Diseases Society of America. Clin Infect Dis. 2006;43(12):1499–539.

2

The Pre-Travel Consultation

THE PRE-TRAVEL CONSULTATION

Rebecca W. Acosta

The pre-travel consultation is a risk-based assessment process that provides a guide to prioritizing and customizing pre-travel health care to the traveler's itinerary, risks, and needs. The goal of the pre-travel consultation is the effective and efficient preparation of travelers with the appropriate counseling, vaccinations, and medications to help reduce their risk of illness and injury during travel.

To conduct a risk-based assessment, health-care providers involved in preparing travelers must—

- Have a working knowledge of destination-specific disease and health risks and standard recommendations to promote health and prevent illness among travelers. The information and recommendations presented in this publication, the Body of Knowledge in Travel Medicine (as published by the International Society of Travel Medicine [ISTM]), and other authoritative sources (see Appendix B) form the basis for this knowledge.
- Understand the standard for and expectations of conducting a pre-travel consultation and gain expertise in the process. The well-organized and well-executed pre-travel consultation supports consistent, appropriate, and efficient pre-travel health preparation with the following three essential elements:
    1. Risk Assessment
    2. Risk Communication
    3. Risk Management

Risk Assessment

The risk assessment provides the foundation for the recommendations given during the consultation. A risk assessment involves gathering pertinent information about the itinerary ("where and when") and traveler ("who, why, what, and how") to highlight the traveler's risks and alert the provider to any contraindications and precautions to vaccinations or medications that may be indicated. A questionnaire designed to collect and organize the itinerary and traveler data is an essential tool to help support the risk assessment process and facilitate consistent practice (see Box 1-1).

The most important information to gather includes the following:

- **Itinerary data**
  o Countries and regions to be visited; urban versus rural
  o Dates and length of travel
  o Purpose of travel (e.g., business, vacation, visiting friends and relatives)
  o Mode(s) of transportation
  o Planned and possible activities
  o Types of accommodations
- **Traveler demographic and health/medical history**
  o Age, sex
  o Vaccination history, including prior adverse events
  o Medical and psychiatric history (past and current)
  o Medications
  o Allergies
  o Pregnancy and breastfeeding status (current status and plans)

A basic example of using the itinerary and traveler data includes determining if there will be a risk of yellow fever disease or a requirement for yellow fever vaccination based on the itinerary, and if there is a contraindication (e.g., egg allergy) or a precaution (e.g., >60 years of age) to the traveler's receiving the vaccine. Malaria risk is another important consideration. Will the traveler be going to a region endemic for malaria, and what are the appropriate measures to help prevent malaria based on the details of the itinerary and traveler's medical history?

During the risk assessment, the provider must remain alert to other factors about "who" will be traveling. Such factors include the traveler's previous travel experience, perception of risk, cultural background, peer group(s), and possible barriers to care, such as economic issues, attitudes regarding vaccine safety, and fear of vaccines. These factors may greatly affect the traveler's ability and willingness to accept and adhere to the recommendations, and therefore affect the pre-travel consultation.

Anticipating the unique needs of high-risk travelers and preparing them for healthy travel will help prevent illness and injury. The following travelers may be considered high risk:

- Travelers visiting friends and relatives (VFRs). These individuals have typically migrated from a less-developed area to a developed area and are now returning to the region of their birth. This is especially important when these individuals are traveling with new family members or children. The traveler returning to his or her country of origin may not understand the dynamics of risk and waning immunity (see the VFR section in Chapter 8).
- The elderly
- Families with young children
- Persons traveling to adopt children abroad
- Persons with weakened immune systems
- Women who are pregnant or breastfeeding

Risk Communication

The next phase of the consultation process is focused on risk communication and includes the presentation of reliable, evidence-based information in a context appropriate for the individual traveler. Time should be allocated for discussion of the risks with the traveler to promote informed decision making about risk avoidance and prevention measures, such as vaccinations and malaria chemoprophylaxis. Risk communication depends heavily upon the risk assessment for the individual traveler, as well as that traveler's perception of risk. For example, three travelers may be going to the same country: one for a week-long, urban-based, business visit; the next on an adventure-seeking, backpack trip to rural areas over several months; and the third is a pregnant VFR traveler. The recommendations and preparation for each of these travelers will vary, even though the destination country is the same.

It is important to give both verbal and written information to the traveler to help guide and focus the discussion and reinforce important issues based on his or her risk assessment. Examples include information pamphlets, malaria risk maps, and vaccine information statements (VISs). Through careful risk assessment and thoughtful risk communication, a risk management plan (i.e., vaccinations, medications, and targeted risk-avoidance education) takes shape.

Risk Management

The essential elements of risk management include the following:

- Selection, administration, and documentation of vaccinations
  - Required, recommended, and routine vaccinations should all be considered (see below)
  - Providers should consider indications, contraindications, precautions, and timing of dosages
- Prescribing and advising about preventive medications
  - Where appropriate according to risk, antimalarial chemoprophylaxis and medications for travelers' diarrhea, motion sickness, and altitude sickness
- Education related to malaria prevention and adherence to chemoprophylaxis (if indicated by the risk assessment)
- Information on risk and prevention of other insect-borne diseases
- Instruction on methods to reduce foodborne and waterborne illness and the self-management of travelers' diarrhea
- Instruction about animal avoidance and rabies
- Information to help reduce the negative effect of
  - Other itinerary risks (e.g., altitude, pollution)
  - Activity-specific risks (e.g., diving, rafting, rural road travel)
  - Personal behavior risks (e.g., sexually transmitted diseases)
- General guidance on
  - Symptoms (e.g., fever, gastrointestinal or dermatologic symptoms) that may require medical attention during or after travel
  - Preparing a travel health kit (see the Travel Health Kits section later in this chapter)
  - Accessing medical care abroad and obtaining medical/evacuation insurance

When considering vaccinations, common terms used include "required," "recommended," and "routine." Required vaccines are those needed when a destination country requires documentation of vaccine administration or some sort of medical waiver. Recommended vaccines are those vaccines that are considered based on the actual disease risk the traveler may encounter during travel. Routine vaccines refer to those vaccines that are recommended in the United States, regardless of travel. These routine vaccines are an important part of pre-travel care because many of the diseases they protect against are more common in countries outside the United States.

Careful documentation of all vaccinations, medications, and specific recommendations given to the traveler helps to complete the care plan record. Providers who are registered to give yellow fever vaccine should be familiar with properly completing the International Certificate of Vaccination or Prophylaxis (ICVP) to ensure that this documentation will be accepted at the borders of destination countries (see the Yellow Fever section later in this chapter). Using an electronic record or standardized form facilitates documentation and helps ensure consistency of practice.

Providers should plan to spend an average of 30–45 minutes conducting a complete pre-travel consultation, based on the risk assessment, given the potential complexities in preparing the traveler. Providers with limited knowledge and expertise in travel medicine and the pre-travel consultation should consider referring travelers with complex itineraries or special needs (see Chapters 7 and 8) to a travel medicine clinic or travel medicine specialist through CDC's Travelers' Health website at www.cdc.gov/travel. References 1–4 can assist those providers interested in gaining a more in-depth perspective on the expectations for providing pre-travel health care and the pre-travel consultation process.

References

1. Kozarsky PE. The body of knowledge for the practice of travel medicine. J Travel Med. 2006;13(5):251–4.
2. Hill DR, Ericsson CD, Pearson RD, et al. The practice of travel medicine: guidelines by the Infectious Diseases Society of America. Clin Infect Dis. 2006; 43(12):1499–539.
3. Spira A. Setting the standard. J Travel Med. 2003;10(1):1–3.
4. Acosta RW, Wolfe MS. Structure and organization of the pre-travel consultation and general advice for travelers. In: Keystone JS,

Kozarsky PE, Freedman DO, Nothdurft HD, Connor BA, editors. Travel medicine. 2nd ed. Philadelphia: Mosby; 2008: p. 35–45.
5. Crockett M, Keystone J. "I hate needles" and other factors impacting on travel vaccine uptake. J Travel Med. 2005; 12(Suppl 1):S41–6.
6. Edwards A, Elwyn G, Mulley A. Explaining risks: turning numerical data into meaningful pictures. BMJ 2002; 324:827–30.
7. Gherardin T. The pre-travel consultation—an overview. Australian Fam Phys. 2007; 36(5):300–3.

GENERAL RECOMMENDATIONS FOR VACCINATION AND IMMUNOPROPHYLAXIS

William Atkinson, Andrew Kroger

Recommendations for the use of vaccines and other biologic products (e.g., immune globulin products) in the United States are developed by the Advisory Committee on Immunization Practices (ACIP) and other groups, such as the American Academy of Pediatrics. These recommendations are based on scientific evidence of benefits (immunity to the disease) and risks (vaccine adverse reactions) and, where few or no data are available, on expert opinion. The recommendations include information on general immunization issues and the use of specific vaccines. When these recommendations are issued or revised, they are published in CDC's Morbidity and Mortality Weekly Report (MMWR) (www.cdc.gov/mmwr). This section is based primarily on the ACIP General Recommendations on Immunization.

Vaccinations against diphtheria, tetanus, pertussis, measles, mumps, rubella, varicella, poliomyelitis, hepatitis A, hepatitis B, *Haemophilus influenzae* type b, rotavirus, influenza, human papillomavirus, and pneumococcal and meningococcal invasive disease are routinely administered in the United States, usually in childhood or adolescence. If persons do not have a history of adequate protection against these diseases, immunizations appropriate to their age and previous immunization status should be obtained, whether or not international travel is planned. A visit to a provider for immunizations for travel should be seen as an opportunity to bring an incompletely vaccinated person up-to-date on his or her routine vaccinations.

Both the child and adolescent vaccination schedule and an adult vaccination schedule are published annually in the MMWR. Vaccine providers should obtain the most current schedules from the CDC Vaccines and Immunization website at www.cdc.gov/vaccines/. The text and Tables 2-1–2-7, 2-9–2-10, 2-18–2-19, 2-21, 5-2, 7-2–7-5, 8-1, 8-7 and 8-8 of this publication present recommendations for the use, number of doses, dose intervals, adverse reactions, precautions, and contraindications for vaccines and toxoids that may be indicated for travelers. For specific vaccines and toxoids, additional details on background, adverse reactions, precautions, and contraindications are found in the respective ACIP statements.

Spacing of Immunobiologics

Simultaneous Administration

All commonly used vaccines can safely and effectively be given simultaneously (i.e., on the same day) at separate sites without impairing antibody responses or increasing rates of adverse reactions. This knowledge is particularly helpful for international travelers, for whom exposure to several infectious diseases might be imminent. Simultaneous administration of all indicated vaccines is encouraged for persons who are the recommended age to receive these vaccines and for whom no contraindications exist. If not administered on the same day, an inactivated vaccine may be given at any time before or after a different inactivated vaccine or a live-virus vaccine.

The immune response to an injected or intranasal live-virus vaccine (e.g., measles, mumps and rubella (MMR); varicella; yellow fever; or live attenuated influenza vaccine) might be impaired if administered within 28 days of another live-virus vaccine. Whenever possible, injected live-virus vaccines administered on different days should be given at least 28 days apart. If two injected or intranasal live-virus vaccines are not administered on the same day but less than 28 days apart, the second vaccine should be readministered at least 4 weeks after the first vaccine was administered.

Live-virus vaccines can interfere with the response to tuberculin testing. Tuberculin testing, if otherwise indicated, can be done either on the day that live-virus vaccines are administered or 4–6 weeks later. Tuberculin skin testing is not a prerequisite for administration of any vaccine.

Missed Doses and Boosters

Travelers may forget to return for a follow-up dose of vaccine or booster at the specified time. Occasionally the demand for a vaccine may exceed its supply, and providers may have difficulty obtaining vaccines. (Information on vaccine shortages and recommendations can be found on the CDC Vaccines and Immunization website at www.cdc.gov/vaccines/vac-gen/shortages/default.htm.) It is unnecessary in these cases to restart the interrupted series or to add any extra doses except for oral typhoid. The next scheduled dose should be given when the patient presents. (There are no data for interrupted dosing with oral typhoid vaccine; thus, a travel medicine specialist should be consulted.) Some vaccines require periodic booster doses to maintain protection (Table 2-1).

Antibody-Containing Blood Products

When MMR and varicella vaccines are given shortly before, simultaneously with, or after an antibody-containing blood product, such as immune globulin (IG) or a blood transfusion, response to the vaccine can be diminished. Antibody-containing blood products from the United States do not interfere with the immune response to yellow fever vaccine and are not believed to interfere with the response to live attenuated influenza vaccine or rotavirus vaccine. The duration of inhibition of MMR and varicella vaccines is related to the dose of IG in the product. MMR or its components and varicella vaccines either should be administered at least 2 weeks before receipt of a blood product or should be delayed 3–11 months after receipt of the blood product, depending on the vaccine (Table 2-2).

Immunoglobulin (IG) administration may become necessary for another indication after MMR or its individual components or varicella vaccines have been given. In such a situation, the IG may interfere with the immune response to the MMR or varicella vaccines. Vaccine virus replication and stimulation of immunity usually occur 2–3 weeks after vaccination. If the interval between administration of one of these vaccines and the subsequent administration of an IG preparation is 14 days or more, the vaccine need not be readministered. If the interval is less than 14 days, the vaccine should be readministered after the interval shown in Table 2-2, unless serologic testing indicates that antibodies have been produced. If administration of IG becomes necessary,

MMR or its components or varicella vaccines can be administered simultaneously with IG, with the recognition that vaccine-induced immunity can be compromised. The vaccine should be administered at a body site different from that chosen for the IG injection. Vaccination should be repeated after the interval noted in Table 2-2, unless serologic testing indicates antibodies have been produced.

When IG is given with the first dose of hepatitis A vaccine, the proportion of recipients who develop a protective level of antibody is not affected, but antibody concentrations are lower. Because the final concentrations of antibody are many times higher than those considered protective, this reduced immunogenicity is not expected to be clinically important. IG preparations interact minimally with other inactivated vaccines and toxoids. Other inactivated vaccines may be given simultaneously or at any time interval after or before an antibody-containing blood product is used. However, such vaccines should be administered at different sites from the IG.

Table 2-1. Revaccination (booster) schedules

Vaccine	Recommendation
Japanese encephalitis	Full duration of protection unknown. Neutralizing antibodies may persist at least 2 years after primary immunization.
Hepatitis A (HAV)	Booster doses not recommended for adults and children who have completed the primary series (2 doses) according to the routine schedule
Hepatitis B (HBV)	Booster doses not recommended for adults and children who have completed the primary series (3 doses) according to the routine schedule[1]
Influenza	1 annual dose (children 6 months to 9 years of age and certain incompletely vaccinated children should receive 2 doses separated by at least 4 weeks the first time that influenza vaccine is administered). Live attenuated influenza vaccine is approved only for healthy nonpregnant persons 2–49 years of age.
Measles–mumps–rubella (MMR)	2 doses of MMR vaccine separated by at least 4 weeks or other evidence of immunity (e.g., serologic testing) is recommended for persons born after 1956 who travel outside the United States. Revaccination is not recommended.
Meningococcal Quadrivalent A,C,Y, W-135	Revaccination after 5 years is recommended for persons who received meningococcal polysaccharide vaccine and who remain at increased risk for meningococcal disease (including some international travelers). Revaccination is not recommended after receipt of meningococcal conjugate vaccine.
Pneumococcal (polysaccharide)	One-time revaccination 5 years after original dose for persons with certain underlying medical conditions (e.g., asplenia) or persons who were first vaccinated at younger than 65 years of age
Rotavirus	Booster doses not recommended
Polio (IPV)	A single lifetime booster dose is recommended for adults who have written documentation of having completed a primary series.
Rabies pre-exposure vaccine	No serologic testing or boosters recommended for travelers. For persons in higher risk groups (e.g., rabies laboratory workers) serologic testing and booster doses are recommended. See Table 2-17.
Tetanus/diphtheria, and acellular pertussis (Tdap)	Tetanus and diphtheria booster dose is recommended every 10 years. A single dose of adolescent/adult formulation Td that includes acellular pertussis vaccine (Tdap) is recommended to replace one Td booster dose for persons 11–64 years of age. See ACIP statement for details.
Typhoid oral	Repeat series every 5 years.
Typhoid IM	Booster dose every 2 years
Varicella	Revaccination is not recommended.
Yellow fever	Repeat vaccination every 10 years.

1 Booster dosing may be appropriate for certain populations, such as hemodialysis patients.

Table 2-2. Recommended intervals between administration of antibody-containing products and measles-containing vaccine or varicella-containing vaccine[1]

Indication	Dose	Recommended Interval Before Measles or Varicella Vaccination
Tetanus (TIG)	250 units (10 mg IgG/kg) IM[2]	3 months
Hepatitis A (IG), duration of international travel		
<3-month stay	0.02 mL/kg (3.3 mg IgG/kg) IM	3 months
>3-month stay	0.06 mL/kg (10 mg IgG/kg) IM	3 months
Hepatitis B prophylaxis (HBIG)	0.06 mL/kg (10 mg IgG/kg) IM	3 months
Rabies prophylaxis (HRIG)	20 IU/kg (22 mg IgG/kg) IM	4 months
Varicella prophylaxis (VZIG)	125 units/10 kg (20–40 mg IgG/kg) IM (maximum 625 units)	5 months
Measles prophylaxis (IG)		
Immunocompetent contact	0.25 mL/kg (40 mg IgG/kg) IM	5 months
Immunocompromised contact	0.50 mL/kg (80 mg IgG/kg) IM	6 months
Blood transfusion		
Red blood cells (RBCs), washed	10 mL/kg (negligible IgG/kg) IV	None
RBCs, adenine-saline added	10 mL/kg (10 mg IgG/kg) IV	3 months
Packed RBCs (Hct 65%)[3]	10 mL/kg (60 mg IgG/kg) IV	6 months
Plasma/platelet products	10 mL/kg (160 mg IgG/kg) IV	7 months
Cytomegalovirus prophylaxis (CMV IGIV)	150 mg/kg maximum	6 months
Respiratory syncytial virus (RSV) monoclonal antibody (Synagis)[4]	15 mg/kg IM	None
Intravenous immune globulin (IGIV)		
Replacement therapy	300–400 mg/kg IV	8 months
Immune thrombocytopenic purpura (ITP)	400 mg/kg IV	8 months
ITP	1 gm/kg IV	10 months
ITP or Kawasaki disease	1.6–2 gm/kg IV	11 months

1 Adapted from General Recommendations on Immunization, MMWR, 2006. This table is not intended for determining the correct indications and dosage for the use of IG preparations. Unvaccinated people may not be fully protected against measles during the entire recommended interval, and additional doses of immune globulin (IG) or measles vaccine may be indicated after measles exposure. Concentrations of measles antibody in an IG preparation can vary by manufacturer's lot. For example, fourfold or greater variation in the amount of measles antibody titers has been demonstrated in different IG preparations. Rates of antibody clearance after receipt of an IG preparation can also vary. Recommended intervals are extrapolated from an estimated half-life of 30 days for passively acquired antibody and an observed interference with the immune response to measles vaccine for 5 months after a dose of 80 mg IgG/kg.

2 IG, immune globulin; IM, intramuscular; IV, intravenous.

3 Assumes a serum IgG concentration of 16 mg/mL..

4 Contains only antibody to respiratory syncytial virus.

Vaccination of Persons with Acute Illnesses

Every opportunity should be taken to provide appropriate vaccinations. The decision to delay vaccination because of a current or recent acute illness depends on the severity of the symptoms and their cause. Although a moderate or severe acute illness is sufficient reason to postpone vaccination, minor illnesses (e.g., diarrhea, mild upper respiratory infection with or without low-grade fever, other low-grade febrile illness) are not contraindications to vaccination.

Persons with moderate or severe acute illness, with or without fever, should be vaccinated as soon as the condition has improved. This precaution is to avoid superimposing adverse effects from the vaccine on underlying illness or mistakenly attributing a manifestation of underlying illness to the vaccine. Antimicrobial therapy is not a contraindication to vaccination, with three exceptions. Antibacterial agents may interfere with the response to oral typhoid vaccine. Antiviral agents active against herpesviruses (e.g., acyclovir) may interfere with the response to varicella-containing vaccines (varicella, MMRV, zoster). Antiviral agents active against influenza virus (e.g., zanamivir, oseltamivir) may interfere with the response to live attenuated influenza vaccine.

A physical examination or temperature measurement is not a prerequisite for vaccinating a person who appears to be in good health. Asking if a person is ill, postponing a vaccination for someone with moderate or severe acute illness, and vaccinating someone without contraindications are appropriate procedures for clinic immunizations.

Altered Immunocompetence

Altered immunocompetence is a general term that is often used interchangeably with the terms immunosuppression and immunodeficiency. It can be caused either by a disease (e.g., leukemia, HIV infection) or by drugs or other therapies (e.g., cancer chemotherapy, prolonged high dose corticosteroids). It can also include conditions such as asplenia and chronic renal disease.

Determination of altered immunocompetence is important because the incidence or severity of some vaccine-preventable diseases is higher in persons with altered immunocompetence. Therefore, certain vaccines (e.g., inactivated influenza vaccine, pneumococcal vaccines) are recommended specifically for persons with these diseases. Inactivated vaccine may be safely administered to a person with altered immunocompetence, although response to the vaccine may be suboptimal. The vaccine may need to be repeated after immune function has improved.

Persons with altered immunocompetence may be at increased risk for an adverse reaction following administration of live attenuated vaccines because of reduced ability to mount an effective immune response. Live vaccines should generally be deferred until immune function has improved. This is particularly important when planning to give yellow fever vaccine (see the Yellow Fever section later in this chapter). MMR and varicella vaccines are recommended for persons with mild or moderate immunosuppression.

For an in-depth discussion, see The Immunocompromised Traveler section in Chapter 8.

Vaccination Scheduling for Last-Minute Travelers

As noted in the Simultaneous Administration section, most vaccine products can be given during one visit for persons anticipating imminent travel. Unless the vaccines given are booster doses of those typically given during childhood, vaccines may require a month or more to induce a sufficient immune response, depending on the vaccine and the number of doses in the series.

Some vaccines require more than one dose for best protection. Recommended spacing should be maintained between doses (Table 2-3). Doses given at less than minimum intervals can lessen the antibody response. Administration of a vaccine earlier than the recommended minimum age or at an interval shorter than the recommended minimum is discouraged. Table 2-3 lists the minimum age and minimum interval between doses for vaccines routinely recommended in the United States. Because some travelers visit their health-care providers without ample time for administration of the vaccine doses recommended for optimal protection against certain diseases, studies have been performed and others are ongoing to determine whether accelerated scheduling is adequate. This concern is primarily the case for hepatitis B vaccine or the combined hepatitis A and B vaccine. An accelerated schedule for combined hepatitis A and hepatitis B vaccine has been approved by the U.S. Food and Drug Administration (FDA). It is unclear what level of protection any given traveler will have if a full series of multidose vaccination is not completed.

Table 2-3. Recommended and minimum ages and intervals between vaccine doses[1]

Vaccine and Dose Number	Recommended Age for this Dose	Minimum Age for this Dose	Recommended Interval to Next Dose	Minimum Interval to Next Dose
Hepatitis B (HepB)-1[2]	Birth	Birth	1–4 months	4 weeks
Hep B-2	1–2 months	4 weeks	2–17 months	8 weeks
Hep B-3[3]	6–18 months	24 weeks	NA	NA
Diphtheria–tetanus–acellular pertussis (DTaP)-1[2]	2 months	6 weeks	2 months	4 weeks
DTaP-2	4 months	10 weeks	2 months	4 weeks
DTaP-3	6 months	14 weeks	6–12 months	6 months[4,5]
DTaP-4	15–18 months	12 months	3 years	6 months[4]
DTaP-5	4–6 years	4 years	NA	NA
Haemophilus influenzae type b (Hib)-1[2,6]	2 months	6 weeks	2 months	4 weeks
Hib-2	4 months	10 weeks	2 months	4 weeks
Hib-3[7]	6 months	14 weeks	6–9 months	8 weeks
Hib-4	12–15 months	12 months	NA	NA
Inactivated poliovirus (IPV)-1[2]	2 months	6 weeks	2 months	4 weeks
IPV-2	4 months	10 weeks	2–14 months	4 weeks
IPV-3	6–18 months	14 weeks	3–5 years	4 weeks
IPV-4	4–6 years	18 weeks	NA	NA
Pneumococcal conjugate (PCV)-1[6]	2 months	6 weeks	2 months	4 weeks
PCV-2	4 months	10 weeks	2 months	4 weeks
PCV-3	6 months	14 weeks	6 months	8 weeks
PCV-4	12–15 months	12 months	NA	NA
Measles–mumps–rubella (MMR)-1[8]	12–15 months	12 months	3–5 years	4 weeks
MMR-2[8]	4–6 years	13 months	NA	NA
Varicella (Var)-1	12–15 months	12 months	3–5 years	12 weeks[9]
Var-2	4–6 years	15 months	NA	NA
Hepatitis A (HepA)-1	12–23 months	12 months	6–18 months[4]	6 months[4]
HepA-2	18–41 months	18 months	NA	NA
Influenza, inactivated[10]	6–18 years	6 months	4 weeks	4 weeks
Influenza, live attenuated[10]	NA	2 years	4 weeks	4weeks
Meningococcal conjugate (MCV)	11–12 years	11 years	NA	NA
Meningococcal polysaccharide (MPSV)-1	NA	2 years	5 years[11]	5 years[11]
MPSV-2[12]	NA	7 years	NA	NA
Td	11–12 years	7 years	10 years	5 years
Tdap[13]	≥11 years	10 years	NA	NA
Pneumococcal polysaccharide (PPV)-1	NA	2 years	5 years	5 years
PPV-2[14]	NA	7 years	NA	NA
Human papillomavirus (HPV)-1[15]	11–12 years	9 years	2 months	4 weeks

(Continued over)

Table 2-3. Recommended and minimum ages and intervals between vaccine doses[1] (Continued)

Vaccine and Dose Number	Recommended Age for This Dose	Minimum Age for this Dose	Recommended Interval to Next Dose	Minimum Interval to Next Dose
HPV-2	2 months after dose 1	9 years, 4 weeks	4 months	12 weeks[15]
HPV-3	6 months after dose 1	9 years, 24 weeks	NA	NA
Rotavirus (RV)-1[16]	2 months	6 weeks	2 months	4 weeks
RV-2	4 months	10 weeks	2 months	4 weeks
RV-3[16]	6 months	14 weeks	NA	NA
Herpes zoster[17]	60 years	60 years	NA	NA
Typhoid, inactivated (ViCPS)	≥2 years	≥2 years	NA	NA
Typhoid, live attenuated (Ty21a)	≥6 years	≥6 years	See footnote 18	See footnote 18
Yellow Fever	>9 months[19]	>9 months[19]	10 years	10 years
Japanese encephalitis (JE)-1	≥1 year	1 year	7 days	7 days
JE-2	7 days after dose 1	1 year, 7 days	30 days	14 days
JE-3	30 days after dose 1	1 year, 21 days	NA	NA
Rabies-1 (pre-exposure)	See footnote 20	See footnote 20	7 days	7 days
Rabies-2	7 days after dose 1	7 days after dose 1	21 days	14 days
Rabies-3	21 days after dose 1	21 days after dose 1	NA	NA

DtaP, diphtheria and tetanus toxoids and acellular pertussis vaccine, pediatric (6 weeks through 6 years); MMR, measles, mumps and rubella; TIV, trivalent (inactivated) influenza vaccine; LAIV, live, attenuated (intranasal) influenza vaccine; Td, tetanus and reduced diphtheria toxoids, Tdap, tetanus toxoid, reduced diphtheria toxoid, and reduced acellular pertussis vaccine.

1 Combination vaccines are available. Use of licensed combination vaccines is generally preferred over separate injections of their equivalent component vaccines (CDC. Combination vaccines for childhood immunization: recommendations of the Advisory Committee on Immunization Practices (ACIP), the American Academy of Pediatrics (AAP), and the American Academy of Family Physicians (AAFP). MMWR Recomm Rep. 1999;48(RR-5):5). When administering combination vaccines, the minimum age for administration is the oldest age for any of the individual components; the minimum interval between doses is equal to the greatest interval of any of the individual components.
2 Combination vaccines containing the HepB component are available (HepB-Hib, DTaP-HepB-IPV, HepA-HepB). These vaccines should not be administered to infants younger than 6 weeks of age because of the other components (i.e., Hib, DTaP, IPV). HepA-HepB is not licensed for persons <18 years of age in the United States.
3 HepB-3 should be administered at least 8 weeks after Hep B-2 and at least 16 weeks after Hep B-1; it should not be administered before age 24 weeks.
4 Calendar months.
5 The minimum recommended interval between DTaP-3 and DTaP-4 is 6 months. However, DTaP-4 need not be repeated if administered at least 4 months after DTaP-3. Adapted from Table 1, CDC. General recommendations on immunization. Recommendations of the Advisory Committee on Immunization Practices (ACIP). MMWR Recomm Rep. 2006; 55(RR-15):1–48.
6 For Hib and PCV, children receiving the first dose of vaccine at ≥7 months of age require fewer doses to complete the series (see the current childhood and adolescent immunization schedule at www.cdc.gov/vaccines/).
7 If PRP-OMP (Pedvax-Hib, Merck Vaccine Division) was administered at 2 and 4 months of age, a dose at 6 months of age is not indicated. Adapted from Table 1, CDC. General recommendations on immunization. Recommendations of the Advisory Committee on Immunization Practices (ACIP). MMWR Recomm Rep. 2006; 55(RR-15):1–48.
8 Combination MMR-varicella can be used for children 12 months through 12 years of age. Also see footnote 9.
9 The minimum interval from VAR-1 to VAR-2 for persons beginning the series at ≥13 years of age is 4 weeks.
10 Two doses of influenza vaccine are recommended only for children <9 years of age who are receiving the vaccine for the first time and for certain incompletely vaccinated children. See reference 5.
11 Some experts recommend that a second dose of MPSV be given 3 years after the first dose for persons at increased risk for meningococcal disease.
12 A second dose of meningococcal vaccine is recommended for persons previously vaccinated with MPSV who remain at high risk for meningococcal disease. MCV is preferred when revaccinating persons 2–55 years of age (CDC. Prevention and control of meningococcal disease. Recommendations of the Advisory Committee on Immunization Practices (ACIP). MMWR Recomm Rep. 2005;54(RR07);1–21.) Adapted from Table 1, CDC. General recommendations on immunization. Recommendations of the Advisory Committee on Immunization Practices (ACIP). MMWR Recomm Rep. 2006; 55(RR-15):1–48.
13 Only one dose of Tdap is recommended. Subsequent doses should be given as Td. If vaccination to prevent tetanus and/or diphtheria disease is required for children 7–9 years of age, Td should be given (minimum age for Td is

7 years). For one brand of Tdap, the minimum age is 11 years. The preferred interval between Tdap and a previous dose of Td is 5 years, but Tdap may be administered earlier if pertussis immunity is needed. For management of a tetanus-prone wound, the minimum interval after a previous dose of any tetanus-containing vaccine is 5 years.

14 A second dose of PPV is recommended for persons at highest risk for serious pneumococcal infection and those who are likely to have a rapid decline in pneumococcal antibody concentration. (CDC. Prevention of pneumococcal disease. Recommendations of the Advisory Committee on Immunization Practices (ACIP). MMWR Recomm Rep. 1997; 46(RR-8):1–24.)

15 HPV is approved only for females 9–26 years of age. HPV-3 should be administered at least 12 weeks after HPV-2 and at least 24 weeks after HPV-1.

16 The first dose of RV must be administered by 14 weeks and 6 days of age. The vaccine series should not be started at 15 weeks of age or older. The final dose in the series should be administered by age 8 months 0 days. If Rotarix rotavirus vaccine is administered at 2 and 4 months of age, a dose at 6 months of age is not indicated.

17 Herpes zoster vaccine is approved as a single dose for persons 60 years of age and older.

18 Oral typhoid vaccine is recommended to be administered 1 hour before a meal with a cold or lukewarm drink (temperature not to exceed body temperature) (i.e., 98.6° F (37° C)) on alternate days, for a total of 4 doses.

19 Yellow fever vaccine may be administered to children younger than 9 months of age in certain situations. (CDC. Yellow Fever Vaccine Recommendations of the Advisory Committee on Immunization Practices (ACIP), 2002. MMWR Recomm Rep. 2002;51(RR-17):6–7.)

20 There is no minimum age for pre-exposure immunization for rabies. (CDC. Human rabies prevention— United States, 2008: recommendations of the Advisory Committee on Immunization Practices. MMWR Recomm Rep. 2008; 57(RR-3):1–28.)

Adapted from Table 1, CDC. General recommendations on immunization. Recommendations of the Advisory Committee on Immunization Practices (ACIP). MMWR Recomm Rep. 2006; 55(RR-15):1–48.

Allergy to Vaccine Components

Vaccine components can cause allergic reactions in some recipients. These reactions can be local or systemic and can include anaphylaxis or anaphylactic-like responses. The vaccine components responsible can include the vaccine antigen, animal proteins, antibiotics, preservatives (e.g., thimerosal), or stabilizers (e.g., gelatin). The most common animal protein allergen is egg protein in vaccines prepared by using embryonated chicken eggs (influenza and yellow fever vaccines). Generally, persons who can eat eggs or egg products safely may receive these vaccines, while those with histories of anaphylactic allergy (e.g., hives, swelling of the mouth and throat, difficulty breathing, hypotension, shock) to eggs or egg proteins ordinarily should not. Screening persons by asking whether they can eat eggs without adverse effects is a reasonable way to identify those who might be at risk from receiving yellow fever and influenza vaccines. Recent studies have indicated that other components in vaccines in addition to egg proteins (e.g., gelatin) may cause allergic reactions, including anaphylaxis in rare instances. Protocols have been developed for testing and vaccinating persons with anaphylactic reactions to egg ingestion.

Some vaccines contain a preservative or trace amounts of antibiotics to which people might be allergic. Those administering the vaccine(s) should carefully review the information provided in the package insert before deciding if the rare person with such an allergy should receive the vaccine. No currently recommended vaccine contains penicillin or penicillin derivatives. Some vaccines (e.g., MMR and its individual component vaccines, inactivated polio vaccine [IPV], varicella, rabies) contain trace amounts of neomycin or other antibiotics; the amount is less than would normally be used for the skin test to determine hypersensitivity. However, persons who have experienced anaphylactic reactions to this antibiotic generally should not receive these vaccines. Most often, neomycin allergy is a contact dermatitis—a manifestation of a delayed-type (cell-mediated) immune response rather than anaphylaxis. A history of delayed-type reactions to neomycin is not a contraindication to receiving these vaccines.

Thimerosal, an organic mercurial compound in use since the 1930s, has been added to certain immunobiologic products as a preservative. Thimerosal is present at preservative concentrations (trace quantities) in multidose vials of some brands of inactivated influenza vaccine, pediatric DT, single-antigen tetanus toxoid, meningococcal polysaccharide vaccine, and Japanese encephalitis vaccine. Receiving thimerosal-containing vaccines has been postulated to lead to induction of allergy. However, there is limited scientific evidence for this assertion. Allergy to thimerosal usually consists of local delayed-type hypersensitivity reactions. Thimerosal elicits positive delayed-type hypersensitivity patch tests in 1%–18% of persons tested, but these tests have limited or no clinical relevance. The majority of persons do not experience reactions to thimerosal administered as a component of vaccines, even when patch or intradermal tests for thimerosal indicate hypersensitivity. A localized or delayed-type hypersensitivity reaction to thimerosal is not a contraindication to receipt of a vaccine that contains thimerosal.

Since mid-2001, vaccines routinely recommended for infants have been manufactured without thimerosal as a preservative. Additional information about thimerosal and the thimerosal content of vaccines is available on the FDA website at www.fda.gov/cber/vaccine/thimerosal.htm.

Reporting Adverse Events Following Immunization

Modern vaccines are extremely safe and effective. Benefits and risks are associated with the use of all immunobiologics—no vaccine is completely effective or completely free of side effects. Adverse events following immunization have been reported with all vaccines, ranging from frequent, minor, local reactions to extremely rare, severe, systemic illness, such as that associated with yellow fever vaccine (see Yellow Fever section later in this chapter). Side effects and adverse events following specific vaccines and toxoids are discussed in detail in each ACIP statement. Health-care providers are required by law to report selected adverse events occurring after vaccination with tetanus vaccine in any combination; pertussis in any combination; measles, mumps or rubella alone or in any combination, oral polio vaccine (OPV), IPV, hepatitis B; varicella; *Haemophilus influenzae* type b (conjugate); pneumococcal conjugate; and rotavirus vaccines. In addition, CDC strongly recommends that all vaccine adverse events be reported to the Vaccine Adverse Event Reporting System (VAERS), even if a causal relation to vaccination is not certain. VAERS reporting forms and information are available electronically at www.vaers.hhs.gov or may be requested by telephone: 800-822-7967. Health-care providers are encouraged to report electronically at https://secure.vaers.org/VaersDataEntryintro.htm.

Injection Route and Injection Site

Injectable vaccines are administered by intramuscular and subcutaneous routes. The method of administration of injectable vaccines depends in part on the presence of an adjuvant in some vaccines. The term adjuvant refers to a vaccine component distinct from the antigen, which enhances the immune response to the antigen. Vaccines containing an adjuvant (i.e., DTaP, DT, human papillomavirus, Td, Tdap, pneumococcal conjugate, Hib, hepatitis A, hepatitis B) should be injected into a muscle mass because administration subcutaneously or intradermally can cause local irritation, induration, skin discoloration, inflammation, and granuloma formation. Routes of administration are recommended by the manufacturer for each immunobiologic. Deviation from the recommended route of administration may reduce vaccine efficacy or increase local adverse reactions. Detailed recommendations on the appropriate route and site for all vaccines have been published in ACIP recommendations; a compiled list of these publications is available on the CDC website at www.cdc.gov/vaccines/pubs/ACIP-list.htm (also see Appendix C: Travel Vaccine Summary Table).

References

1. CDC. General recommendations on immunization. Recommendations of the Advisory Committee on Immunization Practices (ACIP). MMWR Recomm Rep. 2006;55(RR-15):1–48.

2. CDC. Prevention and control of influenza. Recommendations of the Advisory Committee on Immunization Practices (ACIP). MMWR Recomm Rep. 2008;57(RR-7):1–60.

3. CDC. Measles, mumps, and rubella—vaccine use and strategies for elimination of measles, rubella, and congenital rubella syndrome and control of mumps. Recommendations of the Advisory Committee on Immunization Practices (ACIP). MMWR Recomm Rep. 1998;47(RR-8);1–57.

4. CDC. Prevention and control of meningococcal disease. Recommendations of the Advisory Committee on Immunization Practices (ACIP). MMWR Recomm Rep. 2005;54(RR07);1–21.

5. CDC. Preventing tetanus, diphtheria, and pertussis among adults: use of tetanus toxoid,

reduced diphtheria toxoid and acellular pertussis vaccines. Recommendations of the Advisory Committee on Immunization Practices (ACIP). MMWR Recomm Rep. 2006;55(RR 17);1–59.

6. Plotkin SA. Correlates of vaccine-induced immunity. Clin Infect Dis 2008; 47(3):401–9.

7. Murphy KR, Strunk RC. Safe administration of influenza vaccine in asthmatic children hypersensitive to egg proteins. J Pediatr. 1985; 106(6):931–3.

8. Ball LK, Ball R, Pratt RD. An assessment of thimerosal use in childhood vaccines. Pediatrics 2001;107(5):1147–54.

9. Varricchio F, Iskander J, Destefano F, et al. Understanding vaccine safety information from the Vaccine Adverse Event Reporting System. Pediatr Infect Dis J. 2004; 23(4):287–94.

Travel-Related Vaccine-Preventable Diseases

HEPATITIS A

Steven T. Wiersma

Infectious Agent

Hepatitis A virus (HAV), a 27-nm RNA virus classified as a picornavirus.

Mode of Transmission

- Transmission can occur through direct person-to-person contact; through exposure to contaminated water, ice, or shellfish harvested from sewage-contaminated water; or from fruits, vegetables, or other foods that are eaten uncooked and that were contaminated during harvesting or subsequent handling.
- HAV is shed in the feces of persons with HAV infection. The virus reaches peak levels the week or two before onset of symptoms and diminishes rapidly after liver dysfunction or symptoms appear, which is concurrent with the appearance of circulating antibodies to HAV. Infants and children, however, may shed virus for up to 6 months following infection.

Occurrence

- Worldwide, geographic areas can be characterized by high, intermediate, or low levels of endemicity (Map 2-1). Levels of endemicity are related to hygienic and sanitary conditions in the geographic areas.
- HAV infection is common (high or intermediate endemicity) throughout the developing world, where infections most frequently are acquired during early childhood and usually are asymptomatic or mild.
- In areas of high endemicity, adults are usually immune and epidemics of hepatitis A are uncommon.
- In developed countries, HAV infection is less common (low endemicity), but community-wide outbreaks may occur.
- Map 2-1 indicates the seroprevalence of antibody to HAV (total anti-HAV) as measured in selected cross-sectional studies among each country's residents. The seroprevalence of anti-HAV provides an estimate of the endemicity of HAV infections, including asymptomatic infections, within a population.

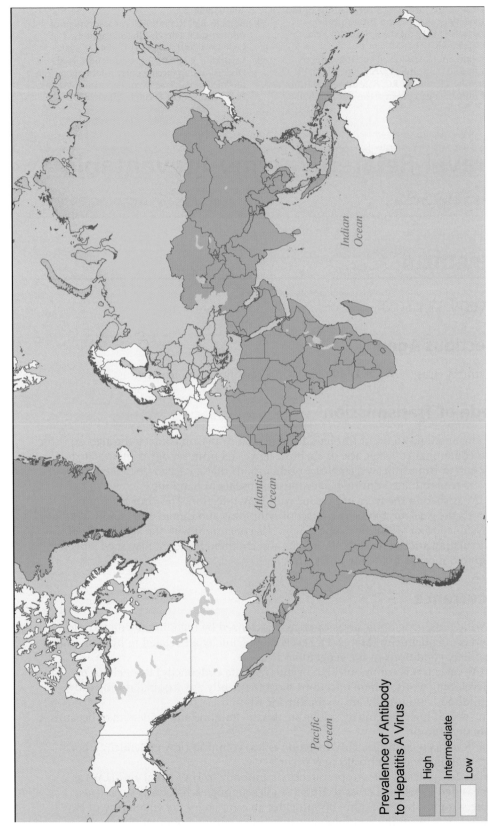

Prevalence of Antibody
to Hepatitis A Virus

■ High

Intermediate

□ Low

Map 2-1. Prevalence of antibody to hepatitis A virus, 2006.[1]
(*See note 1 on opposite page.*)

Box 2-1. Hepatitis A pre-travel case study

Case study: You are a travel medicine professional preparing a group for travel to an eastern European country that is shown in Map 2-1 to have an intermediate prevalence of antibody to hepatitis A virus (anti-HAV). You have recommended that all members of the group take precautions to prevent hepatitis A. The leader of the group questions your advice on the basis of an editorial from a major newspaper written by the ambassador to the U.S. from this country. The editorial claims that her country is stigmatized in the U.S. and cites the example of the Yellow Book, which indicates that travelers from the U.S. to this country are at risk for hepatitis A. The editorial states that cases of hepatitis A are at very low levels in this country and seem to be declining over time. How would you respond to the members of the group?

Points to consider in your response:

- In most intermediate and high anti-HAV-endemic countries, many long-term residents are infected as children, at a time when they may not get symptoms. Cases of hepatitis A in the resident population will be very low; however, travelers from low endemic settings such as the United States are at risk for HAV infection and should be protected.
- The determination of risk is based on CDC estimates of prevalence of anti-HAV, a marker of previous HAV infection. This country-level estimate is based on limited data and might not reflect the current prevalence.
- Prevention of hepatitis A in travelers with vaccination should be used liberally because the vaccine is safe and effective and will give long-term benefits that go beyond the risk posed by any specific trip.

Risk for Travelers

- Hepatitis A is one of the most common vaccine-preventable infections acquired during travel.
- In 2006 in the United States, among cases for which information regarding exposures during the incubation period was collected, the most frequently identified risk factor for hepatitis A was international travel (reported by 15% of case-patients overall).
- As in previous years, most travel-related cases (72%) were associated with travel to Mexico and Central/South America. As HAV transmission in the United States has decreased, cases among travelers to countries in which hepatitis is endemic have accounted for an increased proportion of all cases.
- The risk of acquiring HAV infection for U.S. residents traveling abroad varies with living conditions, length of stay, and the incidence of HAV infection in the area visited. For travelers to other countries, risk for infection increases with duration of travel and is highest for those who live in or visit rural areas, trek in back-country areas, or frequently eat or drink in settings of poor sanitation.
- Nevertheless, many cases of travel-related hepatitis A occur in travelers to developing countries with "standard" tourist itineraries, accommodations, and food consumption behaviors.

Clinical Presentation

- HAV infection may be asymptomatic, or its clinical manifestations may range in severity from a mild illness lasting 1–2 weeks to a severely disabling disease lasting several months.
- Clinical manifestations of hepatitis A often include the abrupt onset of fever, malaise, anorexia, nausea, and abdominal discomfort, followed within a few days by jaundice.

[1]Estimates of prevalence of antibody to hepatitis A virus (anti-HAV), a marker of previous HAV infection, are based on limited data and might not reflect current prevalence. In addition, anti-HAV prevalence might vary within countries by subpopulation and locality. As used on this map, the terms "high," "medium," and "low" endemicity reflect available evidence of how widespread HAV infection is within each country, rather than precise quantitative assessments.

- The incubation period for hepatitis A averages 28 days (range: 15–50 days).
- The likelihood of having symptoms with HAV infection is related to the infected person's age. In children <6 years of age, most (70%) infections are asymptomatic; if illness does occur, its duration is usually less than 2 months.
- No chronic or long-term infection is associated with hepatitis A, but 10% of infected persons will have prolonged or relapsing symptoms over a 6- to 9-month period.
- The overall case–fatality rate among cases reported to CDC is 0.3%; however, the rate is 1.8% among adults >50 years of age.

Diagnosis

- Demonstration of IgM antibodies against hepatitis A virus (IgM anti-HAV) in the serum of acutely or recently ill patients establishes the diagnosis.
- IgM anti-HAV becomes detectable 5–10 days after exposure. A fourfold or greater rise in specific antibodies in paired sera, detected by commercially available EIA, also establishes the diagnosis.
- If laboratory tests are not available, epidemiologic evidence may provide support for the diagnosis in a clinically compatible case.
- HAV RNA can be detected in blood and stools of most persons during the acute phase of infection through nucleic acid amplification methods, but these are not generally used for diagnostic purposes.

Treatment

No specific treatment is available for persons with hepatitis A. Treatment is supportive.

Preventive Measures for Travelers

Health-care providers should administer hepatitis A vaccination for persons traveling for any purpose, frequency, or duration to countries that have high or intermediate endemicity of HAV infection. Providers may also consider its administration to persons for travel to any destination.

Vaccine and Immune Globulin

Monovalent Vaccines

- Two monovalent hepatitis A vaccines are currently licensed in the United States for persons at least 12 months of age:
  - HAVRIX, manufactured by GlaxoSmithKline (Table 2-4), and
  - VAQTA manufactured by Merck & Co., Inc. (Table 2-5).
- Both vaccines are made of inactivated HAV adsorbed to aluminum hydroxide as an adjuvant. HAVRIX is prepared with 2-phenoxyethanol as a preservative, while VAQTA is formulated without a preservative.
- All hepatitis A vaccines should be administered intramuscularly in the deltoid muscle.

Combination Vaccine

- TWINRIX, manufactured by GlaxoSmithKline, is a combined hepatitis A and hepatitis B vaccine licensed for persons ≥18 years of age, containing 720 EL.U. of hepatitis A antigen (50% of the HAVRIX adult dose) and 20 µg of recombinant hepatitis B surface antigen protein (the same as the ENGERIX-B adult dose) (Table 2-6).
- Primary immunization consists of three doses, given on a 0-, 1-, and 6-month schedule, the same schedule as that commonly used for monovalent hepatitis B vaccine.

Table 2-4. Licensed schedule for HAVRIX[1]

Age Group (YRS)	Dose (EL.U.)[2]	Volume	No. of Doses	Schedule (Months)
1–18	720	0.5 mL	2	0, 6–2
≥19	1440	1.0 mL	2	0, 6–12

1 Hepatitis A vaccine, inactivated, GlaxoSmithKline.
2 EL.U., enzyme-linked immunosorbent assay (ELISA) units of inactivated hepatitis A virus.

Table 2-5. Licensed schedule for VAQTA[1]

Age Group (YRS)	Dose (U.)[2]	Volume	No. of Doses	Schedule (Months)
1–18	25	0.5 mL	2	0, 6–18
≥19	50	1.0 mL	2	0, 6–18

1 Hepatitis A vaccine, inactivated, Merck & Co., Inc.
2 U., units of hepatitis A virus antigen.

Table 2-6. Licensed schedule for TWINRIX[1]

Age Group (YRS)	Dose (EL.U./20 μg)[2]	Volume	No. of Doses	Schedule (Months)
≥18	720	1.0 mL	3	0, 1, 6 months
≥18	720	1.0 mL	4	0, 7, 21 days +1 year

1 Combined hepatitis A and hepatitis B vaccine, GlaxoSmithKline.
2 EL.U., enzyme-linked immunosorbent assay (ELISA) units of inactivated hepatitis A virus/micrograms hepatitis B surface antigen.

- TWINRIX contains aluminum phosphate and aluminum hydroxide as adjuvants and 2-phenoxyethanol as a preservative.
- An accelerated schedule of TWINRIX (i.e., doses at days 0, 7, and 21) for travelers has been approved by the FDA. A booster dose should be given at 1 year.
- The immunogenicity of TWINRIX is equivalent to that of the monovalent hepatitis vaccines when tested after completion of the licensed schedule.

Vaccination of Travelers

- All susceptible persons traveling to or working in countries that have high or intermediate hepatitis A endemicity should be vaccinated or receive IG before departure. Hepatitis A vaccine at the age-appropriate dose is preferred to IG. The first dose of hepatitis A vaccine should be administered as soon as travel to countries with high or intermediate endemicity is considered.
- One dose of monovalent hepatitis A vaccine administered at any time before departure can provide adequate protection for most healthy persons <40 years of age.
- Completion of the vaccine series according to the licensed schedule is necessary for long-term protection.
- Many persons will have detectable anti-HAV in response to the monovalent vaccine by 2 weeks after the first vaccine dose. The proportion of persons who develop a detectable antibody response at 2 weeks may be lower when smaller vaccine dosages are used, such as with the use of TWINRIX.
- For optimal protection, older adults, immunocompromised persons, and persons with chronic liver disease or other chronic medical conditions planning to depart to an area in <2 weeks should receive the initial dose of vaccine along with IG (0.02 mL/kg) at a separate anatomic injection site.
- Travelers who receive hepatitis A vaccine less than 2 weeks before traveling to an endemic area and who do not receive IG (either by choice or because of lack of availability) will be at lower risk for infection than those who do not receive hepatitis A vaccine or IG.

- Although vaccination of an immune traveler is not contraindicated and does not increase the risk for adverse effects, screening for total anti-HAV before travel can be useful in some circumstances to determine susceptibility and eliminate unnecessary vaccination or IG prophylaxis of immune travelers. Such serologic screening for susceptibility might be indicated for adult travelers who are >40 years of age and those born in areas of the world with intermediate or high endemicity who are likely to have had prior HAV infection, if the cost of screening (laboratory and office visit) is less than the cost of vaccination or IG prophylaxis and if testing will not delay vaccination and interfere with timely receipt of vaccine or IG before travel. Postvaccination testing for serologic response is not indicated.
- Travelers who are <12 months of age, are allergic to a vaccine component, or who otherwise elect not to receive vaccine should receive a single dose of IG (0.02 mL/kg), which provides effective protection against HAV infection for up to 3 months (Table 2-7).
- Those who do not receive vaccination and plan to travel for >3 months should receive an IG dose of 0.06 mL/kg, which must be repeated if the duration of travel is >5 months.
- In addition, health-care providers should be alert to opportunities to provide vaccination for all travelers whose plans might include travel at some time in the future to an area of high or intermediate endemicity, including those whose current medical evaluation is for travel to an area where hepatitis A vaccination is not currently recommended.
- Those who refuse vaccine and IG should be advised to closely adhere to prevention tips listed below.

Other Vaccine Considerations

- Using the vaccines according to the licensed schedules is preferable. However, an interrupted series does not need to be restarted.
- Given their similar immunogenicity, a series that has been started with one brand of monovalent vaccine (i.e., HAVRIX or VAQTA) may be completed with the other brand.
- Hepatitis A vaccine may be administered at the same time as IG or other commonly used vaccines for travelers, at different injection sites.
- In adults and children who have completed the vaccine series, anti-HAV has been shown to persist for at least 5–12 years after vaccination. Results of mathematical models indicate that, after completion of the vaccination series, anti-HAV will likely persist for 20 years or more. For children and adults who complete the primary series, booster doses of vaccine are not recommended.

Vaccine Safety and Adverse Reactions

- Among adults, the most frequently reported side effects occurring 3–5 days after a vaccine dose are tenderness or pain at the injection site (53%–56%) or headache (14%–16%).
- Among children, the most common side effects reported are pain or tenderness at the injection site (15%–19%), feeding problems (8% in one study), or headache (4% in one study).

Table 2-7. Recommended doses of immune globulin (IG) for protection against hepatitis A

Setting	Duration of Coverage	Dose (Ml/Kg)[1]
Pre-exposure	Short-term (1–2 months)	0.02
	Long-term (3–5 months)	0.06[2]
Postexposure	NA	0.02

1 IG should be administered by intramuscular injection into either the deltoid or gluteal muscle. For children <12 months of age, IG can be administered in the anterolateral thigh muscle.
2 Repeat every 5 months if continued exposure to hepatitis A virus occurs.

- No serious adverse events in children or adults that could be definitively attributed to the vaccine or to increases in serious adverse events among vaccinated persons compared with baseline rates have been identified.
- IG for intramuscular administration prepared in the United States has few side effects (primarily soreness at the injection site) and has never been shown to transmit infectious agents (hepatitis B virus, hepatitis C virus [HCV], or HIV).
- Since December 1994, all IG products commercially available in the United States have had to undergo a viral inactivation procedure or be negative for HCV RNA before release.

Precautions and Contraindications

- These vaccines should not be administered to travelers with a history of hypersensitivity to any vaccine component.
- HAVRIX or TWINRIX should not be administered to travelers with a history of hypersensitivity reactions to the preservative 2-phenoxyethanol.
- TWINRIX should not be administered to persons with a history of hypersensitivity to yeast.
- Because hepatitis A vaccine consists of inactivated virus and hepatitis B vaccine consists of a recombinant protein, no special precautions need to be taken for vaccination of immunocompromised travelers.

Pregnancy

- The safety of hepatitis A vaccine for pregnant women has not been determined.
- However, because hepatitis A vaccine is produced from inactivated HAV, the theoretical risk to either the pregnant woman or the developing fetus is thought to be very low.
- The risk of vaccination should be weighed against the risk of hepatitis A in female travelers who might be at high risk for exposure to HAV.
- Pregnancy is not a contraindication to using IG.

Other Prevention Tips

- Boiling or cooking food and beverage items for at least 1 minute to 185° F (85° C) inactivates HAV. Foods and beverages heated to this temperature and for this length of time cannot serve as vehicles for HAV infection unless they become contaminated after heating.
- Adequate chlorination of water as recommended in the United States will inactivate HAV.
- Travelers should be advised that, to minimize their risk of hepatitis A and other enteric diseases in developing countries, they should avoid potentially contaminated water or food.
- Travelers should also be advised to avoid drinking beverages (with or without ice) of unknown purity, eating uncooked shellfish, and eating uncooked fruits or vegetables that are not peeled or prepared by the traveler personally.

References

1. CDC. Prevention of hepatitis A through active or passive immunization: Recommendations of the Advisory Committee on Immunization Practices (ACIP). MMWR Recomm Rep. 2006; 55(RR07):1–23.

2. CDC. Update: Prevention of hepatitis A after exposure to hepatitis A virus and in international travelers. Updated Recommendations of the Advisory Committee on Immunization Practices (ACIP). MMWR Morbid Mortal Wkly Rep. 2007;56(41):1080–4.

3. Bell BP, Feinstone SM. Hepatitis A vaccine. In: Plotkin SA, Orenstein WA, editors. Vaccines. 4th ed. Philadelphia: W.B. Saunders, 2004. p. 269–97.

4. Mutsch M, Spicher VM, Gut C, Steffen R. Hepatitis A virus infections in travelers, 1988–2004. Clin Infect Dis. 2006;42(4):490–7.

5. Bacaner N, Stauffer B, Boulware DR, et.al. Travel medicine considerations for North American immigrants visiting friends and relatives. JAMA. 2004;291(23):2856–64.

6. CDC. Surveillance for acute viral hepatitis – United States, 2006. MMWR Surv Summ. 2008; 57(SS02):1–24.

7. Van Damme P, Banatvala J, Fay O, et al. Hepatitis A booster vaccination: is there a need? Lancet. 2003;362(9389):1065–71.

8. Winokur PL, Stapleton JT. Immunoglobulin prophylaxis for hepatitis A. Clin Infect Dis. 1992;14(2):580–6.

9. Fiore AE. Hepatitis A transmitted by food. Clin Infect Dis. 2004;38(5):705–15.

HEPATITIS B

Sandra S. Chaves

Infectious Agent

Hepatitis B is caused by the hepatitis B virus (HBV), a small, circular, partially double-stranded DNA molecule in the *Hepadnaviridae* family.

Mode of Transmission

HBV is transmitted through activities that involve contact with blood or blood-derived fluids. Such activities include the following:

- Unprotected sex with an HBV-infected partner
- Shared needles used for injection of illegal drugs
- Shared glucose-monitoring equipment
- Work in health-care fields (e.g., medical, dental, laboratory) that entails direct exposure to potentially infected human blood
- Transfusions with blood or blood products that have not been screened for HBV
- Dental, medical, or cosmetic (e.g., tattooing, body piercing) procedures with needles or other equipment that are contaminated with HBV

In addition, open skin lesions, such as those due to impetigo, scabies, or scratched insect bites, can play a role in HBV transmission if direct exposure to wound exudates from HBV-infected persons occurs.

Occurrence

- The prevalence of chronic HBV infection is low (<2%) in the general population in Northern and Western Europe, North America, Australia, New Zealand, Mexico, and southern South America (Map 2-2).
- The prevalence of chronic HBV infection is intermediate (2%–7%) in South, Central, and Southwest Asia, Israel, Japan, Eastern and Southern Europe, Russia, most areas surrounding the Amazon River basin, Honduras, and Guatemala (see Map 2-2).
- The prevalence of chronic HBV infection is high (≥8%) in all socioeconomic groups in: all of Africa; Southeast Asia, including China, Korea, Indonesia, and the Philippines; the Middle East, except Israel; South and Western Pacific islands; the interior Amazon River basin; and certain parts of the Caribbean (Haiti and the Dominican Republic) (see Map 2-2).

Risk for Travelers

There are no data with which to assess the risk for HBV infection among U.S. travelers. The risk for HBV infection for international travelers is considered generally low, except for travelers to countries where the prevalence of chronic HBV infection is intermediate or high. Some travelers, such as adventure travelers, Peace Corps volunteers, missionaries, and military personnel, may be at increased risk for infection.

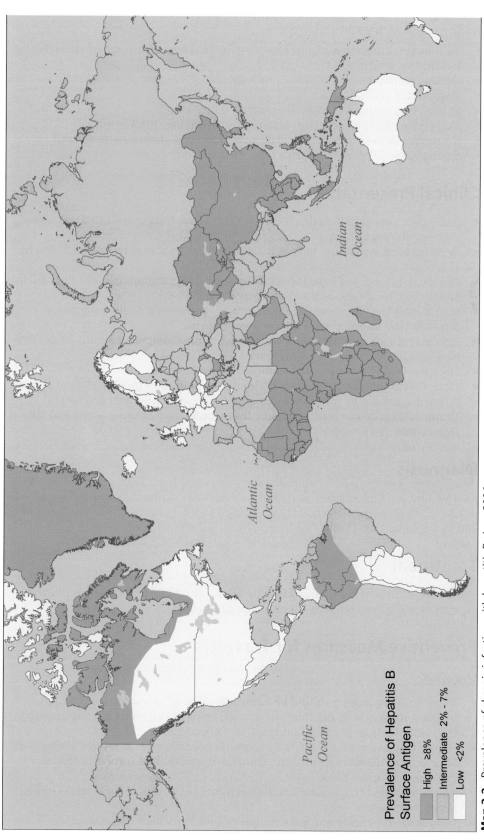

Map 2-2. Prevalence of chronic infection with hepatitis B virus, 2006.

Prevalence of Hepatitis B
Surface Antigen

High ≥8%

Intermediate 2% - 7%

Low <2%

Pacific
Ocean

Atlantic
Ocean

Indian
Ocean

Situations or activities that may carry increased risk for HBV infection for travelers while overseas include the following:

- An injury or illness that requires invasive medical attention (e.g., injection, IV drip, transfusion, stitching)
- Dental treatment
- Unprotected sexual contact
- Sharing illegal drug injection equipment
- Skin-perforation practices (e.g., tattooing, ear piercing, acupuncture)
- Cosmetic practices with risk for skin perforation (e.g., manicure/pedicure)
- Sharing personal grooming items (e.g., earrings, toothbrush, razor)

Clinical Presentation

- Incubation period of hepatitis B is typically 90 days (range: 60–150 days) from exposure to onset of jaundice.
- Constitutional symptoms such as malaise and anorexia may precede jaundice by 1–2 weeks.
- Clinical symptoms and signs include nausea, vomiting, abdominal pain, and jaundice.
- Skin rashes, joint pain, and arthritis may occur.
- Infants, children <5 years of age, and immunosuppressed adults with newly acquired HBV infection typically are asymptomatic.
- Infected persons ≥5 years of age, including immunocompetent adults, 30%–50% have initial clinical signs or symptoms.
- The case–fatality rate of acute hepatitis B is approximately 1%.
- Acute HBV infection causes chronic (long-term) infection in 30%–90% of persons infected as infants or young children and in <5% of adolescents and adults.
- Chronic infection can lead to chronic liver disease, liver scarring (cirrhosis), and liver cancer.

Diagnosis

At least one serologic marker is present during each of the different phases of HBV infection. The serologic markers are typically used to differentiate between acute, resolving, and chronic infection (Table 2-8).

Treatment

No specific treatment is available for acute illness caused by hepatitis B. Antiviral drugs are approved for the treatment of chronic hepatitis B.

Preventive Measures for Travelers

Vaccine

- Hepatitis B vaccination should be administered to all unvaccinated persons traveling to areas with intermediate to high levels of endemic HBV transmission (i.e., with hepatitis B surface antigen [HBsAg] prevalence ≥2%).
- Hepatitis B vaccination is currently recommended for all U.S. residents who work in health-care fields (e.g., medical, dental, laboratory) that involve potential exposure to human blood.
- All unvaccinated U.S. children and adolescents (<19 years of age) should receive hepatitis B vaccine.
- Unvaccinated persons who have indications for hepatitis B vaccination independent of travel should be vaccinated (e.g., men who have sex with men,

Table 2-8. Typical interpretation of serologic test results for hepatitis B virus infection

HBsAg[1]	Total anti-HBc[2]	IgM[3] anti-HBc	Anti-HBs[4]	Interpretation
−[5]	−	−	−	Never infected
+[6,7]	−	−	−	Early acute infection; transient (up to 18 days) after vaccination
+	+	+	−	Acute infection
−	+	+	+ or −	Acute resolving infection
−	+	−	+	Recovered from past infection and immune
+	+	−	−	Chronic infection
−	+	−	−	False-positive (i.e., susceptible); past infection; "low-level" chronic infection;[8] or passive transfer of anti-HBc to infant born to HBsAg-positive mother
−	−	−	+	Immune if concentration is ≥10 mIU/mL after vaccine series completion;[9] passive transfer after hepatitis B immune globulin administration

From CDC. MMWR Recomm Rep. 2006; 55(RR-16):1–25.

1 Hepatitis B surface antigen.
2 IgG antibody to hepatitis B core antigen.
3 Immunoglobulin M.
4 Antibody to HBsAg.
5 Negative test result.
6 Positive test result.
7 To ensure that an HBsAg-positive test result is not a false-positive, samples with reactive HBsAg results should be tested with a licensed neutralizing confirmatory test if recommended in the manufacturer's package insert.
8 Persons positive only for anti-HBc are unlikely to be infectious except under unusual circumstances in which they are the source for direct percutaneous exposure of susceptible recipients to large quantities of virus (e.g., blood transfusion or organ transplant).
9 Milli-international units per milliliter.

injection drug users, anyone who has recently had a sexually transmitted disease or has had more than one sex partner in the previous 6 months).

Vaccine Dose and Administration

- The vaccine is usually administered as a three-dose series on a 0-, 1-, and 6-month schedule (see Table 2-9). The second dose should be given 1 month after the first dose; the third dose should be given at least 2 months after the second dose and at least 4 months after the first dose.
- Alternatively, the vaccine ENGERIX-B, manufactured by GlaxoSmithKline, is also approved for administration on a four-dose schedule at 0, 1, 2, and 12 months.
- There is also a two-dose schedule for RECOMBIVAX HB, a vaccine produced by Merck & Co., Inc., which has been licensed for children and adolescents 11–15 years of age. Using the two-dose schedule, the adult dose of RECOMBIVAX HB is administered, with the second dose given 4–6 months after the first dose.
- A three-dose series that has been started with one brand of vaccine may be completed with the other brand.
- TWINRIX, manufactured by GlaxoSmithKline, is a combined hepatitis A and hepatitis B vaccine licensed for persons 18 years of age or older. Primary immunization consists of three doses, given on a 0-, 1-, and 6-month schedule.

Special Situations

- Ideally, vaccination should begin at least 6 months before travel so the full vaccine series can be completed before departure. Because some protection is provided by one or two doses, the vaccine series should be initiated, if indicated, even if it cannot be completed before departure. Optimal protection, however, is not conferred until after the final vaccine dose. Travelers should be advised to return for completion of the vaccine series.

Table 2-9. Recommended doses of currently licensed formulations of hepatitis B vaccine

Group	Single-Antigen Vaccine				Combination Vaccine					
	RECOMBIVAX HB		ENGERIX-B		COMVAX[1]		PEDIARIX[2]		TWINRIX[3]	
	Dose (μg)[4]	Volume (ml)	Dose (μg)[4]	Volume (ml)	Dose (μg)[4]	Volume (ml)	Dose (μg)[4]	Volume (ml)	Dose (μg)[4]	Volume (ml)
Infants (<1 year)	5[7]	0.5	10[7]	0.5	5	0.5	10	0.5	NA[5]	NA
Children (1–10 years)	5	0.5	10	0.5	5	0.5	10	0.5	NA	NA
Adolescents 11–15 years	10[6]	1.0	NA	NA	NA	NA	NA	NA	NA	NA
11–19 years	5	0.5	10	0.5	NA	NA	NA	NA	20[3]	1.0[3]
Adults (>20 years)	10	1.0	20	1.0	NA	NA	NA	NA	20	1.0
Hemodialysis patients and other immunocompromised persons[7]										
<20 years[7]	5	0.5	10	0.5	NA	NA	NA	NA	NA	NA
≥20 years	40[8]	10	40[9]	2.0	NA	NA	NA	NA	NA	NA

1 Combined hepatitis B–*Haemophilus influenzae* type b conjugate vaccine. This vaccine cannot be administered before age 6 weeks or after age 71 months.
2 Combined hepatitis B–diphtheria, tetanus, pertussis-inactivated poliovirus vaccine. This vaccine cannot be administered at birth, before age 6 weeks, or after age 7 years.
3 Combined hepatitis A and hepatitis B vaccine. This vaccine is recommended for persons ≥18 years who are at increased risk for both hepatitis A virus and hepatitis B virus infections.
4 Recombinant hepatitis B surface antigen dose.
5 Not applicable.
6 Adult formulation administered on a 2-dose schedule.
7 Higher doses might be more immunogenic, but no specific recommendations have been made.
8 Dialysis formulation administered on a 3-dose schedule at 0, 1, and 6 months.
9 Two 1.0-mL doses administered at one site, on a 4-dose schedule at 0, 1, 2, and 6 months.

- An accelerated vaccine schedule could be used for those traveling to endemic areas at short notice and facing imminent exposure because of behavioral risks or to emergency responders to disaster areas. The monovalent hepatitis B vaccines can be used at 0, 7, and 14 days. If an accelerated schedule is used, the patient should receive a booster dose at least 6 months after the start of the series to promote long-term immunity.
- An accelerated vaccine schedule with TWINRIX (hepatitis A and hepatitis B vaccine) can also be used (doses at 0, 7, and 21–30 days). In this situation, a booster dose should be given at 12 months to promote long-term immunity.
- For children and adults whose immune status is normal, booster doses of vaccine are not recommended. Serologic testing to assess antibody levels is not necessary for most vaccinees (see the Vaccine Recommendations for Infants and Children section in Chapter 7).

Vaccine Safety and Adverse Reactions

- Hepatitis B vaccines have been shown to be safe for persons of all ages. Pain at the injection site (3%–29%) and elevated temperature higher than 37.7° C (99.9° F) (1%–6%) are the most frequently reported side effects among vaccine recipients.
- These vaccines should not be administered to persons with a history of hypersensitivity to any vaccine component, including yeast. The vaccine contains a recombinant protein (HBsAg) that is noninfectious. Limited data indicate that there is no apparent

risk of adverse events to the developing fetus when hepatitis B vaccine is administered to pregnant women. HBV infection affecting a pregnant woman can result in serious disease for the mother and chronic infection for the newborn. Neither pregnancy nor lactation should be considered a contraindication for vaccination.

Other Preventive Measures

- As part of the pre-travel education process, all travelers should be given information about the risks for hepatitis B and other bloodborne pathogens from contaminated medical equipment, injection drug use, or sexual activity and informed of prevention measures (see below), including hepatitis B vaccination, that can be used to prevent transmission of HBV.
- Regardless of destination, all persons who may engage in practices that put them at risk for HBV infection during travel should receive hepatitis B vaccination if previously unvaccinated.
- Any adult seeking protection from HBV infection should be vaccinated. Acknowledgment of a specific risk factor is not a requirement for vaccination.
- Behavioral preventive measures for HBV infection are similar to those for HIV infection and AIDS.
- When seeking medical or dental care, travelers should be advised to be alert to the use of medical, surgical, and dental equipment that has not been adequately sterilized or disinfected, reuse of contaminated equipment, and unsafe injecting practices (e.g., reuse of disposable needles and syringes).
- HBV and other bloodborne pathogens (e.g., HIV and hepatitis C) can be transmitted if tools are not sterile or if the tattoo artist or piercer does not follow other proper infection-control procedures (e.g., washing hands, using latex gloves, and cleaning and disinfecting surfaces and instruments).
- Travelers should be advised to consider the health risks in deciding to get a tattoo or body piercing in areas where adequate sterilization or disinfection procedures might not be available or practiced.

References

1. CDC. A comprehensive immunization strategy to eliminate transmission of hepatitis B virus infection in the United States: recommendations of the Advisory Committee on Immunization Practices (ACIP) Part II: immunization of adults. MMWR Recomm Rep. 2006;55(RR-16):1–25.
2. CDC. A comprehensive immunization strategy to eliminate transmission of hepatitis B virus infection in the United States: recommendations of the Advisory Committee on Immunization Practices (ACIP) Part 1: immunization of infants, children, and adolescents. MMWR Recomm Rep. 2005;54(RR-16):1–23.
3. Mast E, Goldstein S, Ward JL. Hepatitis B vaccine. In: Plotkin SA, Orenstein WA, editors. Vaccines. 5th ed. Philadelphia: W.B. Saunders; 2004. p. 299–337.
4. Simonsen L, Kane A, Lloyd J, et al. Unsafe injections in the developing world and transmission of bloodborne pathogens: a review. Bull World Health Organ. 1999;77(10):789–800.
5. Sagliocca L, Stroffolini T, Amoroso P, et al. Risk factors for acute hepatitis B: a case–control study. J Viral Hepat. 1997;4(1):63–6.
6. Lok AS, McMahon BJ. Practice Guidelines Committee, American Association for the Study of Liver Diseases (AASLD). Chronic hepatitis B: update of recommendations. Hepatology. 2004;39(3):857–61.
7. CDC. Updated U.S. Public Health Service guidelines for the management of occupational exposures to HBV, HCV and HIV and recommendations for postexposure prophylaxis. MMWR Recomm Rep. 2001;50(RR-11):1–42.
8. Bock HL, Loscher T, Scheiermann N, et al. Accelerated schedule for hepatitis B immunization. J Travel Med. 1995;2(4):213–7.
9. Long GE, Rickman LS. Infectious complications of tattoos. Clin Infect Dis. 1994;18(4):610–9. Review.
10. Mariano A, Mele A, Tosti ME, et al. Role of beauty treatment in the spread of parenterally transmitted hepatitis viruses in Italy. J Med Virol. 2004;74(2):216–20.
11. CDC. Provisional Recommendations for Hepatitis B vaccination of adults – October 2005. [cited 2006 Oct 31]. Available from: http://www.cdc.gov/nip/recs/provisional_recs/hepB_adult.pdf.

TYPHOID AND PARATYPHOID FEVER

Eric Mintz

Infectious Agent

Typhoid fever is an acute, life-threatening febrile illness caused by the bacterium *Salmonella enterica* serotype Typhi. Paratyphoid fever is a similar illness caused by *S*. Paratyphi A, B, or C.

Mode of Transmission

- Humans are the only source. No animal or environmental reservoirs have been identified.
- Typhoid and paratyphoid fever are most often acquired through consumption of water or food that have been contaminated by feces of an acutely infected or convalescent individual or a chronic asymptomatic carrier.
- Transmission through sexual contact, especially among men who have sex with men, has rarely been documented.

Occurrence

- An estimated 22 million cases of typhoid fever and 200,000 related deaths occur worldwide each year; an additional 6 million cases of paratyphoid fever are estimated to occur annually.
- Approximately 400 cases of typhoid fever and 150 cases of paratyphoid fever are reported to CDC each year among persons with onset of illness in the United States, most of whom are recent travelers.

Risk for Travelers

- Risk is greatest for travelers to South Asia (6 to 30 times higher than all other destinations). Other areas of risk include East and Southeast Asia, Africa, the Caribbean, and Central and South America.
- Travelers to South Asia are at highest risk for infections that are nalidixic acid-resistant or multidrug-resistant (i.e., resistant to ampicillin, chloramphenicol, and trimethoprim–sulfamethoxazole).
- Travelers who are visiting friends or relatives are at increased risk (see the VFR section in Chapter 8).
- Although the risk of acquiring typhoid or paratyphoid fever increases with the duration of stay, travelers have acquired typhoid fever even during visits of less than 1 week to countries where the disease is endemic.

Clinical Presentation

- The incubation period of typhoid and paratyphoid infections is 6–30 days. The onset of illness is insidious, with gradually increasing fatigue and a fever that increases daily from low-grade to as high as 102° F–104° F (38.5° C–40° C) by the third to fourth day of illness. Headache, malaise, and anorexia are nearly universal. Hepatosplenomegaly can often be detected. A transient, macular rash of rose-colored spots can occasionally be seen on the trunk.
- Fever is commonly lowest in the morning, reaching a peak in late afternoon or evening. Untreated, the disease can last for a month. The serious complications of

typhoid fever generally occur only after 2–3 weeks of illness, mainly intestinal hemorrhage or perforation, which can be life threatening.

Diagnosis

- Infection with typhoid or paratyphoid fever results in a very low-grade septicemia. Blood culture is usually positive in only half the cases. Stool culture is not usually positive during the acute phase of the disease. Bone-marrow culture increases the diagnostic yield to about 80% of cases.
- The Widal test is an old serologic assay for detecting IgM and IgG antibodies to the O and H antigens of *Salmonella*. The test is unreliable, but is widely used in developing countries because of its low cost. Newer serologic assays are somewhat more sensitive and specific than the Widal test, but are infrequently available.
- Because there is no definitive test for typhoid or paratyphoid fever, the diagnosis often has to be made clinically. The combination of a history of being at risk for infection and a gradual onset of fever that increases in severity over several days should raise suspicion of typhoid or paratyphoid fever.

Treatment

- Specific antimicrobial therapy shortens the clinical course of typhoid fever and reduces the risk for death.
- Empiric treatment of typhoid or paratyphoid fever in most parts of the world would utilize a fluoroquinolone, most often ciprofloxacin. However, resistance to fluoroquinolones is highest in the Indian subcontinent and increasing in other areas. Injectable third-generation cephalosporins are often the empiric drug of choice when the possibility of fluoroquinolone resistance is high.
- Patients treated with an appropriate antibiotic still require 3–5 days to defervesce completely, although the height of the fever decreases each day. Patients may actually feel worse during the time that the fever is starting to go away. If fever does not subside within 5 days, alternative antimicrobial agents or other foci of infection should be considered.

Preventive Measures for Travelers

Vaccine

- CDC recommends typhoid vaccine for travelers to areas where there is a recognized increased risk of exposure to S. Typhi.
- The typhoid vaccines currently available do not offer protection against S. Paratyphi infection.
- Travelers should be reminded that typhoid immunization is not 100% effective, and typhoid fever could still occur.
- Two typhoid vaccines are currently available in the United States.
  - Oral live, attenuated vaccine (Vivotif Berna vaccine, manufactured from the Ty21a strain of S. Typhi by the Swiss Serum and Vaccine Institute)
  - Vi capsular polysaccharide vaccine (ViCPS) (Typhim Vi, manufactured by Sanofi Pasteur) for intramuscular use
- Both vaccines protect 50%–80% of recipients.
- Table 2-10 provides information on vaccine dosage, administration, and revaccination. The time required for primary vaccination differs for the two vaccines, as do the lower age limits.
- Primary vaccination with oral Ty21a vaccine consists of four capsules, one taken every other day. The capsules should be kept refrigerated (not frozen), and all four doses must be taken to achieve maximum efficacy. Each capsule should be taken

Table 2-10. Dosage and schedule for typhoid fever vaccination

Vaccination	Age (Years)	Dose/Mode of Administration	No. of Doses	Dosing Interval	Boosting Interval
Oral, live, attenuated Ty21a vaccine (Vivotif)					
Primary series	≥6	1 capsule,[1] oral	4	48 hours	Not applicable
Booster	≥6	1 capsule,[1] oral	4	48 hours	Every 5 years
Vi Capsular polysaccharide vaccine (Typhim Vi)					
Primary series	≥2	0.50 mL, intramuscular	1	Not applicable	Not applicable
Booster	≥2	0.50 mL, intramuscular	1	Not applicable	Every 2 years

1 Administer with cool liquid no warmer than 98.6° F (37° C).

with cool liquid no warmer than 37° C (98.6° F), approximately 1 hour before a meal. This regimen should be completed 1 week before potential exposure. The vaccine manufacturer recommends that Ty21a not be administered to infants or children <6 years of age.

- Primary vaccination with ViCPS consists of one 0.5-mL (25-µg) dose administered intramuscularly. One dose of this vaccine should be given at least 2 weeks before expected exposure. The manufacturer does not recommend the vaccine for infants and children <2 years of age.

Vaccine Safety and Adverse Reactions

Information on adverse reactions is presented in Table 2-11. Information is not available on the safety of these vaccines in pregnancy; it is prudent on theoretical grounds to avoid vaccinating pregnant women. Live, attenuated Ty21a vaccine should not be given to immunocompromised travelers, including those infected with HIV. The intramuscular vaccine presents a theoretically safer alternative for this group. The only contraindication to vaccination with ViCPS vaccine is a history of severe local or systemic reactions after a previous dose. Neither of the available vaccines should be given to persons with an acute febrile illness.

Precautions and Contraindications

Theoretical concerns have been raised about the immunogenicity of live, attenuated Ty21a vaccine in persons concurrently receiving antimicrobials (including antimalarial chemoprophylaxis), IG, or viral vaccines. The growth of the live Ty21a strain is inhibited in vitro by various antibacterial agents. Vaccination with Ty21a should be delayed for >72 hours after the administration of any antibacterial agent. Available data do not suggest that simultaneous administration of oral polio or yellow fever vaccine decreases the immunogenicity of Ty21a. If typhoid vaccination is warranted, it should not be delayed because of administration of viral vaccines. Simultaneous administration of Ty21a and IG does not appear to pose a problem.

Table 2-11. Common adverse reactions to typhoid fever vaccines

Vaccine	Reactions		
	Fever	**Headache**	**Local Reactions**
Ty21a[1]	0%–5%	0%–5%	Not applicable
Vi Capsular polysaccharide	0%–1%	16%–20%	7% erythema or induration 1 cm

1 The side effects of Ty21a are rare and mainly consist of abdominal discomfort, nausea, vomiting, and rash or urticaria.

References

1. Gupta, S, Medalla F, Omondi M, et al. Laboratory-based surveillance of paratyphoid fever in the United States: travel and antimicrobial resistance. Clin Infect Dis. In press 2008.
2. Ackers ML, Puhr ND, Tauxe RV, et al. Laboratory-based surveillance of *Salmonella* serotype Typhi infections in the United States: antimicrobial resistance on the rise. JAMA. 2000;283(20):2668–73.
3. Steinberg EB, Bishop R, Haber P, et al. Typhoid fever in travelers: who should be targeted for prevention? Clin Infect Dis. 2004;39(2):186–91.
4. Parry CM, Hien TT, Dougan G, et al. Typhoid fever. N Engl J Med. 2002;347(22):1770–82.
5. Klugman KP, Gilbertson IT, Koornhof HJ, et al. Protective activity of Vi capsular polysaccharide vaccine against typhoid fever. Lancet. 1987;2(8569):1165–9.
6. Simanjuntak CH, Paleologo FP, Punjabi NH, et al. Oral immunisation against typhoid fever in Indonesia with Ty21a vaccine. Lancet. 1991;338(8774):1055–9.
7. CDC. Typhoid immunization: Recommendations of the Advisory Committee on Immunization Practices (ACIP). MMWR Morbid Mortal Wkly Rep. 1994;43(RR-14):1–7.
8. Crump JA, Luby SP, Mintz ED. The global burden of typhoid fever. Bull World Health Organ. 2004;82(5):346–53.
9. Beeching NJ, Clarke PD, Kitchin NR, et al. Comparison of two combined vaccines against typhoid fever and hepatitis A in healthy adults. Vaccine. 2004;23(1):29–35.
10. Kollaritsch H, Que JU, Kunz C, et al. Safety and immunogenicity of live oral cholera and typhoid vaccines administered alone or in combination with antimalarial drugs, oral polio vaccine, or yellow fever vaccine. J Infect Dis. 1997;175(4):871–5.

YELLOW FEVER

Mark Gershman, Betsy Schroeder, J. Erin Staples

Infectious Agent

Yellow fever virus (YFV) is a single-stranded RNA virus that belongs to the genus *Flavivirus*.

Mode of Transmission

- Vector-borne transmission occurs via the bite of an infected mosquito, primarily *Aedes* or *Haemagogus* spp.
- Nonhuman and human primates are the main reservoirs of the virus, with anthroponotic (human-to-vector-to-human) transmission occurring.
- There are three transmission cycles for yellow fever: sylvatic (jungle), intermediate (savannah), and urban.
  - The sylvatic (jungle) transmission cycle involves transmission of the virus between nonhuman primates and mosquito species found in the forest canopy. The virus is transmitted via mosquitoes from monkeys to humans when the humans encroach into the jungle during occupational or recreational activities.
  - In Africa, an intermediate (savannah) cycle involves transmission of YFV from tree hole-breeding *Aedes* spp. to humans living or working in jungle border areas. In this cycle, the virus may be transmitted from monkeys to humans or from human to human via these mosquitoes.
  - The urban transmission cycle involves transmission of the virus between humans and urban mosquitoes, primarily *Ae. aegypti*.
- Humans infected with YFV experience the highest levels of viremia and can transmit the virus to mosquitoes shortly before onset of fever and for the first 3–5 days of illness.
- Given the high level of viremia attained in humans, bloodborne transmission can also occur (via transfusion, needlestick, and intravenous drug abuse).

Occurrence

- Yellow fever occurs in sub-Saharan Africa and tropical South America (Maps 2-3 and 2-4), where it is endemic and intermittently epidemic (see Table 2-12 for a list of countries with risk of yellow fever transmission).
- In Africa, natural immunity accumulates with age, and thus infants and children are at greatest risk for disease.
- In South America, yellow fever occurs most frequently in unimmunized young men who are exposed to mosquito vectors through their work in forested or transitional areas.
- Most yellow fever disease in humans is due to sylvatic or intermediate transmission cycles. However, urban yellow fever does occur periodically in Africa and sporadically in the Americas.

Risk for Travelers

General

A traveler's risk for acquiring yellow fever is determined by various factors, including immunization status, location of travel, season, duration of exposure, occupational and recreational activities while traveling, and local rate of virus transmission at the time of travel. Although reported cases of human disease are the principal indicator of disease risk, case reports may be absent because of a low level of transmission, a high level of immunity in the population (e.g., due to vaccination), or failure of local surveillance systems to detect cases. This "epidemiologic silence" does not equate to absence of risk and should not lead to travel without the protection provided by vaccination.

Africa

YFV transmission in rural West Africa is seasonal, with an elevated risk during the end of the rainy season and the beginning of the dry season (usually July–October). However, YFV may be episodically transmitted by *Ae. aegypti* even during the dry season in both rural and densely settled urban areas.

South America

- The risk for infection for South America is highest during the rainy season (January–May, with a peak incidence in February and March).

Table 2-12. Countries with risk of yellow fever transmission[1]

Africa			Central and South America
Angola	Ethiopia	Nigeria	Argentina[2]
Benin	Gabon	Rwanda	Bolivia[2]
Burkina Faso	The Gambia	Sierra Leone	Brazil[2]
Burundi	Ghana	São Tomé and Príncipe	Colombia
Cameroon	Guinea	Senegal	Ecuador[2]
Central African Republic	Guinea-Bissau	Somalia	French Guiana
Chad[2]	Kenya	Sudan[2]	Guyana
Congo, Republic of the	Liberia	Tanzania	Panama[2]
Côte d'Ivoire	Mali[2]	Togo	Paraguay
Democratic Republic of the Congo	Mauritania[2]	Uganda	Peru[2]
Equatorial Guinea	Niger[2]		Suriname
			Trinidad and Tobago[2]
			Venezuela[2]

1 Countries/areas where "a risk of yellow fever transmission is present," as defined by the World Health Organization, are countries or areas where "yellow fever has been reported currently or in the past, plus vectors and animal reservoirs currently exist" (see www.who.int/ith/countries/2008_country_list.pdf).

2 These countries are not holoendemic (i.e., only a portion of the country has risk of yellow fever transmission). Please see Maps 2-3 and 2-4 and yellow fever vaccine recommendations (Table 2-14) for details.

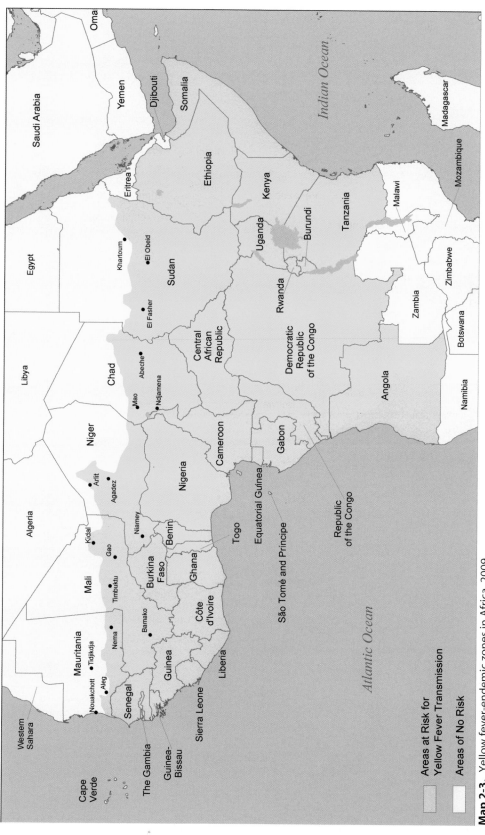

Map 2-3. Yellow fever-endemic zones in Africa, 2009.

Areas at Risk for
Yellow Fever Transmission

Areas of No Risk

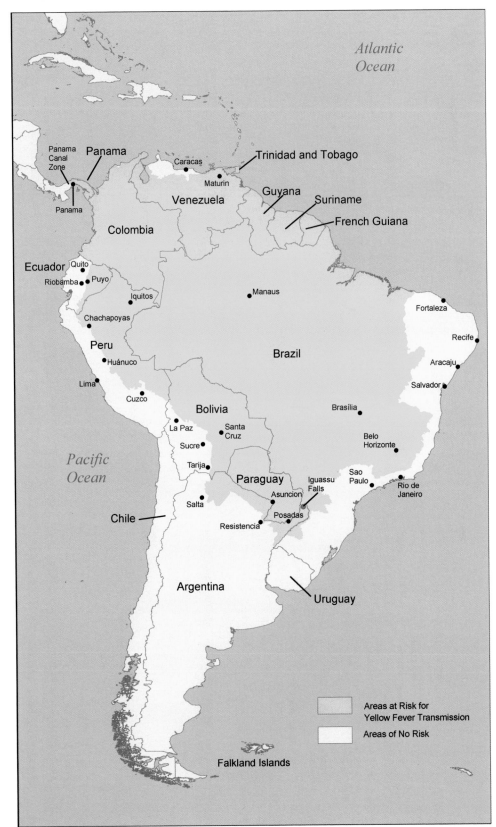

Map 2-4. Yellow fever-endemic zones in the Americas, 2009.

- Given the high level of viremia in humans and the widespread distribution of *Ae. aegypti* in many towns and cities, South America is at risk for a large-scale urban epidemic.

Yellow Fever Cases in Travelers

- During 1970–2002, a total of nine cases of yellow fever were reported in unvaccinated travelers from the United States and Europe who traveled to West Africa (five cases) or South America (four cases). Eight of these nine travelers died.
- Only one documented case of yellow fever has occurred, which was in a vaccinated traveler from Spain, who visited several West African countries during 1988.

Risk Estimates for Travelers

- The risk of acquiring yellow fever is difficult to predict because of variations in ecologic determinants of virus transmission. For a 2-week stay, the risks for illness and death due to yellow fever for an unvaccinated traveler traveling to an endemic area of
  - West Africa are 50 per 100,000 and 10 per 100,000, respectively
  - South America are 5 per 100,000 and 1 per 100,000, respectively
- These estimates are a rough guideline based on the risk to indigenous populations, often during peak transmission season. Thus, these risk estimates may not accurately reflect the true risk to travelers, who may have a different immunity profile, take precautions against getting bitten by mosquitoes, and have less outdoor exposure.
- The risk of acquiring yellow fever in South America is lower than that in Africa because the mosquitoes that transmit the virus between monkeys in the forest canopy do not often come in contact with humans, and there is a relatively high level of immunity in local residents secondary to vaccine use.

Clinical Presentation

- Asymptomatic or clinically inapparent infection is believed to occur in the majority of persons infected with YFV.
- The incubation period is typically 3–6 days.
- The initial illness presents as a nonspecific influenza-like syndrome with sudden onset of fever, chills, headache, backache, myalgias, prostration, nausea, and vomiting. Most patients improve after the initial presentation.
- After a brief remission of hours to a day, approximately 15% of cases progress to develop a more serious or toxic form of the disease characterized by jaundice, hemorrhagic symptoms, and eventually shock and multisystem organ failure.
- The overall case–fatality ratio for cases with jaundice is 20%–50%.

Diagnosis

- The preliminary diagnosis is based on the patient's clinical features, places and dates of travel, and activities.
- Laboratory diagnosis is generally accomplished by testing serum to detect virus-specific IgM and IgG antibodies by serologic assays. Due to cross-reactivity between antibodies raised against other flaviviruses, more specific antibody testing, such as a neutralization test, should be done to confirm the infection.
- Early in the illness, YFV or yellow fever viral RNA can often be detected in serum samples by virus isolation or nucleic acid amplification tests (NAAT). However, by the time more overt symptoms are recognized, the virus or viral RNA is usually undetectable. Therefore, virus isolation and NAAT should not be used for ruling out a diagnosis of yellow fever.

- Health-care providers should contact their state or local health department or call 800-CDC-INFO (800-232-4636) for assistance with diagnostic testing for yellow fever infections and for questions about antibody response to vaccination.

Treatment

- No specific treatments have been found to benefit patients with yellow fever.
- Treatment is symptomatic. Rest, fluids, and use of analgesics and antipyretics may relieve symptoms of fever and aching. Care should be taken to avoid certain medications, such as aspirin or other nonsteroidal anti-inflammatory drugs, which may increase the risk for bleeding.
- Infected persons should be protected from further mosquito exposure (staying indoors and/or under a mosquito net) during the first few days of illness, so they do not contribute to the transmission cycle.

Preventive Measures for Travelers

Personal Protection Measures

- No drugs for preventing infection are available.
- The best way to prevent mosquito-borne diseases, including yellow fever, is to avoid mosquito bites (see the Protection Against Mosquitoes, Ticks, and Other Insects and Arthropods section later in this chapter):
  - Use insect repellent containing DEET, Picaridin, oil of lemon eucalyptus, or IR3535 on exposed skin. Always follow the directions on the package.
  - Wear long sleeves, pants, and socks. If possible, treat clothes with permethrin.
  - Stay in screened or air-conditioned accommodations to keep mosquitoes out.
  - Get rid of mosquito sources by emptying standing water from flowerpots, buckets, car tires and barrels.

Yellow Fever Vaccine

- Yellow fever is preventable by a relatively safe, effective vaccine.
- All yellow fever vaccines currently manufactured are live attenuated viral vaccines.
- YF-VAX, the only yellow fever vaccine approved for use in the United States, is manufactured by sanofi pasteur.
- Studies comparing the reactogenicity and immunogenicity of various yellow fever vaccines, including those manufactured outside of the United States, suggest that there is no significant difference in the reactogenicity or immune response generated by the various vaccines. Thus, individuals who receive yellow fever vaccines in other countries should be considered protected against yellow fever.

Recommendations for the Use of Yellow Fever Vaccine for Travelers

- Persons aged ≥9 months of age who are traveling to or living in areas with risk of yellow fever transmission in South America and Africa should be vaccinated. In addition, some countries require proof of yellow fever vaccination for entry. See the following section in this chapter (Yellow Fever Vaccine Requirements and Recommendations, by Country) for more detailed information on the requirements and recommendations for yellow fever vaccination for specific countries.
- However, because severe adverse events (see below) can follow yellow fever vaccination, physicians should be careful to administer the vaccine only to persons truly at risk of exposure to YFV.
- Refer to Yellow Fever Vaccine Recommendations of the Advisory Committee on Immunization Practices (ACIP) for additional information at www.cdc.gov/vaccines/pubs/ACIP-list.htm.

Vaccine Dose and Administration

- For all eligible persons, a single injection of 0.5 mL of reconstituted vaccine should be administered subcutaneously.
- The International Health Regulations (IHR) published by WHO require revaccination at 10-year intervals.

Vaccine Safety and Adverse Reactions

Common Adverse Events

- Reactions to yellow fever vaccine are generally mild, with 10%–30% of vaccinees reporting mild systemic adverse events.
- Reported events typically include low-grade fever, headache, and myalgias that begin within days after vaccination and last 5–10 days.
- Approximately 1% of vaccinees temporarily curtail their regular activities because of these reactions.

Severe Adverse Events

Hypersensitivity

Immediate hypersensitivity reactions, characterized by rash, urticaria, or asthma or a combination of these, are uncommon. Anaphylaxis following yellow fever vaccine is reported to occur at a rate of 1.8 cases per 100,000 doses administered.

Yellow Fever Vaccine-Associated Neurologic Disease (YEL-AND)

- YEL-AND represents a conglomerate of different clinical syndromes, including meningoencephalitis, Guillain–Barré syndrome (GBS), acute disseminated encephalomyelitis (ADEM), bulbar palsy, and Bell's palsy.
- Historically, YEL-AND was seen primarily among infants as encephalitis, but more recent reports have been among persons of all ages.
- The onset of illness for documented cases ranges 3–28 days after vaccination, and almost all cases were in first-time vaccine recipients.
- YEL-AND is rarely fatal.
- The incidence of YEL-AND in the United States is 0.8 per 100,000 doses administered. The rate is higher in persons ≥60 years of age, with a rate of 1.6 per 100,000 doses in persons 60–69 years of age and 2.3 per 100,000 doses in persons ≥70 years of age.

Yellow Fever Vaccine-Associated Viscerotropic Disease (YEL-AVD)

- YEL-AVD is a severe illness similar to wild-type disease, with vaccine virus proliferating in multiple organs and often leading to multisystem organ failure and death.
- Since the initial cases of YEL-AVD were published in 2001, more than 40 confirmed and suspected cases have been reported throughout the world.
- The onset of illness for YEL-AVD cases averaged 3.5 days (range: 1–8 days) after vaccination. YEL-AVD appears to occur after the first dose of yellow fever vaccine rather than with booster doses.
- The case–fatality ratio for reported YEL-AVD cases is 53%.
- The incidence of YEL-AVD in the United States is 0.4 cases per 100,000 doses of vaccine administered. The rate is higher for persons ≥60 years of age, with a rate of 1 per 100,000 doses in persons 60–69 years of age and 2.3 per 100,000 doses in persons aged ≥70 years of age.

Contraindications

Infants <9 Months of Age

- The vaccine is contraindicated for routine use in infants <9 months of age by the manufacturer and the FDA because of the increased risk of postvaccine encephalitis. However, ACIP and WHO recognize that situations occur in which vaccination of an infant 6–8 months of age might be considered, such as residence in or unavoidable travel to a yellow fever endemic or epidemic zone. The decision to immunize infants who are 6–8 months of age must balance the infant's risk for exposure with the risk for vaccine-associated encephalitis. **YF vaccine should never be administered to infants <6 months of age.**

- Physicians considering vaccinating infants aged <9 months of age should contact their state health department or call 800-CDC-INFO (800-232-4636) for further advice.

Hypersensitivity

- Yellow fever vaccine is contraindicated in anyone with a history of acute hypersensitivity reaction to any of the vaccine components, including gelatin. Because the yellow fever vaccine is produced in chicken embryos, vaccine should not be administered to anyone with a history of acute hypersensitivity to egg or chicken proteins.
- If vaccination of a person with a questionable history of hypersensitivity to one of the vaccine components is considered essential because of a high risk for acquiring yellow fever, desensitizing and vaccinating procedures are described in the vaccine package insert and should be performed under close medical supervision.

Immunosuppression

- The vaccine is contraindicated in persons with immunocompromising conditions, including symptomatic HIV infection or AIDS, malignancy, or diseases of the thymus (e.g., thymectomy) or those receiving immunosuppressant therapy (e.g., corticosteroids, alkylating agents, antimetabolites) or radiation therapy.
- Immunosuppressed persons should not be immunized, and travel to yellow fever-endemic areas should be postponed or avoided.
- If travel to yellow fever endemic areas is unavoidable, persons who cannot be immunized because of their immunosuppressive condition should be advised of the risk for acquiring yellow fever disease, instructed in methods for avoiding vector mosquitoes, and, if warranted, issued a medical waiver to fulfill international health regulations (see information in Exemption from Vaccination and Waiver Letters in this section).
- Physicians considering vaccinating an immunosuppressed individual can contact their state health department or call for more information.
- Family members of immunosuppressed or HIV-infected persons who themselves have no contraindications can receive yellow fever vaccine.

AIDS or Symptomatic HIV

No large-scale trials have been done to evaluate the safety of the yellow fever vaccine in individuals with HIV or AIDS. However, because yellow fever vaccine is a live, viral vaccine, it is contraindicated in persons with symptomatic HIV infection or AIDS. (For persons with asymptomatic HIV infection, see Precautions below.)

History of Thymus Disease

- A history of thymus disease is a contraindication to yellow fever vaccine.
- Four persons with a history of thymectomy for a thymoma were noted among the first 23 cases of YEL-AVD, suggesting that compromised thymus function is an independent risk factor for YEL-AVD.
- Health-care providers should be careful to ask about a history of thymus disorder, including myasthenia gravis, thymoma, or prior thymectomy, when screening a patient before administering yellow fever vaccine.

Immunosuppressive Medication

- Although no studies have been done to evaluate the safety of yellow fever vaccine in persons receiving immunosuppressive or immunomodulating medicines, the vaccine is contraindicated in those receiving medications that alter the ability to resist viral infections. The vaccine should not be given to individuals who are taking medications with a warning in the package insert against the use of live viral vaccines.
- Low-dose (i.e., 20 mg or less of prednisone or equivalent/day); short-term (i.e., <2 weeks) systemic corticosteroid therapy or intra-articular, bursal, or tendon

injections with corticosteroids; and intranasal corticosteroids are not thought to be sufficiently immunosuppressive to constitute an increased hazard to recipients of yellow fever vaccine (see The Immunocompromised Traveler section in Chapter 8).

Precautions

Adults 60 Years of Age or Older

- Analysis of adverse events passively reported to the Vaccine Adverse Event Reporting System (VAERS) indicate that persons 60 years of age or older may be at increased risk for systemic adverse events following vaccination compared with younger persons.
- The rate of any serious adverse event following vaccination is 1.5 times higher than the average rate for persons 60–69 years of age and 3 times higher for persons 70 years or older.
- To determine if vaccination should be administered to travelers 60 years of age or older, the risks and benefits of vaccination should be weighed against their destination-specific risk for exposure to YFV.

Asymptomatic HIV

- Persons who are HIV-infected but who do not have AIDS or other symptomatic manifestations of HIV infection, who have established laboratory verification of adequate immune system function (e.g., CD4+ T cell counts >200/mm^3), and who cannot avoid potential exposure to YFV should be offered the choice of vaccination.
- If international travel requirements are the only reason to vaccinate an asymptomatic HIV-infected person, rather than an increased risk for acquiring yellow fever, the person should be excused from immunization and issued a medical waiver to fulfill health regulations (see information in Exemption from Vaccination and Waiver Letters in this section).
- Data are limited regarding seroconversion rates after yellow fever vaccination among asymptomatic HIV-infected persons, but indicate that the seroconversion rate among such persons may be reduced. Because vaccination of asymptomatic HIV-infected persons might be less effective than that of persons not infected with HIV, measurement of the neutralizing antibody response to vaccination should be considered before travel.

Pregnancy

- The safety of yellow fever vaccination during pregnancy has not been studied in a large prospective trial. However, a recent study of women who were vaccinated with yellow fever vaccine early in their pregnancies found no major malformations in their infants. There was slight increased risk noted for minor, mostly skin, malformations.
- In a similar study, a higher rate of spontaneous abortions in pregnant women receiving the vaccine was reported but not substantiated.
- The proportion of women vaccinated during pregnancy who develop YF IgG-specific antibodies is variable depending on the study (38.6% or 98.2%) and may be correlated with the trimester in which they received the vaccine. Because pregnancy may affect immunologic function, serologic testing can be considered to document a protective immune response to the vaccine.
- For pregnant women, if travel is unavoidable and the vaccination risks are felt to outweigh the risks of YF exposure, these women should be excused from immunization and, if applicable, issued a medical waiver to fulfill international health regulations (see information in Exemption from Vaccination and Waiver Letters in this section). Pregnant women who must travel to areas where the risk of yellow fever infection is high should be vaccinated, and their infants should be monitored after birth for evidence of congenital infection and other possible adverse effects resulting from yellow fever vaccination.
- Although there are no specific data, it is recommended that a woman wait 4 weeks after receiving the live virus yellow fever vaccine before conceiving.

Breastfeeding
- Whether the yellow fever vaccine is excreted in breast milk is not known.
- One suspect case of YEL-AND has been reported in a 1-month old infant whose mother was vaccinated with yellow fever vaccine and the infant was exclusively breastfed. Testing was unable to determine if the breast milk was the mode of transmission.
- It is recommended that vaccination of nursing mothers should be avoided. However, when travel of nursing mothers to high-risk yellow fever-endemic areas cannot be avoided or postponed, these women should be vaccinated.

Simultaneous Administration of Other Vaccines and Drugs
- One study suggested that the immune response to yellow fever vaccine is not inhibited by administration of measles vaccine (also a live, attenuated vaccine) given concurrently or at various intervals of a few days to 1 month prior. However, to minimize the potential risk for interference, injectable or nasally administered live vaccines not administered on the same day should be given at least 4 weeks apart.
- A prospective study of persons given yellow fever vaccine along with 5 mL of commercially available IG showed no alteration of the immunologic response to yellow fever vaccine when compared with controls.

International Certificate of Vaccination or Prophylaxis (ICVP)

Background
- The International Health Regulations (IHR) allow countries to require proof of yellow fever vaccination for entry and from travelers arriving from certain countries, even if only in transit, to prevent importation and indigenous transmission of YFV.
- Some countries require evidence of vaccination from all entering travelers, which includes direct travel from the United States (Table 2-13).
- Travelers who arrive in a country with a yellow fever vaccination entry requirement without proof of yellow fever vaccination may be quarantined up to 6 days.
- Travelers with a specific contraindication to yellow fever vaccine should request a waiver from a physician before traveling to countries requiring vaccination (see below).

Authorization to Provide Vaccinations and to Validate the ICVP
- Under the revised IHR (2005), effective December 15, 2007, all state parties (countries) are required to issue a new ICVP. This is intended to replace the former International Certificate of Vaccination against Yellow Fever (ICV).
  - Persons who received a yellow fever vaccination after December 15, 2007, must provide proof of vaccination on an ICVP.

Table 2-13. Countries that require proof of yellow fever vaccination for all arriving travelers[1]

Angola	French Guiana
Benin	Gabon
Bolivia (or signed affidavit at point of entry)	Ghana
Burkina Faso	Liberia
Burundi	Mali
Cameroon	Niger
Central African Republic	Rwanda
Congo, Republic of the	São Tomé and Príncipe
Côte d'Ivoire	Sierra Leone
Democratic Republic of the Congo	Togo

1 Country requirements for yellow fever vaccination are subject to change at any time; therefore, CDC encourages travelers to check with the destination country's embassy or consulate before departure.

- If the person received the vaccine before December 15, 2007, the original ICV is still valid, provided that the vaccination was given less than 10 years previously.
- Vaccinees should receive a completed ICVP (Figure 2-1), validated (stamped and signed) with the center's stamp where the vaccine was given (see below).
  - An ICVP must be complete in every detail; if incomplete or inaccurate, it is not valid.
  - Failure to secure validations can cause a traveler to be quarantined, denied entry, or possibly revaccinated at the point of entry to a country. This is not a recommended option for the traveler.
- A copy of the ICVP, CDC 731 (formerly PHS 731) may be purchased from the U.S. Government Printing Office, Washington, D.C., http://bookstore.gpo.gov/, telephone 866-512-1800. The stock number is 017-001-00567-3 for 25 copies and 017-001-00566-5 for 100 copies.
- This certificate of vaccination is valid for a period of 10 years, beginning 10 days after vaccination. With booster doses of the vaccine, the certificate is considered valid from the day of vaccination.

Persons Authorized to Sign the Certificate and Designated Yellow Fever Vaccination Centers

- The ICVP must be signed by a licensed physician or by a health-care worker designated by the physician supervising the administration of the vaccine (Figure 2-1). A signature stamp is not acceptable.
- Yellow fever vaccination must be given at a certified center in possession of an official "Uniform Stamp," which can be used to validate the ICVP.
- State health departments are responsible for designating nonfederal yellow fever vaccination centers and issuing Uniform Stamps to physicians.
- Information about the location and hours of yellow fever vaccination centers may be obtained by visiting CDC's Travelers' Health website at wwwn.cdc.gov/travel/yellowfever.aspx.

Exemption from Vaccination and Waiver Letters

- Some countries do not require an ICVP for infants younger than a certain age (e.g., <6 months, <9 months, or <1 year of age, depending on the country). Age requirements for vaccination for individual countries can be found in the Yellow Fever Vaccine Requirements and Recommendations section in this chapter.
- For medical contraindications, a physician who has decided to issue a waiver should fill out and sign the Medical Contraindications to Vaccination section of the ICVP (Figure 2-2). The physician should also—

INTERNATIONAL CERTIFICATE OF VACCINATION OR PROPHYLAXIS
Certificat international de vaccination ou de prophylaxie

This is to certify that
Nous certifions que ______ (name – nom) ______ (date of birth – né(e) le) ______ (sex – de sexe) ______ (nationality – et de nationalité)

______ (national identification document, if applicable – document d'identificaion nationale, le cas échéant)) whose signature follows / dont la signature suit ______

has on the date indicated been vaccinated or received prophylaxis against
a été vacciné(e) ou a reçu une prophylaxie à la date indiquée ______ (name of disease or condition – nom de la maladie ou de l'affection) in accordance with the International Health Regulations. conformément au Règlement sanitaire international.

Vaccine or prophylaxis Vaccin ou agent prophylactique	Date	Signature and professional status of supervising clinician Signature et titre du professionel de santé responsable	Manufacturer and batch no. of vaccine or prophylaxis Fabricant du vaccin ou de l'agent prophylactique et numéro du lot	Certificate valid from: until: Certificat valable à partir du: jusqu'au:	Official stamp of administering center Cachet officiel du centre habilité

Figure 2-1. Example International Certificate of Vaccination or Prophylaxis (ICVP).

MEDICAL CONTRAINDICATION TO VACCINATION
Ceontre-indication médicale à la vaccination

This is to certify that immunization against
Je soussigné(e) certifie que la vaccination contre

_____ for
(Name of disease – Nom de la maladie)   pour

_____ is medically
(Name of traveler – Nom du voyageur)   est médicalement

contraindicated because of the following conditions:
contre-indiquée pour les raisons suivantes:

_____

_____

_____

_____
(Signature and address of physician)
(Signature et adresse du médecin)

Figure 2-2.
Example International Certificate of Vaccination or Prophylaxis (ICVP) medical contraindication to vaccination.

- Give the traveler a signed and dated exemption letter on the physician's letterhead stationery, clearly stating the contraindications to vaccination and bearing the stamp used by the yellow fever vaccination centers to validate the ICVP.
- Inform the traveler of any increased risk of yellow fever infection associated with nonvaccination and how to minimize this risk by using mosquito protection measures.
- Reasons other than medical contraindications are not acceptable for exemption from vaccination.
- The traveler should be advised that issuance of a waiver does not guarantee its acceptance by the destination country. On arrival at the destination, the traveler may be faced with quarantine, refusal of entry, or vaccination on site.
- To potentially improve the likelihood of acceptance of a waiver upon arrival at the destination country, the provider can suggest that the traveler take the following additional measures before initiating travel:
  - Obtain specific and authoritative advice from the embassy or consulate of the country or countries he or she plans to visit.
  - Request documentation of requirements for waivers from embassies or consulates and retain these along with the completed Medical Contraindication to Vaccination section of the ICVP.

Requirements Versus Recommendations

- Country entry **requirements** for proof of yellow fever vaccination under the IHRs are different from CDC's **recommendations**.
- Yellow fever vaccine entry **requirements** are established by countries in order to prevent the importation and transmission of YFV, and are allowed under the IHRs. Travelers must comply with these to enter the country, unless they have been issued a medical waiver. Certain countries require vaccination from travelers arriving from all countries, while some countries require vaccination only for travelers coming from "a country with risk of yellow fever transmission" (Table 2-14). WHO defines those areas "at risk of yellow fever transmission" as countries or areas where yellow fever has been reported currently or in the past, plus where vectors and animal reservoirs currently exist. Country requirements are subject to change at any time; therefore, CDC encourages travelers to check with the appropriate embassy or consulate before departure.
- The information in the section on yellow fever vaccine **recommendations** is advice given by CDC to prevent yellow fever infections among travelers. **Recommendations**

are subject to change at any time if disease conditions change; therefore, CDC encourages travelers to check for relevant travel notices on the CDC website www.cdc.gov/travel before departure.

Vaccination for Travel on Military Orders

Because military requirements may exceed those indicated in this publication, any person who plans to travel on military orders (civilians and military personnel) should be advised to contact the nearest military medical facility to determine the requirements for the trip.

References

1. Monath TP, Teuwen D, Cetron MS. Yellow fever vaccine. In: Plotkin S, Orenstein WA, Offit PA, editors. Vaccines. 5th ed. Philadelphia: W.B. Saunders; 2008. p. 959–1055.

2. Monath TP, Cetron MS. Prevention of yellow fever in persons traveling to the tropics. Clin Infect Dis. 2002;34(10):1369–78.

3. Van der Stuyft P, Gianella A, Pirard M, et al. Urbanisation of yellow fever in Santa Cruz, Bolivia. Lancet. 1999;353(9164):1558–62.

4. Pan American Health Organization. EID Updates: Emerging and Reemerging Infectious Diseases, Region of the Americas. Vol. 5, No. 6 (25 Feb. 2008) Yellow fever in Paraguay: Mobilization continues. [cited 2008 Jun 8]. Available from: http://www.paho.org/english/AD/DPC/CD/eid-eer-2008-02-25.htm.

5. Tomori O. Yellow fever: The recurring plague. Crit Rev Clin Lab Sci. 2004;41(4):391–427.

6. World Health Organization. Yellow fever vaccine: WHO position paper. Wkly Epidemiol Rec. 2003;40:349–60.

7. Monath TP, Nichols R, Archambault WT, et al. Comparative safety and immunogenicity of two yellow fever 17D vaccines (Arilvax and YF-Vax) in a phase III multicenter, double-blind clinical trial. Am J Trop Med Hyg. 2002;66(5):553–41.

8. Pfsiter M, Kuersteiner O, Hilfiker H, et al. Immunogenicity and safety of Berna-YF compared with two other 17D yellow fever vaccines in a phase 3 clinical trial. Am J Trop Med Hyg. 2005;72(3):339–46.

9. Ripoll C, Ponce A, Wilson MM, et al. Evaluation of two yellow fever vaccines for routine immunization programs in Argentina. Hum Vaccin. 2008;4(2):121–6.

10. CDC. Yellow fever vaccine: recommendations of the Advisory Committee on Immunization Practices (ACIP). MMWR Morb Mortal Wkly Rep. 2002;51(RR-17):1–12.

11. World Health Organization. International Health Regulations. 2005. Geneva. [cited 2008 Jun 9]. Available from: http://www.who.int/csr/ihr/en/index.html.

12. Lindsey NP, Schroeder BA, Miller ER, et al. Adverse event reports following yellow fever vaccination. Vaccine. 2008;26(48):6077–82.

13. McMahon AW, Eidex RB, Marfin AA, et al. Neurologic disease associated with 17D-204 yellow fever vaccination: a report of 15 cases. Vaccine. 2007;25(10):1727–34.

14. CDC. Adverse events associated with 17D-derived yellow fever vaccination— United States, 2001–2002. MMWR Morb Mortal Wkly Rep. 2002;51(44):989–93.

15. Marfin AA, Eidex Barwick R, Monath TP. Yellow fever. In: Guerrant RL, Walker DH, Weller PF, editors. Tropical infectious diseases: principles, pathogens, & practice. 2nd ed. Philadelphia: Mosby Elsevier; 2005: p.797–812.

16. Hayes EB. Acute viscerotropic disease following vaccination against yellow fever. Trans R Soc Trop Med Hyg. 2007;101(10):967–71.

17. Muñoz J, Vilella A, Domingo C, et al. Yellow fever-associated viscerotropic disease in Barcelona, Spain. J Travel Med. 2008;15(3):202–5.

18. Barwick R. History of thymoma and yellow fever vaccination. Lancet. 2004;364(9438):936.

19. Cavalcanti DP, Salomao MA, Lopez-Camelo J, et al. Early exposure to yellow fever vaccine during pregnancy. Trop Med Int Health. 2007;12(7):833–7.

20. Nishioka Sde A, Nunes-Araujo FRF, Pires WP, et al. Yellow fever vaccination during pregnancy and spontaneous abortion: a case-control study. Trop Med Int Health. 1998;3(1):29–33.

21. Suzano CE, Amaral E, Sato HK, et al. The effects of yellow fever immunization (17DD) inadvertently used in early pregnancy during a mass campaign in Brazil. Vaccine. 2006;24(9):1421–6.

22. Nasidi A, Monath TP, Vandenberg J, et al. Yellow fever vaccination and pregnancy: a four-year prospective study. Trans R Soc Trop Med Hyg. 1993;87(3):337–9.

23. CDC. General recommendations on immunization: recommendations of the Advisory Committee on Immunization Practices (ACIP). MMWR Recomm Rep. 2006;55(RR-15):1–48.

24. Kaplan JE, Nelson DB, Schonberger LB, et al. The effect of immune globulin on the response to trivalent oral poliovirus and yellow fever vaccinations. Bull World Health Organ. 1984;62(4):585–90.

YELLOW FEVER VACCINE REQUIREMENTS AND RECOMMENDATIONS, BY COUNTRY

Mark Gershman, Betsy Schroeder, Emily S. Jentes, Nina Marano

Table 2-14. Yellow fever vaccine requirements and recommendations, by country

Country	Yellow Fever Vaccine Requirements[1,2]	CDC Yellow Fever Vaccine Recommendations[2,3,4]
Afghanistan	If traveling from a country with risk of yellow fever transmission	None
Albania	If traveling from a country with risk of yellow fever transmission and ≥1 year of age	None
Algeria	If traveling from a country with risk of yellow fever transmission and ≥1 year of age	None
Andorra	Not required	None
Angola	Required upon arrival from all countries if traveler is ≥1 year of age	For all travelers ≥9 months of age
Anguilla (U.K.)	If traveling from a country with risk of yellow fever transmission and ≥1 year of age	None
Antarctica	Not required	None
Antigua and Barbuda	If traveling from a country with risk of yellow fever transmission and ≥1 year of age	None
Argentina	Not required	Yellow fever vaccination is recommended for all travelers ≥9 months of age who are going to the northern and northeastern forested areas of Argentina, including Iguassu Falls and all areas bordering Paraguay and Brazil. These areas include all departments of Misiones and Formosa Provinces; and the Department of Bermejo in Chaco Province; Departments of Berón de Astrada, Capital, General Alvear, General Paz, Ituzaingó, Itatí, Paso de los Libres, San Cosme, San Miguel, San Martín, and Santo Tomé in Corrientes Province; Departments of Valle Grande, Ledesma, Santa Bárbara, and San Pedro in Jujuy Province; and Departments of General José de San Martín, Oran, Rivadavia, and Anta in Salta Province.
Armenia	Not required	None
Aruba	If traveling from a country with risk of yellow fever transmission and ≥6 months of age[5]	None
Australia	All persons ≥1 year of age who, within 6 days of arrival in Australia, have been in or have passed through a country with risk of yellow fever transmission	None

Please note: Country requirements for yellow fever vaccine are subject to change at any time, and CDC vaccine recommendations are subject to change at any time if disease conditions change; therefore, CDC encourages health-care providers and travelers to check for updates on the CDC website www.cdc.gov/travel, and with the destination country's embassy or consulate in sufficient time to receive yellow fever vaccination or to obtain a waiver if recommendations or requirements have changed.

Country	Yellow Fever Vaccine Requirements[1,2]	CDC Yellow Fever Vaccine Recommendations[2,3,4]
Austria	Not required	None
Azerbaijan	Not required	None
Azores (Portugal)	If traveling from a country with risk of yellow fever transmission and ≥1 year of age	None
Bahamas, The	If traveling from a country with risk of yellow fever transmission and ≥1 year of age	None
Bahrain	If traveling from a country with risk of yellow fever transmission and ≥1 year of age	None
Bangladesh	If traveling from a country with risk of yellow fever transmission and ≥1 year of age	None
Barbados	If traveling from a country with risk of yellow fever transmission and ≥1 year of age	None
Belarus	Not required	None
Belgium	Not required	None
Belize	If traveling from a country with risk of yellow fever transmission and ≥1 year of age	None
Benin	Required upon arrival from all countries if traveler is ≥1 year of age	For all travelers ≥9 months of age
Bermuda (U.K.)	Not required	None
Bhutan	If traveling from a country with risk of yellow fever transmission	None
Bolivia	Required for all travelers ≥1 year of age For U.S. citizens: Medical waivers must be translated into Spanish and accompany the International Certificate of Vaccination or Prophylaxis (ICVP). Travelers who do not have a valid ICVP will still be allowed to enter Bolivia if they agree to sign an affidavit exempting the Bolivian state from any liability in the event the traveler gets sick with yellow fever within the Bolivian territory. This last option may cause delays at the point of entry.	For all travelers ≥9 months of age traveling to areas east of the Andes Mountains (see Map 2-4). Vaccination is NOT recommended for travel only to the cities of La Paz or Sucre.
Bosnia and Herzegovina	Not required	None
Botswana	If traveling from a country with risk of yellow fever transmission and ≥1 year of age	None
Brazil	Not required	For all travelers ≥9 months of age going to the following areas at risk of yellow fever transmission, including the ENTIRE states of Acre, Amapá, Amazonas, Distrito Federal (including the capital city of Brasilia), Goiás, Maranhão, Mato Grosso, Mato Grosso do Sul, Minas Gerais, Pará, Rondônia, Roraima, and Tocatins; and the designated areas of the following states: northwest and west Bahia, central and west Paraná, southwest Piauí, northwest and west central Rio Grande do Sul, far west Santa Catarina, and north and west São Paulo. *(Continued)*

The Pre-Travel Consultation

Travel-Related Vaccine-Preventable Diseases

Country	Yellow Fever Vaccine Requirements[1,2]	CDC Yellow Fever Vaccine Recommendations[2,3,4]
Brazil *(Continued)*		Vaccination is recommended for travelers visiting Iguassu Falls. Vaccination is NOT recommended for travel to the following coastal cities: Rio de Janeiro, São Paulo, Salvador, Recife, and Fortaleza.
British Indian Ocean Territory, includes **Diego Garcia** (U.K.)	Not required	None
Brunei	Required from travelers ≥1 year of age arriving within 6 days from countries with risk of yellow fever transmission or having passed through areas partly or wholly at risk of yellow fever transmission within the preceding 6 days.	None
Bulgaria	Not required	None
Burkina Faso	Required upon arrival from all countries if traveler is ≥1 year of age	For all travelers ≥9 months of age
Burma (Myanmar)	If traveling from a country with risk of yellow fever transmission. Required also for nationals and residents of Burma (Myanmar) departing for a country with risk of yellow fever transmission	None
Burundi	Required upon arrival from all countries if traveler is ≥1 year of age	For all travelers ≥9 months of age
Cambodia	If traveling from a country with risk of yellow fever transmission	None
Cameroon	Required upon arrival from all countries if traveler is ≥1 year of age	For all travelers ≥9 months of age
Canada	Not required	None
Canary Islands (Spain)	Not required	None
Cape Verde	If traveling from a country with risk of yellow fever transmission and ≥1 year of age	None
Cayman Islands (U.K.)	Not required	None
Central African Republic	Required upon arrival from all countries if traveler is ≥1 year of age	For all travelers ≥9 months of age
Chad	If traveling from a country with risk of yellow fever transmission	For all travelers ≥9 months of age traveling to areas south of the Sahara Desert
Chile	Not required	None
China	If traveling from a country with risk of yellow fever transmission	None
Christmas Island (Australia)	All travelers ≥1 year of age, who within the past 6 days have traveled or passed through an endemic area, as listed by WHO	None

Please note: Country requirements for yellow fever vaccine are subject to change at any time, and CDC vaccine recommendations are subject to change at any time if disease conditions change; therefore, CDC encourages health-care providers and travelers to check for updates on the CDC website www.cdc.gov/travel, and with the destination country's embassy or consulate in sufficient time to receive yellow fever vaccination or to obtain a waiver if recommendations or requirements have changed.

Country	Yellow Fever Vaccine Requirements[1,2]	CDC Yellow Fever Vaccine Recommendations[2,3,4]
Cocos (Keeling) Islands	All persons ≥1 year of age who, within 6 days of arrival, have been in or have passed through a country with risk of yellow fever transmission	None
Colombia	Not required	For all travelers ≥9 months of age. Travelers whose itinerary is limited to the cities of Bogotá, Cali, or Medellín are at lower risk and may consider foregoing vaccination.
Comoros	Not required	None
Congo, Republic of the (Congo-Brazzaville)	Required upon arrival from all countries if traveler is ≥1 year of age	For all travelers ≥9 months of age
Cook Islands (New Zealand)	Not required	None
Costa Rica	Required from travelers coming from countries with risk of yellow fever transmission. No certificate is required for travelers <9 months of age and ≥60 years of age, pregnant or lactating women, persons with allergy to eggs or gelatin, immunosuppression, thymus disease, a personal or family history of adverse reactions associated with the yellow fever vaccine, or asymptomatic HIV infection with laboratory evidence of satisfactory immune functions. The following countries are considered at risk of yellow fever transmission: *South America:* Boliva, Brazil, Colombia, Ecuador, French Guyana, Peru, Venezuela *Africa:* Angola, Benin, Burkina Faso, Cameroon, Gabon, The Gambia, Ghana, Guinea, Liberia, Nigeria, Democratic Republic of the Congo, Sierra Leone, Sudan	None
Côte d'Ivoire (Ivory Coast)	Required upon arrival from all countries if traveler is ≥1 year of age	For all travelers ≥9 months of age
Croatia	Not required	None
Cuba	Not required	None
Cyprus	Not required	None
Czech Republic	Not required	None
Democratic Republic of the Congo (Congo-Kinshasa)	Required upon arrival from all countries if traveler is ≥1 year of age	For all travelers ≥9 months of age
Denmark	Not required	None
Djibouti	If traveling from a country with risk of yellow fever transmission and ≥1 year of age	None
Dominica	If traveling from a country with risk of yellow fever transmission and ≥1 year of age	None
Dominican Republic	Not required	None
Easter Island (Chile)	Required for travelers coming from a country with risk of yellow fever transmission	None

The Pre-Travel Consultation

Travel-Related Vaccine-Preventable Diseases

Country	Yellow Fever Vaccine Requirements[1,2]	CDC Yellow Fever Vaccine Recommendations[2,3,4]
Ecuador (including the **Galápagos Islands**)	Required from travelers ≥1 year of age coming from countries with risk of yellow fever transmission. Nationals and residents of Ecuador are required to possess certificates of vaccination on their departure to an area with risk of yellow fever transmission.	For all travelers ≥9 months of age who are traveling to the following provinces in the Amazon Basin: Morona-Santiago, Napo, Orellana, Pastaza, Sucumbíos, and Zamora-Chinchipe, and all other areas in the eastern part of the Andes Mountains, NOT including the cities of Quito and Guayaquil or the Galápagos Islands
Egypt	If traveling from countries with risk of yellow fever transmission and ≥1 year of age. Air passengers without a certificate in transit, but coming from these countries or areas, will be detained in the precincts of the airport until they resume their journey. All travelers arriving from Sudan are required to have a vaccination certificate or a location certificate issued by a Sudanese official center, stating that they have not been in Sudan south of 15° N within the previous 6 days. Required also for travelers arriving or transiting from: *Africa:* Angola, Benin, Burkina Faso, Burundi, Cameroon, Central African Republic, Chad, Congo, Côte d'Ivoire, Democratic Republic of the Congo, Equatorial Guinea, Ethiopia, Gabon, The Gambia, Ghana, Guinea, Guinea-Bissau, Kenya, Liberia, Mali, Niger, Nigeria, Rwanda, São Tomé and Príncipe, Senegal, Sierra Leone, Somalia, Sudan (south of 15° N), Tanzania, Togo, Uganda, and Zambia *Americas:* Belize, Bolivia, Brazil, Colombia, Costa Rica, Ecuador, French Guiana, Guyana, Panama, Peru, Suriname, Trinidad and Tobago, and Venezuela	None
El Salvador	If traveling from a country with risk of yellow fever transmission and ≥6 months of age[5]	None
Equatorial Guinea	If traveling from a country with risk of yellow fever transmission	For all travelers ≥9 months of age
Eritrea	If traveling from a country with risk of yellow fever transmission	None
Estonia	Not required	None
Ethiopia	If traveling from a country with risk of yellow fever transmission and ≥1 year of age	For all travelers ≥9 months of age
Falkland Islands (U.K.)	Not required	None
Faroe Islands (Denmark)	Not required	None

Please note: Country requirements for yellow fever vaccine are subject to change at any time, and CDC vaccine recommendations are subject to change at any time if disease conditions change; therefore, CDC encourages health-care providers and travelers to check for updates on the CDC website www.cdc.gov/travel, and with the destination country's embassy or consulate in sufficient time to receive yellow fever vaccination or to obtain a waiver if recommendations or requirements have changed.

Country	Yellow Fever Vaccine Requirements[1,2]	CDC Yellow Fever Vaccine Recommendations[2,3,4]
Fiji	If traveling from a country with risk of yellow fever transmission within 10 days of having stayed overnight or longer and ≥1 year of age	None
Finland	Not required	None
France	Not required	None
French Guiana	Required upon arrival from all countries if traveler is ≥1 year of age	For all travelers ≥9 months of age
French Polynesia, includes the island groups of Society Islands (Tahiti, Moorea, and Bora-Bora), Marquesas Islands (Hiva Oa and Ua Huka), and Austral Islands (Tubuai and Rurutu)	If traveling from a country with risk of yellow fever transmission and ≥1 year of age	None
Gabon	Required upon arrival from all countries if traveler is ≥1 year of age	For all travelers ≥9 months of age
Gambia, The	If traveling from a country with risk of yellow fever transmission and ≥1 year of age	For all travelers ≥9 months of age
Georgia	Not required	None
Germany	Not required	None
Ghana	Required upon arrival from all countries	For all travelers ≥9 months of age
Gibraltar (U.K.)	Not required	None
Greece	Not required	None
Greenland (Denmark)	Not required	None
Grenada	If traveling from a country with risk of yellow fever transmission and ≥1 year of age	None
Guadeloupe, including St. Barthelemy and Saint Martin (France)	If traveling from a country with risk of yellow fever transmission and ≥1 year of age	None
Guam (U.S.)	Not required	None
Guatemala	If traveling from a country with risk of yellow fever transmission and ≥1 year of age	None
Guinea	If traveling from a country with risk of yellow fever transmission and ≥1 year of age	For all travelers ≥9 months of age
Guinea-Bissau	If traveling from a country with risk of yellow fever transmission and ≥1 year of age Required also for travelers arriving from: *Africa:* Angola, Benin, Burkina Faso, Burundi, Cape Verde, Central African Republic, Chad, Congo, Côte d'Ivoire, Democratic Republic of the Congo, Djibouti, Equatorial Guinea, Ethiopia, Gabon, The Gambia, Ghana, Guinea, Kenya, Liberia, Madagascar, Mali, Mauritania, Mozambique, Niger, Nigeria, Rwanda,	For all travelers ≥9 months of age

(Continued)

Guinea-Bissau *(Continued)* to **India**

Country	Yellow Fever Vaccine Requirements[1,2]	CDC Yellow Fever Vaccine Recommendations[2,3,4]
Guinea-Bissau *(Continued)*	São Tomé and Príncipe, Senegal, Sierra Leone, Somalia, Tanzania, Togo, Uganda, and Zambia *Americas:* Bolivia, Brazil, Colombia, Ecuador, French Guiana, Guyana, Panama, Peru, Suriname, and Venezuela	
Guyana	If traveling from a country with risk of yellow fever transmission Required also for travelers arriving from: *Africa:* Angola, Benin, Burkina Faso, Burundi, Cameroon, Central African Republic, Chad, Congo, Côte d'Ivoire, Democratic Republic of the Congo, Equatorial Guinea, Ethiopia, Gabon, The Gambia, Ghana, Guinea, Guinea-Bissau, Kenya, Liberia, Mali, Mauritania, Niger, Nigeria, Rwanda, São Tomé and Príncipe, Senegal, Sierra Leone, Somalia, Sudan, Tanzania, Togo, and Uganda *Americas:* Belize, Bolivia, Brazil, Colombia, Ecuador, French Guiana, Guyana, Panama, Peru, Suriname, and Venezuela	For all travelers ≥9 months of age
Haiti	If traveling from a country with risk of yellow fever transmission	None
Holy See	Not required	None
Honduras	Required from travelers ≥1 year of age coming from countries with risk of yellow fever transmission. The Government of Honduras is also recommending vaccine for travelers coming from Panama.	None
Hong Kong SAR (China)	Not required	None
Hungary	Not required	None
Iceland	Not required	None
India	Required from travelers ≥6 months of age coming from a country with risk of yellow fever transmission Specifically, per the Government of India, anyone (except infants ≤6 months old) arriving by air or sea without a certificate is detained in isolation for up to 6 days if that person (i) arrives within 6 days of departure from an area with risk of yellow fever transmission, or (ii) has been in such an area in transit (except those passengers and members of crew who, while in transit through an aiport situated in an area with risk of yellow fever transmission, remained within the airport premises during the period of their entire stay and the Health Officer agrees to such an	None

(Continued)

Please note: Country requirements for yellow fever vaccine are subject to change at any time, and CDC vaccine recommendations are subject to change at any time if disease conditions change; therefore, CDC encourages health-care providers and travelers to check for updates on the CDC website www.cdc.gov/travel, and with the destination country's embassy or consulate in sufficient time to receive yellow fever vaccination or to obtain a waiver if recommendations or requirements have changed.

Country	Yellow Fever Vaccine Requirements[1,2]	CDC Yellow Fever Vaccine Recommendations[2,3,4]
India *(Continued)*	exemption), or (iii) has come on a ship that started from or touched at any port in a yellow fever area with risk of yellow fever transmission up to 30 days before its arrival into India, unless such a ship has been disinsected in accordance with the procedure laid down by WHO, or (iv) has come by an aircraft which has been in an area with risk of yellow fever transmission and has not been disinsected in accordance with the provisions laid down in the Indian Aircraft Public Health Rules, 1954, or those recommended by WHO. The following countries and areas are regarded as at risk of yellow fever transmission: *Africa:* Angola, Benin, Burkina Faso, Burundi, Cameroon, Central African Republic, Chad, Congo, Côte d'Ivoire, Democratic Republic of the Congo, Equatorial Guinea, Ethiopia, Gabon, The Gambia, Ghana, Guinea, Guinea-Bissau, Kenya, Liberia, Mali, Niger, Nigeria, Rwanda, São Tomé and Principe, Senegal, Sierra Leone, Somalia, Sudan, Togo, Uganda, Tanzania, and Zambia *Americas:* Bolivia, Brazil, Colombia, Ecuador, French Guiana, Guyana, Panama, Peru, Suriname, Trinidad and Tobago, and Venezuela *Note:* When a case of yellow fever is reported from any country, that country is regarded by the Government of India as a country with risk of yellow fever and is added to the above list.	
Indonesia	If traveling from a country with risk of yellow fever transmission and ≥9 months of age	None
Iran	If traveling from a country with risk of yellow fever transmission	None
Iraq	If traveling from a country with risk of yellow fever transmission	None
Ireland	Not required	None
Israel	Not required	None
Italy	Not required	None
Jamaica	If traveling from a country with risk of yellow fever transmission and ≥1 year of age	None
Japan	Not required	None
Jordan	If traveling from a country with risk of yellow fever transmission and ≥1 year of age	None
Kazakhstan	If traveling from a country with risk of yellow fever transmission	None
Kenya	If traveling from a country with risk of yellow fever transmission and ≥1 year of age	For all travelers ≥9 months of age. The cities of Nairobi and Mombasa have lower risk of transmission than rural areas.

Kiribati (formerly **Gilbert Islands**) to **Malta**

Country	Yellow Fever Vaccine Requirements[1,2]	CDC Yellow Fever Vaccine Recommendations[2,3,4]
Kiribati (formerly **Gilbert Islands**), includes **Tarawa, Tabuaeran (Fanning Island)**, and **Banaba (Ocean Island)**	If traveling from a country with risk of yellow fever transmission and ≥1 year of age	None
Korea, North	If traveling from a country with risk of yellow fever transmission and ≥1 year of age	None
Korea, South	Not required	None
Kosovo	Not required	None
Kuwait	Not required	None
Kyrgyzstan	Not required	None
Laos	If traveling from a country with risk of yellow fever transmission	None
Latvia	Not required	None
Lebanon	If traveling from a country with risk of yellow fever transmission and ≥6 months of age[5]	None
Lesotho	If traveling from a country with risk of yellow fever transmission	None
Liberia	Required upon arrival from all countries if traveler is ≥1 year of age	For all travelers ≥9 months of age
Libya	If traveling from a country with risk of yellow fever transmission	None
Liechtenstein	Not required	None
Lithuania	Not required	None
Luxembourg	Not required	None
Macau SAR (China)	Not required	None
Macedonia	Not required	None
Madagascar	If traveling from a country with risk of yellow fever transmission	None
Madeira Islands (Portugal)	If traveling from a country with risk of yellow fever transmission and ≥1 year of age	None
Malawi	If traveling from a country with risk of yellow fever transmission	None
Malaysia	Required from travelers ≥1 year of age arriving within 6 days from countries with risk of yellow fever transmission	None
Maldives	If traveling from a country with risk of yellow fever transmission	None
Mali	Required upon arrival from all countries if traveler is ≥1 year of age	For all travelers ≥9 months of age going to areas south of the Sahara Desert
Malta	If traveling from a country with risk of yellow fever transmission and ≥9 months of age If indicated on epidemiological grounds, infants <9 months of age are subject to isolation or surveillance if coming from an area with risk of yellow fever transmission.	None

Please note: Country requirements for yellow fever vaccine are subject to change at any time, and CDC vaccine recommendations are subject to change at any time if disease conditions change; therefore, CDC encourages health-care providers and travelers to check for updates on the CDC website www.cdc.gov/travel, and with the destination country's embassy or consulate in sufficient time to receive yellow fever vaccination or to obtain a waiver if recommendations or requirements have changed.

Country	Yellow Fever Vaccine Requirements[1,2]	CDC Yellow Fever Vaccine Recommendations[2,3,4]
Marshall Islands	Not required	None
Martinique (France)	Not required	None
Mauritania	If traveling from a country with risk of yellow fever transmission and ≥1 year of age	For all travelers ≥9 months of age traveling to areas south of the Sahara Desert
Mauritius	If traveling from a country with risk of yellow fever transmission and ≥1 year of age	None
Mayotte (French territorial collectivity)	Not required	None
Mexico	Not required	None
Micronesia, Federated States of; includes **Yap Islands**, **Pohnpei**, **Chuuk**, and **Kosrae**	Not required	None
Moldova	Not required	None
Monaco	Not required	None
Mongolia	Not required	None
Montenegro	Not required	None
Montserrat (U.K.)	If traveling from a country with risk of yellow fever transmission and ≥1 year of age	None
Morocco	Not required	None
Mozambique	If traveling from a country with risk of yellow fever transmission and ≥1 year of age	None
Namibia	If traveling from a country with risk of yellow fever transmission The countries, or parts of countries, included in the endemic zones in Africa and South America are regarded as areas with risk of yellow fever transmission. Travelers on scheduled flights that originated outside the countries with risk of yellow fever transmission, but who have been in transit through these areas, are not required to possess a certificate provided that they remained at the scheduled airport or in the adjacent town during transit. All passengers whose flights originated in countries with risk of yellow fever transmission or who have been in transit through these countries on unscheduled flights are required to possess a certificate. The certificate is not insisted upon in the case of children <1 year of age, but such infants may be subject to surveillance.	None
Nauru	If traveling from a country with risk of yellow fever transmission and ≥1 year of age	None
Nepal	If traveling from a country with risk of yellow fever transmission	None
Netherlands	Not required	None

CHAPTER

2

The Pre-Travel Consultation

Travel-Related Vaccine-Preventable Diseases

Country	Yellow Fever Vaccine Requirements[1,2]	CDC Yellow Fever Vaccine Recommendations[2,3,4]
Netherlands Antilles (Bonaire, **Curaçao**, **Saba**, **St. Eustasius**, and **St. Maarten)**	If traveling from a country with risk of yellow fever transmission and ≥6 months of age[5]	None
New Caledonia (France)	If traveling from a country with risk of yellow fever transmission and ≥1 year of age Note: In the event of an epidemic threat to the territory, a specific vaccination certificate may be required.	None
New Zealand	Not required	None
Nicaragua	If traveling from a country with risk of yellow fever transmission and ≥1 year of age	None
Niger	Required upon arrival from all countries if traveler is ≥1 year of age. The Government of Niger recommends vaccine for travelers leaving Niger.	For all travelers ≥9 months of age traveling to areas south of the Sahara Desert
Nigeria	If traveling from a country with risk of yellow fever transmission and ≥1 year of age	For all travelers ≥9 months of age
Niue (New Zealand)	If traveling from a country with risk of yellow fever transmission and ≥1 year of age	None
Norfolk Island (Australia)	If traveling from a country with risk of yellow fever transmission and ≥1 year of age	None
Northern Mariana Islands (U.S.), includes **Saipan**, **Tinian**, and **Rota Island**	Not required	None
Norway	Not required	None
Oman	If traveling from a country with risk of yellow fever transmission and ≥1 year of age	None
Pakistan	Required from travelers coming from any part of a country in which there is a risk of yellow fever transmission; infants <6 months of age are exempt if the mother's vaccination certificate shows that she was vaccinated before the birth of the child.[5]	None
Palau	Required from all travelers ≥1 year of age coming from countries with risk of yellow fever transmission or from countries in any part of which there is a risk of yellow fever transmission	None
Panama	If traveling from a country with risk of yellow fever transmission	For all travelers ≥9 months of age traveling to the provinces of Darien, Kuna Yala (old San Blas), Comarca Emberá, and Panama east of the Canal Zone, EXCLUDING the Canal Zone, Panama City, and San Blas Islands

Please note: Country requirements for yellow fever vaccine are subject to change at any time, and CDC vaccine recommendations are subject to change at any time if disease conditions change; therefore, CDC encourages health-care providers and travelers to check for updates on the CDC website www.cdc.gov/travel, and with the destination country's embassy or consulate in sufficient time to receive yellow fever vaccination or to obtain a waiver if recommendations or requirements have changed.

Country	Yellow Fever Vaccine Requirements[1,2]	CDC Yellow Fever Vaccine Recommendations[2,3,4]
Papua New Guinea	If traveling from a country with risk of yellow fever transmission and ≥1 year of age	None
Paraguay	If traveling from a country with risk of yellow fever transmission and ≥1 year of age	For all travelers ≥9 months of age
Peru	Not required	For all travelers ≥9 months of age traveling to the areas east of the Andes Mountains (see Map 2-4) and for those who intend to visit any jungle areas of the country <2,300 m (<7,546 ft). Travelers who are limiting travel to the cities of Cuzco and Machu Picchu do NOT need vaccination.
Philippines	If traveling from a country with risk of yellow fever transmission and ≥1 year of age	None
Pitcairn Islands (U.K.)	If traveling from a country with risk of yellow fever transmission and ≥1 year of age	None
Poland	Not required	None
Portugal	Required only for travelers ≥1 year of age arriving from a country with risk of yellow fever transmission and destined for the Azores and Madeira. However, no certificate is required for travelers in transit at Funchal, Santa Maria, and Porto Santo.	None
Puerto Rico (U.S.)	Not required	None
Qatar	Not required	None
Réunion (France)	If traveling from a country with risk of yellow fever transmission and ≥1 year of age	None
Romania	Not required	None
Russia	Not required	None
Rwanda	Required upon arrival from all countries if traveler is ≥1 year of age	For all travelers ≥9 months of age
Saint Helena (U.K.)	If traveling from a country with risk of yellow fever transmission and ≥1 year of age	None
Saint Kitts (Saint Christopher) and Nevis (U.K.)	If traveling from a country with risk of yellow fever transmission and ≥1 year of age	None
Saint Lucia	If traveling from a country with risk of yellow fever transmission and ≥1 year of age	None
Saint Pierre and Miquelon (France)	Not required	None
Saint Vincent and the Grenadines	If traveling from a country with risk of yellow fever transmission and ≥1 year of age	None
Samoa (formerly Western Somoa)	If traveling from a country with risk of yellow fever transmission and ≥1 year of age	None
Samoa, American (U.S.)	Not required	None
San Marino	Not required	None
São Tomé and Príncipe	Required upon arrival from all countries if traveler is ≥1 year of age	For all travelers ≥9 months of age
Saudi Arabia	If traveling from a country with risk of yellow fever transmission	None

Country	Yellow Fever Vaccine Requirements[1,2]	CDC Yellow Fever Vaccine Recommendations[2,3,4]
Senegal	If traveling from a country with risk of yellow fever transmission	For all travelers ≥9 months of age
Serbia	Not required	None
Seychelles	If traveling from a country with risk of yellow fever transmission within the preceding 6 days and ≥1 year of age	None
Sierra Leone	Required upon arrival from all countries	For all travelers ≥9 months of age
Singapore	If traveling from a country with risk of yellow fever transmission within the preceding 6 days and ≥1 year of age	None
Slovakia	Not required	None
Slovenia	Not required	None
Solomon Islands	If traveling from a country with risk of yellow fever transmission	None
Somalia	If traveling from a country with risk of yellow fever transmission	For all travelers ≥9 months of age
South Africa	If traveling from a country with risk of yellow fever transmission and ≥1 year of age	None
South Georgia	Not required	None
South Sandwich Islands	Not required	None
Spain	Not required	None
Sri Lanka	If traveling from a country with risk of yellow fever transmission and ≥1 year of age	None
Sudan	If traveling from a country with risk of yellow fever transmission and ≥9 months of age. A certificate may be required for travelers leaving Sudan.	For all travelers ≥9 months of age traveling to areas south of the Sahara Desert, EXCLUDING the city of Khartoum
Suriname	If traveling from a country with risk of yellow fever transmission and ≥1 year of age	For all travelers ≥9 months of age
Swaziland	If traveling from a country with risk of yellow fever transmission	None
Sweden	Not required	None
Switzerland	Not required	None
Syria	If traveling from a country with risk of yellow fever transmission	None
Taiwan	If traveling from a country with risk of yellow fever transmission	None
Tajikistan	Not required	None
Tanzania	If traveling from a country with risk of yellow fever transmission and ≥1 year of age	For all travelers ≥9 months of age. The city of Dar es Salaam has a lower risk of transmission than rural areas.
Thailand	If traveling from a country with risk of yellow fever transmission and ≥9 months of age	None
Timor-Leste (East Timor)	If traveling from a country with risk of yellow fever transmission and ≥1 year of age	None
Togo	Required upon arrival from all countries if traveler is ≥1 year of age	For all travelers ≥9 months of age

Please note: Country requirements for yellow fever vaccine are subject to change at any time, and CDC vaccine recommendations are subject to change at any time if disease conditions change; therefore, CDC encourages health-care providers and travelers to check for updates on the CDC website www.cdc.gov/travel, and with the destination country's embassy or consulate in sufficient time to receive yellow fever vaccination or to obtain a waiver if recommendations or requirements have changed.

Country	Yellow Fever Vaccine Requirements[1,2]	CDC Yellow Fever Vaccine Recommendations[2,3,4]
Tokelau (New Zealand)	Not required	None
Tonga	If traveling from a country with risk of yellow fever transmission and ≥1 year of age	None
Trinidad and Tobago	If traveling from a country with risk of yellow fever transmission and ≥1 year of age	For all travelers ≥9 months of age whose itinerary includes Trinidad. Port of Spain has lower risk of transmission than rural or forested areas. Cruise ship passengers who do not disembark from the ship or travelers visiting only the urban area of Port of Spain (including passengers in-transit only) may consider foregoing vaccination. Vaccination is NOT recommended for those visiting only Tobago.
Tunisia	If traveling from a country with risk of yellow fever transmission and ≥1 year of age	None
Turkey	Not required	None
Turkmenistan	Not required	None
Turks and Caicos Islands (U.K.)	If traveling from a country with risk of yellow fever transmission and ≥1 year of age	None
Tuvalu	Not required	None
Uganda	If traveling from a country with risk of yellow fever transmission and ≥1 year of age	For all travelers ≥9 months of age
Ukraine	Not required	None
United Arab Emirates	Not required	None
United Kingdom (with **Channel Islands** and **Isle of Man**)	Not required	None
United States	Not required	None
Uruguay	If traveling from a country with risk of yellow fever transmission	None
Uzbekistan	Not required	None
Vanuatu	Not required	None
Venezuela	Not required	For all travelers ≥9 months of age traveling to Venezuela, EXCEPT the northern coastal area (see Map 2-4). The cities of Caracas and Valencia are NOT in the endemic zone.
Vietnam	If traveling from a country with risk of yellow fever transmission and ≥1 year of age	None
Virgin Islands, British	Not required	None
Virgin Islands, U.S.	Not required	None
Wake Island, U.S.	Not required	None
Western Sahara	Not required	None
Yemen	If traveling from a country with risk of yellow fever transmission and ≥1 year of age	None
Zambia	Not required	None
Zimbabwe	If traveling from a country with risk of yellow fever transmission	None

(See next page for table footnotes)

Table 2-14—footnotes

1 Yellow fever vaccine entry requirements are established by countries to prevent the importation and transmission of yellow fever virus, and are allowed under the International Health Regulations (IHR). Travelers must comply with these to enter the country, unless they have been issued a medical waiver. Certain countries require vaccination from travelers arriving from all countries, while some countries require vaccination only for travelers coming from "a country with risk of yellow fever transmission" (see Table 2-12). Country requirements are subject to change at any time; therefore, CDC encourages travelers to check with the destination country's embassy or consulate prior to departure.

2 As a part of an ongoing project, CDC, WHO, and other partners have made every effort to harmonize the listed yellow fever vaccine requirements and recommendations wherever possible. These efforts will continue, and will likely result in further changes to the printed version of this table. Please check the online version of the Yellow Book (www.cdc.gov/yellowbook) for the latest information on country requirements and vaccine recommendations.

3 The information in the section on yellow fever vaccine recommendations is advice given by CDC to prevent yellow fever infections among travelers. Note: CDC recommendations and country requirements may not be the same.

4 Recommendations are subject to change at any time if disease conditions change; therefore, CDC encourages travelers to check for relevant travel notices on the website (www.cdc.gov/travel) prior to departure.

5 Please note, the U.S. Advisory Committee on Immunization Practices (ACIP) recommends avoiding vaccination of infants <9 months of age.

JAPANESE ENCEPHALITIS (JE)

Marc Fischer, Anne Griggs, J. Erin Staples

Infectious Agent

Japanese encephalitis virus (JEV) is a single-stranded RNA virus that belongs to the genus *Flavivirus* and is closely related to West Nile and St. Louis encephalitis viruses.

Mode of Transmission

- JEV is transmitted to humans through the bite of an infected mosquito, primarily *Culex* species. Wading birds are the main animal reservoir for the virus, but the presence of pigs greatly amplifies the transmission of JEV.
- Humans are a dead-end host in the JEV transmission cycle.

Occurrence

- JEV is the most common cause of encephalitis in Asia, occurring throughout most of Asia and parts of the western Pacific (Map 2-5). JEV has not been locally transmitted in Africa, Europe, or the Americas.
- JEV transmission principally occurs in rural agricultural areas, often associated with rice production and flooding irrigation. In some areas of Asia, these ecologic conditions may occur near or occasionally within urban centers.
- In temperate areas of Asia, transmission is seasonal, and human disease usually peaks in summer and fall. In the subtropics and tropics, seasonal transmission varies with monsoon rains and irrigation practices and may be extended or even occur year-round.
- In endemic countries, JE is primarily a disease of children. However, travel-associated JE can occur among persons of any age.

Risk for Travelers

- The risk for JE for most travelers to Asia is extremely low but varies according to season, destination, duration, and activities. Fewer than 40 cases of confirmed JE have been reported in travelers in the last 40 years.
- The overall incidence of JE reported among people from nonendemic countries traveling to Asia is <1 case per 1 million travelers. However, expatriates and travelers staying for prolonged periods in rural areas with active JEV transmission are likely at similar risk as the susceptible resident population (0.1–2 cases per 100,000 persons per week).

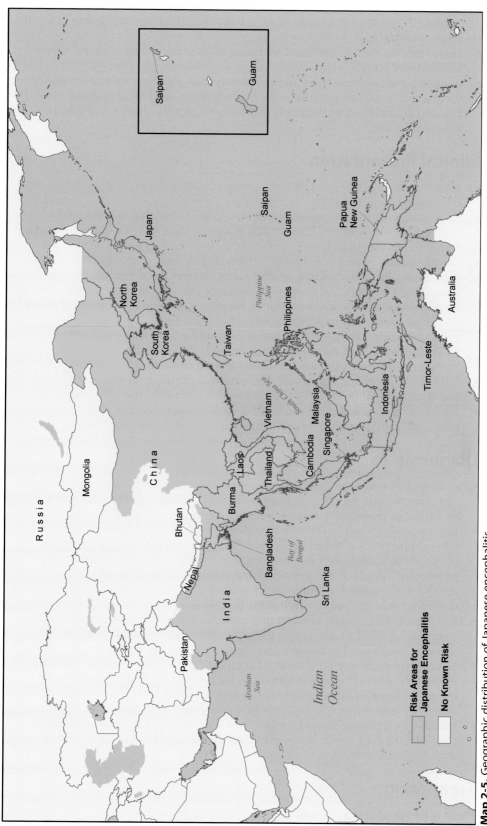

Map 2-5. Geographic distribution of Japanese encephalitis.

- Travelers on even brief trips are probably at increased risk if they have extensive outdoor or nighttime exposure in rural areas, including persons staying in resort areas or with family.
- Short-term travelers whose visits are restricted to major urban areas are at very minimal risk for JE.
- In endemic areas where there are few human cases among residents because of vaccination or natural immunity, JEV is often maintained in an enzootic cycle between animals and mosquitoes. Therefore, susceptible visitors still may be at risk for infection.

Clinical Presentation

- Most human infections with JEV are asymptomatic; <1% of people infected with JEV develop clinical disease.
- Acute encephalitis is the most commonly recognized clinical manifestation of JEV infection. Milder forms of disease such as aseptic meningitis or undifferentiated febrile illness can also occur.
- The incubation period is 5–15 days. Illness usually begins with sudden onset of fever, headache, and vomiting. Mental status changes, focal neurologic deficits, generalized weakness, and movement disorders may develop over the next few days.
  - ○ A parkinsonian syndrome resulting from extrapyramidal involvement is a very distinctive clinical presentation of JE.
  - ○ Acute flaccid paralysis, with clinical and pathological features similar to poliomyelitis, has also been associated with JEV infection.
  - ○ Seizures are very common, especially among children.
- Clinical laboratory findings include moderate leukocytosis, mild anemia, hyponatremia, and cerebrospinal fluid (CSF) pleocytosis with a lymphocytic predominance.
- Case–fatality ratio is approximately 20%–30%. Among survivors, 30%–50% may still have significant neurologic or psychiatric sequelae, even years after their acute illness.

Diagnosis

- JE should be suspected in a patient with evidence of a neurologic infection (e.g., encephalitis, meningitis, or acute flaccid paralysis) who has recently traveled or resided in an endemic country in Asia or the western Pacific.
- Laboratory diagnosis of JEV infection should be performed by using JE-specific IgM-capture enzyme-linked immunosorbent assay (ELISA) on CSF or serum. JE-specific IgM antibodies will be present in the CSF or blood of almost all patients by 7 days following onset of symptoms. A fourfold or greater rise in JEV-specific neutralizing antibodies between acute- and convalescent-phase serum specimens may be used to confirm the diagnosis.
- Vaccination history, date of onset of symptoms, and information regarding other flaviviruses known to circulate in the geographic area that may cross-react in serologic assays need to be considered when interpreting results.
- Humans have low levels of transient viremia and usually have neutralizing antibodies by the time distinctive clinical symptoms are recognized. Virus isolation and nucleic-acid amplification tests (NAATs) are insensitive for the detection of JEV or JE viral RNA in blood or CSF and should not be used for ruling out a diagnosis of JE.
- Health-care providers should contact their state or local health department or CDC's Division of Vector Borne Infectious Diseases at 970-221-6400 for assistance with diagnostic testing.

Treatment

There is no specific antiviral treatment for JE; therapy consists of supportive care and management of complications.

Preventive Measures for Travelers

Personal Protection Measures

- No drugs for preventing JEV infection are available.
- The best way to prevent mosquito-borne diseases, including JE, is to avoid mosquito bites (see the Protection Against Mosquitoes, Ticks, and Other Insects and Arthropods section later in this chapter).

JE Vaccines

- An inactivated mouse brain-derived JE vaccine (JE-VAX, manufactured by sanofi pasteur) has been licensed for use in adult and pediatric travelers (≥1 year of age) in the United States since 1992. Although production of JE-VAX was discontinued in 2006, stockpiles of the vaccine will be used for U.S. travelers until they are depleted.
- An inactivated cell culture-derived JE vaccine (IXIARO, manufactured by Intercell) was approved for adult travelers (≥18 years of age) in the United States on March 30, 2009. Recommendations for its use will be available at www.cdc.gov/travel. Other inactivated and live attenuated JE vaccines are manufactured and used in Asia but not licensed for use in the United States.

Inactivated Mouse Brain-Derived JE Vaccine (JE-VAX)

- A randomized controlled trial among 65,000 children in Thailand showed an efficacy of 91% (95% CI 70%–97%) after two doses.
- From 88% to 100% of adults from nonendemic settings developed neutralizing antibodies after receiving three doses of vaccine.
- The duration of protection after primary immunization is unknown, but circulating neutralizing antibodies appear to last for at least 2–3 years.
- Booster doses produce an anamnestic response in neutralizing antibody titers.

Recommendations for the Use of JE Vaccine for Travelers

- Decisions regarding the use of JE vaccine for travelers must balance the low risk for disease and the small chance of an adverse event following immunization.
- The U.S. Advisory Committee on Immunization Practices (ACIP) currently recommends JE vaccine for travelers who plan to spend a month or longer in endemic areas or areas with ongoing transmission. Vaccine should also be considered for shorter-term travelers whose itineraries may put them at increased risk for JEV exposure, such as rural stays during the rainy season.
- Evaluation of an individual traveler's risk should take into account itinerary, activities, and best-available information on the current level of JE activity in the travel area (Table 2-15). Complicating the concept of risk assessment, however, is the fact that sporadic cases of JE have very rarely occurred in travelers whose itineraries would not ordinarily have indicated a risk for JE (e.g., a resort hotel in Bali, a standard tour of China).

Vaccine Safety and Adverse Events

- Inactivated mouse brain-derived JE vaccine has been associated with localized erythema, tenderness, and swelling at the injection site in about 20% of recipients.
- Mild systemic side effects (e.g., fever, chills, headache, rash, myalgia, gastrointestinal symptoms) have been reported in approximately 10% of vaccinees.
- Serious allergic hypersensitivity reactions, including generalized urticaria and angioedema of the extremities, face, and oropharynx, have been reported. Accompanying bronchospasm, respiratory distress, and hypotension have been observed in some of these patients, although there have been no fatalities among vaccine recipients with these symptoms.

Table 2-15. Risk for Japanese encephalitis, by country[1]

Country	Affected Areas	Transmission Season	Comments
Australia	Outer islands of Torres Strait	December to May; all human cases reported from February to April	One human case reported from north Queensland mainland
Bangladesh	Limited data; probably widespread	Unknown; most human cases reported from May to October	One outbreak of human disease reported from Tangail District in 1977. Sentinel surveillance has identified human cases in Chittagong, Khulna, and Rajshahi divisions, and Mymensingh district.
Bhutan	No data	No data	
Brunei	No data; presumed to be endemic countrywide	Unknown; presumed year-round transmission	
Burma (Myanmar)	Limited data; presumed be endemic countrywide	Unknown; most human cases reported from May to October	Outbreaks of human disease documented in Shan State. JEV antibodies documented in animals and humans in other areas
Cambodia	Presumed to be endemic countrywide	Probably year round with peaks reported from May to October	Sentinel surveillance has identified human cases in at least 14 provinces including Phnom Penh, Takeo, Kampong, Cham, Battambang, Svay Rieng, and Siem Reap.
China	Human cases reported from all provinces except Xizang (Tibet), Xinjiang, and Qinghai *Hong Kong and Macau:* Not considered endemic. Rare cases reported from the New Territories	Most human cases reported from April to October	Highest rates reported from the southwest and south central provinces Vaccine not routinely recommended for travel limited to Beijing or other major cities
India	Human cases reported from all states except Dadra, Daman, Diu, Gujarat, Himachal, Jammu, Kashmir, Lakshadweep, Meghalaya, Nagar Haveli, Punjab, Rajasthan, and Sikkim	Most human cases reported from May to October especially in northern India. The season may be extended or year round in some areas especially in southern India.	Highest rates of human disease reported from the states of Andhra Pradesh, Assam, Bihar, Goa, Haryana, Karnataka, Kerala, Tamil Nadu, Uttar Pradesh, and West Bengal
Indonesia	Presumed to be endemic countrywide	Human cases reported year round; peak season varies by island	Sentinel surveillance has identified human cases in Bali, Kalimantan, Java, Nusa Tenggara, Papua, and Sumatra.
Japan[2]	Rare sporadic human cases on all islands except Hokkaido. Enzootic activity ongoing	Most human cases reported from May to October	Large number of human cases reported until routine JE vaccination introduced in 1968. Most recent small outbreak reported from Chugoku district in 2002. Sporadic cases reported among U.S. military personnel on Okinawa. Enzootic transmission without human cases observed on Hokkaido Vaccine not routinely recommended for travel limited to Tokyo or other major cities

Table 2-15. Risk for Japanese encephalitis, by country[1] *(Continued)*

Country	Affected Areas	Transmission Season	Comments
Korea, North	No data	No data	
Korea, South[2]	Rare sporadic human cases countrywide. Enzootic activity ongoing	Most human cases reported from May to October	Large number of human cases reported until routine JE vaccination introduced in 1968. Highest rates of disease were reported from the southern provinces. Last major outbreak reported in 1982 Vaccine not routinely recommended for travel limited to Seoul or other major cities
Laos	No data; presumed to be endemic countrywide	Presumed to be May to October	
Malaysia	Endemic in Sarawak; sporadic cases or outbreaks reported from all states of Peninsula, and probably Sabah	Year-round transmission	Most human cases reported from Penang and Sarawak Vaccine not routinely recommended for travel limited to Kuala Lumpur or other major cities
Mongolia	Not considered endemic		
Nepal	Endemic in southern lowlands (Terai). Sporadic cases or outbreaks reported from the Kathmandu valley	Most human cases reported from May to November	Highest rates of human disease reported from western Terai districts, including Bankey, Bardia, Dang, and Kailali Vaccine not routinely recommended for travel limited to high-altitude areas
Pakistan	Limited data; human cases reported from around Karachi	Most human cases reported from May to October	
Papua New Guinea	Limited data; sporadic human cases reported from Western, Gulf, and South Highland Provinces	Unknown	A case of JE was reported from near Port Moresby in 2004. Human cases documented in Papua Indonesia
Philippines	Limited data; presumed to be endemic on all islands	Unknown; probably year-round	Outbreaks reported in Nueva Ecija, Luzon, and Manila
Russia	Rare human cases reported from the Far Eastern maritime areas south of Khabarousk	Most human cases reported from July to September	
Singapore	Rare sporadic human cases reported	Year-round transmission	Vaccine not routinely recommended
Sri Lanka	Endemic countrywide except in mountainous areas	Year-round with variable peaks based on monsoon rains	Highest rates of human disease reported from Anuradhapura, Gampaha, Kurunegala, Polonnaruwa, and Puttalam districts
Taiwan[2]	Rare sporadic human cases island-wide	Most human cases reported from May to October	Large number of human cases reported until routine JE vaccination introduced in 1968 Vaccine not routinely recommended for travel limited to Taipei or other major cities

(Continued)

Table 2-15. Risk for Japanese encephalitis, by country[1] (Continued)

Country	Affected Areas	Transmission Season	Comments
Thailand	Endemic countrywide; seasonal epidemics in the northern provinces	Year-round with seasonal peaks from May to October, especially in the north	Highest rates of human disease reported from the Chiang Mai Valley. Sporadic human cases reported from Bangkok suburbs
Timor-Leste	Limited data; anecdotal reports of sporadic human cases	No data	
Vietnam	Endemic countrywide; seasonal epidemics in the northern provinces	Year-round with seasonal peaks from May to October, especially in the north	Highest rates of disease in the northern provinces around Hanoi and northwestern provinces bordering China
Western Pacific Islands	Outbreaks of human disease reported in Guam in 1947–1948 and Saipan in 1990	Unknown; most human cases reported from October to March	Enzootic cycle might not be sustainable; outbreaks may follow introductions of JE virus.

1 Data are based on published reports and personal correspondence. Risk assessments should be performed cautiously because risk can vary within areas and from year to year, and surveillance data regarding human cases and JE virus transmission are incomplete.

2 In some endemic areas, human cases among residents are limited because of vaccination or natural immunity. However, because JE virus is maintained in an enzootic cycle between animals and mosquitoes, susceptible visitors to these areas still may be at risk for infection.

- Estimates of the frequency of these reactions range from 20 to 600 cases per 100,000 vaccinees and vary by country, year, case definition, surveillance method, and vaccine lot.
- Most hypersensitivity reactions occur within 24–48 hours after the first dose, when they occur following a subsequent dose, the onset of symptoms is often delayed (median: 3 days; range: up to 2 weeks).
- Most reactions can be treated with antihistamines or corticosteroids on an outpatient basis; however, up to 10% of vaccinees with rare severe reactions are hospitalized.
- At least four deaths due to anaphylactic shock temporally associated with receipt of this vaccine have been reported in the world literature, which includes endemic country national vaccine programs. None of these patients had evidence of urticaria or angioedema, and two had received other vaccines simultaneously.
- Moderate to severe neurologic symptoms, including encephalitis, seizures, gait disturbances, and parkinsonian syndrome have been reported, with an incidence of 0.1 to 2 cases per 100,000 vaccinees.
- In addition, there have been case reports of children in Japan and Korea with severe or fatal acute disseminated encephalomyelitis (ADEM) temporally associated with JE vaccination.

Vaccine Dose and Administration

- For travelers ≥3 years of age, the recommended primary immunization series for JE-VAX is three doses of 1.0 mL each, administered subcutaneously on days 0, 7, and 30.
- An abbreviated schedule (days 0, 7, and 14) provides similar rates of seroconversion but significantly lower neutralizing antibody titers.
- Immunization routes and schedules for children 1 and 2 years of age are identical except that 0.5-mL doses should be administered.
- Vaccine recipients should be observed for a minimum of 30 minutes after immunization and warned about the possibility of delayed allergic reactions.
- The last dose should be administered at least 10 days before beginning travel to ensure an adequate immune response and access to medical care in the event of any delayed adverse reactions.
- Booster doses may be administered 2–3 years after the primary series. The timing and immune response of subsequent boosters have not been studied in travelers.

Precautions and Contraindications

- A history of allergy or hypersensitivity reaction to a previous dose of mouse brain-derived JE vaccine is a contraindication to receiving additional doses.
- Proven or suspected hypersensitivity to thimerosal or proteins of rodent or neural origin is a contraindication to vaccination.
- Persons with a previous history of urticaria are more likely to develop a hypersensitivity reaction following receipt of JE vaccine. This history should be considered when weighing the risks and benefits of the vaccine for an individual patient.
- No specific information is available on the safety of JE vaccine in pregnancy. Therefore, the vaccine should not be routinely administered during pregnancy. Pregnant women who must travel to an area where risk for JE is high should be vaccinated when the theoretical risk for immunization is outweighed by the risk for infection.
- No data are available on vaccine safety and efficacy in infants <1 year of age.
- Two small studies of inactivated JE vaccine in children with underlying medical conditions did not show a change in the adverse reactions or immune response after vaccination.

References

1. CDC. Inactivated Japanese encephalitis virus vaccine: Recommendations of the Advisory Committee on Immunization Practices (ACIP). MMWR Recomm Rep. 1993;42(RR-01):1–16.
2. Marfin AA, Eidex RS, Kozarsky PE, et al. Yellow fever and Japanese encephalitis vaccines: indications and complications. Infect Dis Clin North Am. 2005;19(1):151–68.
3. Shlim DR, Solomon T. Japanese encephalitis vaccine for travelers: exploring the limits of risk. Clin Infect Dis. 2002;35(2):183–8.
4. Halstead SB, Tsai TF. Japanese encephalitis vaccine. In: Plotkin SA, Orenstein WA, editors. Vaccines, 4th edition. Philadelphia: WB Saunders; 2004. p. 919–58.
5. Solomon T. Flavivirus encephalitis. N Engl J Med. 2004;351(4):370–8.
6. Tauber E, Kollaritsch H, Korinek M, et al. Safety and immunogenicity of a Vero-cell-derived, inactivated Japanese encephalitis vaccine: a non-inferiority, phase III, randomised controlled trial. Lancet. 2007;370(9602):1847–53.
7. Gambel JM, DeFraites R, Hoke C, et al. Japanese encephalitis vaccine: Persistence of antibody up to 3 years after a three-dose primary series. J Infect Dis. 1995;171(4):1074.
8. WHO. Japanese encephalitis vaccines. weekly Epidemiol Rec. 2006;81(34/35):331–340.
9. Martin DA, Biggerstaff BJ, Allen B, et al. Use of immunoglobulin M cross-reactions in differential diagnosis of human flaviviral encephalitis infections in the United States. Clin Diag Lab Immunol. 2002;9(3):544–549.
10. Burke DS, Nisalak A, Ussery MA, et al. Kinetics of IgM and IgG responses to Japanese encephalitis virus in human serum and cerebrospinal fluid. J Infect Dis. 1985;151(6):1093–9.
11. Beasley DWC, Lewthwaite P, Solomon T. Current use and development of vaccines for Japanese encephalitis. Expert Opin Biol Ther. 2008;8(1):95–106.
12. Hoke CH, Nisalak A, Sangawhipa N, et al. Protection against Japanese encephalitis by inactivated vaccines. N Engl J Med. 1988;319(10):608–14.
13. Defraites RF, Gambel JM, Hoke CH Jr, et al. Japanese encephalitis vaccine (inactivated, BIKEN) in U.S. soldiers: Immunogenicity and safety of vaccine administered in two dosing regimens. Am J Trop Med Hyg. 1999;61(2):288–93.
14. Monath TP. Japanese encephalitis vaccines: current vaccines and future prospects. In: Current topics in microbiology and immunology: Japanese encephalitis and West Nile virus infections. In: Mackenzie JS, Barrett AD, Deubel V, editors. Berlin: Springer-Verlag 2002. p. 105–38.
15. Plesner AM. Allergic reactions to Japanese encephalitis vaccine. Immunol Allergy Clin North Am. 2003;23(4):665–97.
16. Takahashi H, Pool V, Tsai T, et al. Adverse events after Japanese encephalitis vaccination: review of post-marketing surveillance data from Japan and the United States. The VAERS Working Group. Vaccine. 2000;18(26):2963–9.
17. Berg SW, Mitchell BS, Hanson RK, et al. Systemic reactions in U.S. Marine Corps personnel who received Japanese encephalitis vaccine. Clin Infect Dis. 1997;24(2):265–6.
18. Sohn YM. Japanese encephalitis immunization in Korea: past, present and future. Emerg Infect Dis. 2000;6(1):17–24.
19. Puthanakit T, Aurpibul L, Yoksan S, et al. Japanese encephalitis vaccination in HIV-infected children with immune recovery after highly retroactive antiretroviral therapy. Vaccine. 2007;25(49):8257–61.
20. Yamada A, Imanishi J, Juang R-F, et al. Trial of inactivated Japanese encephalitis vaccine in children with underlying diseases. Vaccine. 1986;4(1):32–4.

MENINGOCOCCAL DISEASE

Amanda Cohn, Michael L. Jackson

Infectious Agent

- The infectious agent is a gram-negative diplococci, *Neisseria meningitidis*. Meningococci are classified into serogroups on the basis of the composition of the capsular polysaccharide.
- The five major meningococcal serogroups associated with disease are A, B, C, Y, and W-135.

Mode of Transmission

Person-to-person transmission occurs by close contact with respiratory secretions or saliva.

Occurrence

- *Neisseria meningitidis* is found worldwide. At any time, 5%–10% of the population may be carriers of *N. meningitidis*.
- Invasive disease is much rarer, occurring at a rate of 0.5–10 cases per 100,000 population in nonepidemic areas and up to 1,000 cases per 100,000 population in epidemic regions.
- The incidence of meningococcal disease is highest in the "meningitis belt" of sub-Saharan Africa (Map 2-6). The incidence of meningococcal disease is several times higher in the meningitis belt than in the United States, with periodic epidemics during the dry season (December–June). During nonepidemic periods the rate of meningococcal disease is roughly 5–10 cases per 100,000 population per year. During epidemics the rate can be as high as 1,000 cases per 100,000 population.
- Serogroup A predominates in the meningitis belt, although serogroups C, X, and W-135 are also found.
- Young children have the highest risk for meningococcal disease.

Risk for Travelers

- Travelers to the meningitis belt may be at risk for meningococcal disease, particularly during the dry season.
- Risk is likely highest in travelers who will have prolonged contact with local populations in the meningitis belt during an epidemic.
- The incidence of meningococcal disease in international travelers who acquire sporadic disease is very low, estimated at 0.4 per 100,000 in one retrospective study.
- The Hajj pilgrimage to Saudi Arabia has been associated with outbreaks of meningococcal disease in returning pilgrims and their contacts.

Clinical Presentation

- Meningococcal disease generally occurs 1–14 days after exposure.
- Meningococcal disease presents as meningitis in 50% or more of cases. Meningococcal meningitis is characterized by sudden onset of headache, fever, and stiffness of the neck, sometimes accompanied by nausea, vomiting, photophobia, and/or altered mental status.
- Up to 20% of persons with meningococcal disease present with meningococcal sepsis. Meningococcal sepsis is characterized by an abrupt onset of fever and a

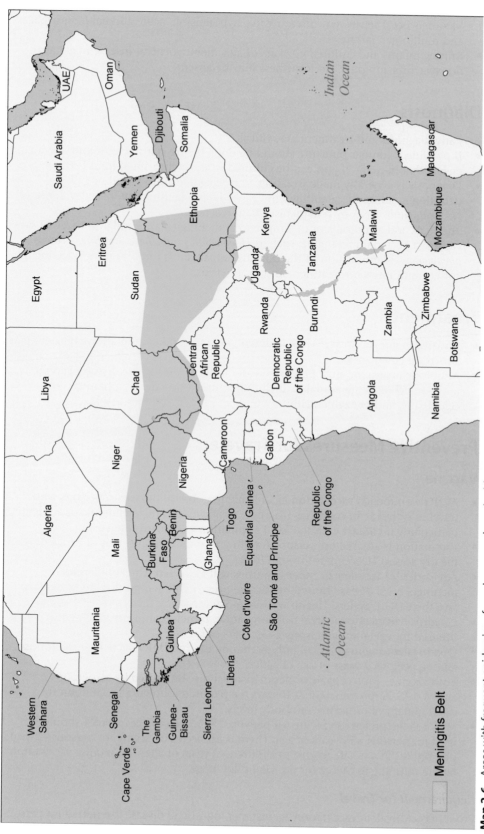

Map 2-6. Areas with frequent epidemics of meningococcal meningitis.

Meningitis Belt

petechial or purpuric rash. The rash may progress to purpura fulminans. Meningococcal sepsis may often involve hypotension, acute adrenal hemorrhage, and multiorgan failure.
- Among infants and children <2 years of age, meningococcal disease may have nonspecific symptoms. Neck stiffness may be absent.

Diagnosis

- Early diagnosis and treatment are critical.
- If possible, a lumbar puncture should be done before starting antibiotic therapy to ensure that bacteria, if any, can be cultured from cerebrospinal fluid (CSF).
- Diagnosis is generally made isolating *N. meningitidis* from blood or CSF, by detecting meningococcal antigen in CSF by latex agglutination, or by evidence of *N. meningitidis* DNA by polymerase chain reaction.
- The signs and symptoms of meningococcal meningitis are similar to those of other causes of bacterial meningitis, such as *Haemophilus influenzae* and *Streptococcus pneumoniae*. Identification of the causative organism is important for selecting the correct antibiotics for treatment and prophylaxis.

Treatment

- Invasive meningococcal disease is potentially fatal and should always be viewed as a medical emergency.
- Antibiotic treatment must be started early in the course of the disease. Several antibiotic choices are available, including ceftriaxone, chloramphenicol, cefotaxime, and benzylpenicillin.

Preventive Measures for Travelers

Vaccine

- ACIP recommends vaccination against meningococcal disease to persons who travel to or reside in countries where *N. meningitidis* is hyperendemic or epidemic, particularly if contact with the local population will be prolonged.
- Vaccination is advised for persons traveling to the meningitis belt of Africa during the dry season (December through June).
- Advisories for travelers to other countries will be issued when epidemics of meningococcal disease caused by vaccine-preventable serogroups are recognized (see the CDC Travelers' Health website at www.cdc.gov/travel).
- Quadrivalent meningococcal polysaccharide–protein conjugate vaccine (MCV4) is licensed for use among persons 2–55 years of age.
- Quadrivalent meningococcal polysaccharide vaccine (MPVS4) is licensed for use among persons 2 years of age or older.
- Both vaccines protect against meningococcal disease caused by serogroups A, C, Y, and W-135. Approximately 7–10 days are required following vaccination for development of protective antibody levels.
- MCV4 is the preferred vaccine for persons 2–55 years of age; MPSV4 should be used for persons >55 years of age. There is no licensed vaccine for persons <2 years old, but MPSV4 is safe to give to children <2 years of age who require vaccination before traveling to Mecca for the Hajj pilgrimage.

Requirement for Travel

Proof of quadrivalent vaccination against meningococcal disease is required for persons traveling to Mecca during the annual Hajj and Umrah pilgrimage.

Antibiotic Chemoprophylaxis

- Antibiotic chemoprophylaxis among close contacts of a patient with invasive meningococcal disease is recommended for prevention of secondary cases in the United States and most industrialized countries.
- Antibiotic regimens for prophylaxis include rifampin, ciprofloxacin, and ceftriaxone. Ceftriaxone is recommended for pregnant women.

References

1. Raghunathan PL, Bernhardt SA, Rosenstein NE. Opportunities for control of meningococcal disease in the United States. Ann Rev Med. 2004;55:333–53.
2. Rosenstein NE, Perkins BA, Stephens DS, et al. Meningococcal disease. N Engl J Med. 2001;344(18):1378–88.
3. Greenwood B. Manson Lecture. Meningococcal meningitis in Africa. Trans R Soc Trop Med Hyg. 1999;93(4):341–53.
4. Stephens DS, Greenwood B, Brandtzaeg P. Epidemic meningitis, meningococcaemia, and *Neisseria meningitidis*. Lancet. 2007;369(9580):2196–210
5. American Academy of Pediatrics. Meningococcal infections. In: Pickering LK, ed. Red book: 2003 Report of the Committee on Infectious Disease. 26th ed. Elk Grove Village, IL: American Academy of Pediatrics; 2003. p. 430–6.
6. CDC. Prevention and control of meningococcal disease: recommendations of the Advisory Committee on Immunization Practices (ACIP). MMWR Recomm Rep. 2005;54(RR07):1–21.
7. Koch S, Steffen R. Meningococcal disease in travelers: vaccination recommendations. J Travel Med. 1994;1(1):4–7.
8. Wilder-Smith A. Meningococcal disease: risk for international travellers and vaccine strategies. Travel Med Infect Dis. 2008;6(4):182–6.

RABIES

Charles E. Rupprecht, David R. Shlim

Infectious Agent

Rabies is an acute, progressive, fatal encephalomyelitis caused by neurotropic viruses in the family *Rhabdoviridae*, genus *Lyssavirus*. Regardless of the viral variant found throughout the world, all lyssaviruses cause rabies.

Mode of Transmission

- The disease is almost always transmitted by an animal bite that inoculates virus into wounds.
- Very rarely, rabies virus has been transmitted by exposures other than bites that introduce the virus into open wounds or mucous membranes.
- All mammals are believed to be susceptible, but reservoirs are carnivores and bats.
- Although dogs are the main reservoir in developing countries, the epidemiology of the disease differs sufficiently enough from one region or country to another to warrant the medical evaluation of all mammal bites.
- Bat bites anywhere in the world are a cause of concern and an indication for prophylaxis.

Pathophysiology of Rabies

- Rabies virus is present in the saliva of the biting mammal.
- The virus that is inoculated into the wound does not enter the bloodstream. The virus must be taken up at a nerve synapse to travel to the brain, where it causes a

fatal encephalitis. The virus may enter a nerve rapidly, or it may remain at the bite site for an extended period before gaining access to the nervous system. The density of nerve endings in the region of the bite increases the risk of developing rabies encephalitis more rapidly. The hands and face, because of the density of nerve endings, are considered higher-risk exposures.

- Prevention of rabies encephalitis is dependent upon preventing the virus from entering a peripheral nerve. This can be accomplished by wound cleansing and disinfection, instillation of rabies virus neutralizing antibodies into the wound, and stimulating an active immune response with a series of rabies vaccine injections.

Occurrence

- Rabies is found on all continents except Antarctica.
- In certain areas of the world, canine rabies remains highly endemic, including but not limited to parts of Africa, Asia, and Central and South America. Table 2-16 lists countries that have reported no cases of rabies during the most recent period for which information is available (formerly referred to as "rabies-free" countries).
- Additional information about the global occurrence of rabies can be obtained from:
  ○ The World Health Organization (www.who.int/rabies/rabnet/en/)
  ○ The Pan American Health Organization (www.paho.org/english/ad/dpc/vp/rabia.htm)
  ○ The Rabies Bulletin—Europe (www.rbe.fli.bund.de)
  ○ The World Organization for Animal Health (www.oie.int/eng/en_index.htm)
  ○ Other sources are local health authorities of the country, the embassy, or the local consulate's office in the United States.

Lists are provided only as a guide, because up-to-date information may not be available, surveillance standards vary, and reporting status can change suddenly as a result of disease re-introduction or emergence.

Risk for Travelers

- The actual rate of possible rabies exposure in tourists has not been calculated with accuracy. However, studies have found a range of roughly 16 to 200 per 100,000 based on differing criteria.

Table 2-16. Countries and political units reporting no indigenous cases of rabies during 2005[1]

Region	Countries
Africa	Cape Verde, Libya, Mauritius, Réunion, São Tomé and Príncipe, and Seychelles
Americas	**North:** Bermuda, St. Pierre and Miquelon
	Caribbean: Antigua and Barbuda, Aruba, Bahamas, Barbados, Cayman Islands, Dominica, Guadeloupe, Jamaica, Martinique, Montserrat, Netherlands Antilles, Saint Kitts (Saint Christopher) and Nevis, Saint Lucia, Saint Martin, Saint Vincent and Grenadines, Turks and Caicos, and Virgin Islands (UK and US)
	South: Uruguay
Asia	Hong Kong, Japan, Kuwait, Lebanon, Malaysia (Sabah), Qatar, Singapore, United Arab Emirates
Europe	Austria, Belgium, Cyprus, Czech Republic,[2] Denmark,[2] Finland, France,[2] Gibraltar, Greece, Iceland, Ireland, Isle of Man, Italy, Luxemburg, Netherlands,[2] Norway, Portugal, Spain[2] (except Ceuta/Melilla), Sweden, Switzerland, and United Kingdom[2]
Oceania[3]	Australia,[2] Northern Mariana Islands, Cook Islands, Fiji, French Polynesia, Guam, Hawaii, Kiribati, Micronesia, New Caledonia, New Zealand, Palau, Papua New Guinea, Samoa, and Vanuatu

1 Bat rabies may exist in some areas that are reportedly free of rabies in other animals.
2 Bat lyssaviruses are known to exist in these areas that are reportedly free of rabies in other animals.
3 Most of Pacific Oceania is reportedly rabies-free.

- Travelers to rabies-endemic countries should be warned about the risk of acquiring rabies and educated in animal bite prevention strategies.
- Street dogs represent the most frequent risk for bite exposure to travelers, followed by monkeys, especially those that live near temples in parts of Asia. Travelers should be instructed not to approach these animals and to be aware of their surroundings so that they do not surprise a dog in a confined space. If a dog is charging at a person, stooping to pick up a rock (or pretending to pick up a rock) can often make the dog turn and run away.
- Monkeys are attracted to food and may jump on travelers' backs if there is food in their backpacks.
- Children are considered to be at high risk from rabies virus exposures because their small stature makes extensive bites more likely, they are attracted to animals, and there is the remote possibility that they may not report a possible exposure.
- Casual exposure to cave air is not a concern, but cavers should be warned not to handle bats. Noncavers can occasionally encounter a bat. Many bats have tiny teeth, and not all wounds may be appreciated compared with the lesions caused by carnivores. Any suspected or documented bite or scratch from a bat should be grounds for seeking postexposure rabies immunoprophylaxis.

Clinical Presentation

- After infection, the incubation period is highly variable, but lasts approximately 1–3 months.
- The disease progresses from a nonspecific prodromal phase to paresis or paralysis; spasms of swallowing muscles can be stimulated by the sight, sound, or perception of water (hydrophobia); and delirium and convulsions can develop, followed rapidly by coma and death.

Diagnosis

- Definitive diagnosis can be made by demonstrating the presence of the rabies virus in corneal impressions or nuchal biopsy, either through staining or polymerase chain reaction.
- A serologic response to rabies virus can also prove the diagnosis.

Treatment

No treatment is effective after the development of clinical signs, but the extremely rare case of recovery after extensive medical intervention offers hope that future experimental therapeutics may be developed.

Preventive Measures for Travelers

- Prevention of possible exposures to rabies virus is best accomplished by avoiding bites from mammals (mainly dogs, monkeys, bats, and cats in some countries).
- Although licks from animals to fresh wounds or mucus membranes of humans are a theoretical risk of acquiring rabies and postexposure prophylaxis should be considered, there are no examples of rabies in travelers who were exposed in this way.
- Travelers should be counseled to avoid approaching stray animals, to be aware of their surroundings so that they do not accidentally surprise a stray dog, to avoid contact with bats, and not to carry or eat food while walking among monkeys.
- In addition to avoiding bite exposures, two strategies are available to travelers for the prevention of rabies: vaccination and management of a possible rabies exposure (see sections below for more specific details).

- For certain international travelers, pre-exposure rabies vaccine may be recommended, based on the local incidence of rabies in the country to be visited, the availability of appropriate anti-rabies biologicals, and the intended activity and duration of stay of the traveler.
  - A decision to receive pre-exposure rabies immunization may also be based on the likelihood of repeat travel to at-risk destinations over time or taking up residence in a high-risk destination.
  - Pre-exposure vaccination may be recommended for veterinarians, animal handlers, field biologists, cavers, missionaries, and certain laboratory workers. Table 2-17 provides criteria for pre-exposure vaccination.
- Immediate and adequate medical care after an animal bite is critical to preventing rabies (see Management of a Possible Rabies Exposure below). Regardless of whether or not pre-exposure vaccine is administered, travelers going to areas with a high risk for rabies should be especially encouraged to purchase medical evacuation insurance (see the Travel Insurance and Evacuation Insurance section later in this chapter).

Vaccine

Pre-Exposure Vaccination

- In the United States, pre-exposure vaccination consists of a series of three injections with human diploid cell rabies vaccine (HDCV) or purified chick embryo cell (PCEC) vaccine.
- The schedule for this series in given in Table 2-18.
- In the event of a possible rabies exposure in someone who has received pre-exposure rabies immunization, rabies immune globulin (RIG) is not given, and two boosters of an acceptable rabies vaccine are given on days 0 and 3. The booster doses need to be modern cell culture vaccines, but they do not need to be the same brand as the vaccine given in the pre-exposure immunization series.
- Pre-exposure immunization does not eliminate the need for additional medical attention after a rabies exposure, but it greatly simplifies postexposure prophylaxis.
- Pre-exposure vaccination may also provide some degree of protection when there is an unapparent or unrecognized exposure to rabies virus and when postexposure prophylaxis might be delayed.
- Travelers should receive all three pre-exposure immunizations before travel. If three doses of rabies vaccine cannot be completed prior to travel, the traveler should not start the series, as it would be problematic to plan postexposure prophylaxis after a partial immunization series.

Beginning in 2007 and anticipated to continue through 2009, the United States has experienced a limitation in supply of rabies vaccine. As a result, during this time, pre-exposure rabies vaccination has not been available to international travelers, except under special circumstances. The existing supplies of rabies vaccine are being reserved for postexposure prophylaxis.

Postexposure Vaccination

- If pre-exposure rabies immunization is not given, the traveler will need to obtain full postexposure rabies prophylaxis in the event of a possible rabies virus exposure. This consists of injections of RIG (20 IU/kg) and a series of five injections of rabies vaccine over a 1-month period.
- Because RIG or rabies vaccine may not be available in the destination country, travelers should have a strategy in place before travel as to how to respond to a possible exposure. This strategy may require the traveler to fly to a different country to obtain the appropriate prophylaxis.
- Different postexposure vaccine schedules, alternative routes of administration and other rabies vaccines besides HDCV and PCEC may be found abroad. Although not approved for sale in the United States, purified vero cell rabies vaccine and purified chick embryo cell vaccine (manufactured abroad) are acceptable alternatives if available in a destination country.

Table 2-17. Criteria for pre-exposure immunization for rabies

Risk Category	Nature of Risk	Typical Populations	Pre-exposure Regimen
Continuous	Virus present continuously, often in high concentrations Specific exposures likely to go unrecognized Bite, nonbite, or aerosol exposure	Rabies research laboratory workers,[1] rabies biologics production workers	Primary course: serologic testing every 6 months; booster vaccination if antibody titer is below acceptable level[2]
Frequent	Exposure usually episodic with source recognized, but exposure might also be unrecognized Bite, nonbite, or aerosol exposure possible	Rabies diagnostic laboratory workers,[1] cavers, veterinarians and staff, and animal control and wildlife workers in rabies-epizootic areas	Primary course: serologic testing every 2 years; booster vaccination if antibody titer is below acceptable level[2]
Infrequent (greater than general population)	Exposure nearly always episodic with source recognized Bite or nonbite exposure	Veterinarians, animal control and wildlife workers in areas with low rabies rates; veterinary students; and travelers visiting areas where rabies is enzootic and immediate access to appropriate medical care, including biologics, is limited	Primary course: no serologic testing or booster vaccination
Rare (general population)	Exposure always episodic, with source recognized	U.S. population at large, including individuals in rabies-epizootic areas	No pre-exposure immunization necessary

1 Judgment of relative risk and extra monitoring of vaccination status of laboratory workers is the responsibility of the laboratory supervisor (see U.S. Department of Health and Human Services' Biosafety in Microbiological and Biomedical Laboratories, 1999).
2 Pre-exposure booster immunization consists of one dose of human diploid cell (rabies) vaccine (HDCV) or purified chick embryo cell (PCEC) vaccine, 1.0-mL dose, intramuscular (IM) (deltoid area). Minimum acceptable antibody level is complete virus neutralization at a 1:5 serum dilution by the rapid fluorescent focus inhibition test. A booster dose should be administered if titer falls below this level.

Table 2-18. Pre-exposure immunization for rabies[1]

Vaccine	Dose (MI)	No. of Doses	Schedule (Days)	Route
HDCV	1.0	3	0, 7, and 21 or 28	Intramuscular
PCEC	1.0	3	0, 7, and 21 or 28	Intramuscular

1 HDCV, human diploid cell vaccine; PCEC, purified chick embryo cell. Patients who are immunosuppressed by disease or medications should postpone pre-exposure vaccinations and consider avoiding activities for which rabies pre-exposure prophylaxis is indicated. When this course is not possible, immunosuppressed persons who are at risk for rabies should have their antibody titers checked after vaccination.

- Historically, rabies vaccine was once manufactured from viruses grown in animal brains, and some of these vaccines are still in use in developing countries. The brain-derived vaccines can be identified if the traveler is offered a large injection (5 mL) daily for 14–21 days. The traveler should not accept these vaccines, but rather travel to where acceptable vaccines and immune globulin are available.

Management of a Possible Rabies Exposure

- Travelers should be advised that any animal bite or scratch should receive prompt local first aid by thorough cleansing of the wound with copious amounts of soap and water and povidone iodine, if available. This local care will substantially reduce the risk for rabies.

- Wounds that might require suturing should have the suturing delayed for a few days. If suturing is necessary for control of bleeding or for functional or cosmetic reasons, RIG should be administered into the wound before closing the wound. The use of local anesthetic is not contraindicated in wound management.
- Human rabies immune globulin (HRIG) is manufactured by plasmaphoresis of hyperimmunized volunteers. The manufactured quantity of HRIG falls short of world-wide requirements, and the substance is not available in many developing countries. Equine rabies immune globulin (ERIG) or purified fractions of ERIG have been used effectively in some developing countries where HRIG might not be available. If necessary, such heterologous products are preferable to no RIG administration in human rabies postexposure prophylaxis.
- The incidence of adverse reactions after the use of these products has been low (0.8%–6.0%), and most of those reactions were minor. However, such products are neither evaluated by U.S. standards nor regulated by the FDA, and their use cannot be unequivocally recommended at this time. In addition, unpurified antirabies serum of equine origin might still be used in some countries where neither HRIG nor ERIG is available. The use of this antirabies serum is associated with higher rates of serious adverse reactions, including anaphylaxis.
- After wound cleansing, as much of the calculated amount of RIG (see Table 2-19) as is anatomically feasible is infiltrated around the wound. The dose injected around the wound may be as small as 0.5 mL if the wound is small or on a finger. If the wounds are extensive, the calculated dose of RIG must not be exceeded. If the calculated dose is inadequate to inject all the wounds, the RIG should be diluted with normal saline to extend the number of wounds that can be injected. This is a particular issue in children, whose body weight may be small in relation to the size and number of wounds.
- The remainder of the RIG dose, if any, should be injected intramuscularly. Care should be taken to guarantee that this remaining amount of RIG is deposited in a muscle and not injected subcutaneously, which may decrease its effectiveness. The remaining RIG can be given in the deltoid muscle, on the opposite side of the initial vaccine dose. The anterior thigh is also an alternative site.
- RIG should not be given more than 7 days after the start of the postexposure vaccine series. This 7-day period does not relate to the time of the bite exposure itself.
- Postexposure prophylaxis, including RIG, should be initiated after a possible bite exposure even if there has been a considerable delay between the exposure and the traveler presenting for evaluation.
- Travelers who have completed a three-dose pre-exposure rabies immunization series or have received the full postexposure prophylaxis are considered pre-immunized and do not require routine boosters, except after a possible rabies exposure.
- Periodic serum testing for rabies antibody is not necessary in routine international travelers.

Table 2-19. Postexposure immunization for rabies[1]

Immunization Status	Vaccine/Product	Dose	No. of Doses	Schedule (Days)	Route
Not previously immunized	RIG plus	20 IU/kg body weight	1	0	Infiltrated at bite site (if possible possible); remainder intramuscular
	HDCV or PCEC	1.0 mL	5	0, 3, 7, 14, 28	Intramuscular
Previously immunized[2,3]	HDCV or PCEC	1.0 mL	2	0, 3	Intramuscular

RIG, rabies immune globulin; HDCV, human diploid cell (rabies) vaccine; PCEC, purified chick embryo cell.

1 All postexposure prophylaxis should begin with immediate, thorough cleansing of all wounds with soap and water.
2 Pre-exposure immunization with HDCV or PCEC, prior postexposure prophylaxis with HDCV or PCEC, or persons previously immunized with any other type of rabies vaccine and a documented history of positive antibody response to the prior vaccination.
3 RIG should not be administered.

Vaccine Safety and Adverse Reactions

- Travelers should be advised that they may experience local reactions after vaccination, such as pain, erythema, swelling, or itching at the injection site, or mild systemic reactions, such as headache, nausea, abdominal pain, muscle aches, and dizziness.
- Approximately 6% of persons receiving booster vaccinations with HDCV may experience an immune complex-like reaction characterized by urticaria, pruritus, and malaise. The likelihood of these reactions is less with PCECV.
- Once initiated, rabies postexposure prophylaxis should not be interrupted or discontinued because of local or mild systemic reactions to rabies vaccine.

Precautions and Contraindications

- Pregnancy is not a contraindication to postexposure prophylaxis.
- In infants and children, the dose of HDCV or PCEC for pre-exposure or postexposure prophylaxis is the same as that recommended for adults. The dose of RIG for postexposure prophylaxis is based on body weight (Table 2-19).

References

1. Warrell MJ, Warrell DA. Rabies and other lyssavirus diseases. Lancet. 2004;363(9413):959–69.
2. Strauss R, Granz A, Wassermann-Neuhold M, et al. A human case of travel-related rabies in Austria, September 2004. Euro Surveill. 2005;10(11):225–6.
3. Smith A, Petrovic M, Solomon T, et al. Death from rabies in a UK traveller returning from India. Euro Surveill. 2005;10(30):2761.
4. Jackson AC, Warrell MJ, Rupprecht CE, et al. Management of rabies in humans. Clin Infect Dis. 2003;36(1):60–3.
5. CDC. Human Rabies Prevention—United States, 2008: Recommendations of the Advisory Committee on Immunization Practices. MMWR Recomm Rep. 2008;57(RR-03):1–28.
6. World Health Organization Expert Consultation on Rabies. World Health Organ Tech Rep Ser. 2005;931:1–88.
7. Rupprecht CE, Gibbons RV. Clinical practice. Prophylaxis against rabies. N Engl J Med. 2004;351(26):2626–35.

Routine Vaccine-Preventable Diseases

DIPHTHERIA

Tejpratap S. P. Tiwari

Infectious Agent

- Diphtheria is caused by toxigenic strains of *Corynebacterium diphtheriae* biotype mitis, gravis, intermedius, or belfanti.
- The bacteria produce an exotoxin which, if absorbed in the bloodstream, may damage organs such as the heart, kidneys, and nerves.

Mode of Transmission

- Humans are the only known reservoir of *C. diphtheriae*.

- Person-to-person transmission occurs through oral or respiratory droplets, close physical contact, and rarely by fomites.
- Cutaneous diphtheria is common in tropical countries, and contact with discharge from skin lesions may play an important role in transmission of infection in these environments.

Occurrence

- Diphtheria is found worldwide. Countries with endemic diphtheria are shown in Table 2-20.
- Diphtheria causes significant morbidity and mortality in developing countries where vaccination coverage is low.
- During the 1990s, large epidemics occurred in the newly independent states of the former Soviet Union. More recently in the Americas, diphtheria outbreaks occurred in Paraguay, the Dominican Republic, and Haiti.
- Diphtheria is uncommon in industrialized countries because of long-standing routine use of DTP (diphtheria and tetanus toxoids and pertussis vaccine). Diphtheria is uncommon in the United States; and the last case occurred in an elderly traveler returning from Haiti in 2003.

Risk for Travelers

- Symptomatic infection is extremely rare in adequately immunized persons, although active immunization with diphtheria toxoid does not prevent colonization or transient carriage of *C. diphtheriae*.
- Exposure and higher risk of acquiring disease and potentially life-threatening complications are possible in inadequately immunized or unimmunized travelers to countries with endemic diphtheria.

Clinical Presentation

- The incubation period is 2–5 days (range 1–10 days).
- Nasal diphtheria can be asymptomatic or mild, with a blood-tinged discharge.
- Affected anatomic sites include the mucous membrane of the upper respiratory tract (nose, pharynx, tonsils, larynx, and trachea [respiratory diphtheria]), skin (cutaneous diphtheria), or rarely, mucous membranes at other sites (eye, ear, vulva).
- Respiratory diphtheria has a gradual onset and is characterized by a mild fever (rarely >101° F or >38.3° C), sore throat, difficulty in swallowing, malaise, loss of appetite, and if the larynx is involved, hoarseness may occur.
- The hallmark of respiratory diphtheria is the presence of a membrane that appears within 2–3 days of illness over the mucous membrane of the tonsils, pharynx, larynx, or nares, and which can extend into the trachea. The membrane is firm, fleshy, grey, and adherent, and bleeds following attempts to remove or dislodge it.

Table 2-20. Countries with endemic diphtheria

Regions	Countries
Africa	Algeria, Angola, Egypt, Niger, Nigeria, Sudan, and sub-Saharan countries
Americas	Bolivia, Brazil, Colombia, Dominican Republic, Ecuador, Haiti, and Paraguay
Asia/South Pacific	Afghanistan, Bangladesh, Bhutan, Burma (Myanmar), Cambodia, China, India, Indonesia, Laos, Malaysia, Mongolia, Nepal, Pakistan, Papua New Guinea, Philippines, Thailand, and Vietnam
Middle East	Iran, Iraq, Saudi Arabia, Syria, Turkey, and Yemen
Europe	Albania, Russia, and countries of the former Soviet Union

- Local complications such as life-threatening or fatal airway obstruction can result from extension of the membrane or dislodgement of a piece of the membrane into the larynx or trachea.
- In severe respiratory diphtheria, cervical lymphadenopathy and soft-tissue swelling in the neck give rise to a "bull-neck" appearance.
- The case–fatality rate of respiratory diphtheria is 5%–10%.
- Systemic complications, including myocarditis, and polyneuropathies, can result from absorption of diphtheria toxin from the infection site. However, cutaneous and nasal diphtheria are localized and rarely associated with systemic toxicity.

Diagnosis

- A presumptive diagnosis is usually based on clinical features.
- A confirmed diagnosis is made by isolation of *C. diphtheriae* from culture of nasal or throat swabs, or membrane tissue.
- Toxin production is confirmed by performing a modified Elek test.
- Polymerase chain reaction assays can also be performed on isolates, swabs, or membrane specimens to rapidly confirm the presence of tox gene responsible for production of diphtheria toxin, but the test is available only in research or reference laboratories.

Treatment

- Patients with respiratory diphtheria require hospitalization to monitor response to treatment and manage complications.
- Equine diphtheria antitoxin (DAT) is the mainstay of treatment and is administered after sensitivity testing, without waiting for laboratory confirmation. In the United States, DAT is available to physicians under an FDA-approved Investigational New Drug protocol by contacting CDC at 770-488-7100.
- An appropriate antibiotic (erythromycin or penicillin) to eliminate the causative organisms, stop exotoxin production, and reduce communicability.
- Supportive care (airway, cardiac monitoring) is required.
- Antimicrobial prophylaxis (erythromycin or penicillin) is recommended for close contacts of patients.

Preventive Measures for Travelers

Vaccine

- For protection against diphtheria, all travelers should be up-to-date with diphtheria toxoid vaccine before departure. Diphtheria toxoid is not manufactured as a monovalent vaccine but is available in pediatric (D) and adult formulations (d) that are combined with other vaccines such as tetanus toxoid (DT, Td), or tetanus toxoid and acellular or whole-cell pertussis antigens (DTaP, DTwP, Tdap), or as a DTwP/DTaP combination with other antigens (e.g., hepatitis B, inactivated poliovirus vaccines, or Hib vaccine).
- In the United States, infants and children <7 years of age are vaccinated with diphtheria toxoid in combination with tetanus toxoid and acellular pertussis vaccine (DTaP) according to a routine childhood immunization schedule as recommended by the ACIP (see the Vaccine Recommendations for Infants and Children section in Chapter 7).
- Immunization for infants and children <7 years of age consists of five doses of DTaP vaccine. The first three doses are usually given at ages 2, 4, and 6 months, followed by booster doses at ages 12–18 months and 4–6 years (see Table 7-2).

- Adolescents 11–18 years of age should receive a dose of Tdap instead of Td for booster immunization against tetanus, diphtheria, and pertussis if they have completed the recommended childhood DTwP/DTaP vaccination series (see Table 7-3).
- Adults 19–64 years of age should receive a single dose of age-appropriate Tdap to replace a single dose of Td for active booster immunization against tetanus, diphtheria and pertussis. Thereafter, routine booster doses with Td should be given every 10 years to maintain seroprotection against diphtheria as well as tetanus. This booster is particularly important for travelers who will live or work with local populations in countries where diphtheria is endemic.
- Adults >65 years of age should receive Td; Tdap is not licensed for this age group.
- Persons >7 years of age and with uncertain vaccination history or who have never been vaccinated against tetanus, diphtheria, or pertussis should receive three doses of an age-appropriate tetanus and diphtheria toxoid-containing vaccine. If a person is 10–65 years old, a single dose of Tdap may be substituted for one Td dose for added protection against pertussis.

References

1. American Academy of Pediatrics. Diphtheria. In: Pickering LK, Baker CJ, Long SS, McMillan JA, editors. Red book: 2006 Report of the Committee on Infectious Diseases. 27th ed. Elk Grove Village, IL: American Academy of Pediatrics; 2006:p.277–81.
2. World Health Organization. WHO vaccine-preventable diseases monitoring system: 2005 global summary. Geneva, Switzerland: World Health Organization; 2005 Dec. 333 p. Report No.: WHO/IVB/2005.
3. Galazka A. The changing epidemiology of diphtheria in the vaccine era. J Infect Dis. 2000 Feb;181 Suppl 1:S2–9.
4. CDC. Fatal respiratory diphtheria in a U.S. traveler to Haiti—Pennsylvania, 2003. MMWR Morbid Mortal Wkly Rep. 2004;52(53):1285–6.
5. Wharton M, Vitek CR. Diphtheria toxoid. In: Plotkin SA, Orenstein WA, editors. Vaccines. 4th ed. Philadelphia: W.B. Saunders; 2004:211–28.
6. Bisgard KM, Hardy IRB, Popovic T, et al. Respiratory diphtheria in the United States, 1980 through 1995. Am J Public Health. 1998;88(5):787–91.
7. CDC. Diphtheria acquired by U.S. citizens in the Russian Federation and Ukraine—1994. MMWR Morbid Mortal Wkly Rep. 1995;44(12):237, 243–4.
8. Farizo KM, Strebel PM, Chen RT, et al. Fatal respiratory disease due to *Corynebacterium diphtheriae*: case report and review of guidelines for management, investigation, and control. Clin Infect Dis. 1993;16(1):59–68.
9. CDC. Availability of diphtheria antitoxin through an Investigational New Drug protocol. MMWR Morb Mortal Wkly Rep. 2004;53(19);413.
10. Kretsinger K, Broder KR, Cortese MM, et al. Preventing tetanus, diphtheria, and pertussis among adults: use of tetanus toxoid, reduced diphtheria toxoid and acellular pertussis vaccine. Recommendations of the Advisory Committee on Immunization Practices (ACIP) and recommendation of ACIP, supported by the Healthcare Infection Control Practices Advisory Committee (HICPAC) for use of Tdap among health-care personnel. MMWR Recomm. Rep. 2006;55(RR-17):1–37.

HUMAN PAPILLOMAVIRUS (HPV)

Eileen F. Dunne

Infectious Agent

- Human papillomavirus (HPV) is in the family Papillomaviridae, a family of DNA viruses that has a double-stranded, closed, circular genome of ~8 kb and a nonenveloped icosahedral capsid.
- Infection with human papillomavirus is specific to humans.

Mode of Transmission

- There are more than 100 HPV types. Some types cause infection on the skin and others cause infection on the mucosa. More than 40 mucosal HPV types are commonly found on the genitals and are transmitted primarily by sexual contact, most commonly sexual intercourse.
- Sometimes transmission of genital HPV types occurs by other routes (e.g., mother-to-child transmission).

Occurrence

- HPV is common worldwide.
- Studies in multiple countries demonstrate prevalence of HPV from 3% to 70%.

Risk for Travelers

There are no inherent risks for travelers. HPV is ubiquitous and common worldwide. Risk depends on the behavior of the traveler.

Clinical Presentation

- HPV infection is usually subclinical and asymptomatic.
- HPV infection with cutaneous types can cause the common skin wart.
- HPV infection with mucosal types is presumed when anogenital warts or cervical cell changes are detected in screening.
- HPV rarely causes recurrent respiratory papillomatosis (RRP); anogenital cancers such as vaginal, vulvar, anal, penile cancers; and some oral cancers.

Diagnosis

- Infection is most commonly asymptomatic and transient.
- When clinical disease occurs, diagnosis is usually made by detection of the lesion by visual inspection, and in women by a Papanicolaou test (Pap test), HPV test (done in similar fashion to a Pap test), or by colposcopy. Definitive diagnosis is made by biopsy.
- Laboratory diagnosis of HPV in the clinical setting can be made by using the Digene hybrid capture 2 test (hc2); this test is recommended only in the setting of cervical cancer screening. Other DNA and serologic tests are available in research settings.

Treatment

There is no treatment for HPV, but there are treatments for HPV-associated conditions such as genital warts and cervical cell changes.

Preventive Measures for Travelers

- There are no recommendations for preventive measures for travelers beyond abstinence or engaging in safe sexual behaviors.
- The quadrivalent HPV vaccine prevents four HPV types (types 6, 11, 16, 18) commonly associated with genital warts and cervical cancers. Cervical cancer screening with the Pap test should be continued because the vaccine does not prevent all types associated with cancers.

- ACIP recommendations for HPV vaccine are that 11- and 12-year-old girls should be routinely vaccinated, and the vaccine series can be started as young as 9 years of age. Girls and young women 13–26 years of age should be vaccinated if they have not received the vaccine or have not completed the series.
- Vaccination consists of three intramuscular doses, on day 0, at 2 months, and 6 months; see product insert for some variability in administration timing. The vaccine is generally well tolerated, although pain at the injection site is common.

References

1. Franceschi S, Herrero R, Clifford GM, et al. Variations in the age-specific curves of human papillomavirus prevalence in women worldwide. Int J Cancer. 2006;119(11):2677–84.

2. Markowitz LE, Dunne EF, Saraiya MD, et al. Quadrivalent human papillomavirus vaccine: Recommendations of the Advisory Committee for Immunization Practices (ACIP). MMWR Morbid Mortal Wkly Rep. 2007;56(RR-2):1–24.

INFLUENZA (SEASONAL, AVIAN, AND PANDEMIC)

Margaret McCarron, David K. Shay

Infectious Agent

- Influenza is caused by infection with influenza viruses.
- Human influenza viruses can be divided into three types: A, B, and C. Only types A and B cause widespread illness in humans.
- Influenza A viruses are further classified into subtypes on the basis of two surface proteins: hemagglutinin (H) and neuraminidase (N). There are 16 different hemagglutinin subtypes and 9 different neuraminidase subtypes.

Mode of Transmission

- Person-to-person transmission results from respiratory droplets of coughs and sneezes.
  - Most healthy adults can infect others beginning 1 day before symptoms develop and up to 5 days after becoming sick.
  - Children can pass the virus for longer than 7 days.
  - Fomite transmission is also possible.

Occurrence

Seasonal Influenza

- Infection with seasonal influenza viruses is common.
- In temperate climates in the Northern Hemisphere, annual seasonal epidemics of influenza generally occur during the winter months, while in the temperate regions of the Southern Hemisphere most activity occurs from April through September.
- In tropical and subtropical areas, influenza can occur throughout the year.
- CDC has estimated that U.S. epidemics during the 1990s were associated with an annual average of 36,000 influenza-related deaths.
- Influenza virus infections cause disease in all age groups. Rates of infection are highest among infants and children, but rates of serious morbidity and mortality are highest among persons ≥65 years of age and persons of any age who have medical conditions (e.g., chronic cardiopulmonary disease) that place them at

increased risk for complications from influenza. Children <2 years of age have rates of influenza-related hospitalization that are as high as those in the elderly.

Avian Influenza

- Avian influenza refers to influenza A viruses usually found in birds. Influenza A viruses infect a broad range of avian species and several mammalian species, including humans, swine, and horses.
    - Most cases of avian influenza infection in humans have resulted from contact with infected poultry (e.g., domesticated chickens, ducks, and turkeys) or surfaces contaminated with secretions or excretions from infected birds.
    - The spread of avian influenza viruses from one ill person to another has been reported very rarely and has thus far been limited, inefficient, and unsustained.
- H5N1 is an influenza A virus, which is a type characterized by the ability to constantly undergo change. H5N1 virus has caused serious disease among wild birds and poultry on multiple continents. Human cases of H5N1 are very rare but have occurred in countries in Asia, Africa, Eastern Europe, and the Middle East since 2003. As of June 2008, only 385 human cases of H5N1 infection have been reported worldwide. These cases, however, are a concern because the mortality rate is high. There is a concern that H5N1 may gain the ability to spread easily between people. Vigilant monitoring for human infection and person-to-person transmission has become an important component of pandemic preparedness. For a current list of countries reporting outbreaks of H5N1 among birds, see the World Organization for Animal Health (OIE) website at www.oie.int/.
- The global influenza research community conducts surveillance for novel influenza viruses in travelers. In a 2007 review of returned U.S. travelers suspected of having H5N1 infection, no evidence of infection with novel viruses was reported. Surveillance continues for human infection with H5N1 in travelers.
- For current, continuously updated information, see CDC's Avian Influenza website (www.cdc.gov/flu/avian/index.htm).

Pandemic Influenza

- The emergence of a novel human influenza A virus could lead to a global pandemic, during which rates of morbidity and mortality from influenza-related complications could increase dramatically. The public health threat of a pandemic arising from novel influenza A viruses, including influenza A (H5N1), becomes imminent only if the virus gains the ability to spread efficiently from one human to another.
- Such transmission has not yet been observed with the currently circulating A (H5N1) viruses. Although a few cases of limited person-to-person spread of H5N1 viruses have been reported as of June 2008, no instances of transmission continuing beyond one person are thought to have occurred.
- Because the situation has and may continue to evolve, for current information see the official U.S. government website for pandemic influenza (www.pandemicflu.gov/).

Risk for Travelers

Seasonal Influenza

- The risk for exposure to seasonal influenza during international travel depends on the time of year and destination. In the tropics, influenza can occur throughout the year, while in the temperate regions of the Southern Hemisphere most activity occurs from April through September.
- In temperate climates, travelers can also be exposed to influenza during the summer, especially when traveling as part of large tourist groups with travelers from areas of the world where influenza viruses are circulating.

Avian Influenza

- In those countries where H5N1 has occurred most people become infected through direct contact with birds (e.g., domesticated chickens, ducks, and turkeys) that were carrying the H5N1 virus or from surfaces contaminated with secretions or excretions from these birds. Direct contact could happen during activities such as—
  - o Visiting poultry farms
  - o Visiting live bird or poultry markets
  - o Preparing or consuming uncooked or undercooked bird products (such as meat, eggs, or blood).
- Because the situation has and may continue to evolve, travelers can stay abreast of new developments by checking the following websites that are updated regularly:
  - o U.S. government website for pandemic influenza (www.pandemicflu.gov/)
  - o CDC's Travelers' Health website (wwwn.cdc.gov/travel/contentAvianFluInformation.aspx)
  - o CDC's Avian Influenza website (www.cdc.gov/flu/avian/)
  - o WHO website (www.who.int/csr/disease/avian_influenza/en/index.html).

Clinical Presentation

- Onset of symptoms typically occurs 1–4 days after infection.
- Uncomplicated influenza illness is characterized by the abrupt onset of constitutional and respiratory signs and symptoms (e.g., fever, myalgia, headache, malaise, nonproductive cough, sore throat, and rhinitis). Among children, otitis media, nausea, and vomiting are also commonly reported with influenza illness.
- Influenza illness typically resolves within 1 week for most persons, although cough and malaise can persist for >2 weeks. However, influenza virus infections can cause primary influenza viral pneumonia; exacerbate underlying medical conditions (e.g., pulmonary or cardiac disease); lead to secondary bacterial pneumonia, sinusitis, or otitis; or contribute to co-infections with other viral or bacterial pathogens. Influenza-related deaths can result from primary illnesses, secondary bacterial pneumonia, or exacerbations of chronic cardiac or pulmonary conditions.
- Young children with influenza virus infection may have initial symptoms mimicking bacterial sepsis with high fevers, and febrile seizures have been reported in 6%–20% of children hospitalized with influenza virus infection. Population-based studies among hospitalized children with laboratory-confirmed influenza have demonstrated that, although the majority of hospitalizations are brief (2 days or less), 4%–11% of children hospitalized with laboratory-confirmed influenza required treatment in the intensive-care unit and 3% required mechanical ventilation. Among 1,308 hospitalized children in one study, 80% were <5 years of age and 27% were <6 months of age. Influenza virus infection also has been uncommonly associated with encephalopathy, transverse myelitis, myositis, myocarditis, pericarditis, and Reye syndrome.

Diagnosis

- Respiratory illnesses caused by influenza virus infection are difficult to distinguish from illnesses caused by other respiratory pathogens on the basis of signs and symptoms alone. Sensitivity and predictive value of clinical definitions can vary, depending on the degree of circulation of other respiratory pathogens and the level of influenza activity. Among studies conducted with children and adults, the positive predictive value of clinical signs and symptoms for laboratory-confirmed influenza virus infection has ranged from 30% to 88%.

- Laboratory testing can aid in diagnosis. Diagnostic tests available for influenza include viral culture, serology, rapid antigen testing, polymerase chain reaction, and immunofluorescence assays.
- Respiratory specimens obtained via nasopharyngeal swabs typically yield better detection of influenza than specimens obtained via oropharyngeal swabs.
- Commercial rapid diagnostic tests are available that can detect influenza viruses within 30 minutes. Some tests are approved for use in any outpatient setting, whereas others must be used in a moderately complex clinical laboratory. These rapid tests differ in the types of influenza viruses they can detect and whether they can distinguish between influenza types. Some tests can detect only influenza A viruses, some detect both influenza A and B viruses, but cannot distinguish between the two types, and some detect both influenza A and B and can distinguish between the two.
- None of the commercially available rapid tests provides any information about influenza A subtypes. The types of specimens acceptable for use (i.e., throat, nasopharyngeal, or nasal aspirates, swabs, or washes) also vary by test. The specificity and, in particular, the sensitivity of rapid tests are lower than for viral culture and vary by test. Because of the lower sensitivity of the rapid tests, physicians should consider confirming negative tests with viral culture or other means because of the possibility of false-negative rapid test results.

Treatment

- Influenza-specific antiviral drugs for chemoprophylaxis of influenza are important adjuncts to the influenza vaccine.
- The four currently licensed U.S. antiviral agents are amantadine, rimantadine, zanamivir, and oseltamivir. Amantadine and rimantadine have a mechanism of action effective only against influenza A viruses, while the neuraminidase inhibitors oseltamivir and zanamivir are effective against both influenza A and B viruses.
- Antiviral drug testing results conducted at CDC during the 2005–2006 influenza season, indicated 79% resistance among influenza A H3N2 viruses and 10% among H1N1. CDC recommends that neither amantadine nor rimantadine be used for the treatment or chemoprophylaxis of influenza A in the United States until susceptibility to these antiviral medications has been re-established among circulating influenza A viruses.
- Oseltamivir or zanamivir can be prescribed if antiviral treatment of influenza is indicated. Oseltamivir is approved for treatment of persons aged ≥1 year, and zanamivir is approved for treatment of persons ≥7 years of age. Oseltamivir and zanamivir can be used for chemoprophylaxis of influenza; oseltamivir is licensed for use in persons ≥1 year of age, and zanamivir is licensed for use in persons ≥5 years of age. These two drugs differ in dosing, approved age groups for use, side effects, and cost. The package inserts should be consulted for more information.

Antiviral Resistance

- In the winter of 2007–2008, oseltamivir-resistant influenza A (H1N1) viruses were found to be circulating in several countries, including the United States, but the highest rates of resistance were found in Northern Europe. Oseltamivir resistance appears to be geographically variable, both within Europe and globally. In the United States, approximately 12% of H1N1 viruses from the 2007–2008 season were resistant to oseltamivir, resistance was highest in Europe at 26%, and overall global resistance was approximately 16%. The oseltamivir-resistant H1N1 viruses remained sensitive to amantadine and rimantadine. This strain of oseltamivir-resistant influenza A (H1N1) may continue to circulate in future seasons or may spread geographically. Oseltamivir and zanamivir remain the preferred antiviral drugs to be used in the treatment of influenza virus infection, given their relatively low levels of resistance compared with the high resistance found to amantadine and rimantadine among currently circulating influenza A viruses.

- Some H5N1 viruses currently infecting birds and humans are resistant to amantadine and rimantadine. Most of the H5N1 viruses tested have been susceptible to the antiviral medications oseltamivir and zanamivir, but resistance has been reported. The effectiveness of antivirals for treating H5N1 virus infections is unknown. For more information about influenza antiviral drugs, see www.cdc.gov/flu/avian/gen-info/avian-flu-humans.htm#antiviral.

- For more detailed information on influenza vaccines, treatment, and general prevention and control, please refer to "Prevention and Control of Influenza: Recommendations of the Advisory Committee on Immunization Practices (ACIP)" (the most recent version is available at: www.cdc.gov/vaccines/pubs/ACIP-list.htm).

Preventive Measures for Travelers

- Handwashing and cough hygiene can play important roles in limiting person-to-person transmission of influenza. Where handwashing is not available, use of hand sanitizing gels containing greater than 60% alcohol can be used.

- Annual vaccination of persons at high risk for complications and vaccination of health-care workers and close contacts of high risk persons before the influenza season are the most effective measure for preventing seasonal influenza and associated complications.

- Vaccination of travelers is recommended when the vaccine is available and if there are no contraindications.

Vaccine

- Two types of influenza vaccines are currently available for use in the United States: trivalent inactivated vaccine (TIV), administered by intramuscular injection; and live, attenuated influenza vaccine (LAIV), administered by nasal spray. LAIV is approved currently for use only in healthy persons 2–49 years of age who are not pregnant.

- In the United States, annual influenza vaccination is recommended by CDC and ACIP for certain groups of people, primarily those who are at high risk of having serious flu complications or those who live with or care for those at high risk for serious complications. Annual recommendations are published by CDC and ACIP, including information about the season's vaccine composition, dosage and administration, and recommendations for specific populations. The current version of these routine recommendations is available at www.cdc.gov/vaccines/pubs/ACIP-list.htm.

- The influenza vaccine must be administered annually to optimize protection because vaccine-derived immunity declines over time and because the vaccine strains must be updated regularly to reflect ongoing antigenic changes among circulating influenza viruses.

- Dosages differ according to age group and type of vaccine used. For inactivated vaccines, two doses administered at least 1 month apart are required for previously unvaccinated infants and children through 8 years of age. In adults, studies have indicated little or no improvement in antibody response when a second dose of inactivated vaccine is administered during the same season; therefore, a booster is not recommended. Inactivated vaccine should be administered in infants and young children in the anterolateral aspect of the thigh; all other recipients should be vaccinated in the deltoid muscle.

- The age groups for which influenza and pneumococcal vaccination are recommended overlap considerably. For travelers at high risk who have not previously been vaccinated with pneumococcal vaccine, health-care providers should strongly consider administering pneumococcal and influenza vaccines concurrently. Both vaccines can be administered at the same time at different sites without increasing side effects. Infants and children can receive influenza vaccine at the same time they receive other routine vaccinations.

- Both influenza vaccines contain three strains of influenza viruses. Viruses in inactivated vaccines are killed, while those in LAIV are live. These live viruses are attenuated and do not cause influenza illnesses. The viruses used in both vaccines are representative of viruses likely to circulate in the upcoming season, and usually one or more vaccine strains are updated annually. Because the vaccine is grown in hen eggs, the vaccine may contain small amounts of egg protein. The package insert should be consulted regarding the use of other compounds to inactivate the viruses or to limit bacterial contamination.

Avian Influenza

- H5N1 infections in humans, though rare, can cause serious disease and death.
- CDC advises travelers to countries with known outbreaks of H5N1 to avoid—
  - Poultry farms
  - All poultry, whether or not symptomatic, and especially contact with sick or dead poultry
  - Contact with surfaces that may have been contaminated by poultry feces or secretions
  - Contact with animals in live food markets
- Since transmission of H5N1 viruses to two persons through consumption of uncooked duck blood may have occurred in Vietnam in 2005, uncooked poultry or poultry products, including blood, should not be consumed. Care should be taken when preparing these foods.
- For more information, see Human Infection with Avian Influenza A (H5N1) Virus Advice for Travelers (wwwn.cdc.gov/travel/contentAvianFluAsia.aspx) and the WHO Avian Influenza Fact Sheet (www.who.int/mediacentre/factsheets/avian_influenza/en/index.html#humans).
- A vaccine to protect humans against influenza A (H5N1) is not yet available commercially, but candidate vaccines are undergoing human clinical trials in the United States, with one vaccine currently licensed in the United States. This vaccine is approved by the U.S. FDA for stockpiling purposes only.

References

1. Fiore AES, Shay DK, Broder K, et al. Prevention and control of influenza: recommendations of the Advisory Committee on Immunization Practices (ACIP), 2008. MMWR Morbid Mortal Wkly Rep. 2008;57(RR-7):1–60.

2. Ortiz JR, Wallis TR, Katz MA, et al. No evidence of avian influenza A (H5N1) among returning US travelers. Emerg Infect Dis. 2007;13(2):294–7.

3. Uyeki TM, Zane SB, Bodnar UR, et al. Large summertime influenza A outbreak among tourists in Alaska and the Yukon Territory. Clin Infect Dis. 2003;36(9):1095–102.

4. Juurlink DN, Stukel TA, Kwong J, et al. Guillain–Barré syndrome after influenza vaccination in adults: a population-based study. Arch Intern Med. 2006;166(20):2217–21.

5. Naleway AL, Smith WJ, Mullooly JP. Delivering influenza vaccine to pregnant women. Epidemiol Rev. 2006;28:47–53.

6. Kroon FP, van Dissel JT, de Jong JC, et al. Antibody response after influenza vaccination in HIV-infected individuals: a consecutive 3-year study. Vaccine. 2000;18(26):3040–9.

7. CDC. Avian Influenza A virus infections of humans [Internet]. Atlanta: Centers for Disease Control and Prevention. [updated 2008 May 23; cited 2008 Nov 30]. Available from: http://www.cdc.gov/flu/avian/gen-info/avian-flu-humans.htm.

8. CDC. Diganosis: clinical signs and symptoms of influenza [Internet]. Atlanta: Centers for Disease Control and Prevention. [updated 2008 Sep 12; cited 2008 Jul 28]. Available from: http://www.cdc.gov/flu/professionals/acip/clinical.htm.

9. Heinonen OS, Shapiro S, Monson RR, et al. Immunization during pregnancy against poliomyelitis and influenza in relation to childhood malignancy. Int J Epidemiol. 1973;2(3):229–35.

10. NIH, CDC, HIVMA/IDSA. Guidelines for prevention and treatment of opportunistic infections in HIV-infected adults and adolescents [Internet]. Rockville (MD): AIDS*Info*; 2008. [cited 25 Jul 2008]. Available from: http://www.aidsinfo.nih.gov/contentfiles/Adult_OI.pdf

11. Lin JC, Nichol KL. Excess mortality due to pneumonia or influenza during influenza seasons among persons with acquired immunodeficiency syndrome. Arch Intern Med. 2001;161:441–446.

12. Miotti PG., Nelson KE, Dallabetta GA, et al. The influence of HIV infection on antibody responses to a two-dose regimen of influenza vaccine. JAMA. 1989;262(6):779–83.

13. Bright RA, Shay DK, Shu B, et al. Adamantane resistance among influenza A viruses isolated early during the 2005–2006 influenza season in the United States. JAMA. 2006;295(8):891–4.

14. WHO. Influenza A(H1N1) virus resistance to oseltamivir—2008 influenza season, southern hemisphere [Internet]. Geneva: World Health Organization; 2008. [cited 2008 Nov 30]. Available from: http://www.who.int/csr/ disease/ influenza/H1N1webupdate20082008_kf.pdf.

15. CDC. Questions & answers: Influenza antiviral drug resistance [Internet]. Atlanta: Centers for Disease Control and Prevention. [updated 2008 Jul 17; cited 2008 Nov 30]. Available from: http://www.cdc.gov/flu/ about/qa/antiviralresistance.htm.

16. European Centre for Disease Prevention and Control (ECDC). Antivirals and antiviral resistant influenza [Internet]. Stockholm: ECDC; 2008 [cited 2008 Nov 30]; Available from: http://ecdc.europa.eu/Health%5Ftopics/ influenza/antivirals.html.

17. WHO. WHO/ECDC frequently asked questions for Oseltamivir resistance [Internet]. Geneva: WHO; 2008 [cited 2008 Nov 30]. Available from: http://www.who.int/ csr/disease/influenza/oseltamivir_faqs/en/ index.html.

MEASLES (RUBEOLA)

Amy A. Parker, Amra Uzicanin

Infectious Agent

- Measles virus is a member of the genus *Morbillivirus* of the family Paramyxoviridae.
- Humans are the only known natural host for the measles virus.
- Measles, also known as rubeola, is one of the most highly communicable infectious diseases.

Mode of Transmission

- Measles spreads by airborne droplets.
- Direct contact with nasal or throat secretions of infected persons.
- Less commonly it is spread by articles freshly soiled with nose and throat secretions.
- Infected persons are usually contagious from 4 days before onset of signs or symptoms, and until 4 days after the onset of signs or symptoms.

Occurrence

- An estimated 20 million measles cases still occur globally every year, and travelers could be exposed in almost any country they visit. However, the risks are greater in countries where measles remains endemic or where large outbreaks are occurring.
- In the Americas, indigenous measles circulation was interrupted in 2002, but risk of measles due to virus importations from other parts of the world still remains.
- The number of reported measles cases in the United States has declined from 894,134 in 1941 to fewer than 150 cases each year since 1997. However, from January 1 through April 25, 2008, a total of 64 confirmed measles cases were reported to CDC, which is the largest number of cases reported in the United States for the corresponding period for any year since 2001. Ten of these cases were acquired abroad by unvaccinated travelers (five in visitors to the United States and five in U.S. residents) and the remaining cases were considered to be associated with these importations of measles.

Risk for Travelers

- All persons who do not have evidence of measles immunity are at risk for contracting measles during international travel.
- Acceptable presumptive evidence of immunity to measles for international travelers includes—
  - For infants 6–11 months of age, documented administration of one dose of live measles-containing vaccine[1] and, for persons ≥12 months of age, two doses of MMR[2] vaccine at least 28 days apart, on or after the first birthday
  - Laboratory evidence of immunity
  - Birth before 1957
  - Documented physician-diagnosed measles

Clinical Presentation

- Incubation period is ~10 days (range 7–18 days) from exposure to onset of fever, usually 14 days before appearance of rash.
- Symptoms include prodromal fever, conjunctivitis, coryza, cough, and small spots with white or bluish white centers on an erythematous base on the buccal mucosa (Koplik spots).
- Characteristic red, blotchy (maculopapular) rash appears on third to seventh day that begins on the face, becomes generalized, and lasts 4–7 days.
- Complications include diarrhea (8%), middle ear infection (7%–9%), and pneumonia (1%–6%). Encephalitis, frequently resulting in permanent brain damage, occurs in approximately 1 per 1,000–2,000 cases of measles. Subacute sclerosing panencephalitis (SSPE), a rare but serious degenerative central nervous system disease, is thought to occur in 1 per 100,000 cases, although a risk of 22 cases of SSPE per 100,000 measles cases was found during the 1989–1991 measles resurgence in the United States. SSPE, which is caused by a persistent infection with a defective measles virus, is manifested by mental and motor deterioration that starts an average of 7 years after measles virus infection (most frequently in children <2 years of age), progressing to coma and death.
- The risk of serious complications and death is highest for children ≤5 years of age and adults ≥20 years of age. It is also higher in populations with poor nutritional status.

Diagnosis

- A clinical case of measles illness is characterized by all of the following:
  - Generalized maculopapular rash lasting ≥3 days
  - Temperature ≥101° F (≥38.3° C)
  - Cough, coryza, or conjunctivitis
- Laboratory criteria for diagnosis is a positive serologic test for measles immunoglobulin M (IgM) antibody, seroconversion or significant rise in measles IgG antibody level by any standard serologic assay, or isolation of measles virus or identification by PCR of measles virus RNA from a clinical specimen.
- A confirmed case is either laboratory confirmed or meets the clinical case definition and is epidemiologically linked to a confirmed case. A laboratory-confirmed case does not need to meet the clinical case definition.

Treatment

- There is no specific antiviral therapy or treatment for measles.
- Supportive therapy includes hydration, antipyretics, and treating complications such as pneumonia.

- The WHO currently recommends vitamin A for all children with acute measles, regardless of their country of residence, to reduce morbidity and mortality. Vitamin A is administered once a day for 2 days, at the following doses:
    - ○ 50,000 IU for infants <6 months of age
    - ○ 100,000 IU for infants 6–11 months of age
    - ○ 200,000 IU for children ages 12 months or older
- A third age-specific dose of vitamin A is to be given 2–4 weeks later to case-patients with clinical signs and symptoms of vitamin A deficiency. Parenteral and oral formulations of vitamin A are available in the United States.

Preventive Measures for Travelers

Vaccine

- Measles vaccine contains live, attenuated measles virus. It is available as a monovalent formulation and in combination formulations, such as measles–rubella (MR), measles–mumps–rubella (MMR), and measles–mumps–rubella–varicella (MMRV).
- Ensure that all travelers who do not have evidence of measles immunity (see Risk for Travelers earlier in this section) are up to date on measles vaccination prior to departure.
    - ○ Infants 6–11 months of age should have at least one dose of measles-containing vaccine.[1]
    - ○ Preschool children ≥12 months of age should have two doses of MMR[2] vaccine separated by at least 28 days.
    - ○ School-age children should have two doses of MMR.[2]
    - ○ Adults born in or after 1957 should have two doses of measles-containing vaccine.
    - ○ If administered at ≥12 months of age, one dose of measles-containing vaccine or MMR is 95% effective in preventing measles disease and two doses are 99% effective. One dose of measles-containing vaccine or MMR is approximately 85% effective if administered at 9 months of age.
- For persons ≥12 months of age, combined MMR vaccine is recommended whenever one or more of the individual components is indicated to provide optimal protection against mumps and rubella. For infants <12 months of age, measles vaccine alone is recommended if it is available; otherwise MMR should be used.
- MMR vaccine, if administered within 72 hours of initial measles exposure, may provide some protection. If the exposure does not result in infection, the vaccine should induce protection against subsequent measles virus infection.
- Immune globulin (IG) can be used to prevent or mitigate measles in a susceptible person when administered within 6 days of exposure. However, any immunity conferred is temporary unless modified or typical measles occurs, and the person should receive measles-containing vaccine 5–6 months after IG administration.

Adverse Reactions, Precautions, and Contraindications to Measles Vaccine

Allergy

Persons with severe allergy (i.e., hives, swelling of the mouth or throat, difficulty breathing, hypotension, and shock) to gelatin or neomycin or who have had a severe allergic reaction to a prior dose of MMR or MMRV should not be revaccinated except with extreme caution. MMR or MMRV vaccines may be administered to egg-allergic persons without prior routine skin testing or the use of special protocols.

Immunosuppression

Replication of vaccine viruses can be potentiated in persons who have immune deficiency disorders. Death related to vaccine-associated measles infection has been reported among severely immunocompromised persons. Therefore, severely immunosuppressed individuals should not be vaccinated with MMR or MMRV vaccines

- MMR or MMRV should be avoided for at least 1 month after cessation of high-dose corticosteroid therapy. Some experts, however, recommend waiting only 2 weeks after completion of therapy among individuals receiving high doses of systemic corticosteroids daily or on alternate days even if they were receiving therapy for less than 14 days.
- Other immunosuppressive therapy: MMR or MMRV vaccines in general should be withheld for at least 3 months. This interval is based on the assumption that the immunologic responsiveness will have been restored in 3 months and the underlying disease for which the therapy was given is in remission.

Thrombocytopenia

The benefits of primary immunization are usually greater than the potential risks. However, avoiding a subsequent dose of MMR or MMRV vaccine may be prudent if an episode of thrombocytopenia occurred within approximately 6 weeks after a previous dose of vaccine.

Footnotes:

1 Measles vaccine alone is recommended for infants vaccinated before 12 months of age if it is available, otherwise MMR should be administered. Infants vaccinated before 12 months of age must be revaccinated on or after the first birthday with two doses of measles-containing vaccine separated by at least 28 days. MMRV is not licensed for children <12 months of age.
2 MMRV vaccine is licensed for children 12 months to 12 years of age and may be used in place of MMR vaccine if vaccination for measles, mumps, rubella and varicella are needed.

References

1. American Academy of Pediatrics. Measles. In: Pickering LK, Baker CJ, Long SS, McMillan JA, editors. Red book: 2006 report of the Committee on Infectious Diseases. 27th ed. Elk Grove Village, IL: American Academy of Pediatrics; 2006. p. 441–52.
2. WHO. Measles fact sheet. 2007 Nov [cited 2008 Nov 25] Available from: http://www.who.int/mediacentre/factsheets/fs286/en/.
3. CDC. Progress toward measles elimination—Region of the Americas, 2002–2003. MMWR. Morbid Mortal Wkly Rep. 2004;53(14):304–6.
4. CDC. Measles—United States, January 1–April 25, 2008. MMWR Morb Mortal Wkly Rep. 2008;57:1–4.
5. CDC. Measles, mumps, and rubella-vaccine use and strategies for elimination of measles, rubella, and congenital rubella syndrome and control of mumps: Recommendations of the Advisory Committee on Immunization Practices (ACIP). MMWR Morbid Mortal Wkly Rep. 1998;47(RR-8):1–57.
6. CDC. Update: recommendations from the Advisory Committee on Immunization Practices (ACIP) regarding administration of combination MMRV vaccine. MMWR Morbid Mortal Wkly Rep. 2008;57(10);258–60.
7. Strebel PM, Papania MJ, dayan GH, et al. Measles vaccine. In: Plotkin SA, Orenstein WA, Offit PA, editors. Vaccines. 5th ed. Philadelphia: Saunders Elsevier; 2008. p. 353–98.
8. Bellini WJ, Rota JS, Lowe LE, et al. Subacute sclerosing panencephalitis: more cases of this fatal disease are prevented by measles immunization than was previously recognized. J Infect Dis. 2005;192(10):1686–93.
9. Perry RT, Halsey NA. The clinical significance of measles: a review. J Infect Dis. 2004;189 Suppl 1;S4–16.
10. CDC. Measles (rubeola) 2007 case definition. 2008 Jan 9 [cited 2008 Nov 25]. Available from: http://www.cdc.gov/ncphi/disss/nndss/casedef/measles_current.htm.
11. American Academy of Pediatrics. Measles. In: Pickering LK, Baker CJ, Long SL, Kimberlin DW, editors. Red book: 2006 report of the Committee on Infectious Diseases. 27th ed. Elk Grove Village, IL: American Academy of Pediatrics; 2006.
12. CDC. Recommended childhood and adolescent immunization schedule—United States, 2006. MMWR Morb Mortal Wkly Rep. 2006;54(52):Q1–4.

MUMPS

Preeta K. Kutty, Albert E. Barskey IV, Kathleen M. Gallagher

Infectious Agent

- Mumps virus is an enveloped, negative-strand RNA virus, a member of the genus *Rubulavirus*.
- Humans are the only known natural host for mumps virus.

Mode of Transmission

- Transmission is by respiratory droplets, saliva, or contact with contaminated fomites.
- Patients are usually contagious 1–2 days (occasionally as long as 7 days) before symptom onset until 5 days afterward.

Occurrence

- With the exception of the multistate outbreak in 2006, mumps is an uncommon disease in the United States because of a successful vaccination program.
- Mumps virus remains endemic in many countries throughout the world because mumps vaccine is used in only 57% of the World Health Organization member countries.

Risk for Travelers

- The risk of exposure to mumps among travelers can be high in most countries of the world, especially for travelers >12 months of age who do not have evidence of mumps immunity (see Preventive Measures for Travelers later in this section). Although some countries have had variable successes with a national vaccination program—including Finland, which has declared elimination—the risk of contacting imported mumps in these countries is still a concern.
- Acceptable presumptive evidence of immunity to mumps for international travelers includes—
  - Documented administration of two doses of live mumps virus vaccine at least 28 days apart, on or after the first birthday
  - Laboratory evidence of immunity
  - Birth before 1957
  - Documentation of physician-diagnosed mumps

Clinical Presentation

- Incubation period from exposure to onset of symptoms is generally 16–18 days (range 12–25 days).
- Onset of illness is usually nonspecific, with symptoms of fever, headache, malaise, myalgia, and anorexia.
- Mumps is characterized by parotitis, either unilateral or bilateral.
- Although mumps is generally a mild and self-limited disease, complications of mumps infection can include deafness; orchitis, oophoritis, or mastitis (inflammation of the testicles, ovaries or breasts, respectively); pancreatitis; and meningitis or encephalitis. With the exception of deafness, these complications are more frequent in adults than in children.

Diagnosis

- Mumps may occur in epidemics; mumps virus is the only cause of epidemic parotitis.
- Diagnosis is usually clinical, based on the presence of parotitis and associated signs, symptoms, or complications.
- Clinical case definition: An illness with acute onset of unilateral or bilateral tender, self-limited swelling of the parotid glands, other salivary gland(s), or both, lasting at least 2 days, and without other apparent cause.
- Laboratory criteria include—
  - Isolation of mumps virus from clinical specimen
  - Detection of mumps nucleic acid (e.g., standard or real-time RT-PCR assays)
  - Detection of mumps IgM antibody
  - Demonstration of specific mumps antibody response in the absence of recent vaccination, either a fourfold increase in IgG titer as measured by quantitative assays, or seroconversion from negative to positive by using a standard serologic assay of paired acute- and convalescent-phase serum specimens
- Laboratory specimens that can be collected are serum for serology (IgM, IgG) and a buccal swab (or a throat swab) for viral specimens. For more information see www.cdc.gov/vaccines/vpd-vac/mumps/outbreak/faqs-lab-spec-collect.htm.
- Laboratory confirmation is more challenging in highly vaccinated populations. Serologic tests should be interpreted with caution. A negative laboratory test should not rule out a clinically compatible case, especially in a two-dose vaccine recipient.

Treatment

There is no specific antiviral therapy for mumps, and the basic treatment consists of supportive care.

Preventive Measures for Travelers

Vaccine

- Although vaccination against mumps is not a requirement for entry into any country (including the United States), travelers leaving the United States or living abroad should ensure they are immune to mumps.
- Mumps vaccine contains live, attenuated mumps virus. It is available as a monovalent formulation and in combination formulations, such as MMR. Combined MMR vaccine is recommended whenever one or more of the individual components is indicated to provide optimal protection against measles and rubella. Mumps vaccine is highly, but not 100%, effective in preventing mumps. One dose of mumps vaccine is approximately 80%–85% effective in preventing clinical mumps with parotitis, and two doses are approximately 90% effective.
- Mumps vaccine has not been demonstrated to be effective in preventing infection after exposure; however, it can be administered postexposure to provide protection against subsequent exposures. Immune globulin is not effective in preventing mumps infection following an exposure and is not recommended.

Adverse Reactions, Precautions, and Contraindications to Mumps Vaccine

- Refer to the Measles (Rubeola) section earlier in this chapter for information on reactions following MMR vaccine and additional precautions and contraindications.

General Vaccine Recommendations, Pediatric and Catch-Up Schedules, and Recommendations for Special Populations

- Refer to Chapters 7 and 8.

References

1. American Academy of Pediatrics. Mumps. In: Pickering LK, Baker CJ, Long SS, McMillan JA, editors. Red book: 2006 report of the Committee on Infectious Diseases. 27th ed. Elk Grove Village, IL: American Academy of Pediatrics; 2003. p. 464–8.

2. CDC. Updated recommendations for isolation of persons with mumps. MMWR Morbid Mortal Wkly Rep. 2008;57(40):1103–5.

3. World Health Organization. Global status of mumps immunization and surveillance. Wkly Epidemiol Rec. 2005;80(48):417–24.

4. CDC. Measles, mumps, and rubella-vaccine use and strategies for elimination of measles, rubella, and congenital rubella syndrome and control of mumps. Recommendations of the Advisory Committee on Immunization Practices (ACIP). MMWR Morbid Mortal Wkly Rep. 1998;47(RR-8):1–57.

5. CDC. Notice to readers: Updated recommendations of the Advisory Committee on Immunization Practices (ACIP) for the control and elimination of mumps. MMWR Morbid Mortal Wkly Rep. 2006;55(22):629–30.

6. CDC. Measles prevention: recommendations of the Immunization Practices Advisory Committee on Infectious Diseases (ACIP). MMWR Morbid Mortal Wkly Rep. 1989;38(No. S-9):1–18.

7. Plotkin SA, Rubin S. Mumps Vaccine. In: Plotkin SA, Orenstein WA, Offit PA, editors. Vaccines. 5th ed. Philadelphia: Elsevier Saunders; 2008. p. 436–65.

8. Watson JC, Hadler SC, Dykewicz CA, et al.; CDC. Measles, mumps and rubella vaccine use and strategies for elimination of measles, rubella, and congenital rubella syndrome and control of mumps: recommendations of the Advisory Committee on Immunization Practices (ACIP). MMWR Morbid Mortal Wkly Rep. 1998;47(RR-8):1–57.

9. Council of State and Territorial Epidemiologists. Infectious Disease Committee. Revision of the surveillance case definition for mumps. [cited 2008 Nov 25] Available from: http://www.cste.org/PS/2007ps/2007psfinal/ID/07-ID-02.pdf.

10. Harling R, White JM, Ramsay ME, et al. The effectiveness of the mumps component of the MMR vaccine: a case control study. Vaccine. 2005;23(31):4070–4.

PERTUSSIS

Tami H. Skoff, Cynthia G. Thomas

Infectious Agent

Pertussis is caused by fastidious gram-negative coccobacillus, *Bordetella pertussis.*

Mode of Transmission

It is spread by person-to-person transmission via aerosolized respiratory droplets or by direct contact with respiratory secretions.

Occurrence

- *B. pertussis* circulates worldwide, but disease rates are highest among young children in countries where vaccination coverage is low, which is primarily in the developing world.
- In developed countries, the incidence of pertussis is highest among unvaccinated infants and increases again among adolescents.
- Immunity from childhood vaccination and natural disease wanes with time; therefore, adolescents and adults who have not received a Tdap booster vaccination can become infected or re-infected.

Risk for Travelers

- Pertussis remains endemic worldwide, even in areas with high vaccination rates.

- Travelers who come in close contact with infected persons are at risk for disease. Infants too young to be protected by a complete vaccination series are at greatest risk for severe pertussis requiring hospitalization.

Clinical Presentation

- In classic disease, mild upper respiratory tract symptoms begin 7–10 days (range 6–21 days) after exposure, followed by a cough that becomes paroxysmal. Coughing paroxysms may be frequent or relatively infrequent and are often followed by vomiting. Fever is absent or minimal. The CDC/Council of State and Territorial Epidemiologists' clinical case definition for pertussis includes cough for ≥2 weeks with paroxysms, whoop, and/or post-tussive vomiting.
- Disease in infants <6 months of age can be atypical with a short catarrhal stage, gagging, gasping, or apnea as early manifestations; among infants <2 months of age, the case–fatality rate is approximately 1%.
- Recently immunized children may have mild cough illness; older children and adults may have prolonged cough with or without paroxysms. The cough gradually wanes over several weeks to months.

Diagnosis

- Factors such as prior vaccination status, stage of disease, antibiotic use, specimen collection and transport conditions, and nonstandardized tests may affect the sensitivity, specificity, and interpretation of available diagnostic tests for *B. pertussis*.
- Current CDC guidelines for the laboratory confirmation of pertussis cases include culture and PCR (when the above clinical case definition is met); serology and direct fluorescent antibody (DFA) tests are not confirmatory tests included in the case definition.

Treatment

- Macrolide antibiotics (azithromycin, clarithromycin, and erythromycin) are recommended for the treatment of pertussis in persons ≥1 month of age; for infants <1 month of age, azithromycin is the preferred antibiotic.
- Antimicrobial therapy with a macrolide antibiotic administered <3 weeks after cough onset can limit transmission to others.
- Postexposure prophylaxis is recommended for close contacts of cases and for individuals at high risk of developing severe disease. The recommended agents and dosing regimens for prophylaxis are the same as those indicated for the treatment of pertussis.

Preventive Measures for Travelers

Vaccine

- Travelers should be up to date with pertussis vaccinations prior to departure.
- Complete vaccination of children <7 years of age with five doses of acellular pertussis vaccine in combination with diphtheria and tetanus toxoids (DTaP) is recommended; an accelerated schedule of doses may be used to complete the DTaP series.
- There is no pertussis-containing vaccine licensed for children 7–9 years of age. If a child turns 10 years old during the vaccination series with Td (tetanus and diphtheria toxoids vaccine), a single dose of Tdap may be substituted for one of the Td doses.

- Adolescents aged 11–18 years should receive a single dose of Tdap instead of Td for booster immunization against tetanus, diphtheria, and pertussis if they have completed the recommended childhood DTwP/DTaP vaccination series. Adolescents who received their last Td (tetanus and diphtheria toxoids vaccine) 5 years or more previously should also receive a single dose of Tdap.
- Adults 19–64 years of age should receive a single dose of Tdap to replace a single dose of Td for booster immunization against tetanus, diphtheria, and pertussis if their last tetanus toxoid-containing vaccine (e.g., Td) was administered 10 years or more prior. Tdap is not licensed for adults 65 years of age or older.
- Tdap can be given in intervals <10 years from the last Td to provide pertussis protection prior to travel, except in those individuals with a contraindication to vaccination.
- Adolescents and adults who have never been immunized against pertussis, tetanus, or diphtheria, have incomplete immunization, or whose immunity is uncertain should follow the catch-up schedule established for Td/Tdap. Tdap can be substituted for any one of the Td doses in the series.

References

1. Edwards KM, Decker MD. Pertussis vaccines. In: Plotkin SA, Orenstein WA, editors. Vaccines. 4th ed. Philadelphia: W.B. Saunders; 2004: p. 471–528.
2. CDC. Preventing tetanus, diphtheria, and pertussis among adolescents: Use of tetanus toxoid, reduced diptheria toxoid and acellular pertussis vaccines. Recommendations of the Advisory Committee on Immunization Practices (ACIP). MMWR Recomm Rep. 2006;55(RR-17):1–37.
3. American Academy of Pediatrics. Pertussis. In: Pickering LK, Baker CJ, Long SS, McMillan JA, editors. Red book: 2006 report of the

Committee on Infectious Diseases. 27th ed. Elk Grove Village, IL: American Academy of Pediatrics; 2006. p. 498–520.
4. Tiwari T, Murphy TV, Moran J. Recommended antimicrobial agents for the treatment and postexposure prophylaxis of pertussis: 2005 CDC guidelines. MMWR Recomm Rep. 2005;54(RR-14):1–16.
5. CDC. Pertussis vaccination: Use of acellular pertussis vaccines among infants and young children. Recommendations of the Advisory Committee on Immunization Practices (ACIP). MMWR Recomm Rep. 1997;46(RR-7):1–25.

PNEUMOCOCCAL DISEASE (*STREPTOCOCCUS PNEUMONIAE*)

J. Pekka Nuorti

Infectious Agent

- *Streptococcus pneumoniae* (pneumococcus) is a bacterium that frequently colonizes the nasopharynx of healthy persons, particularly young children, without causing illness.
- There are 91 known pneumococcal serotypes.
- The major clinical syndromes include life-threatening infections such as meningitis, bacteremia, and pneumonia.
- Pneumococcus is the most commonly identified cause of community-acquired pneumonia. It is also a major cause of milder but more common illnesses, such as sinusitis and otitis media.

Mode of Transmission

- Direct person-to-person transmission is through close contact via respiratory droplets.
- Transmission is thought to be common, but clinical illness occurs infrequently among casual contacts.

Occurrence

- Pneumococcal disease occurs worldwide, and the reported incidence varies by geographic region.
- Rates are higher in developing countries than in industrialized countries.
- Pneumococcal disease is more common during winter and early spring, when respiratory viruses such as influenza are circulating. Most illnesses are sporadic.
- Outbreaks of pneumococcal disease are uncommon but may occur in closed populations such as nursing homes, childcare centers or other institutions.
- In the United States, most deaths from pneumococcal disease occur in older adults, although in developing countries, many children die of pneumococcal pneumonia.
- Routine use of the 7-valent pneumococcal conjugate vaccine (PCV7) in the United States since 2000 has dramatically reduced the incidence of pneumococcal disease in both children and adults. Because the vaccine interrupts transmission of vaccine-type pneumococci, rates of pneumococcal disease in unvaccinated older children and adults have also decreased.
- As of 2008, 18 industrialized countries are routinely using pneumococcal conjugate vaccines, including Canada, Australia, the United Kingdom, and other Western European and Middle Eastern countries.

Risk for Travelers

- The risk for pneumococcal disease is generally highest among young children, the elderly, and persons of any age who have chronic medical conditions, such as heart disease, lung disease, diabetes or asplenia, or conditions that suppress the immune system, such as HIV.
- Cigarette smokers are also at increased risk.
- Most travelers, however, are not in these categories. It is important to recognize that healthy travelers in their twenties or thirties have developed pneumococcal pneumonia while traveling in developing countries.

Clinical Presentation

- Sudden onset with fever and malaise are typical symptoms for all forms of pneumococcal infections and may be the only symptoms in young children with bacteremia.
- In pneumococcal pneumonia, fever may precede the usual symptoms of cough, pleuritic chest pain, and the production of purulent or blood-tinged sputum.
- In elderly persons, the onset of pneumococcal pneumonia may be less abrupt, with fever, shortness of breath, or altered mental status as the initial symptoms; sputum production may be absent.
- Pneumococcal meningitis may present with a stiff neck, headache, lethargy, or seizures; otitis media or sinusitis typically cause pain in the ears or sinuses.

Diagnosis

- A definitive diagnosis of pneumococcal infection can be made by isolation of the bacterium from blood or other normally sterile body sites, such as cerebrospinal fluid. Most patients with pneumococcal pneumonia, however, do not have detectable bacteremia.
- The diagnosis of pneumococcal pneumonia can be suspected if on microscopy a sputum specimen contains many gram-stain positive diplococci and polymorphonuclear leukocytes and very few epithelial cells.
- Typical chest radiography may show lobar, segmental, or multilobar consolidation.

- Pneumococcal pneumonia is usually, but not always, associated with a high white blood cell count. High white blood cell counts should raise suspicion for this diagnosis, since other serious travel-related diseases causing fever, such as hepatitis, typhoid fever, malaria, dengue fever, or typhus, all have normal or low white blood cell counts.

Treatment

- All types of pneumococcal infections are usually treated with antibiotics.
- Worldwide, many strains are increasingly resistant to penicillin, cephalosporin, and macrolides, and some are resistant to multiple classes of drugs, complicating treatment choices. Antimicrobial susceptibility of strains isolated from blood and cerebrospinal fluid should be determined, and treatment should be targeted based on the susceptibility results.
- In 2008, the Clinical and Laboratory Standards Institute adopted new susceptibility breakpoints for penicillin treatment of nonmeningitis cases of pneumococcal disease. However, empiric antibiotic therapy should not be delayed and should begin before microbiological confirmation of etiology.
- In the United States and other countries where beta-lactam resistance among pneumococcal isolates is common, the initial regimen for suspected pneumococcal meningitis should include vancomycin until the antimicrobial susceptibility pattern of the organism is available.

Preventive Measures for Travelers

Vaccine

- No specific recommendations for the use of pneumococcal vaccines in travelers have been formulated.
- Currently, two vaccines are available for prevention of pneumococcal disease in the United States.
  - *Pneumococcal conjugate vaccine*—The 7-valent pneumococcal conjugate vaccine (PCV7) (Prevnar, Wyeth Vaccines) is mainly used in children. It is part of the routine infant immunization schedule in the United States and is now recommended for all children <5 years of age (see the Vaccine Recommendations for Infants and Children section in Chapter 7). The infant schedule consists of a three-dose primary series at ages 2, 4, and 6 months and a booster dose at 12–15 months of age. Fewer doses are required for children who begin the series after 7 months of age.
  - *Pneumococcal polysaccharaide vaccine*—A 23-valent pneumococcal polysaccharide vaccine (PPV23) (Pneumovax, Merck) is mainly used in older adults and persons with underlying medical conditions. PPV23 is recommended for all adults ≥65 years of age and for persons 2–64 years of age with underlying medical conditions at the time the condition is recognized. In 2006, only about 57% of adults aged ≥65 years of age had received the vaccine. Children 2–4 years of age who have underlying medical conditions that are indications for PPV23 should also receive polysaccharide vaccine after receiving the conjugate vaccine series.
- Both vaccines induce antibodies to the specific types of pneumococcal capsule and have been shown to be effective against invasive disease.
- Additional pneumococcal conjugate vaccine formulations are expected to be licensed soon. The WHO recommends that inclusion of pneumococcal conjugate vaccines in all national immunization programs should be a priority.
- Routine revaccination is not recommended for most people. A second dose of PPV23 is recommended 5 years after the first dose for the following groups:

○ Persons with sickle cell disease, asplenia, renal disease, hematologic or generalized malignancy, or other immunocompromising condition

○ Persons ≥65 years of age who received PPV23 before age 65 years for an underlying medical condition, if at least 5 years have passed since their previous dose

• Because of limited data regarding the duration of protection provided by PPV23 and the safety of multiple doses, only a single revaccination is recommended. Persons should receive one dose if they have an indication for polysaccharide vaccine and their vaccination history is unknown.

Safety and Side Effects

• After receipt of PCV7, mild local reactions, such as redness, swelling, or tenderness, occur in 10%–23% of infants. Larger areas of redness or swelling or limitations in arm movement may occur in 1%–9% of infants. Low-grade fever can occur in up to 24% and fever higher than 102.2° F may occur in up to 2.5% of vaccinees.

• After receipt of PPV23, self-limiting local side effects occur in approximately half of vaccine recipients and are more common after revaccination than with first dose. These reactions usually resolve within 48 hours. More severe local reactions and systemic symptoms, including myalgias and fever, are rare.

Precautions and Contraindications

• PCV7 is contraindicated for children known to have hypersensitivity to any component of the vaccine.

• Health-care providers may delay vaccination of children with moderate or severe illness until the child has recovered, although minor illnesses, such as mild upper-respiratory tract infection with or without low-grade fever, are not contraindications.

• Revaccination with PPV23 is contraindicated for persons who had a severe reaction (e.g., anaphylactic reaction or localized arthus-type reaction) to the initial dose.

Additional Preventive Measures

• The following may reduce the risk of pneumococcal disease:
  ○ improving control of chronic conditions that predispose to pneumococcal disease, such as diabetes and HIV,
  ○ stopping smoking, and
  ○ avoiding crowded living conditions.

• Chemoprophylaxis is not routinely recommended for close contacts of pneumococcal meningitis or other cases of invasive disease or for travelers unless otherwise recommended by the health-care practitioner supervising their care.

References

1. CDC. Prevention of pneumococcal disease. Recommendations of the Advisory Committee on Immunization Practices (ACIP). MMWR Morbid Mortal Wkly Rep. 1997;46(RR-8):1–24.

2. CDC. Preventing pneumococcal disease among infants and young children: Recommendations of the Advisory Committee on Immunization Practices (ACIP). MMWR Recomm Rep. 2000;49(No. RR-9):1–38.

3. American Academy of Pediatrics. Pneumococcal infections. In: Pickering LK, Baker CJ, Long SS, McMillan JA, editors. Red book: 2006 Report of the Committee on Infectious Diseases. Elk Grove Village, IL: American Academy of Pediatrics; 2006. p. 525–37.

4. CDC. Invasive pneumococcal disease in children 5 years after routine conjugate vaccine introduction—eight states, 1998–2005. MMWR Morb Mortal Wkly Rep. 2008;57(6):144–8.

5. Fedson DS, Scott JAG. The burden of pneumococcal disease among adults in developed and developing countries: what is and is not known. Vaccine. 1999;17(Supplement 1):S11–18.

6. WHO. Pneumococcal conjugate vaccine for childhood immunisation—WHO position paper. Wkly Epidemiol Rec. 2007;82(12):93–104.

7. Whitney CG, Farley MM, Hadler J, et al. Decline in invasive pneumococcal disease after

the introduction of protein–polysaccharide conjugate vaccine. N Engl J Med. 2003;348(18):1737–46.

8. Greenwood B. The epidemiology of pneumococcal infection in children in the developing world. Phil Trans R Soc Lond B Biol Sci. 1999;354(1384):777–85.

9. Clinical and Laboratory Standards Institute. Performance standards for antimicrobial susceptibility testing; eighteenth informational supplement. Wayne, PA: Clinical and Laboratory Standards Institute; 2008 Jan. CLSI Document M100-S18.

10. Tunkel AR, Hartman BJ, Kaplan SL, et al. Practice guidelines for the management of bacterial meningitis. Clin Infect Dis. 2004;39(9):1267–84.

POLIOMYELITIS

James P. Alexander, Steven Wassilak

Infectious Agent

- The infectious agent is poliovirus (genus Enterovirus) types 1, 2, and 3.
- Polioviruses are small (27–30 nm), nonenveloped viruses with capsids enclosing a single-stranded, positive-sense RNA genome about 7,500 nucleotides long.
- Most of the properties of polioviruses are shared with the other enteroviruses.

Mode of Transmission

Fecal–oral or oral transmission. Acute infection involves the gastrointestinal tract and occasionally the central nervous system.

Occurrence

- In the prevaccine era, infection with poliovirus was common worldwide, with seasonal peaks and epidemics in the summer and fall in temperate areas.
- The incidence of poliomyelitis in the United States declined rapidly after the licensure of inactivated polio vaccine (IPV) in 1955 and live oral polio vaccine (OPV) in the 1960s. The last cases of indigenously acquired polio in the United States occurred in 1979.
- The Global Polio Eradication Initiative (GPEI) subsequently led to elimination of polio in the Americas, where the last wild poliovirus (WPV)-associated polio case was detected in 1991.
- In 1999, a change in vaccination policy in the United States from use of OPV to exclusive use of IPV resulted in the elimination of the 8–10 vaccine-associated paralytic poliomyelitis (VAPP) cases that had occurred annually since the introduction of OPV in the 1960s.
- In the United States, two events that occurred in 2005 highlighted the continuing but low risk for poliovirus infection for unvaccinated persons, whether residing in the United States or traveling.
  - A case of imported VAPP occurred in an unvaccinated U.S. adult who had traveled abroad, likely from contact with an infant recently vaccinated with OPV.
  - An unvaccinated immunocompromised infant and four children in two other families in the same small rural community were found to be asymptomatically infected with a vaccine-derived poliovirus, presumably originating outside the United States in a country that uses OPV.
- The GPEI has built upon the success in the Americas and made great progress in eradicating wild polioviruses. There are only four countries where wild poliovirus

circulation has never been interrupted: Afghanistan, India, Nigeria, and Pakistan. WPV type 2 has not been detected since October 1999.

- During 2002–2006, 22 previously polio-free countries were affected by importations of WPV type 1 from the remaining polio-endemic countries, primarily Nigeria. In 2007–2008, polio cases occurred in 12 countries following importations of WPV originating from Nigeria or India.
- In spite of recent WPV outbreaks and continued circulation in the four countries where WPV circulation has never been interrupted, the GPEI has reduced the number of reported polio cases worldwide by more than 99% since the mid-1980s. With intensified efforts, worldwide eradication of polio appears feasible in the future.

Risk for Travelers

- Because of polio eradication efforts, the number of countries where travelers are at risk for polio has decreased dramatically.
- At the time of publication, most of the world's population resides in areas considered free of WPV circulation, including the Western Hemisphere, the Western Pacific region (which encompasses China), and the European region.
- Vaccination is recommended for all travelers to polio-endemic or epidemic areas, including countries with recent proven WPV circulation and neighboring countries. As of September 2008, these areas include some but not all countries in Africa, South Asia, Southeast Asia, and the Middle East. For current information on the status of polio eradication efforts and vaccine recommendations, consult the Travel Notices on the CDC Travelers' Health website (www.cdc.gov/travel/) or the GPEI website (www.polioeradication.org/).

Clinical Presentation

Clinical manifestations of poliovirus infection range from asymptomatic (most infections) to symptomatic, including acute flaccid paralysis of a single limb to quadriplegia, respiratory failure, and, rarely, death.

Diagnosis

The diagnosis is made by the identification of poliovirus in clinical specimens (usually stool) obtained from an acutely ill patient. Poliovirus may be detected from stool specimens for up to 4 weeks after onset of illness.

Treatment

Only symptomatic treatment is available, ranging from pain and fever relief to intubation and mechanical ventilation for those with respiratory insufficiency.

Preventive Measures for Travelers

- A person is considered to be fully immunized if he or she has received a primary series of at least three doses of IPV, three doses of OPV, or four doses of any combination of IPV and OPV.
- To eliminate the risk for VAPP, OPV has not been recommended for routine immunization in the United States since January 1, 2000, and is no longer available in this country.
- OPV continues to be used in the majority of countries and for global polio eradication activities.

Vaccine

Infants and Children

- Because OPV is no longer recommended for routine immunization in the United States, all infants and children should receive four doses of IPV at 2, 4, and 6–18 months and 4–6 years of age. The fourth (booster) dose is not needed if the third dose of the primary series is administered on or after the fourth birthday.
- If accelerated protection is needed, the minimum interval between doses is 4 weeks, although the preferred interval between the second and third doses is 2 months.
- The minimum age for IPV administration is 6 weeks. Infants and children who have initiated the poliovirus vaccination series with one or more doses of OPV should receive IPV to complete the series.

Adults

- Adults who are traveling to areas where poliomyelitis cases are still occurring and who are unvaccinated, incompletely vaccinated, or whose vaccination status is unknown should receive two doses of IPV administered at an interval of 4–8 weeks; a third dose should be administered 6–12 months after the second.
- If three doses of IPV cannot be administered within the recommended intervals before protection is needed, the following alternatives are recommended:
  - If >8 weeks is available before protection is needed, three doses of IPV should be administered at least 4 weeks apart.
  - If <8 weeks but >4 weeks is available before protection is needed, two doses of IPV should be administered at least 4 weeks apart.
  - If <4 weeks is available before protection is needed, a single dose of IPV is recommended.
- If fewer than three doses are administered, the remaining IPV doses to complete a three-dose series should be administered when feasible, at the intervals recommended above, if the person remains at increased risk for poliovirus exposure.
- Adults (≥18 years of age) who are traveling to areas where poliomyelitis cases are occurring and who have received a primary series with either IPV or OPV in childhood should receive another dose of IPV before departure.
- For adults, available data do not indicate the need for more than a single lifetime booster dose with IPV.

Allergy to Vaccine

- Minor local reactions (pain and redness) can occur following IPV. No serious adverse reactions to IPV have been documented.
- IPV should not be administered to persons who have experienced a severe allergic (anaphylactic) reaction after a previous dose of IPV or after receiving streptomycin, polymyxin B, or neomycin which IPV contains in trace amounts; hypersensitivity reactions can occur following IPV among persons sensitive to these three antibiotics.

Pregnancy and Breastfeeding

- If a pregnant woman is unvaccinated or incompletely vaccinated and requires immediate protection against polio because of planned travel to a country or area where polio cases are occurring, IPV can be administered as recommended for adults.
- Breastfeeding is not a contraindication to immunization of an infant or mother against polio.

Precautions and Contraindications

- IPV may be administered to persons with diarrhea.
- Minor upper respiratory illnesses with or without fever, mild to moderate local reactions to a previous dose of IPV, current antimicrobial therapy, and the convalescent phase of acute illness are not contraindications for vaccination.

Immunosuppression

- IPV may be administered safely to immunodeficient travelers and their household contacts. Although a protective immune response cannot be ensured, IPV might confer some protection to the immunodeficient person.
- Persons with certain primary immunodeficiency diseases should avoid contact with excreted OPV virus (e.g., exposure to a child vaccinated with OPV within the previous 6 weeks); however, this situation no longer occurs in the United States unless a child receives OPV overseas.

References

1. Sutter RW, Kew OM, Cochi SL. Poliovirus vaccine—live. In: Plotkin SA, Orenstein WA, Offit PA, editors. Vaccines. 5th ed. Philadelphia: Saunders Elsevier; 2008. p. 631–86.
2. Plotkin SA, Vidor E. Poliovirus Vaccine—Inactivated. In: Plotkin SA, Orenstein WA, Offit PA, editors. Vaccines. 5th ed. Philadelphia: Saunders Elsevier; 2008. p. 605–30.
3. CDC. Poliomyelitis. In: Atkinson W, Hamborsky J, McIntyre L, Wolfe S, editors. Epidemiology and prevention of vaccine-preventable diseases. 9th ed. Washington, DC: Public Health Foundation; 2006. p. 97–110.
4. CDC. Progress toward interruption of wild poliovirus transmission-worldwide, January 2007–April 2008. MMWR Morbid Mortal Wkly Rep. 2008;57(18):489–94.
5. CDC. Resurgence of wild poliovirus type 1 transmission and consequences of importation—21 countries, 2002–2005. MMWR Morbid Mortal Wkly Rep. 2006;55(6):145–50.
6. WHO. Global case count. [cited 2008 Sept 16]. Available from: http://www.polioeradication. org/casecount.asp.
7. CDC. Poliomyelitis prevention in the United States—updated recommendations of the Advisory Committee on Immunization Practices (ACIP). MMWR Recomm Rep. 2000;49 (RR-5):1–22.
8. CDC. Poliomyelitis—United States, 1975–1984. MMWR Morbid Mortal Wkly Rep. 1986;35(11):180–2.
9. CDC. International Notes: Certification of poliomyelitis eradication—the Americas, 1994. MMWR Morbid Mortal Wkly Rep. 1994;43(39):720–2.
10. Alexander LN, Seward JF, Santibanez TA, et al. Vaccine policy changes and epidemiology of polio in the United States. JAMA. 2004;292(14):1696–701.
11. CDC. Imported vaccine-associated paralytic poliomyelitis—United States, 2005. MMWR Morbid Mortal Wkly Rep. 2006;55(4);97–9.
12. CDC. Poliovirus infections in four unvaccinated children—Minnesota, August–October, 2005. MMWR Morbid Mortal Wkly Rep. 2005;54(41);1053–5.
13. CDC. Laboratory surveillance for wild and vaccine-derived polioviruses. MMWR Morbid Mortal Wkly Rep. 2008;57(35):967–70.
14. World Health Organization. Conclusions and recommendations of the Advisory Committee on Poliomyelitis Eradication, Geneva 27–28 November 2007. Wkly Epidemiol Rec. 2008;83(3):25–35.

RUBELLA

Susan E. Reef

Infectious Agent

Rubella virus is a member of *Togaviridae* family and the only member of the genus *Rubivirus*.

Mode of Transmission

- Rubella virus is transmitted through person-to-person contact or droplets shed from the respiratory secretions of infected persons.
- If a woman with rubella is infected during pregnancy, the virus can cross the placenta and infect the fetus.

Occurrence

- Rubella occurs worldwide.

- In the United States, endemic rubella has been eliminated. However, since 2005, an average of 10 cases is reported each year. Of these cases, approximately 33% are imported or linked to importations.

Risk for Travelers

- All susceptible persons are at risk for infection from exposure to rubella during travel outside the United States.
- Because asymptomatic rubella infections are common, travelers may be unaware that they have been in contact with an infected person.

Clinical Presentation

- The average incubation period is 14 days, with a range of 12–23 days.
- Rubella usually presents as a nonspecific, maculopapular, generalized rash lasting 3 days or fewer (hence the term "3-day measles") with generalized lymphadenopathy, particularly of the posterior auricular, suboccipital and posterior cervical lymph nodes.
- Asymptomatic rubella virus infections are common, and up to 50% of infections occur without rash.
- In adults and adolescents, the rash may be preceded by a 1- to 5-day prodrome of low-grade fever, malaise, anorexia, mild conjunctivitis, coryza, sore throat, and lymphadenopathy.
- The most important and serious consequence of rubella is infection during early pregnancy. These consequences may include miscarriages, fetal deaths/stillbirths, and an infant born with constellation of severe birth defects known as congenital rubella syndrome (CRS). The most common congenital defects are cataracts, heart defects, and hearing impairment.

Diagnosis

- Many illnesses can mimic rubella, and up to 50% of rubella infections are asymptomatic. Therefore, the only reliable evidence of acute rubella virus infection is laboratory diagnosis.
- Serologic testing for rubella-specific IgM antibody is the most commonly used for diagnosis of rubella.
- Diagnosis can also be made by demonstration of seroconversion of rubella-specific IgG antibody titers and by detection of virus either through virus culture or PCR.

Treatment

There is no specific antiviral therapy for rubella; basic treatment consists of supportive care.

Preventive Measures for Travelers

Vaccine

- Before international travel, persons should be immune to rubella.
- Acceptable presumptive evidence of immunity to rubella for international travelers includes—
  - Documentation of receipt of one or more doses of rubella-containing vaccine on or after the first birthday
  - Laboratory evidence of rubella immunity (a positive serologic test for rubella-specific IgG antibody)

Adverse Reactions, Precautions, and Contraindications to Rubella Vaccine

- Refer to the Measles (Rubeola) section earlier in this chapter for information on reactions following MMR vaccine and additional precautions and contraindications.

References

1. CDC. Rubella. In: Atkinson W, Hamborsky J, McIntyre L, Wolfe S, editors. Epidemiology and prevention of vaccine-preventable diseases. 10th ed. Washington (DC): Public Health Foundation, 2008. p. 159–74.

2. Reef SE, Redd SB, Abernathy E, et al. The epidemiological profile of rubella and congenital rubella syndrome in the United States, 1998–2004: the evidence for absence of endemic transmission. Clin Infect Dis. 2006;43(Suppl 3):S126–32.

3. Plotkin SA, Reef SE. Rubella vaccine. In: Plotkin SA, Orenstein WA, Offit PA, editors. Vaccines. 5th ed. Philadelphia: Saunders Elsevier; 2008. p. 735–71.

4. Reef SE, Cochi SL. The evidence for the elimination of rubella and congenital rubella syndrome in the United States: a public health achievement. Clin Infect Dis. 2006;43(Suppl 3):S123–5.

5. Meissner HC, Reef SE, Cochi S. Elimination of rubella from the United States: a milestone on the road to global elimination. Pediatrics. 2006;117(3):933–5.

6. Robertson SE, Featherstone DA, Gacic-Dobo M, et al. Rubella and congenital rubella syndrome: global update. Rev Panam Salud Publica. 2003;14(5):306–15.

7. Plotinsky RN, Talbot EA, Kellenberg JE, et al. Congenital rubella syndrome in a child born to Liberian refugees: clinical and public health perspectives. Clin Pediatr (Phila). 2007;46(4):349–55.

8. Watson JC, Hadler SC, Dykewicz CA, et al. Measles, mumps, and rubella-vaccine use and strategies for elimination of measles, rubella, congenital rubella syndrome and control of mumps: recommendations of the Advisory Committee on Immunization Practices (ACIP). MMWR Recomm Rep. 1998;47(RR-8):1–57.

9. Kroger AT, Atkinson WL, Marcuse EK, et al.; CDC. General recommendations on immunization: recommendations of the Advisory Committee on Immunization Practices (ACIP). MMWR Recomm Rep. 2006;55(RR-15):1–48.

TETANUS

M. Patricia Joyce

Infectious Agent

- *Clostridium tetani*, the tetanus bacillus, is a spore-forming, anaerobic gram-positive bacterium.
- Clinical disease is caused by a neurotoxin produced by anaerobic tetanus bacilli growing in contaminated wounds.

Mode of Transmission

- Tetanus is a global health problem because *C. tetani* spores are ubiquitous in the environment.
- Lesions that are considered "tetanus prone" are wounds contaminated with dirt, feces, or saliva, deep wounds, burns, crush injuries, or those with necrotic tissue.
- Tetanus has also been associated with apparently clean superficial wounds, surgical procedures, insect bites, dental infections, chronic sores and infections, and intravenous drug use.
- A reservoir of tetanus bacteria exists in the intestines of horses and other animals, including humans, in which the organism is a harmless normal inhabitant. Soil or fomites contaminated with animal and human feces propagate transmission.
- Tetanus has no direct person-to-person transmission.

Occurrence

- In 2006, an estimated 290,000 people worldwide died of tetanus, most of them in Asia, Africa, and South America.
- The disease occurs almost exclusively in persons who are inadequately immunized.
- Worldwide, the disease is more common in agricultural regions and in areas where contact with animal excreta is more likely and immunization is inadequate.
- In developing countries, tetanus in neonates born to unvaccinated mothers (neonatal tetanus) is the most common form of the disease.
- In 10% of reported cases in the United States, no antecedent wound was identified.

Risk for Travelers

Tetanus can occur anywhere in the world in inadequately vaccinated persons.

Clinical Presentation

- Acute manifestations of tetanus are characterized by muscle rigidity and painful spasms, often starting in the muscles of the jaw and neck. Severe tetanus can lead to respiratory failure and death.
- The incubation period is usually 3–21 days (average 10 days), although it may range from 1 day to several months, depending on the character, extent, and location of the wound. Most cases occur within 14 days. In general, shorter incubation periods are associated with more heavily contaminated wounds, more severe disease, and a worse prognosis.

Clinical Syndromes

Generalized Tetanus

- Generalized tetanus is the most common form, accounting for more than 80% of cases.
- Neonatal tetanus is generalized tetanus in neonates, usually due to umbilical stump infections.
- The average incubation period from injury to symptom onset is 7–8 days (range 3 days–3 weeks).
- The most common initial sign is trismus (spasm of the muscles of mastication or "lockjaw"). Trismus may be followed by painful spasms in other muscle groups in the neck, trunk, and extremities and by generalized, tonic, seizure-like activity or frank convulsions in severe cases.
- Generalized tetanus can be accompanied by autonomic nervous system abnormalities, as well as a variety of complications related to severe spasm and prolonged hospitalization.
- The clinical course of generalized tetanus is variable and depends on the degree of prior immunity, the amount of toxin present, and the age and general health of the patient.
- Even with modern intensive care, generalized tetanus is associated with mortality rates of 10%–20%.

Localized Tetanus

- Localized tetanus is an unusual form of the disease consisting of spasm of muscles in a confined area close to the site of the injury.
- Although localized tetanus often occurs in persons with partial immunity and is usually mild, progression to generalized tetanus can occur.

Cephalic Tetanus

- The rarest form, cephalic tetanus, is associated with lesions of the head or face and has been described in association with ear infections (i.e., otitis media).

- The incubation period is short, usually 1–2 days.
- Unlike generalized and localized tetanus, cephalic tetanus results in flaccid cranial nerve palsies rather than spasm. Trismus may also be present. Like localized tetanus, cephalic tetanus can progress to the generalized form.

Diagnosis

- The diagnosis is almost always made clinically.
- The disease is characterized by painful muscular contractions, primarily of the masseter and neck muscles, secondarily of trunk muscles.
- A common first sign suggestive of tetanus in older children and adults is abdominal rigidity, though rigidity is sometimes confined to the region of injury.
- Generalized spasms occur, frequently induced by sensory stimuli; typical features of the tetanic spasm are the position of opisthotonos and the facial expression known as "risus sardonicus."
- History of an injury or apparent portal of entry may be lacking.
- The organism is rarely recovered from the site of infection, and usually there is no detectable antibody response.

Treatment

- Tetanus is a medical emergency requiring hospitalization, immediate treatment with human tetanus immune globulin (TIG) (or equine antitoxin if human immune globulin is not available), a tetanus toxoid booster, agents to control muscle spasm, and, if indicated, aggressive wound care and antibiotics.
  - ○ Specific treatment: TIG administered intramuscularly in doses of 3000–6000 IU. If immunoglobulin is not available, tetanus antitoxin (equine origin) in a single large dose should be given intravenously, following testing for hypersensitivity.
- Metronidazole is the most appropriate antibiotic. It is associated with the shortest recovery time and lowest case–fatality rate. It should be given for 7–14 days in large doses; this also allows for a reduction in the amount of muscle relaxants and sedatives required.
- The wound should be debrided widely and excised if possible. Wide debridement of the umbilical stump in neonates is not indicated.
- Depending on the severity of disease, mechanical ventilation and agents to control autonomic nervous system instability may be required.
- An adequate airway should be maintained, and sedation should be used as indicated; muscle relaxant drugs, together with tracheostomy or nasotracheal intubation and mechanically assisted respiration, may be lifesaving.
- Active immunization should be initiated concurrently with treatment.

Preventive Measures for Travelers

- Travelers should ensure they have adequate immunity to tetanus.
  - ○ Active immunity is induced by tetanus toxoid and persists for at least 10 years after full immunization; transient passive immunity follows injection of TIG or tetanus antitoxin (equine origin).
  - ○ Infants of actively immunized mothers acquire passive immunity that protects them from neonatal tetanus.
  - ○ Recovery from tetanus may not result in immunity; second attacks can occur, and primary immunization is indicated after recovery.
- Wounded travelers who received their most recent tetanus toxoid-containing vaccine more than 5 years previously or who have not received at least three doses

of tetanus toxoid-containing vaccines may require a dose of tetanus toxoid-containing vaccine (Tdap, Td, or DTaP), depending on the nature of the wound.

- Human tetanus immune globulin (TIG) is indicated in travelers with tetanus-prone wounds who have an unknown or incomplete history of primary tetanus vaccination.

General Preventive Measures

- Universal active immunization with adsorbed tetanus toxoid, gives durable protection for at least 10 years; after the initial basic series has been completed, single booster doses elicit high levels of immunity.
- In children <7 years of age, the toxoid is generally administered together with diphtheria toxoid and pertussis vaccine as a triple (DTP or DTaP) antigen, or as a double (DT) antigen when contraindications to pertussis vaccine exist.
- Td is used for children >7 years of age.
- For adolescents 11–12 years of age, a single dose of Tdap is recommended for routine booster, and for adolescents and adults 13–64 years of age, a single dose of Tdap is recommended to replace the next decennial Td booster or when indicated as part of wound prophylaxis.
- In countries with incomplete immunization programs for children, all pregnant women should receive two doses of tetanus toxoid in the first pregnancy, with an interval of at least 1 month, and with the second dose at least 2 weeks prior to childbirth.
- Vaccine-induced maternal immunity is important in preventing maternal and neonatal tetanus. Active protection should be maintained by administering booster doses of Td every 10 years, preferably before or between pregnancies.
- For children and adults who are severely immunocompromised or infected with HIV, tetanus toxoid is indicated in the same schedule and dose as for immunocompetent persons even though the immune response may be suboptimal.
- Minor local reactions following tetanus toxoid injections are relatively frequent; severe local and systemic reactions are infrequent but do occur, particularly after excessive numbers of prior doses have been given.

Prophylaxis in Wound Management (see Table 2-21)

- Tetanus prophylaxis in patients with wounds is based on careful assessment of whether the wound is clean or contaminated, the immunization status of the patient, proper use of tetanus toxoid and/or TIG, wound cleaning and, where required, surgical debridement and the proper use of antibiotics.
- Those who have been completely immunized and who sustain minor and uncontaminated wounds require a booster dose of toxoid only if more than 10 years have elapsed since the last dose was given. For major or contaminated wounds, a single booster injection of tetanus toxoid (preferably as Td or Tdap) should be administered promptly on the day of injury if the patient has not received tetanus toxoid within the preceding 5 years.
- Persons who have not completed a full primary series of tetanus toxoid require a dose of toxoid as soon as possible following the wound and may require passive immunization with human TIG if the wound is major or if it is contaminated with soil containing animal excreta. DTP/DTaP, DT, or Td, as determined by the age of the patient and previous immunization history, should be used at the time of the wound and ultimately to complete the primary series.
- Passive immunization with at least 250 IU of TIG intramuscularly (or 1,500 to 5,000 IU of antitoxin of animal origin, if globulin is not available), regardless of the patient's age, is indicated for patients with other than clean, minor wounds and a history of no, unknown, or fewer than three previous tetanus toxoid doses. When tetanus toxoid and TIG or antitoxin are given concurrently, separate syringes and separate sites must be used.

Table 2-21. Summary guide to tetanus prophylaxis in routine wound management[1]

History of Tetanus Immunization (Doses)	Clean, Minor Wounds		All Other Wounds	
	Td[2]	TIG	Td[2]	TIG
Uncertain or <3 doses	Yes	No	Yes	Yes
3 or more doses	No[3]	No	No[4]	No

1 Important details in the text.
2 For children <7 years old, DTaP or DTP (DT, if pertussis vaccine contraindicated) preferred to tetanus toxoid alone. For children ≥7 years of age, Td preferred to tetanus toxoid alone. For adolescents and adults to age 64, tetanus toxoid as Tdap is preferred, if the patient has not previously been vaccinated with Tdap.
3 Yes, if more than 10 years since last dose.
4 Yes, if more than 5 years since last dose. More frequent boosters are not needed and can accentuate side effects.

References

1. Kretsinger K, Broder KR, Cortese MM, et al. Preventing tetanus, diphtheria, and pertussis among adults: use of tetanus toxoid, reduced diphtheria toxoid and acellular pertussis vaccine. Recommendations of the Advisory Committee on Immunization Practices (ACIP), supported by the Healthcare Infection Control Practices Advisory Committee (HICPAC), for use of Tdap among health-care personnel. MMWR Recomm Rep. 2006;55(RR-17):1–37.

2. Broder KR, Cortese MM, Iskander JK, et al. Preventing tetanus, diphtheria, and pertussis among adolescents: use of tetanus toxoid, reduced diphtheria toxoid and acellular pertussis vaccines. Recommendations of the Advisory Committee on Immunization Practices (ACIP). MMWR Recomm Rep. 2006;55(RR-3):1–34.

3. Roper MH, Vandelaer JH, Gasse FL. Maternal and neonatal tetanus. Lancet. 2007;370(9603):1947–59.

4. Wassilak SGF, Roper MH, Kretsinger K, Orenstein WA. Tetanus toxoid. In: Plotkin SA, Orenstein WA, Offit PA, editors. Vaccines. 5th ed. Philadelphia: Saunders Elsevier; 2008:805–39.

5. Vandelaer J, Birmingham M, Gasse F, et al. Tetanus in developing countries: an update on the Maternal and Neonatal Tetanus Elimination Initiative. Vaccine. 2003;21(24):3442–5.

6. Murphy TV, Slade BA, Broder KR, et al. Prevention of pertussis, tetanus, and diphtheria among pregnant and postpartum women and their infants. Recommendations of the Advisory Committee on Immunization. Practices (ACIP). MMWR Recomm Rep. 2008;57(RR-4):1–51.

7. Hsu SS, Groleau G. Tetanus in the emergency department: a current review. J Emerg Med. 2001;20(4):357–65.

8. Pascual FB, McGinley EL, Zanardi LR, et al. Tetanus surveillance—United States, 1998–2000. MMWR Surveill Summ. 2003;52(3):1–8.

9. Farrar JJ, Yen LM, Cook T, et al. Tetanus. J Neurol Neurosurg Psychiatry. 2000;69(3):292–301.

10. American Academy of Pediatrics. Tetanus (lockjaw). In: Pickering LK, Baker CH, Long SS, McMillan JA, editors. Red Book: 2006 Report of the Committee on Infectious Diseases. 27th ed. Elk Grove Village, IL: American Academy of Pediatrics; 2006: p. 648–53.

VARICELLA (CHICKENPOX)

Kathleen H. Harriman, Gilberto F. Chavez

Infectious Agent

- Varicella-zoster virus (VZV) is a member of the herpesvirus family.
- Humans are the only reservoir of the virus, and disease occurs only in humans.

Mode of Transmission

- VZV is transmitted from person to person by direct contact, inhalation of aerosols from vesicular fluid of skin lesions of acute varicella or zoster, or infected respiratory tract secretions that might also be aerosolized.
- The virus enters the host through the upper respiratory tract or the conjunctiva.

- In utero infection can also occur as a result of transplacental passage of virus during maternal varicella infection.
- The period of contagiousness is estimated to begin 1–2 days before the onset of rash and to end when all lesions are crusted, typically 4–7 days after onset of rash in immunocompetent persons, but this period may be longer in immunocompromised persons.

Occurrence

- Varicella occurs worldwide. In temperate climates, varicella tends to be a childhood disease, with peak incidence during late winter and early spring. In tropical climates, infection tends to occur at older ages, resulting in higher susceptibility among adults than in temperate climates.
- Before introduction of varicella vaccine in the United States in 1995, varicella was endemic, and virtually all persons were infected by adulthood. Since implementation of the varicella vaccination program, the epidemiology and clinical characteristics of varicella have changed, with substantial declines in morbidity and mortality. The incidence of varicella has steadily declined in all age groups, with the greatest decline among children 1–4 years of age.

Risk for Travelers

- Varicella vaccine is routinely used for vaccination of healthy children in only some countries, including the United States, Uruguay, Qatar, Australia, Canada, Costa Rica, Germany, and South Korea.
- The risk for varicella infection is higher for people traveling to most other parts of the world than it is in the United States. However, VZV is still widely circulating in the United States. Additionally, exposure to herpes zoster (shingles), while less common than varicella, poses a risk for varicella infection in susceptible travelers.
- Travelers at highest risk for severe varicella disease are immunocompromised persons or pregnant women without a history of varicella disease or vaccination.

Clinical Presentation

- Varicella is generally a mild disease in children. It usually lasts 4–7 days and is characterized by a short (1- to 2-day) or absent prodromal period (low-grade fever, malaise) and by a pruritic rash consisting of crops of macules, papules, and vesicles (on average 250–500 lesions), which appear in three or more successive waves and resolve by crusting.
- Serious complications are the exception but can occur, mainly in infants, adolescents, adults, and immunocompromised persons. They include secondary bacterial infections of skin lesions, pneumonia, cerebellar ataxia, and encephalitis.
- The average incubation period for varicella is 14–16 days (range 10–21 days).
- A modified varicella, known as breakthrough disease, can occur in some vaccinated persons, because the vaccine is 70%–90% effective in preventing disease. Breakthrough varicella is most commonly (~70%–80% of cases) mild, with <50 skin lesions, less fever, and shorter duration of rash. The rash may be atypical in appearance with fewer vesicles and predominance of maculopapular lesions. Nevertheless, breakthrough varicella is infectious (although less than varicella in unvaccinated persons). Persons with breakthrough varicella should be isolated for as long as lesions persist.

Diagnosis

- Skin lesions are the preferred specimen for laboratory confirmation of varicella disease.

- Vesicular fluid or a scab can be used to identify VZV by using polymerase chain reaction (PCR). Rapid diagnostic tests (PCR, direct fluorescent antibody) are the methods of choice.
- VZV can also be isolated from scrapings of a vesicle base during the first 3–4 days of the eruption.
- Collecting skin lesion specimens from breakthrough cases can be challenging because the rash is often maculopapular with few or no vesicles. If lesions are not present, scraping of the lesion is recommended.
- Serologic tests for confirmation of disease:
  - A significant rise in serum varicella IgG antibody from acute- and convalescent-phase samples by any standard serologic assay can confirm a diagnosis retrospectively, but may not be reliable in immunocompromised people.
  - Commercially available tests are not sufficiently sensitive to reliably demonstrate vaccine-induced immunity.

Postexposure Prophylaxis

Vaccine

- Varicella vaccine is recommended for postexposure administration for healthy unvaccinated persons without other evidence of immunity.
- Administration of varicella vaccine to exposed susceptible persons ≥12 months of age, as soon as possible within 72 hours and possibly up to 120 hours after exposure, may prevent or modify disease and is recommended if there are no contraindications to use. In several studies, protective efficacy was reported as ≥90% when children were vaccinated within 3 days of exposure.

Use of Varicella Zoster Immune Globulin (VZIG)

- In certain circumstances, postexposure prophylaxis with VZIG is recommended.
- The decision to administer VZIG to a person exposed to varicella should be based on 1) whether the person is susceptible, 2) whether the exposure is likely to result in infection, and 3) whether the person is at greater risk for complications than the general population.
- Persons at greater risk for severe complications who are not candidates for varicella vaccination who may benefit from postexposure prophylaxis with VZIG include:
  - susceptible immunocompromised persons (including people being treated with chronic corticosteroids ≥2 mg/kg of body weight or a total of 20 mg/day of prednisone or equivalent)
  - susceptible pregnant women
  - newborns whose mothers had onset of varicella within 5 days before and 2 days after delivery
  - preterm infants at ≥28 weeks gestation whose mothers are susceptible to varicella
  - preterm infants at <28 weeks gestation or ≤1,000 g birth weight, regardless of maternal history or serostatus.
- VZIG provides maximum benefit when administered as soon as possible after exposure, but may be effective if administered as late as 96 hours after exposure.
- The product currently in use in the United States, VariZIG, is available under an Investigational New Drug protocol and can be obtained from the sole authorized U.S. distributor, FFF enterprises (Temecula, California) (24-hour telephone, 800-843-7477 or www.fffenterprises.com).
- If administration of VariZIG does not appear possible within 96 hours of exposure, administration of immune globulin intravenous (IGIV) should be considered as an alternative (IGIV should also be administered within 96 hours of exposure).

Treatment

- Oral acyclovir is not recommended for routine use in healthy children with varicella but should be considered for otherwise healthy people at increased risk for moderate to severe disease, e.g.: persons aged >12 years; people with chronic cutaneous or pulmonary disorders; receiving long-term salicylate therapy; and receiving short, intermittent or aerosolized courses of corticosteroids.
- Intravenous antiviral therapy, when administered within 24 hours of onset of rash is recommended for immunocompromised persons, including patients being treated with chronic corticosteroids.

Preventive Measures for Travelers

Although vaccination against varicella is not a requirement for entry into any country (including the United States), persons traveling or living abroad should ensure that they are immune.

Vaccine

- Varicella vaccine contains live, attenuated VZV. It is available as a monovalent formulation and in combination formulation, as measles–mumps–rubella–varicella (MMRV) vaccine, which is licensed in the United States for children 1–12 years only.
- Two doses of varicella-containing vaccine are now recommended for all susceptible persons older than one year without contraindications. The first dose should be administered at 12–15 months of age and the second dose at 4–6 years of age. A second catch-up dose of varicella vaccination is recommended for children, adolescents and adults who previously have received one dose. The minimum interval for children younger than 13 years is 3 months. The ACIP now recommends that all others at least 13 years of age without evidence of immunity be vaccinated with two doses of varicella vaccine at an interval of 4–8 weeks. In case of uncertainty, prior varicella disease is not a contraindication to varicella vaccination.
- Evidence of immunity to varicella includes any of the following:
  - Documentation of age-appropriate vaccination:
    - Preschool-age children aged ≥12 months: 1 dose
    - School-age children, adolescents, and adults: 2 doses
  - Laboratory evidence of immunity or laboratory confirmation of disease
  - Birth in the United States before 1980 (not a criterion for health-care personnel, pregnant women, and immunocompromised persons)
  - A health-care provider diagnosis of varicella or a health-care provider verification of a history of varicella disease
  - A health-care provider diagnosis of herpes zoster or a health-care provider verification of a history of herpes zoster disease

Adverse Reactions

- The most common adverse reactions following varicella vaccine are injection site complaints (pain, soreness, redness, and swelling) that are self-limited. Fever was reported in uncontrolled trials in 15% of children and 10% of adolescents and adults. A macular or vaccine rash usually consisting of a few lesions at the injection site was reported in 3% and 1% of persons receiving the first and second dose, respectively. A generalized rash with a small number of lesions may rarely occur, within 3 weeks of vaccination.
- Varicella vaccine is a live-virus vaccine that induces latent infection similar to that caused by wild VZV. Consequently, zoster caused by vaccine virus has been reported. This appears to occur at a lower rate than following natural infection but longer term follow-up is needed.

Contraindications

Allergy

- Persons with severe allergy (hives, swelling of the mouth or throat, difficulty breathing, hypotension, and shock) to gelatin or neomycin or who have had a severe allergic reaction to a prior dose of vaccine should not be vaccinated.
- Single-antigen varicella vaccine does not contain egg protein or preservative. For the combination MMRV vaccine, live measles and live mumps vaccine are produced in chick embryo culture. However, the risk for serious allergic reactions after administration of measles- or mumps-containing vaccines in persons who are allergic to eggs is low.

Altered Immunity

Persons with immunosuppression of cellular immune function resulting from leukemia, lymphomas of any type, generalized malignancy, immunodeficiency disease, or immuno-suppressive therapy should not be vaccinated. Treatment with low-dose prednisone (e.g., <2 mg/kg of body weight/day or <20 mg/day) or aerosolized steroid preparations is not a contraindication to varicella vaccination. Persons whose immunosuppressive therapy with steroids has been stopped for 1 month (3 months for chemotherapy) may be vaccinated. In addition, persons with impaired humoral immunity may now be vaccinated. Because children infected with HIV are at greater risk for morbidity from varicella and herpes zoster than are healthy children, the ACIP recommends that varicella vaccine should be considered for HIV-infected children at least 12 months of age with CD4+ T-lymphocyte percentages ≥15% and without evidence of varicella immunity. Eligible children should receive two doses of single-antigen varicella vaccine, with a minimum 3-month interval between doses. Vaccination (two doses, administered 3 months apart) may be considered for HIV-infected older children, adolescents and adults with CD4+ T-lymphocyte count ≥200 cells/mL, after weighing the risks and benefits.

Pregnancy

Women known to be pregnant or attempting to become pregnant should not receive varicella vaccine. Pregnancy should be avoided for 1 month following varicella vaccination. Breastfeeding is not a contraindication to the varicella vaccination.

Precautions

Illness

Vaccination of persons who have acute severe illness, including untreated, active tuberculosis, should be postponed until recovery.

Recent Administration of Blood, Plasma, or Immune Globulin

The effect of the administration of immune globulin (IG) on the response to varicella virus vaccine is unknown. Because of the potential inhibition of the antibody response by passively transferred antibodies, varicella vaccines should not be administered for 3–11 months, depending on the dosage, after administration of blood (except washed red cells), plasma, or IG.

Use of Salicylates

No adverse events following varicella vaccination related to the use of salicylates (e.g., aspirin) have been reported to date. However, the manufacturer recommends that vaccine recipients avoid the use of salicylates for 6 weeks after receiving varicella vaccine because of the association between aspirin use and Reye syndrome following varicella.

References

1. CDC. Prevention of varicella. Recommendations of the Advisory Committee on Immunization Practices (ACIP). MMWR Morbid Mortal Wkly Rep. 2007;56(RR-4):1–40.
2. Gershon AA, Takahasi M, Seward J. Varicella vaccine. In: Plotkin SA, Orenstein WA, editors. Vaccines. 4th ed. Philadelphia: W.B. Saunders; 2004:783–823.
3. Seward JF, Watson BM, Peterson CL, et al. Varicella disease after introduction of varicella vaccine in the United States, 1995–2000. JAMA. 2002;287(5):606–11.

4. CDC. Decline in annual incidence of varicella-selected states, 1990–2001. MMWR Morbid Mortal Wkly Rep. 2003;52(37):884–5.
5. Guris D, Jumaan AO, Mascola L, et al. Changing varicella epidemiology in active surveillance sites—United States, 1995–2005. J Infect Dis. 2008;197(Suppl 2):S71–5.
6. WHO. Immunization summary: The 2007 edition. [cited 2008 April 14]. Available from: http://www.unicef.org/publications/files/Immunization_Summary_2007.pdf
7. CDC. A new product (VariZIG) for postexposure prophylaxis of varicella available under an Investigational New Drug application expanded access protocol. MMWR Morbid Mortal Wkly Rep. 2006;55:1–2.
8. Kuter B, Matthews H, Shinefield H, et al. Ten year follow-up of healthy children who received one or two injections of varicella vaccine. Pediatr Infect Dis J. 2004;23(2):132–7.
9. Seward JF. Update on varicella. Pediatr Infect Dis J. 2001;20(6):19–21.
10. Harpaz R, Ortega-Sanchez IR, Seward JF. Prevention of herpes zoster. Recommendations of the Advisory Committee on Immunization Practices (ACIP). MMWR Recomm Rep. 2008;57(RR-05):1–30.

Malaria

MALARIA

Paul M. Arguin, Stefanie F. Steele

Infectious Agent

Malaria in humans is caused by one of four protozoan species of the genus *Plasmodium*: *P. falciparum*, *P. vivax*, *P. ovale*, or *P. malariae*. Recently, *P. knowlesi*, a parasite of Old World monkeys, has been documented as a cause of human infections and some fatalities in Southeast Asia. Investigations are ongoing to determine the extent of its transmission to humans.

Mode of Transmission

All species are transmitted by the bite of an infected female *Anopheles* mosquito. Occasionally, transmission occurs by blood transfusion, organ transplantation, needle sharing, or congenitally from mother to fetus.

Occurrence

- Each year malaria causes 350–500 million infections worldwide and approximately 1 million deaths.
- Transmission occurs in large areas of Central and South America, parts of the Caribbean, Africa, Asia (including South Asia, Southeast Asia, and the Middle East), Eastern Europe, and the South Pacific (Maps 2-7 and 2-8).
- Information about malaria transmission in specific countries (see the Malaria Risk Information and Prophylaxis, by Country, section later in this chapter) is derived from various sources, including WHO.
- Tools such as the interactive malaria map can assist in locating more unusual destinations and determining if malaria transmission occurs there (see www.cdc.gov/malaria/risk_map/).

Risk for Travelers

- The risk for a traveler acquiring malaria differs substantially from region to region and from traveler to traveler, even within a single country.

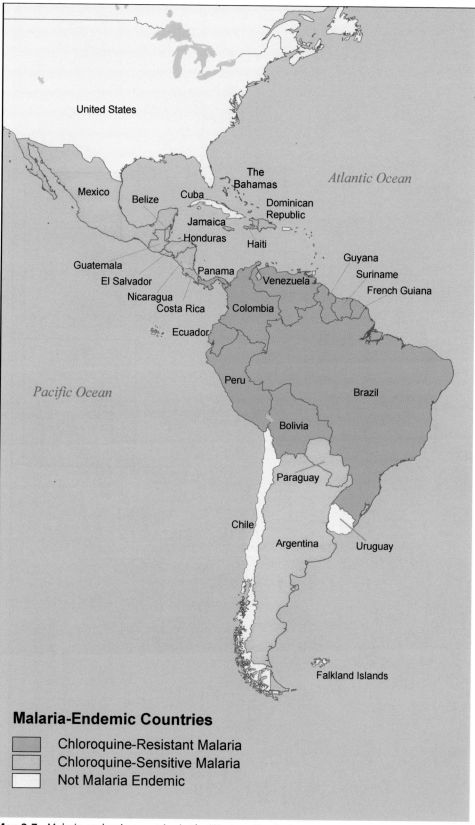

Malaria-Endemic Countries

☐ Chloroquine-Resistant Malaria
☐ Chloroquine-Sensitive Malaria
☐ Not Malaria Endemic

Map 2-7. Malaria-endemic countries in the Western Hemisphere.

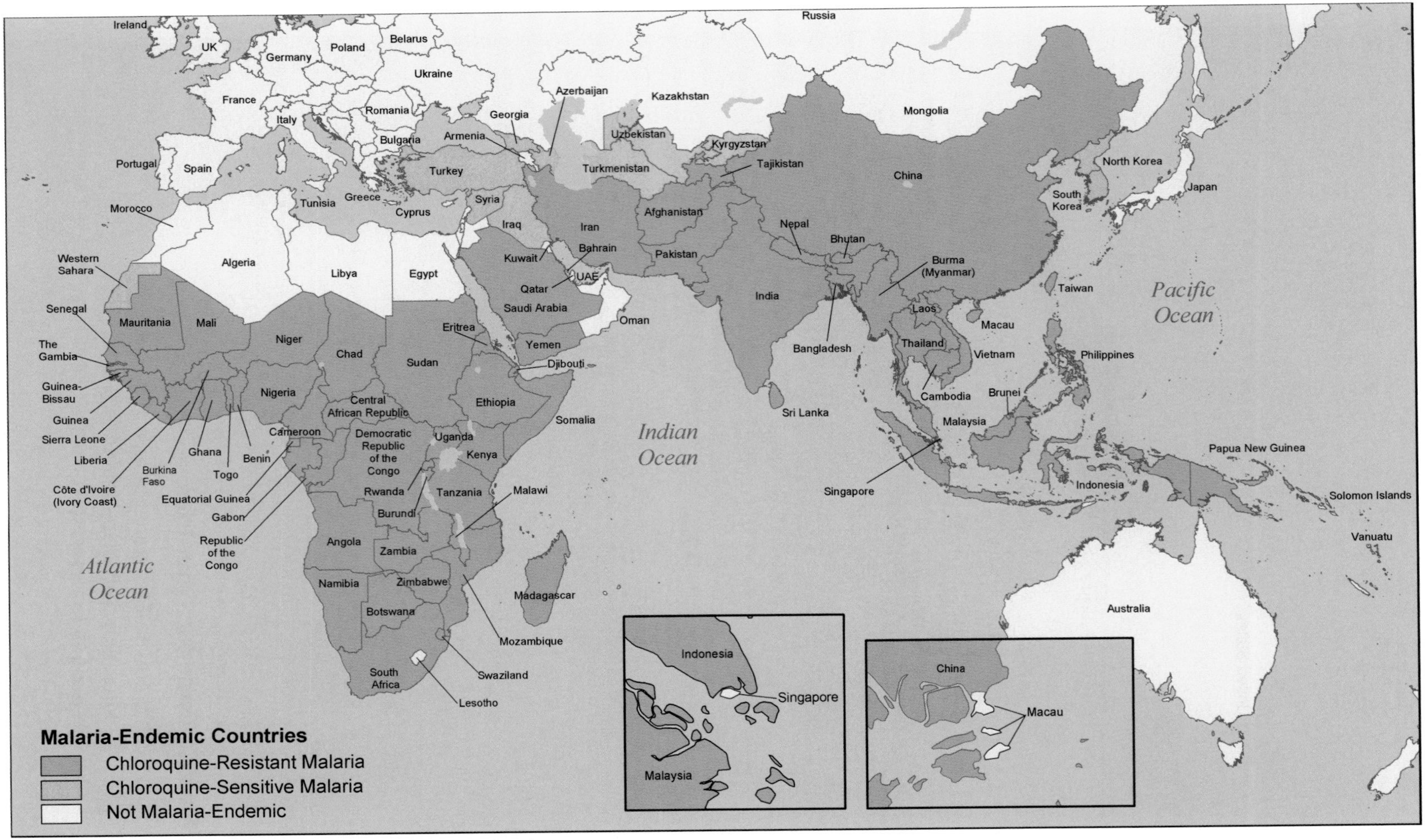

Malaria-Endemic Countries

- � Chloroquine-Resistant Malaria
- ▢ Chloroquine-Sensitive Malaria
- ▢ Not Malaria-Endemic

Map 2-8. Malaria-endemic countries in the Eastern Hemisphere.

- From 1997 through 2006, 10,745 cases of malaria among U.S. residents were reported to CDC. Of these, 6,376 (59.3%) were acquired in sub-Saharan Africa; 1,498 (13.9%) in Asia; 1,427 (13.3%) in the Caribbean and Central and South America; and 278 (0.03%) in Oceania. During this period, 54 fatal malaria infections occurred among U.S. residents; 46 (85.2%) were caused by *P. falciparum*, of which 33 (71.1%) were acquired in sub-Saharan Africa.
- These absolute numbers of cases should be considered within the context of the volume of travel to these locations. Regions with the highest estimated relative risk for infection for travelers are West Africa and Oceania. Regions with moderate estimated relative risk for infection are the other parts of Africa, South Asia, and South America. Regions with lower estimated relative risk are Central America and other parts of Asia. There is considerable country-by-country variation, as well as variable transmission within countries and sometimes seasonal variation.
- Prevention of malaria involves striking a balance between ensuring that all people who will be at risk for infection use the appropriate prevention measures, while preventing adverse effects of those interventions among people using them unnecessarily. An individual risk assessment should be conducted for every traveler, taking into account not only the destination country, but also the detailed itinerary, including specific cities, types of accommodation, season, and style of travel. In addition, conditions such as pregnancy or the presence of antimalarial drug resistance at the destination may modify the risk assessment.
- Depending on level of risk, it may be appropriate to recommend no specific interventions, mosquito avoidance measures only, or mosquito avoidance measures plus chemoprophylaxis.
- For areas of intense transmission, such as West Africa, exposure for even short periods of time can result in transmission, so this area should be considered high risk.
- Malaria risk is not distributed homogeneously throughout all countries. Some destinations have malaria transmission occurring throughout the whole country, while in others it occurs in defined pockets. If travelers are going to the high-risk pockets during peak transmission times, even though the country as a whole may be low risk, this destination for this individual may be high risk.
- Geography is just one part of determining a traveler's risk for infection. Risk can differ substantially for different travelers if their behaviors and circumstances differ. For example, travelers staying in air-conditioned hotels may be at lower risk than backpackers or adventure travelers. Similarly, long-term residents living in screened and air-conditioned housing are less likely to be exposed than are persons living without such amenities.
- The highest risk is associated with first- and second-generation immigrants living in nonendemic countries who return to their countries of origin to visit friends and relatives (VFRs). VFR travelers often consider themselves to be at no risk because they grew up in a malarious country and consider themselves immune. However, acquired immunity is lost very quickly, and VFRs should be considered as having the same risk as otherwise nonimmune travelers.
- Travelers should also be reminded that even if one has had malaria before, one can get it again and preventive measures are still necessary. All travelers going to malaria-endemic countries, even for short periods of time, such as cruise ship passengers, may be at risk for becoming infected with malaria.
- Persons who have been in an area where malaria transmission occurs, either during daytime or nighttime hours, are not permitted to donate blood in the United States for a period of time after returning from the malarious area. Persons who are residents of nonmalarious countries are not permitted to donate blood for 1 year after they have returned from a malarious area. Persons who are residents of malarious countries are not permitted to donate blood for 3 years after leaving a malarious area. Persons who have had malaria are not allowed to donate blood for 3 years after treatment for malaria.

- Risk assessments may differ between travel medicine providers and blood banks. A travel medicine provider advising a traveler going to a relatively low-risk country for a short period of time and engaging in behaviors that place them at lower risk for exposure may choose insect avoidance only and no chemoprophylaxis for the traveler. However, upon the traveler's return, a blood bank may still choose to defer that traveler for 1 year because of the travel to an area where transmission occurs.

Clinical Presentation

- Malaria is characterized by fever and influenza-like symptoms, including chills, headache, myalgias, and malaise; these symptoms can occur at intervals.
- Uncomplicated disease may be associated with anemia and jaundice. In severe disease, most commonly caused by *P. falciparum*, seizures, mental confusion, kidney failure, acute respiratory disease syndrome (ARDS), coma, and death may occur.
- Malaria symptoms can develop as early as 7 days (usually at least 14 days) after initial exposure in a malaria-endemic area and as late as several months or more after departure.

Diagnosis

- Travelers who have symptoms of malaria should be advised to seek medical evaluation **as soon as possible**.
- Smear microscopy remains the gold standard for malaria diagnosis. Microscopy can also be used to determine the species of malaria parasite and quantify the parasitemia—both of which are necessary pieces of information for providing the most appropriate treatment.
- Various test kits are available to detect antigens derived from malaria parasites. Such immunologic (immunochromatographic) tests most often use a dipstick or cassette format and provide results in 2–15 minutes. These rapid diagnostic tests (RDTs) offer a useful alternative to microscopy in situations where reliable microscopic diagnosis is not available. The U.S. Food and Drug Administration (FDA) has approved one RDT for use in the United States by hospital and commercial laboratories, not by individual clinicians or by patients themselves. This RDT, called BinaxNOW Malaria test, is produced by Inverness Medical Professional Diagnostics, located in Scarborough, Maine.
- Polymerase chain reaction (PCR) tests are also available for detecting malaria parasites; however, none are FDA-approved. Although these tests are slightly more sensitive than routine microscopy, results are not usually available as quickly as microscopy results should be, thus limiting the clinical utility of this test. PCR testing can be used to determine the species of the parasite if the microscopic results are ambiguous.
- In sub-Saharan Africa, the rate of false-positive blood films for malaria may be very high. Travelers to this region should be warned they may be diagnosed with malaria incorrectly, even though they are taking a reliable antimalarial regimen. In such cases, acutely ill travelers should be advised to seek the best available medical services and follow the treatment offered locally (except the use of halofantrine which is not recommended; see below), but **not** to stop their chemoprophylaxis regimen.

Treatment

- Malaria can be treated effectively early in the course of the disease, but delay of appropriate therapy can have serious or even fatal consequences.
- Travelers who have symptoms of malaria should be advised to seek medical evaluation **as soon as possible**.

- Specific treatment options depend on the species of malaria, the likelihood of drug resistance (based on the location of acquisition of infection), the age of the patient, pregnancy status, and the severity of infection. If possible, it is advisable to consult with a provider who has specialized travel/tropical medicine expertise or with an infectious disease physician.
- CDC recommendations for malaria treatment can be found at www.cdc.gov/malaria/diagnosis_treatment/treatment.htm.
- Medications that are not used in the United States for the treatment of malaria, such as halofantrine (Halfan), are widely available overseas. CDC does not recommend halofantrine for treatment because of cardiac adverse events, including deaths, which have been documented following treatment doses. These adverse events have occurred in persons with and without pre-existing cardiac problems and both in the presence and absence of other antimalarial drugs (e.g., mefloquine).

Self-Treatment (Table 2-22)

- Travelers who reject the advice to take prophylaxis, who choose a suboptimal drug regimen (e.g., chloroquine in an area with chloroquine-resistant *P. falciparum*), or who require a less-than-optimal drug regimen for medical reasons are at greater risk for acquiring malaria and needing prompt treatment.
- Travelers who are taking effective prophylaxis but who will be in very remote areas may decide, in consultation with their health-care provider, to take along a full course of an approved malaria treatment regimen for self-treatment. This should occur very rarely.
- Travelers should be advised to take their presumptive self-treatment promptly if they have fever, chills, or other influenza-like illness and if professional medical care is not available within 24 hours. **Travelers should be advised that this self-treatment of a possible malarial infection is only a temporary measure and that prompt medical evaluation is imperative**.
- Atovaquone/proguanil may be used for presumptive self-treatment for travelers NOT taking atovaquone/proguanil for prophylaxis. If taking atovaquone/proguanil for prophylaxis, the use of the same drug at therapeutic doses is not recommended to empirically treat fever (suspected malaria). The CDC Malaria Branch (Malaria Hotline 770-488-7788) can provide consultation to health-care providers on other potential options for self-treatment if atovaquone/proguanil cannot be used.

Table 2-22. Presumptive self-treatment of malaria

Drug	Adult Dose	Pediatric Dose	Comments
Atovaquone/proguanil (Malarone). Self-treatment drug to be used if professional medical care is not available within 24 hours. Medical care should be sought immediately after treatment.	4 tablets (each dose contains 1,000 mg atovaquone and 400 mg proguanil) orally as a single daily dose for 3 consecutive days	Daily dose to be taken for 3 consecutive days: 5–8 kg: 2 pediatric tablets; 9–10 kg: 3 pediatric tablets; 11–20 kg: 1 adult tablet; 21–30 kg: 2 adult tablets; 31–40 kg: 3 adult tablets; >41 kg: 4 adult tablets	Contraindicated in persons with severe renal impairment (creatinine clearance <30 mL/min). Not recommended for self-treatment in persons on atovaquone/proguanil prophylaxis. Not currently recommended for children <5 kg, pregnant women, and women breastfeeding infants weighing <5 kg

Malaria Hotline

- Health-care professionals who require assistance with the diagnosis or treatment of malaria should call the CDC Malaria Hotline (770-488-7788) from 8:00 am to 4:30 pm Eastern time. After hours or on weekends and holidays, health-care providers requiring assistance should call the CDC Emergency Operations Center at 770-488-7100 and ask the operator to page the person on call for the Malaria Branch.
- Information on diagnosis and treatment is available at www.cdc.gov/malaria.

Preventive Measures for Travelers

Malaria prevention consists of a combination of mosquito avoidance measures and chemoprophylaxis. Although very efficacious, none of the recommended interventions are 100% effective.

Mosquito Avoidance Measures

- Because of the nocturnal feeding habits of *Anopheles* mosquitoes, malaria transmission occurs primarily between dusk and dawn.
- Contact with mosquitoes can be reduced by remaining in well-screened areas, using mosquito bed nets (preferably insecticide-treated nets), using a pyrethroid-containing flying-insect spray in living and sleeping areas during evening and nighttime hours, and wearing clothes that cover most of the body.
- All travelers should use an effective mosquito repellent.
- The most effective repellent against a wide range of vectors is DEET (*N,N*-diethyl-metatoluamide), an ingredient in many commercially available insect repellents. The actual concentration of DEET varies widely among repellents. DEET formulations as high as 50% are recommended for both adults and children older than 2 months of age (see the Protection Against Mosquitoes, Ticks, and Other Insects and Arthropods section later in this chapter). DEET should be applied to the exposed parts of the skin when mosquitoes are likely to be present.
- In addition to using a topical insect repellent, a permethrin-containing product may be applied to bed nets and clothing for additional protection against mosquitoes.

Chemoprophylaxis

- All currently recommended primary chemoprophylaxis regimens involve taking a medicine before travel, during travel, and for a period of time after leaving the malaria endemic area. Beginning the drug before travel allows the antimalarial agent to be in the blood before the traveler is exposed to malaria parasites.
- Presumptive antirelapse therapy (also known as terminal prophylaxis) uses a medication towards the end of the exposure period (or immediately thereafter) to prevent relapses or delayed-onset clinical presentations of malaria caused by hypnozoites (dormant liver stages) of *P. vivax* or *P. ovale*. Because most malarious areas of the world (except the Caribbean) have at least one species of relapsing malaria, travelers to these areas have some risk for acquiring either *P. vivax* or *P. ovale*, although the actual risk for an individual traveler is difficult to define. Presumptive anti-relapse therapy is generally indicated only for persons who have had prolonged exposure in malaria-endemic areas (e.g., missionaries, volunteers).
- In choosing an appropriate chemoprophylactic regimen before travel, the traveler and the health-care provider should consider several factors. The travel itinerary should be reviewed in detail and compared with the information on where malaria transmission occurs within a given country (see the Malaria Risk Information and Prophylaxis, by Country, section later in this chapter) to determine whether the traveler will actually be traveling in a part of the country

where malaria occurs and if significant antimalarial drug resistance has been reported in that location.

- The resistance of *P. falciparum* to chloroquine has been confirmed in all areas with *P. falciparum* malaria except the Caribbean, Central America west of the Panama Canal, and some countries in the Middle East. In addition, resistance to sulfadoxine–pyrimethamine (e.g., Fansidar) is widespread in the Amazon River Basin area of South America, much of Southeast Asia, other parts of Asia, and in large parts of Africa. Resistance to mefloquine has been confirmed on the borders of Thailand with Burma (Myanmar) and Cambodia, in the western provinces of Cambodia, in the eastern states of Burma (Myanmar), on the border between Burma and China, along the borders of Laos and Burma, and the adjacent parts of the Thailand–Cambodia border, as well as in southern Vietnam (Map 2-9).
- Additional factors to consider are the patient's other medical conditions, medications being taken (to assess potential drug–drug interactions), the cost of the medicines, and the potential side effects.
- The medications recommended for chemoprophylaxis of malaria may also be available at overseas destinations. However, combinations of these medications and additional drugs that are not recommended may be commonly prescribed and used in other countries. Travelers should be strongly discouraged from obtaining chemoprophylactic medications while abroad. The quality of these products is not known, and they may not be protective and may be dangerous. These medications may have been produced by substandard manufacturing practices, may be counterfeit, or may contain contaminants. Additional information on this topic can be found in *Perspectives:* Counterfeit Drugs later in this chapter and in an FDA document Purchasing Medications Outside the United States (www.fda.gov/ora/import/purchasing_medications.htm).

Medications Used for Chemoprophylaxis

Atovaquone/Proguanil (Malarone)

- Atovaquone/proguanil is a fixed combination of the two drugs, atovaquone and proguanil.
- Prophylaxis should begin 1–2 days before travel to malarious areas and should be taken daily, at the same time each day, while in the malarious areas, and daily for 7 days after leaving the area (see Table 2-23 for recommended dosages).
- Malarone is very well tolerated, and side effects are rare. The most common adverse effects reported in persons using atovaquone/proguanil for prophylaxis or treatment are abdominal pain, nausea, vomiting, and headache. Malarone should not be used for prophylaxis in children weighing <5 kg, pregnant women, or patients with severe renal impairment (creatinine clearance <30 mL/min). It should be used with caution by patients taking coumadin (warfarin) for anticoagulation.

Chloroquine (Aralen) and Hydroxychloroquine (Plaquenil)

- Chloroquine phosphate or hydroxychloroquine sulfate can be used for prevention of malaria only in destinations where chloroquine resistance is not present (see Maps 2-7 and 2-8 or the next section in this chapter, Malaria Risk Information and Prophylaxis, by Country).
- Prophylaxis should begin 1–2 weeks before travel to malarious areas. It should be continued by taking the drug once a week, on the same day of the week, during travel in malarious areas and for 4 weeks after a traveler leaves these areas (see Table 2-23 for recommended dosages).
- Reported side effects include gastrointestinal disturbance, headache, dizziness, blurred vision, insomnia, and pruritus, but generally these effects do not require that the drug be discontinued. High doses of chloroquine, such as those used to treat rheumatoid arthritis, have been associated with retinopathy; this serious side effect appears to be extremely unlikely when chloroquine is used for routine weekly malaria prophylaxis. Chloroquine and related compounds have been reported to

Box 2-2. Clinical pearls

- Overdose of antimalarial drugs, particularly chloroquine, can be fatal. Medication should be stored in childproof containers out of the reach of infants and children.
- Chemoprophylaxis can be started earlier if there are particular concerns about tolerating one of the medications. For example, mefloquine can be started 3–4 weeks in advance to allow potential adverse events to occur before travel. If unacceptable side effects develop, there would be time to change the medication before the traveler's departure.
- The drugs used for antimalarial chemoprophylaxis are generally well tolerated. However, side effects can occur. Minor side effects usually do not require stopping the drug. Travelers who have serious side effects should see a health-care provider who can determine if their symptoms are related to the medicine and make an appropriate medication change.
- In comparison with drugs with short half-lives, which are taken daily, drugs with longer half-lives, which are taken weekly, offer the advantage of a wider margin of error if the traveler is late with a dose. For example, if a traveler is 1–2 days late with a weekly drug, prophylactic blood levels can remain adequate; if the traveler is 1–2 days late with a daily drug, protective blood levels are less likely to be maintained.
- In those who are G6PD deficient, primaquine can cause hemolysis, which can be fatal. Be sure to document a normal G6PD level before prescribing primaquine.
- Travelers should be informed that malaria can be fatal if treatment is delayed. Medical help should be sought promptly if malaria is suspected, and a blood sample should be taken and examined for malaria parasites on one or more occasions.
- Malaria smear results or an RDT test must be available immediately. Sending specimens to offsite laboratories where results are not available for extended periods of time (days) is not acceptable. If a patient has an illness suggestive of severe malaria and a compatible travel history in an area where malaria transmission occurs, it is advisable to start treatment as soon as possible, even before the diagnosis is established. CDC recommendations for malaria treatment can be found at www.cdc.gov/malaria/diagnosis_treatment/treatment.htm.

exacerbate psoriasis. Persons who experience uncomfortable side effects after taking chloroquine may tolerate the drug better by taking it with meals. As an alternative, the related compound hydroxychloroquine sulfate may be better tolerated.

Doxycycline (Many Brand Names and Generic)

- Doxycycline prophylaxis should begin 1–2 days before travel to malarious areas. It should be continued once a day, at the same time each day, during travel in malarious areas and daily for 4 weeks after the traveler leaves such areas.
- Insufficient data exist on the antimalarial prophylactic efficacy of related compounds such as minocycline (commonly prescribed for the treatment of acne). Persons on a long-term regimen of minocycline who are in need of malaria prophylaxis should stop taking minocycline 1–2 days before travel and start doxycycline instead. The minocycline can be restarted after the full course of doxycycline is completed (see Table 2-23 for recommended dosages).
- Doxycycline can cause photosensitivity, usually manifested as an exaggerated sunburn reaction. The risk for such a reaction can be minimized by avoiding prolonged, direct exposure to the sun and by using sunscreens. In addition, doxycycline use is associated with an increased frequency of vaginal yeast infections. Gastrointestinal side effects (nausea or vomiting) may be minimized by taking the drug with a meal. To reduce the risk for esophagitis, travelers should be advised not to take doxycycline before going to bed. Doxycycline is contraindicated in persons with an allergy to tetracyclines, during pregnancy, and in infants and children <8 years of age.
- Vaccination with the oral typhoid vaccine Ty21a should be delayed for at least 24 hours after taking a dose of doxycycline.

Mefloquine (Lariam)

- Mefloquine prophylaxis should begin 1–2 weeks before travel to malarious areas. It should be continued once a week, on the same day of the week, during travel in malarious areas and for 4 weeks after a traveler leaves such areas (see Table 2-23 for recommended dosages).

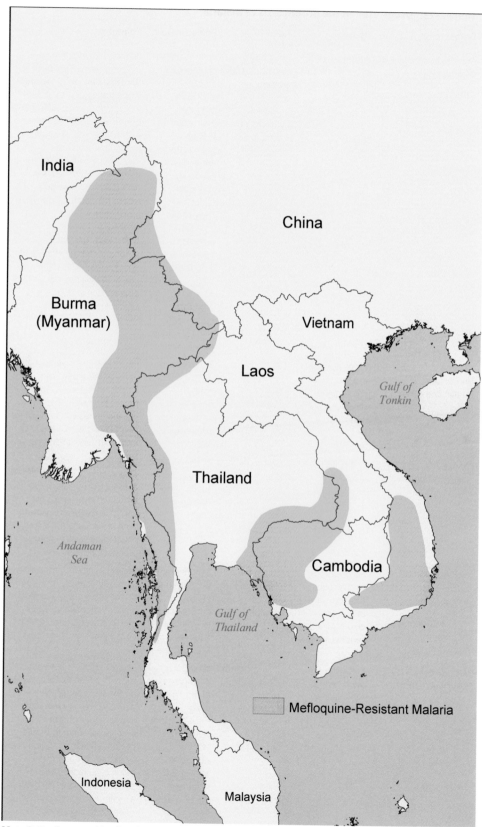

Map 2-9. Geographic distribution of mefloquine-resistant malaria.

Table 2-23. Drugs used in the prophylaxis of malaria

Drug	Usage	Adult Dose	Pediatric Dose	Comments
Atovaquone/proguanil (Malarone)	Prophylaxis in all areas	Adult tablets contain 250 mg atovaquone and 100 mg proguanil hydrochloride. 1 adult tablet orally, daily	Pediatric tablets contain 62.5 mg atovaquone and 25 mg proguanil hydrochloride. 5–8 kg: ½ pediatric tablet daily; >8–10 kg: ¾ pediatric tablet daily; >10–20 kg: 1 pediatric tablet daily; >20–30 kg: 2 pediatric tablets daily; >30–40 kg: 3 pediatric tablets daily; >40 kg: 1 adult tablet daily	Begin 1-2 days before travel to malarious areas. Take daily at the same time each day while in the malarious area and for 7 days after leaving such areas. Contraindicated in persons with severe renal impairment (creatinine clearance <30 mL/min). Atovaquone/proguanil should be taken with food or a milky drink. Not recommended for prophylaxis for children <5 kg, pregnant women, and women breastfeeding infants weighing <5 kg. Partial tablet dosages may need to be prepared by a pharmacist and dispensed in individual capsules, as described in the text.
Chloroquine phosphate (Aralen and generic)	Prophylaxis only in areas with chloroquine-sensitive malaria	300 mg base (500 mg salt) orally, once/week	5 mg/kg base (8.3 mg/kg salt) orally, once/week, up to maximum adult dose of 300 mg base	Begin 1–2 weeks before travel to malarious areas. Take weekly on the same day of the week while in the malarious area and for 4 weeks after leaving such areas. May exacerbate psoriasis
Doxycycline (many brand names and generic)	Prophylaxis in all areas	100 mg orally, daily	≥8 years of age: 2 mg/kg up to adult dose of 100 mg/day	Begin 1–2 days before travel to malarious areas. Take daily at the same time each day while in the malarious area and for 4 weeks after leaving such areas. Contraindicated in children <8 years of age and pregnant women
Hydroxychloroquine sulfate (Plaquenil)	An alternative to chloroquine for prophylaxis only in areas with chloroquine-sensitive malaria	310 mg base (400 mg salt) orally, once/week	5 mg/kg base (6.5 mg/kg salt) orally, once/week, up to maximum adult dose of 310 mg base	Begin 1–2 weeks before travel to malarious areas. Take weekly on the same day of the week while in the malarious area and for 4 weeks after leaving such areas.
Mefloquine (Lariam and generic)	Prophylaxis in areas with mefloquine-sensitive malaria	228 mg base (250 mg salt) orally, once/week	≤9 kg: 4.6 mg/kg base (5 mg/kg salt) orally, once/week; >9–19 kg: ¼ tablet once/week; >19–30 kg: ½ tablet once/week;	Begin 1–2 weeks before travel to malarious areas. Take weekly on the same day of the week while in the malarious area and for 4 weeks after leaving such areas. Contraindicated in persons allergic to mefloquine or related compounds (e.g., quinine, quinidine) and in persons with active depression, a recent history of depression, generalized anxiety disorder, *(Continued)*

Table 2-23. Drugs used in the prophylaxis of malaria *(Continued)*

Drug	Usage	Adult Dose	Pediatric Dose	Comments
Mefloquine (Lariam and generic) *(Continued)*			>31–45 kg: ¾ tablet once/week; >45 kg: 1 tablet once/week	psychosis, schizophrenia, other major psychiatric disorders, or seizures. Use with caution in persons with psychiatric disturbances or a previous history of depression. Not recommended for persons with cardiac conduction abnormalities
Primaquine	Prophylaxis for short-duration travel to areas with principally *P. vivax*	30 mg base (52.6 mg salt) orally, daily	0.5 mg/kg base (0.8 mg/kg salt) up to adult dose orally, daily	Begin 1–2 days before travel to malarious areas. Take daily at the same time each day while in the malarious area and for 7 days after leaving such areas. Contraindicated in persons with G6PD[1] deficiency. Also contraindicated during pregnancy and lactation unless the infant being breastfed has a documented normal G6PD level
Primaquine	Used for presumptive antirelapse therapy (terminal prophylaxis) to decrease the risk for relapses of *P. vivax* and *P. ovale*	30 mg base (52.6 mg salt) orally, once/day for 14 days after departure from the malarious area	0.5 mg/kg base (0.8 mg/kg salt) up to adult dose orally, once/day for 14 days after departure from the malarious area	Indicated for persons who have had prolonged exposure to *P. vivax* and *P. ovale* or both. Contraindicated in persons with G6PD[1] deficiency. Also contraindicated during pregnancy and lactation unless the infant being breastfed has a documented normal G6PD level

1 Glucose-6-phosphate dehydrogenase. All persons who take primaquine should have a documented normal G6PD level before starting the medication.

- Mefloquine has been associated with rare serious adverse reactions (e.g., psychoses, seizures) at prophylactic doses; these reactions are more frequent with the higher doses used for treatment. Other side effects that have occurred in chemoprophylaxis studies include gastrointestinal disturbance, headache, insomnia, abnormal dreams, visual disturbances, depression, anxiety disorder, and dizziness. Other more severe neuropsychiatric disorders occasionally reported during postmarketing surveillance include sensory and motor neuropathies (including paresthesia, tremor, and ataxia), agitation or restlessness, mood changes, panic attacks, forgetfulness, confusion, hallucinations, aggression, paranoia, and encephalopathy. On occasion, psychiatric symptoms have been reported to continue long after mefloquine has been stopped. Mefloquine is contraindicated for use by travelers with a known hypersensitivity to mefloquine or related compounds (e.g., quinine, quinidine) and in persons with active depression, a recent history of depression, generalized anxiety disorder, psychosis, schizophrenia, other major psychiatric disorders, or seizures. It should be used with caution in persons with psychiatric disturbances or a previous history of depression. A review of available data suggests that mefloquine may be used in persons concurrently on beta blockers, if they have no underlying arrhythmia. However, mefloquine is not recommended for persons with cardiac conduction abnormalities.

- Any traveler receiving a prescription for mefloquine must also receive a copy of the FDA Medication Guide, which can be found at the following website: www.fda.gov/cder/foi/label/2003/19591s19lbl_Lariam.pdf.

Primaquine

- Primaquine phosphate has two distinct uses for malaria prevention: primary prophylaxis and presumptive antirelapse therapy (also called terminal prophylaxis).
- When taken for primary prophylaxis, primaquine should be taken 1–2 days before travel to malarious areas, daily, at the same time each day, while in the malarious areas, and daily for 7 days after leaving the areas (see Table 2-23 for recommended dosages). Primary prophylaxis with primaquine obviates the need for presumptive antirelapse therapy.
- When used for presumptive antirelapse therapy, primaquine is administered for 14 days after the traveler has left a malarious area. When chloroquine, doxycycline, or mefloquine is used for primary prophylaxis, primaquine is usually taken during the last 2 weeks of postexposure prophylaxis. When atovaquone/proguanil is used for prophylaxis, primaquine may be taken during the final 7 days of atovaquone/proguanil, and then for an additional 7 days. It is preferable that primaquine be given concurrently with the primary prophylaxis medication. However, if that is not feasible, the primaquine course should still be administered after the primary prophylaxis medication has been completed.
- The most common adverse event in glucose-6-phosphate dehydrogenase (G6PD) in normal persons is gastrointestinal upset if primaquine is taken on an empty stomach. This problem is minimized or eliminated if primaquine is taken with food.
- In G6PD-deficient persons, primaquine can cause hemolysis that can be fatal. **Before primaquine is used, G6PD deficiency MUST be ruled out by appropriate laboratory testing.**

Travel to Areas with Limited Malaria Transmission

For destinations (see the next section in this chapter, Malaria Risk Information and Prophylaxis, by Country) where malaria cases occur sporadically and risk for infection to travelers is assessed as being very low, it is recommended that travelers use mosquito avoidance measures only, and no chemoprophylaxis should be prescribed.

Travel to Areas with Mainly *P. vivax* Malaria

- For destinations where the main species of malaria present is *P. vivax*, in addition to mosquito avoidance measures, primaquine is a good choice for primary prophylaxis for travelers who are not G6PD-deficient. Its use for this indication is considered off-label use in the United States.
- The predominant species of malaria and the recommended chemoprohylaxis medicines are listed in the following section in this chapter, Malaria Risk Information and Prophylaxis, by Country.
- For persons unable to take primaquine, other drugs can be used as described below, depending on the presence of antimalarial drug resistance.

Travel to Areas with Chloroquine-Sensitive Malaria

- For destinations where chloroquine-sensitive malaria is present, in addition to mosquito avoidance measures, the many effective chemoprophylaxis alternatives include chloroquine, atovaquone/proguanil, doxycycline, mefloquine, and in some instances primaquine for travelers who are not G6PD-deficient.
- Longer-term travelers may prefer the convenience of weekly chloroquine, while shorter-term travelers may prefer the shorter course of atovaquone/proguanil or primaquine.

Travel to Areas with Chloroquine-Resistant Malaria

For destinations where chloroquine-resistant malaria is present, in addition to mosquito avoidance measures, chemoprophylaxis options are limited to atovaquone/proguanil, doxycycline, and mefloquine.

Travel to Areas with Mefloquine-Resistant Malaria

For destinations where mefloquine-resistant malaria is present, in addition to mosquito avoidance measures, chemoprophylaxis options are reduced to either atovaquone/proguanil or doxycycline.

Chemoprophylaxis for Infants, Children, and Adolescents

- Infants of any age or weight or children and adolescents of any age can contract malaria. Therefore, all children traveling to malaria-risk areas should take an antimalarial drug.
- In the United States, antimalarial drugs are available only in tablet form and may taste quite bitter. Pediatric dosages should be carefully calculated according to body weight but should never exceed adult dosage. Pharmacists can pulverize tablets and prepare gelatin capsules for each measured dose. If the child is unable to swallow the capsules or tablets, parents should prepare the child's dose of medication by breaking open the gelatin capsule and mixing the drug with a small amount of something sweet, such as applesauce, chocolate syrup, or jelly, to ensure the entire dose is delivered to the child. Giving the dose on a full stomach may minimize stomach upset and vomiting.
- Chloroquine and mefloquine are options for use in infants and children of all ages and weights, depending on the presence of drug resistance at their destination.
- Primaquine can be used for children who are not G6PD-deficient traveling to areas with principally *P. vivax*.
- Doxycycline may be used for children who are at least 8 years of age.
- Atovaquone/proguanil may be used for prophylaxis for infants and children weighing at least 5 kg (11 lbs). Providers should note that this prophylactic dosing for children weighing <11 kg constitutes off-label use in the United States.
- Pediatric dosing regimens are contained in Table 2-23.

Chemoprophylaxis during Pregnancy and Breastfeeding

- Malaria infection in pregnant women can be more severe than in nonpregnant women. Malaria can increase the risk for adverse pregnancy outcomes, including prematurity, abortion, and stillbirth. For these reasons, and because no chemoprophylactic regimen is completely effective, women who are pregnant or likely to become pregnant should be advised to avoid travel to areas with malaria transmission if possible (see the Traveling while Pregnant section in Chapter 8). If travel to a malarious area cannot be deferred, use of an effective chemoprophylaxis regimen is essential.
- Pregnant women traveling to areas where chloroquine-resistant *P. falciparum* has not been reported may take chloroquine prophylaxis. Chloroquine has not been found to have any harmful effects on the fetus when used in the recommended doses for malaria prophylaxis; therefore, pregnancy is not a contraindication for malaria prophylaxis with chloroquine phosphate or hydroxychloroquine sulfate.
- For travel to areas where chloroquine resistance is present, mefloquine is currently the only medication recommended for malaria chemoprophylaxis during pregnancy. A review of mefloquine use in pregnancy from clinical trials and reports of inadvertent use of mefloquine during pregnancy suggests that its use at prophylactic doses during the second and third trimesters of pregnancy is not associated with adverse fetal or pregnancy outcomes. More limited data suggest it is also safe to use during the first trimester.
- Because of insufficient data regarding the use during pregnancy, atovaquone/proguanil is not currently recommended for the prevention of malaria in pregnant women.

- Doxycycline is contraindicated for malaria prophylaxis during pregnancy because of the risk for adverse effects seen with tetracycline, a related drug, on the fetus, which include discoloration and dysplasia of the teeth and inhibition of bone growth.
- Primaquine should not be used during pregnancy because the drug may be passed transplacentally to a G6PD-deficient fetus and cause hemolytic anemia in utero.
- Health-care professionals who require additional assistance with the management of pregnant travelers who are unable to take mefloquine chemoprophylaxis should call the CDC Malaria Hotline (770-488-7788).
- Very small amounts of antimalarial drugs are excreted in the breast milk of lactating women. Because the quantity of antimalarial drugs transferred in breast milk is insufficient to provide adequate protection against malaria, infants who require chemoprophylaxis must receive the recommended dosages of antimalarial drugs listed in Table 2-23.
- Because chloroquine and mefloquine may be safely prescribed to infants, it is also safe for infants to be exposed to the small amounts excreted in breast milk.
- Although data are very limited about the use of doxycycline in lactating women, most experts consider the theoretical possibility of adverse events to the infant to be remote.
- Although no information is available on the amount of primaquine that enters human breast milk, the mother and infant should be tested for G6PD deficiency before primaquine is given to a woman who is breastfeeding.
- Because data are not yet available on the safety of atovaquone/proguanil prophylaxis in infants weighing <5 kg (<11 lbs), CDC does not currently recommend it for the prevention of malaria in women breastfeeding infants weighing <5 kg. However, it can be used for treatment of women who are breastfeeding infants of any weight when the potential benefit outweighs the potential risk to the infant (e.g., treating a breastfeeding woman who has acquired *P. falciparum* malaria in an area of multidrug-resistant strains and who cannot tolerate other treatment options).

Changing Medications during Chemoprophylaxis as a Result of Side Effects

- Medications recommended for prophylaxis against malaria have different modes of action that affect the parasites at different stages of the life cycle. Thus, if the medication needs to be changed because of side effects before a full course has been completed, there are some special considerations.
- If a traveler starts prophylaxis with a medication such as mefloquine or doxycycline and then changes to atovaquone/proguanil during or after travel, the standard duration of prophylaxis for atovaquone/proguanil would be insufficient.
- If the switch occurs 3 weeks or more before departure from the risk area, atovaquone/proguanil should be taken for the remainder of the stay in the risk area and for 1 week thereafter.
- If the switch occurs <3 weeks before departure from the risk area, atovaquone/proguanil should be taken for 4 weeks after the switch.
- If the switch occurs following departure from the risk area, atovaquone/proguanil should be continued until 4 weeks after the date of departure from the risk area.
- Due to their pharmacokinetics, switching from a daily medicine such as doxycycline to a weekly medicine such as mefloquine should be avoided.
- Health-care professionals who require additional assistance with the management of travelers who need to change medications during prophylaxis should call the CDC Malaria Hotline (770-488-7788).

References

1. CDC. Malaria map application. [cited 2008 Nov 26]. Available from: http://www.cdc.gov/malaria/risk_map/.
2. CDC. Malaria website. [cited 2008 Nov 26]. Available from: http://www.cdc.gov/malaria/.
3. Cox-Singh J, Davis TM, Lee KS, et al. *Plasmodium knowlesi* malaria in humans is widely distributed and potentially life threatening. Clin Infect Dis 2008;46(2):165–71.

4. Guinovart C, Navia MM, Tanner M, et al. Malaria: burden of disease. Curr Mol Med. 2006;6(2):137–40.

5. Mali S, Steele S, Slutsker L, et al. Malaria surveillance—United States, 2006. MMWR Surveill Summ. 2008;57(5):24–39.

6. Newman RD, Parise ME, Barber AM, et al. Malaria-related deaths among U.S. travelers, 1963–2001. Ann Intern Med. 2004;141(7):547–55.

7. Leder K, Black J, O'Brien D, et al. Malaria in travelers: a review of the GeoSentinel surveillance network. Clin Infect Dis. 2004;39(8):1104–12.

8. Leder K, Tong S, Weld L, et al. Illness in travelers visiting friends and relatives: a review of the GeoSentinel surveillance network. Clin Infect Dis. 2006; 43:1185–93.

9. Kitchen AD, Chiodini PL. Malaria and blood transfusion. Vox Sanguin. 2006;90(2):77–84.

10. Parise ME, Lewis LS. Severe malaria: North American perspective. In: Feldman C, Sarosi GA, editors. Tropical and parasitic infections in the ICU. New York: Springer Science+ Buisness Media, Inc.; 2005. p. 17–38.

11. Kochar DK, Saxena V, Singh N, et al. Plasmodium vivax malaria. Emerg Infect Dis. 2005;11(1):132–4

12. Reyburn H, Mbatia R, Drakeley C, et al. Overdiagnosis of malaria in patients with severe febrile illness in Tanzania: a prospective study. BMJ. 2004;329(7476):1212.

13. Hill DR, Ericsson CD, Pearson RD, et al. The practice of travel medicine: guidelines by the Infectious Diseases Society of America. Clin Infect Dis. 2006;43(12):1499–539.

14. Fradin MS, day JF. Comparative efficacy of insect repellents against mosquito bites. N Engl J Med. 2002;347(1):13–8.

15. Boggild AK, Parise ME, Lewis LS, et al. Atovaquone-proguanil: report from the CDC expert meeting on malaria chemoprophylaxis (II). Am J Trop Med Hyg. 2007;76(2):208–23.

16. Baird JK, Fryauff DJ, Hoffman SL. Primaquine for prevention of malaria in travelers. Clin Infect Dis. 2003;37(12):1659–67.

17. Hill DR, Baird JK, Parise ME,et al. Primaquine: report from CDC expert meeting on malaria chemoprophylaxis I. Am J Trop Med Hyg. 2006; 75(3):402–15.

18. Schwartz E, Parise M, Kozarsky P, et al. Delayed onset of malaria-implications for chemoprophylaxis in travelers. N Engl J Med. 2003;349(16):1510–6.

19. Whitty CJM, Edmonds S, Mutabingwa TK. Malaria in pregnancy. BJOG. 2005;112(9):1189–95.

MALARIA RISK INFORMATION AND PROPHYLAXIS, BY COUNTRY

Kathrine R. Tan, Sonja Mali, Paul M. Arguin

Table 2-24. Malaria risk information and prophylaxis, by country[1]

Country	Areas with Malaria	Drug Resistance[2]	Malaria Species[3]	Recommended Chemoprophylaxis[4]
Afghanistan	April–December in all areas at altitudes <2,000 m (<6,561 ft)	Chloroquine	*P. vivax* 80%–90% *P. falciparum* 10%–20%	Atovaquone/proguanil, doxycycline, or mefloquine
Albania	None	Not applicable	Not applicable	Not applicable
Algeria	None	Not applicable	Not applicable	Not applicable
Andorra	None	Not applicable	Not applicable	Not applicable
Angola	All	Chloroquine	*P. falciparum* 90% *P. ovale* 5% *P. vivax* 5%	Atovaquone/proguanil, doxycycline, or mefloquine

1 The information presented herein was accurate at the time of publication; however, factors that can change rapidly and from year to year, such as local weather conditions, mosquito vector density, and prevalence of infection, can markedly affect local malaria transmission patterns. Updated information may be found on the CDC Travelers' Health website at www.cdc.gov/travel.

2 Refers to *P. falciparum* malaria.

3 Estimates of malaria species are based on best available data from multiple sources.

4 Several medications are available for chemoprophylaxis. When deciding which drug to use, consider specific itinerary, length of trip, cost of drug, previous adverse reactions to antimalarials, drug allergies, and current medical history. All travelers should seek medical attention in the event of fever during or after return from travel to areas with malaria.

5 Primaquine can cause hemolytic anemia in persons with G6PD deficiency. Patients must be tested and documented to have a normal level of G6PD activity prior to starting primaquine.

Country	Areas with Malaria	Drug Resistance[2]	Malaria Species[3]	Recommended Chemoprophylaxis[4]
Anguilla (U.K.)	None	Not applicable	Not applicable	Not applicable
Antarctica	None	Not applicable	Not applicable	Not applicable
Antigua and Barbuda	None	Not applicable	Not applicable	Not applicable
Argentina	Rural areas of Salta and Jujuy provinces (along Bolivian border) and Misiones and Corrientes provinces (along border of Paraguay). Malaria present in Iguassu Falls	None	*P. vivax* 100%	Atovaquone/proguanil, chloroquine, doxycycline, mefloquine, or primaquine[5]
Armenia	Previously limited to the Ararat Valley in the Ararat and Artashat regions and Masis district. No cases reported since 2006	None	Historically *P. vivax* 100%	Mosquito avoidance only
Aruba	None	Not applicable	Not applicable	Not applicable
Australia, including Cocos (**Keeling**) Islands	None	Not applicable	Not applicable	Not applicable
Austria	None	Not applicable	Not applicable	Not applicable
Azerbaijan	Rural areas <1,500 m (4,921 ft). None in Baku	None	*P. vivax* 100%	Atovaquone/proguanil, chloroquine, doxycycline, mefloquine, or primaquine[5]
Azores (Portugal)	None	Not applicable	Not applicable	Not applicable
Bahamas, The	Present only in Great Exuma Island	None	*P. falciparum* 100%	Atovaquone/proguanil, chloroquine, doxycycline, or mefloquine
Bahrain	None	Not applicable	Not applicable	Not applicable
Bangladesh	All areas, except in city of Dhaka	Chloroquine	*P. falciparum* 77% *P. vivax* 23%	Atovaquone/proguanil, doxycycline, or mefloquine
Barbados	None	Not applicable	Not applicable	Not applicable
Belarus	None	Not applicable	Not applicable	Not applicable
Belgium	None	Not applicable	Not applicable	Not applicable
Belize	All areas, except in Belize City	None	*P. vivax* 95% *P. falciparum* 5%	Atovaquone/proguanil, chloroquine, doxycycline, mefloquine, or primaquine[5]

1 The information presented herein was accurate at the time of publication; however, factors that can change rapidly and from year to year, such as local weather conditions, mosquito vector density, and prevalence of infection, can markedly affect local malaria transmission patterns. Updated information may be found on the CDC Travelers' Health website at www.cdc.gov/travel.

2 Refers to *P. falciparum* malaria.

3 Estimates of malaria species are based on best available data from multiple sources.

4 Several medications are available for chemoprophylaxis. When deciding which drug to use, consider specific itinerary, length of trip, cost of drug, previous adverse reactions to antimalarials, drug allergies, and current medical history. All travelers should seek medical attention in the event of fever during or after return from travel to areas with malaria.

5 Primaquine can cause hemolytic anemia in persons with G6PD deficiency. Patients must be tested and documented to have a normal level of G6PD activity prior to starting primaquine.

Country	Areas with Malaria	Drug Resistance[2]	Malaria Species[3]	Recommended Chemoprophylaxis[4]
Benin	All	Chloroquine	P. falciparum 85% P. ovale 5%–10% P. vivax rare	Atovaquone/proguanil, doxycycline, or mefloquine
Bermuda (U.K.)	None	Not applicable	Not applicable	Not applicable
Bhutan	Rural areas <1,700 m (<5,577 ft) of the southern belt districts along the border with India: Chirang, Geylegphug, Samchi, Samdrup Jongkhar, Sarpang and Shemgang	Chloroquine	P. falciparum 50% P. vivax 50%	Atovaquone/proguanil, doxycycline, or mefloquine
Bolivia	All areas <2,500 m (<8,202 ft) in the following departments: Beni, Chuquisaca, Cochabamba, La Paz, Pando, Santa Cruz, and Tarija. None in city of La Paz	Chloroquine	P. vivax 70%–95% P. falciparum 5%–30%	Atovaquone/proguanil, doxycycline, or mefloquine
Bosnia and Herzegovina	None	Not applicable	Not applicable	Not applicable
Botswana	North of 22° S in the northern provinces of Central, Chobe, Ghanzi, and Ngamiland, including safaris to the Okavango Delta area. None in the city of Gaborone	Chloroquine	P. falciparum 90% P. vivax 5% P. ovale 5%	Atovaquone/proguanil, doxycycline, or mefloquine
Brazil	States of Acre, Rondônia, Amapá, Amazonas, Roraima, and Tocantins. Parts of states of Maranhaõ (western part), Mato Grosso (northern part), and Pará (except Belem City). Also present in urban areas, including large cities such as Porto Velho, Boa Vista, Macapa, Manaus, Santarem, and Maraba, where the transmission occurs on the periphery of these cities Malaria in Iguassu Falls	Chloroquine	P. vivax 75% P. falciparum 25%	Atovaquone/proguanil, doxycycline, or mefloquine
British Indian Ocean Territory, includes Diego Garcia (U.K.)	None	Not applicable	Not applicable	Not applicable
Brunei	None	Not applicable	Not applicable	Not applicable
Bulgaria	None	Not applicable	Not applicable	Not applicable
Burkina Faso	All	Chloroquine	P. falciparum 80% P. ovale 5%–10% P. vivax rare	Atovaquone/proguanil, doxycycline, or mefloquine

Country	Areas with Malaria	Drug Resistance[2]	Malaria Species[3]	Recommended Chemoprophylaxis[4]
Burma (Myanmar)	Rural areas throughout the country at altitudes <1,000 m (<3,281 ft). None in cities of Rangoon (Yangon) and Mandalay	Chloroquine Mefloquine (see Map 2-9)	*P. falciparum* 80% *P. vivax* 20%	In the provinces of Bago, Kayah, Kachin, Kayin, Shan, and Tanintharyi: Atovaquone/proguanil or doxycycline All other areas: Atovaquone/proguanil, doxycycline, or mefloquine
Burundi	All	Chloroquine	*P. falciparum* >85% *P. malariae*, *P. ovale*, and *P. vivax* <15%	Atovaquone/proguanil, doxycycline, or mefloquine
Cambodia	Present throughout country, including the temple complex at Angkor Wat, except none in Phnom Penh and around Lake Tonle Sap	Chloroquine Mefloquine (see Map 2-9)	*P. falciparum* 86% *P. vivax* 12% *P. malariae* 2%	In the provinces of Preah Vihear, Siemreap, Oddar Meanchey, Banteay Meanchey, Battambang, Pailin, Kampot, Koh Kong, and Pursat bordering Thailand: Atovaquone/proguanil or doxycycline All other areas: Atovaquone/proguanil, doxycycline, or mefloquine
Cameroon	All	Chloroquine	*P. falciparum* 80% *P. ovale* 5%–10% *P. vivax* rare	Atovaquone/proguanil, doxycycline, or mefloquine
Canada	None	Not applicable	Not applicable	Not applicable
Canary Islands (Spain)	None	Not applicable	Not applicable	Not applicable
Cape Verde	Limited to Sao Tiago Island	Chloroquine	*P. falciparum* primarily	Atovaquone/proguanil, doxycycline, or mefloquine
Cayman Islands (U.K.)	None	Not applicable	Not applicable	Not applicable
Central African Republic	All	Chloroquine	*P. falciparum* 85% *P. malariae*, *P. ovale*, and *P. vivax* 15%	Atovaquone/proguanil, doxycycline, or mefloquine
Chad	All	Chloroquine	*P. falciparum* 85% *P. malariae*, *P. ovale*, and *P. vivax* 15%	Atovaquone/proguanil, doxycycline, or mefloquine

1   The information presented herein was accurate at the time of publication; however, factors that can change rapidly and from year to year, such as local weather conditions, mosquito vector density, and prevalence of infection, can markedly affect local malaria transmission patterns. Updated information may be found on the CDC Travelers' Health website at www.cdc.gov/travel.
2   Refers to *P. falciparum* malaria.
3   Estimates of malaria species are based on best available data from multiple sources.
4   Several medications are available for chemoprophylaxis. When deciding which drug to use, consider specific itinerary, length of trip, cost of drug, previous adverse reactions to antimalarials, drug allergies, and current medical history. All travelers should seek medical attention in the event of fever during or after return from travel to areas with malaria.
5   Primaquine can cause hemolytic anemia in persons with G6PD deficiency. Patients must be tested and documented to have a normal level of G6PD activity prior to starting primaquine.

Country	Areas with Malaria	Drug Resistance[2]	Malaria Species[3]	Recommended Chemoprophylaxis[4]
Chile	None	Not applicable	Not applicable	Not applicable
China	Rural parts of Anhui, Yunnan, Hainan provinces. Rare cases occur in other rural parts of the country <1,500 m (<4,921 ft) during May–December. None in major river cruises and urban areas	Chloroquine Mefloquine (see Map 2-9)	*P. falciparum* primarily in Hainan and Yunnan. *P. vivax* primarily elsewhere	Along China–Burma border in the western part of Yunnan province: Atovaquone/proguanil or doxycycline Hainan and the other parts of Yunnan province : Atovaquone/proguanil, doxycycline or mefloquine Anhui province: Atovaquone/proguanil, chloroquine, doxycycline, or mefloquine All other areas with malaria transmission: Mosquito avoidance
Christmas Island (Australia)	None	Not applicable	Not applicable	Not applicable
Colombia	All rural areas at altitudes <1,800 m (<5,906 ft). None in Bogota and Cartagena	Chloroquine	*P. falciparum* 50% *P. vivax* 50%	Atovaquone/proguanil, doxycycline, or mefloquine
Comoros	All	Chloroquine	*P. falciparum* primarily	Atovaquone/proguanil, doxycycline, or mefloquine
Congo, Republic of the (Congo-Brazzaville)	All	Chloroquine	*P. falciparum* primarily	Atovaquone/proguanil, doxycycline, or mefloquine
Cook Islands (New Zealand)	None	Not applicable	Not applicable	Not applicable
Costa Rica	Limon province, but not in Limon city (Puerto Limon). Rare cases in Puntarenas, Alajuela, Guanacaste, and Heredia provinces	None	*P. vivax* 90% *P. falciparum* 10%	Limon province: Atovaquone/proguanil, chloroquine, doxycycline, mefloquine, or primaquine[5] All other areas with malaria transmission: Mosquito avoidance
Côte d'Ivoire (Ivory Coast)	All	Chloroquine	*P. falciparum* 85% *P. ovale* 5%–10% *P. vivax* rare	Atovaquone/proguanil, doxycycline, or mefloquine
Croatia	None	Not applicable	Not applicable	Not applicable
Cuba	None	Not applicable	Not applicable	Not applicable
Cyprus	None	Not applicable	Not applicable	Not applicable
Czech Republic	None	Not applicable	Not applicable	Not applicable

Democratic Republic of the Congo (Congo-Kinshasa) to Finland

Country	Areas with Malaria	Drug Resistance[2]	Malaria Species[3]	Recommended Chemoprophylaxis[4]
Democratic Republic of the Congo (Congo-Kinshasa)	All	Chloroquine	*P. falciparum* 90% *P. ovale* 5% *P. vivax* rare	Atovaquone/proguanil, doxycycline, or mefloquine
Denmark	None	Not applicable	Not applicable	Not applicable
Djibouti	All	Chloroquine	*P. falciparum* 90% *P. vivax* 5%–10%	Atovaquone/proguanil, doxycycline, or mefloquine
Dominica	None	Not applicable	Not applicable	Not applicable
Dominican Republic	All areas (including resort areas), except not present in the cities of Santo Domingo and Santiago	None	*P. falciparum* 100%	Atovaquone/proguanil, chloroquine, doxycycline, or mefloquine
Easter Island (Chile)	None	Not applicable	Not applicable	Not applicable
Ecuador, including the Galápagos Islands	All areas at altitudes <1,500 m (<4,921 ft). Not present in the cities of Guayaquil, Quito, and the Galápagos Islands	Chloroquine	*P. vivax* 75% *P. falciparum* 25%	Atovaquone/proguanil, doxycycline, or mefloquine
Egypt	None	Not applicable	Not applicable	Not applicable
El Salvador	Rural areas of Santa Ana, Ahuachapán, La Paz, and La Unión departments	None	*P. vivax* 99% *P. falciparum* <1%	Atovaquone/proguanil, chloroquine, doxycycline, mefloquine or primaquine[5]
Equatorial Guinea	All	Chloroquine	*P. falciparum* 85% *P. malariae, P. ovale,* and *P. vivax* 15%	Atovaquone/proguanil, doxycycline, or mefloquine
Eritrea	All areas at altitudes <2,200 m (<7,218 ft). None in Asmara	Chloroquine	*P. falciparum* 85% *P. vivax* 10%–15% *P. ovale* rare	Atovaquone/proguanil, doxycycline, or mefloquine
Estonia	None	Not applicable	Not applicable	Not applicable
Ethiopia	All areas at altitudes <2,500m (<8,202 ft), except none in Addis Ababa	Chloroquine	*P. falciparum* 85% *P. vivax* 10%–15% *P. malariae* and *P. ovale* <5%	Atovaquone/proguanil, doxycycline, or mefloquine
Falkland, South Georgia & South Sandwich Islands (U.K.)	None	Not applicable	Not applicable	Not applicable
Faroe Islands (Denmark)	None	Not applicable	Not applicable	Not applicable
Fiji	None	Not applicable	Not applicable	Not applicable
Finland	None	Not applicable	Not applicable	Not applicable

1   The information presented herein was accurate at the time of publication; however, factors that can change rapidly and from year to year, such as local weather conditions, mosquito vector density, and prevalence of infection, can markedly affect local malaria transmission patterns. Updated information may be found on the CDC Travelers' Health website at www.cdc.gov/travel.
2   Refers to *P. falciparum* malaria.
3   Estimates of malaria species are based on best available data from multiple sources.
4   Several medications are available for chemoprophylaxis. When deciding which drug to use, consider specific itinerary, length of trip, cost of drug, previous adverse reactions to antimalarials, drug allergies, and current medical history. All travelers should seek medical attention in the event of fever during or after return from travel to areas with malaria.
5   Primaquine can cause hemolytic anemia in persons with G6PD deficiency. Patients must be tested and documented to have a normal level of G6PD activity prior to starting primaquine.

Country	Areas with Malaria	Drug Resistance[2]	Malaria Species[3]	Recommended Chemoprophylaxis[4]
France	None	Not applicable	Not applicable	Not applicable
French Guiana	All areas, except none in city of Cayenne or Devil's Island (Ile du Diable)	Chloroquine	*P. falciparum* >50% *P. vivax*, <50%	Atovaquone/proguanil, doxycycline, or mefloquine
French Polynesia, includes the island groups of **Society Islands** (**Tahiti**, **Moorea**, and **Bora-Bora**), **Marquesas Islands** (**Hiva Oa** and **Ua Huka**), and **Austral Islands** (**Tubuai** and **Rurutu**)	None	Not applicable	Not applicable	Not applicable
Gabon	All	Chloroquine	*P. falciparum* 95% *P. malariae, P. ovale, P. vivax* 5%	Atovaquone/proguanil, doxycycline, or mefloquine
Gambia, The	All	Chloroquine	*P. falciparum* 85% *P. malariae, P. ovale, P. vivax* 15%	Atovaquone/proguanil, doxycycline, or mefloquine
Georgia	Present in the southeastern part of the country near the Azerbaijan border, mainly in the Kakheti and Kveno Kartli regions. None in Tblisi	None	*P. vivax* 100%	Atovaquone/proguanil, chloroquine, doxycycline, mefloquine, or primaquine[5]
Germany	None	Not applicable	Not applicable	Not applicable
Ghana	All	Chloroquine	*P. falciparum* 85% *P. ovale* 5%–10% *P. vivax* rare	Atovaquone/proguanil, doxycycline, or mefloquine
Gibraltar (U.K.)	None	Not applicable	Not applicable	Not applicable
Greece	None	Not applicable	Not applicable	Not applicable
Greenland (Denmark)	None	Not applicable	Not applicable	Not applicable
Grenada	None	Not applicable	Not applicable	Not applicable
Guadeloupe (France)	None	Not applicable	Not applicable	Not applicable
Guam (U.S.)	None	Not applicable	Not applicable	Not applicable
Guatemala	Rural areas only at altitudes <1,500 m (<4,921ft). None in Guatemala City, Antigua or Lake Atitlán	None	*P. vivax* 97% *P. falciparum* 3%	Atovaquone/proguanil, chloroquine, doxycycline, mefloquine, or primaquine[5]
Guinea	All	Chloroquine	*P. falciparum* 85% *P. ovale* 5%–10% *P. vivax* rare	Atovaquone/proguanil, doxycycline, or mefloquine
Guinea-Bissau	All	Chloroquine	*P. falciparum* 85% *P. ovale* 5%–10% *P. vivax* rare	Atovaquone/proguanil, doxycycline, or mefloquine
Guyana	All rural areas <900 m (<2,953 ft)	Chloroquine	*P. falciparum* 60% *P. vivax* 40% *P. malariae* <1%	Atovaquone/proguanil, doxycycline, or mefloquine

Country	Areas with Malaria	Drug Resistance[2]	Malaria Species[3]	Recommended Chemoprophylaxis[4]
Haiti	All (including Port Labadee)	None	*P. falciparum* 100%	Atovaquone/proguanil, chloroquine, doxycycline, or mefloquine
Holy See	None	Not applicable	Not applicable	Not applicable
Honduras	Present throughout the country at altitudes <1000 m (<3,281 ft) and in Roatán and other Bay Island. None in Tegucigalpa and San Pedro Sula	None	*P. vivax* 50%–95% *P. falciparum* 5%–50%	Atovaquone/proguanil, chloroquine, doxycycline, or mefloquine
Hong Kong SAR (China)	None	Not applicable	Not applicable	Not applicable
Hungary	None	Not applicable	Not applicable	Not applicable
Iceland	None	Not applicable	Not applicable	Not applicable
India	All areas throughout country **except** no malaria in areas >2,000 m (>6,561 ft) in Himachal Pradesh, Jammu, Kashmir, and Sikkim. Present in cities of Delhi and Bombay (Mumbai)	Chloroquine	*P. vivax* 40% *P. falciparum* 20%–40% *P. malariae* and *P. ovale* 20%–40%	Atovaquone/proguanil, doxycycline, or mefloquine
Indonesia	Present in rural areas of Sumatra, Sulawesi, Kalimantan (Borneo) and Nusa Tenggara Barat (includes the island of Lombok) All areas of eastern Indonesia (provinces of Papua Indonesia, Irian Jaya Barat, Nusa Tenggara Timur, Maluku, and Maluku Utara) None in Jakarta, resort areas of Bali and the island of Java, except for the Menoreh Hills in central Java. None in urban areas in Sumatra, Kalimantan, Nusa Tenggara Barat and Sulawesi	Chloroquine	*P. falciparum* 66% *P. vivax* 34%	Atovaquone/proguanil, doxycycline, or mefloquine

1 The information presented herein was accurate at the time of publication; however, factors that can change rapidly and from year to year, such as local weather conditions, mosquito vector density, and prevalence of infection, can markedly affect local malaria transmission patterns. Updated information may be found on the CDC Travelers' Health website at www.cdc.gov/travel.
2 Refers to *P. falciparum* malaria.
3 Estimates of malaria species are based on best available data from multiple sources.
4 Several medications are available for chemoprophylaxis. When deciding which drug to use, consider specific itinerary, length of trip, cost of drug, previous adverse reactions to antimalarials, drug allergies, and current medical history. All travelers should seek medical attention in the event of fever during or after return from travel to areas with malaria.
5 Primaquine can cause hemolytic anemia in persons with G6PD deficiency. Patients must be tested and documented to have a normal level of G6PD activity prior to starting primaquine.

Country	Areas with Malaria	Drug Resistance[2]	Malaria Species[3]	Recommended Chemoprophylaxis[4]
Iran	Rural areas of Sistan-Baluchestan, the southern tropical part of Kerman, and Hormozgan province Ardebil and East Azerbijan provinces north of the Zagros mountains during March through November	Chloroquine	*P. vivax* 88% *P. falciparum* 11%	Atovaquone/proguanil, doxycycline, or mefloquine
Iraq	Present in areas at altitudes <1,500 m (<4,921 ft) in provinces of Duhok, Erbil, Ninawa, Sulaimaninya, and Ta'mim. None in Baghdad, Tikrit, and Ramadi	None	*P. vivax* 100%	Atovaquone/proguanil, chloroquine, doxycycline, mefloquine, or primaquine[5]
Ireland	None	Not applicable	Not applicable	Not applicable
Israel	None	Not applicable	Not applicable	Not applicable
Italy	None	Not applicable	Not applicable	Not applicable
Jamaica	Rare local cases in Kingston	None	*P. falciparum* 100%	Mosquito avoidance only
Japan	None	Not applicable	Not applicable	Not applicable
Jordan	None	Not applicable	Not applicable	Not applicable
Kazakhstan	None	Not applicable	Not applicable	Not applicable
Kenya	Present in all areas (including game parks) at altitudes <2,500 m (<8,202 ft). None in Nairobi	Chloroquine	*P. falciparum* 85% *P. vivax* 5%–10% *P. ovale* up to 5%	Atovaquone/proguanil, doxycycline, or mefloquine
Kiribati (formerly **Gilbert Islands**), includes **Tarawa, Tabuaeran (Fanning Island)**, and **Banaba (Ocean Island)**	None	Not applicable	Not applicable	Not applicable
Korea, North	Present in southern provinces	None	Presumed to be *P. vivax* 100%	Atovaquone/proguanil, chloroquine, doxycycline, mefloquine, or primaquine[5]
Korea, South	Limited to rural areas in the northern parts of Kyonggi and Kangwon provinces including the demilitarized zone (DMZ)	None	*P. vivax* 100%	Atovaquone/proguanil, chloroquine, doxycycline, mefloquine, or primaquine[5]
Kosovo	None	Not applicable	Not applicable	Not applicable
Kuwait	None	Not applicable	Not applicable	Not applicable

Country	Areas with Malaria	Drug Resistance[2]	Malaria Species[3]	Recommended Chemoprophylaxis[4]
Kyrgyzstan	Frequent border crossings between neighboring countries with malaria poses a small risk of malaria transmission in the southern and western parts of the country along the borders of Tajikistan and Uzbekistan. No malaria transmission reported in Bishkek	None	P. vivax 99% P. falciparum rare imported cases	Mosquito avoidance only
Laos	All, except none in the city of Vientiane	Chloroquine Mefloquine (see Map 2-9)	P. falciparum 95% P. vivax 4% P. malariae and P. ovale 1%	Along the Laos–Burma border in the provinces of Bokèo and Louang Namtha and along the Laos–Thailand border in the province of Saravane and Champassack: Atovaquone/proguanil or doxycycline

All other areas: Atovaquone/proguanil, doxycycline, or mefloquine |
Latvia	None	Not applicable	Not applicable	Not applicable
Lebanon	None	Not applicable	Not applicable	Not applicable
Lesotho	None	Not applicable	Not applicable	Not applicable
Liberia	All	Chloroquine	P. falciparum 85% P. ovale 5%–10% P. vivax rare	Atovaquone/proguanil, doxycycline, or mefloquine
Libya	None	Not applicable	Not applicable	Not applicable
Liechtenstein	None	Not applicable	Not applicable	Not applicable
Lithuania	None	Not applicable	Not applicable	Not applicable
Luxembourg	None	Not applicable	Not applicable	Not applicable
Macau SAR (China)	None	Not applicable	Not applicable	Not applicable
Macedonia	None	Not applicable	Not applicable	Not applicable
Madagascar	All	Chloroquine	P. falciparum 85% P. vivax 5%–10% P. ovale 5%	Atovaquone/proguanil, doxycycline, or mefloquine
Madeira Islands (Portugal)	None	Not applicable	Not applicable	Not applicable

1   The information presented herein was accurate at the time of publication; however, factors that can change rapidly and from year to year, such as local weather conditions, mosquito vector density, and prevalence of infection, can markedly affect local malaria transmission patterns. Updated information may be found on the CDC Travelers' Health website at www.cdc.gov/travel.
2   Refers to *P. falciparum* malaria.
3   Estimates of malaria species are based on best available data from multiple sources.
4   Several medications are available for chemoprophylaxis. When deciding which drug to use, consider specific itinerary, length of trip, cost of drug, previous adverse reactions to antimalarials, drug allergies, and current medical history. All travelers should seek medical attention in the event of fever during or after return from travel to areas with malaria.
5   Primaquine can cause hemolytic anemia in persons with G6PD deficiency. Patients must be tested and documented to have a normal level of G6PD activity prior to starting primaquine.

Country	Areas with Malaria	Drug Resistance[2]	Malaria Species[3]	Recommended Chemoprophylaxis[4]
Malawi	All	Chloroquine	*P. falciparum* 90% *P. malariae, P. ovale,* and *P. vivax* 10%	Atovaquone/proguanil, doxycycline, or mefloquine
Malaysia	Present in rural areas of Malaysian Borneo, and to a lesser extent in rural areas of peninsular Malaysia	Chloroquine	*P. falciparum* 40% *P. vivax* 50% *P. ovale* <1% *P. knowlesi* reported to cause some human infections here	Atovaquone/proguanil, doxycycline, or mefloquine
Maldives	None	Not applicable	Not applicable	Not applicable
Mali	All	Chloroquine	*P. falciparum* 85% *P. ovale* 5%–10% *P. vivax* rare	Atovaquone/proguanil, doxycycline, or mefloquine
Malta	None	Not applicable	Not applicable	Not applicable
Marshall Islands	None	Not applicable	Not applicable	Not applicable
Martinique (France)	None	Not applicable	Not applicable	Not applicable
Mauritania	Present in southern provinces. None in Dakhlet-Nouadhibou, Inchiri, Adrar and Tiris-Zemmour regions	Chloroquine	*P. falciparum* 85% *P. ovale* 5%–10% *P. vivax* rare	Atovaquone/proguanil, doxycycline, or mefloquine
Mauritius	None	Not applicable	Not applicable	Not applicable
Mayotte (French territorial collectivity)	All	Chloroquine	*P. falciparum* 40%–50% *P. vivax* 35%–40% *P. ovale* <1%	Atovaquone/proguanil, doxycycline, or mefloquine
Mexico	Limited to areas infrequently visited by travelers, including small foci along the Guatemala and Belize borders in the states of Chiapas, Quintana Roo, and Tabasco; rural areas in the states of Nayarit, Oaxaca, and Sinaloa; and in an area between 24° N and 28° N latitude, and 106° W and 110° W longitude, which lies in parts of Sonora, Chihuahua, and Durango. No malaria along the United States–Mexico border and in the major resorts along the Pacific and Gulf coasts	None	*P. vivax* 99% *P. falciparum* 1%	Atovaquone/proguanil, chloroquine, doxycycline, mefloquine, or primaquine[5]
Micronesia, Federated States of; includes **Yap Islands**, **Pohnpei**, **Chuuk**, and **Kosrae**	None	Not applicable	Not applicable	Not applicable
Moldova	None	Not applicable	Not applicable	Not applicable
Monaco	None	Not applicable	Not applicable	Not applicable
Mongolia	None	Not applicable	Not applicable	Not applicable

Country	Areas with Malaria	Drug Resistance[2]	Malaria Species[3]	Recommended Chemoprophylaxis[4]
Montenegro	None	Not applicable	Not applicable	Not applicable
Montserrat (U.K.)	None	Not applicable	Not applicable	Not applicable
Morocco	None	Not applicable	Not applicable	Not applicable
Mozambique	All	Chloroquine	*P. falciparum* 95% *P. malariae* and *P. ovale* 5% *P. vivax* rare	Atovaquone/proguanil, doxycycline, or mefloquine
Namibia	Present in the provinces of Kunene, Ohangwena, Okavango, Omaheke, Omusati, Oshana, Oshikoto, Otjozondjupa, and the Caprivi Strip	Chloroquine	*P. falciparum* 90% *P. malariae*, *P. ovale*, and *P. vivax* 10%	Atovaquone/proguanil, doxycycline, or mefloquine
Nauru	None	Not applicable	Not applicable	Not applicable
Nepal	Present throughout country at altitudes <1,200 m (<3,937 ft). None in Kathmandu and on typical Himalayan treks	Chloroquine	*P. vivax* 88% *P. falciparum* 12%	Atovaquone/proguanil, doxycycline, or mefloquine
Netherlands	None	Not applicable	Not applicable	Not applicable
Netherlands Antilles (Bonaire, Curaçao, Saba, St. Eustasius, and St. Maarten)	None	Not applicable	Not applicable	Not applicable
New Caledonia (France)	None	Not applicable	Not applicable	Not applicable
New Zealand	None	Not applicable	Not applicable	Not applicable
Nicaragua	Present in rural areas. None in Managua	None	*P. vivax* 95% *P. falciparum* 5%	Atovaquone/proguanil, chloroquine, doxycycline, mefloquine, or primaquine[5]
Niger	All	Chloroquine	*P. falciparum* 85% *P. ovale* 5%–10% *P. vivax* rare	Atovaquone/proguanil, doxycycline, or mefloquine
Nigeria	All	Chloroquine	*P. falciparum* 85% *P. ovale* 5%–10% *P. vivax* rare	Atovaquone/proguanil, doxycycline, or mefloquine
Niue (New Zealand)	None	Not applicable	Not applicable	Not applicable
Norfolk Island (Australia)	None	Not applicable	Not applicable	Not applicable

1 The information presented herein was accurate at the time of publication; however, factors that can change rapidly and from year to year, such as local weather conditions, mosquito vector density, and prevalence of infection, can markedly affect local malaria transmission patterns. Updated information may be found on the CDC Travelers' Health website at www.cdc.gov/travel.

2 Refers to *P. falciparum* malaria.

3 Estimates of malaria species are based on best available data from multiple sources.

4 Several medications are available for chemoprophylaxis. When deciding which drug to use, consider specific itinerary, length of trip, cost of drug, previous adverse reactions to antimalarials, drug allergies, and current medical history. All travelers should seek medical attention in the event of fever during or after return from travel to areas with malaria.

5 Primaquine can cause hemolytic anemia in persons with G6PD deficiency. Patients must be tested and documented to have a normal level of G6PD activity prior to starting primaquine.

Country	Areas with Malaria	Drug Resistance[2]	Malaria Species[3]	Recommended Chemoprophylaxis[4]
Northern Mariana Islands (U.S.), includes **Saipan**, **Tinian**, and **Rota Island**	None	Not applicable	Not applicable	Not applicable
Norway	None	Not applicable	Not applicable	Not applicable
Oman	None	Not applicable	Not applicable	Not applicable
Pakistan	All areas (including all cities) at altitudes <2,500 m (<8202 ft)	Chloroquine	*P. falciparum* 70% *P. vivax* 30%	Atovaquone/proguanil, doxycycline, or mefloquine
Palau	None	Not applicable	Not applicable	Not applicable
Panama	Present in rural areas of the provinces of Bocas Del Toro, Darién, Veragaus, San Blas and San Blas Islands. None in Panama City or in the former Canal Zone	Chloroquine	*P. vivax* 90%–95% *P. falciparum* 5%–10%	Bocas Del Toro: Atovaquone/proguanil, chloroquine, doxycycline, mefloquine, or primaquine[5] Darién, San Blas, and Veragaus provinces: Atovaquone/proguanil, doxycycline, mefloquine, or primaquine[5]
Papua New Guinea	Present throughout at altitudes <1,800 m (<5,906 ft)	Chloroquine (both *P. falciparum* and *P. vivax*)	*P. falciparum* 65%–80% *P. vivax* 10%–30% *P. malariae* and *P. ovale* rare	Atovaquone/proguanil, doxycycline, or mefloquine
Paraguay	Present in the departments of Alto Paraná, Caaguazú, and Canendiyú	None	*P. vivax* 95% *P. falciparum* 5%	Atovaquone/proguanil, chloroquine, doxycycline, mefloquine, or primaquine[5]
Peru	All departments <2000 m (6,561 ft) except none in Arequipa, Moquegua, Puno, and Tacna. Present in Puerto Maldonado	Chloroquine	*P. vivax* 70% *P. falciparum* 30% *P. malariae* <1%	Lima, coastal areas south of Lima, or the highland tourist areas (Cuzco, Machu Picchu, and Lake Titicaca): Mosquito avoidance only Other areas: Atovaquone/proguanil, doxycycline, or mefloquine
Philippines	Present in rural areas <600 m (1,969 ft), on islands of Luzon, Palawan, and Mindanao. None in urban areas	Chloroquine	*P. falciparum* 70%–80% *P. vivax* 20%–30%	Atovaquone/proguanil, doxycycline, or mefloquine
Pitcairn Islands (U.K.)	None	Not applicable	Not applicable	Not applicable
Poland	None	Not applicable	Not applicable	Not applicable
Portugal	None	Not applicable	Not applicable	Not applicable
Puerto Rico (U.S.)	None	Not applicable	Not applicable	Not applicable

Qatar to **Seychelles**

Country	Areas with Malaria	Drug Resistance[2]	Malaria Species[3]	Recommended Chemoprophylaxis[4]
Qatar	None	Not applicable	Not applicable	Not applicable
Réunion (France)	None	Not applicable	Not applicable	Not applicable
Romania	None	Not applicable	Not applicable	Not applicable
Russia	Rare local cases by border with Azerbaijan	None	*P. vivax* 100%	By border with Azerbaijan: Mosquito avoidance only
Rwanda	All	Chloroquine	*P. falciparum* >85% *P. vivax* 5% *P. ovale* 5%	Atovaquone/proguanil, doxycycline, or mefloquine
Saint Barthelemy (France)	None	Not applicable	Not applicable	Not applicable
Saint Helena (U.K.)	None	Not applicable	Not applicable	Not applicable
Saint Kitts (Saint Christopher) and Nevis (U.K.)	None	Not applicable	Not applicable	Not applicable
Saint Lucia	None	Not applicable	Not applicable	Not applicable
Saint Martin (France)	None	Not applicable	Not applicable	Not applicable
Saint Pierre and Miquelon (France)	None	Not applicable	Not applicable	Not applicable
Saint Vincent and the Grenadines	None	Not applicable	Not applicable	Not applicable
Samoa (formerly **Western Samoa**)	None	Not applicable	Not applicable	Not applicable
Samoa, American (U.S.)	None	Not applicable	Not applicable	Not applicable
San Marino	None	Not applicable	Not applicable	Not applicable
São Tomé and Príncipe	All	Chloroquine	*P. falciparum* 85% *P. malariae, P. ovale* 15% *P. vivax* rare	Atovaquone/proguanil, doxycycline, or mefloquine
Saudi Arabia	Provinces of Al Madinah, Asir (excluding high-altitude areas >2,000 m), Jazan, and Mecca. None in cities of Jeddah, Mecca, Medina, Riyadh, and Ta'if	Chloroquine	*P. falciparum* predominantly *P. vivax* rare	Atovaquone/proguanil, doxycycline, or mefloquine
Senegal	All	Chloroquine	*P. falciparum* >85% *P. ovale* 5%–10% *P. vivax* rare	Atovaquone/proguanil, doxycycline, or mefloquine
Serbia	None	Not applicable	Not applicable	Not applicable
Seychelles	None	Not applicable	Not applicable	Not applicable

1 The information presented herein was accurate at the time of publication; however, factors that can change rapidly and from year to year, such as local weather conditions, mosquito vector density, and prevalence of infection, can markedly affect local malaria transmission patterns. Updated information may be found on the CDC Travelers' Health website at www.cdc.gov/travel.
2 Refers to *P. falciparum* malaria.
3 Estimates of malaria species are based on best available data from multiple sources.
4 Several medications are available for chemoprophylaxis. When deciding which drug to use, consider specific itinerary, length of trip, cost of drug, previous adverse reactions to antimalarials, drug allergies, and current medical history. All travelers should seek medical attention in the event of fever during or after return from travel to areas with malaria.
5 Primaquine can cause hemolytic anemia in persons with G6PD deficiency. Patients must be tested and documented to have a normal level of G6PD activity prior to starting primaquine.

Country	Areas with Malaria	Drug Resistance[2]	Malaria Species[3]	Recommended Chemoprophylaxis[4]
Sierra Leone	All	Chloroquine	*P. falciparum* 85% *P. malariae*, *P. ovale*, and *P. vivax* 15%	Atovaquone/proguanil, doxycycline, or mefloquine
Singapore	None	Not applicable	Not applicable	Not applicable
Slovakia	None	Not applicable	Not applicable	Not applicable
Slovenia	None	Not applicable	Not applicable	Not applicable
Solomon Islands	All	Chloroquine	*P. falciparum* 60% *P. vivax* 35%–40% *P. ovale* <1%	Atovaquone/proguanil, doxycycline, or mefloquine
Somalia	All	Chloroquine	*P. falciparum* 95% *P. vivax*, *P. malariae*, and *P. ovale* 5%	Atovaquone/proguanil, doxycycline, or mefloquine
South Africa	Present in the Mpumalanga Province, Limpopo (Northern) Province, and northeastern KwaZulu-Natal as far south as the Tugela River. Present in Kruger National Park	Chloroquine	*P. falciparum* 90% *P. vivax* 5% *P. ovale* 5%	Atovaquone/proguanil, doxycycline, or mefloquine
Spain	None	Not applicable	Not applicable	Not applicable
Sri Lanka	All areas, except none in the districts of Colombo, Galle, Gampaha, Kalutara, Matara, and Nuwara Eliya	Chloroquine	*P. vivax* 88% *P. falciparum* 12%	Atovaquone/proguanil, doxycycline, or mefloquine
Sudan	All	Chloroquine	*P. falciparum* 90% *P. malariae*, *P. vivax*, and *P. ovale* 10%	Atovaquone/proguanil, doxycycline, or mefloquine
Suriname	All areas, except none in Paramaribo	Chloroquine	*P. falciparum* 70% *P. vivax* 15%–20%	Atovaquone/proguanil, doxycycline, or mefloquine
Swaziland	Present in the northern and eastern areas bordering Mozambique and Zimbabwe, including all of Lubombo district	Chloroquine	*P. falciparum* 90% *P. vivax* 5% *P. ovale* 5%	Atovaquone/proguanil, doxycycline, or mefloquine
Sweden	None	Not applicable	Not applicable	Not applicable
Switzerland	None	Not applicable	Not applicable	Not applicable
Syria	Rare cases in the northern border in El Hassaka province	None	*P. vivax* predominantly	Mosquito avoidance only
Taiwan	None	Not applicable	Not applicable	Not applicable
Tajikistan	All areas <2,000 m (6562 ft)	Chloroquine	*P. vivax* 90% *P. falciparum* 10%	Atovaquone/proguanil, doxycycline, mefloquine, or primaquine[5]
Tanzania	All areas at altitudes <1,800 m (<5,906 ft)	Chloroquine	*P. falciparum* >85% *P. malariae*, and *P. ovale* >10% *P. vivax* rare	Atovaquone/proguanil, doxycycline, or mefloquine

Country	Areas with Malaria	Drug Resistance[2]	Malaria Species[3]	Recommended Chemoprophylaxis[4]
Thailand	Rural, forested areas that border Cambodia, Laos, and Myanmar (Burma). Rare local cases in Phang Nga and Phuket. None in cities and in major tourist resorts. None in cities of Bangkok, Chiang Mai, Chiang Rai, Pattaya, Koh Samui, and Koh Phangan	Chloroquine Mefloquine (see Map 2-9)	*P. falciparum* 50% (up to 75% some areas) *P. vivax* 50% (up to 60% some areas) *P. ovale*, rare	Phang Nga and Phuket: Mosquito avoidance only All other areas: Atovaquone/proguanil or doxycycline
Timor-Leste (East Timor)	All	Chloroquine	*P. falciparum* 50% *P. vivax* 50% *P. ovale* <1% *P. malariae* <1%	Atovaquone/proguanil, doxycycline, or mefloquine
Togo	All	Chloroquine	*P. falciparum* 85% *P. ovale* 5%–10% *P. vivax* rare	Atovaquone/proguanil, doxycycline, or mefloquine
Tokelau (New Zealand)	None	Not applicable	Not applicable	Not applicable
Tonga	None	Not applicable	Not applicable	Not applicable
Trinidad and Tobago	None	Not applicable	Not applicable	Not applicable
Tunisia	None	Not applicable	Not applicable	Not applicable
Turkey	Present by border with Syria. None on the Incerlik U.S. Air Force base and on typical cruise itineraries	None	*P. vivax* and *P. falciparum* present	Atovaquone/proguanil, chloroquine, doxycycline, or mefloquine
Turkmenistan	Rare local cases by Afghanistan border	None	*P. vivax* 100%	Mosquito avoidance only
Turks and Caicos Islands (U.K.)	None	Not applicable	Not applicable	Not applicable
Tuvalu	None	Not applicable	Not applicable	Not applicable
Uganda	All	Chloroquine	*P. falciparum* >85% *P. malariae, P. ovale,* and *P. vivax* <15%	Atovaquone/proguanil, doxycycline, or mefloquine
Ukraine	None	Not applicable	Not applicable	Not applicable
United Arab Emirates	None	Not applicable	Not applicable	Not applicable
United Kingdom (with **Channel Islands** and **Isle of Man**)	None	Not applicable	Not applicable	Not applicable
United States	None	Not applicable	Not applicable	Not applicable
Uruguay	None	Not applicable	Not applicable	Not applicable

1 The information presented herein was accurate at the time of publication; however, factors that can change rapidly and from year to year, such as local weather conditions, mosquito vector density, and prevalence of infection, can markedly affect local malaria transmission patterns. Updated information may be found on the CDC Travelers' Health website at www.cdc.gov/travel.

2 Refers to *P. falciparum* malaria.

3 Estimates of malaria species are based on best available data from multiple sources.

4 Several medications are available for chemoprophylaxis. When deciding which drug to use, consider specific itinerary, length of trip, cost of drug, previous adverse reactions to antimalarials, drug allergies, and current medical history. All travelers should seek medical attention in the event of fever during or after return from travel to areas with malaria.

5 Primaquine can cause hemolytic anemia in persons with G6PD deficiency. Patients must be tested and documented to have a normal level of G6PD activity prior to starting primaquine.

Country	Areas with Malaria	Drug Resistance[2]	Malaria Species[3]	Recommended Chemoprophylaxis[4]
Uzbekistan	Rare cases along the Afghanistan and Tajikistan border	None	*P. vivax* 100%	Mosquito avoidance only
Vanuatu	All	Chloroquine	*P. falciparum* 60% *P. vivax* 35%–40% *P. ovale* <1%	Atovaquone/proguanil, doxycycline, or mefloquine
Venezuela	Rural areas of the following states: Apure, Amazonas, Barinas, Bolivar, Sucre, Tachira, and Delta Amacuro. Present in Angel Falls. None in Margarita Island	Chloroquine	*P. vivax* 80%–90% *P. falciparum* 10%–20%	Atovaquone/proguanil, doxycycline, or mefloquine
Vietnam	Rural, forested areas, **except** none in the Red River delta and the coast north of Nha Trang. None in Can Tho, Da Nang, Haiphong, Hanoi, Ho Chi Minh City (Saigon), Hue, Nha Trang, and Qui Nhon	Chloroquine Mefloquine (see Map 2-9)	*P. falciparum* 50%–80% *P. vivax* 20%–50%	Southern part of the country in the provinces of Dac Lac, Gia Lai, Khanh Hoa, Kon Tum, Lam Dong, Ninh Thuan, Song Be, Tay Ninh: Atovaquone/proguanil or doxycycline All other areas: Atovaquone/proguanil, doxycycline, or mefloquine
Virgin Islands, British	None	Not applicable	Not applicable	Not applicable
Virgin Islands, U.S.	None	Not applicable	Not applicable	Not applicable
Western Sahara	Rare cases	None	Unknown	Mosquito avoidance only
Yemen	All areas at altitudes <2,000 m (<6,561 ft). None in Sana'a	Chloroquine	*P. falciparum* 95% *P. malariae, P. vivax,* and *P. ovale* 5%	Atovaquone/proguanil, doxycycline, or mefloquine
Zambia	All	Chloroquine	*P. falciparum* >90% *P. vivax* up to 5% *P. ovale* up to 5 %	Atovaquone/proguanil, doxycycline, or mefloquine
Zimbabwe	All	Chloroquine	*P. falciparum* >90% *P. vivax* up to 5% *P. ovale* up to 5 %	Atovaquone/proguanil, doxycycline, or mefloquine

Self-Treatable Diseases

SELF-TREATABLE DISEASES

Alan J. Magill

Despite our best efforts at helping to prevent illness, travelers will often become ill while traveling. Obtaining reliable and timely medical care can be problematic in many destinations. As a result, prescribing certain medications in advance can empower the traveler to self-diagnose and treat common health problems. During an activity in a remote setting, such as trekking, the only alternative to self-treatment would be no treatment. In some developing countries, appropriate pre-travel counseling may result in a more accurate diagnosis and treatment than relying on local medical care. In addition, the increasing awareness of counterfeit drugs in pharmacies in the developing world (as many as 20%–30% of the drugs on the shelves) makes it more important for travelers to carry reliable drugs from their own country.

Providing education and prescriptions is part of the pre-travel consultation. The key aspect to this strategy is to recognize which travelers may be at risk and to educate them as to the diagnosis and treatment of the particular illness. The keys to successful self-treatment strategies are providing a simple disease definition, providing one choice of treatment, and educating the traveler about the expected outcome of treatment. Using travelers' diarrhea as an example, one could provide the following advice:

- Travelers' diarrhea is defined as "the sudden onset of relatively uncomfortable diarrhea."
- The treatment is ciprofloxacin 500 mg every 12 hours for 1 day (two doses).
- The traveler should feel better within 6 to 24 hours.

To minimize the potential negative effects of a self-treatment strategy, the recommendations should follow a few key points:

- Drugs used must be safe, well tolerated, and effective for use as self-treatment.
- A drug's toxicity or potential for harm, if used incorrectly or in an overdose situation, should be minimal.
- Good directions are critical. Consider providing simple but clear handouts describing how to use the drugs. Keeping the directions simple will greatly increase the effectiveness of the strategy.

Following are some of the most common situations in which people would find self-treatment useful. The extent of self-treatment recommendations offered to the traveler should reflect the remoteness and difficulty of travel and the availability of reliable medical care at the particular destination. The recommended self-treatment options for each disease are provided in the designated section of the Yellow Book.

Travelers' diarrhea (TD) is perhaps most frequent indication for self-treatment. The success of this strategy is based on the epidemiologic evidence that bacterial pathogens account for more than 90% of TD in short-term travelers. The recognition of antibiotic resistance for certain organisms in specific destinations has made the empiric choice of treatment somewhat more problematic in recent times (see the Travelers' Diarrhea section next in this chapter).

Altitude illness or acute mountain sickness (AMS) is a risk for travelers who ascend rapidly to altitudes >8,000 ft (2,440 m). Certain common travel destinations, such as Cuzco, Peru, or Lhasa, Tibet, involve flying to altitudes of 11,300 ft (3,445 m) or 12,700 ft (3,870 m). The symptoms of headache, anorexia, nausea, fatigue, lassitude, and poor sleep can largely be prevented or treated with acetazolamide (see the Altitude Illness section later in this chapter).

Jet lag affects almost everyone who crosses three or more time zones. There is no consensus on the optimal pharmacologic treatment or prevention of the symptoms of jet lag, but sleeping medication taken at the destination may help regularize sleep patterns (see the Jet Lag section later in this chapter).

Motion sickness can be a major deterrent to enjoyment for any susceptible person on a boat or a winding road. Premedication may help alleviate or ameliorate this bothersome syndrome (see the Motion Sickness section later in this chapter).

The self-treatment of suspected **respiratory infections** with empiric antibiotics is controversial. Almost all upper respiratory tract infections are initially caused by viruses. However, these viral infections, under the stress of travel, can lead to bacterial sinusitis, bronchitis or pneumonia. Respiratory infections that last longer than a week without signs of improvement may require empiric antibiotics for recovery. Prolonged respiratory infections may have more of a negative impact on a trip than diarrheal disease (see the Respiratory Infections section later in this chapter).

Bacterial skin infections are not common among travelers, but when they occur, they can be particularly distressing. Bacterial abscesses or cellulitis can worsen rapidly and be very painful. If the traveler is in a remote area or even more than a day's travel from medical care, the use of empiric antibiotic treatment can be extremely beneficial (see the Skin and Soft Tissue Infections in Returned Travelers section in Chapter 4).

Urinary tract infections are common among many women, and carrying an antibiotic for empiric treatment of this condition may be valuable in many circumstances.

Vaginal yeast infections in women can be a very annoying and debilitating problem. For women who know they are prone to infections, all sexually active women, and those who may be receiving antibiotics for other reasons, including doxycycline for antimalarial prophylaxis, a self-treatment course of their preferred antifungal medication can be prescribed.

Occupational/HIV needlestick is a particular risk to those participating in medical-related activities. Every year thousands of such individuals are now working in areas of sub-Saharan Africa, where the HIV prevalence may be higher than 15%–20%. A significant needlestick in this setting should prompt immediate wound care and the possible use of antiretroviral medications (see the Occupational Exposure to HIV section later in this chapter).

Malaria self-treatment is often referred to as stand-by emergency treatment (SBET). This strategy asks the traveler to use a therapeutic dose of an appropriate antimalarial drug when the traveler has a significant fever accompanied by systemic illness, and then proceed to reliable medical care within 24 hours. The goal is to prevent death or severe malaria. Since most travelers at risk of malaria should be advised to use prophylactic medication, this strategy is usually discouraged and reserved for a specific type of traveler under certain defined circumstances (see the Malaria section earlier in this chapter).

TRAVELERS' DIARRHEA

Bradley A. Connor

Description

Travelers' diarrhea (TD) is the most predictable travel-related illness. Attack rates range from 30% to 70% of travelers, depending on the destination. Traditionally, it was thought that TD could be prevented by following eating rules, but studies have found that people who follow the rules still get ill. Poor hygiene practice in local restaurants is likely the largest contributor to the risk for TD.

TD itself is a clinical syndrome that can result from a variety of intestinal pathogens. Bacterial pathogens are the predominant risk, thought to account for 80%–90% of TD. Intestinal viruses have been isolated in studies of TD, but they usually account for 5%–8% of illnesses. Protozoal pathogens are slower to manifest symptoms, and collectively account for about 10% of diagnoses in longer-term travelers. What is commonly known as "food poisoning" involves the ingestion of preformed toxins in food. In this syndrome, vomiting and diarrhea may both be present, but symptoms usually resolve spontaneously within 12 hours.

Infectious Agent

- Bacteria are the most common cause of TD. The most common pathogen is enterotoxigenic *Escherichia coli*, followed by *Campylobacter jejuni*, *Shigella* sp., and *Salmonella* sp. Enteroadherent and other *E. coli* species have been found to also be common pathogens in bacterial diarrhea.
- Viral diarrhea can be caused by a number of viral pathogens, including norovirus, rotavirus, and astrovirus.

- *Giardia* is the main protozoal pathogen found in travelers. *Entamoeba histolytica* is a relatively uncommon pathogen in travelers. *Cryptosporidium* is also relatively uncommon. The risk for *Cyclospora* is highly geographic and seasonal, with the most well-known risks in Nepal, Peru, Haiti, and Guatemala. *Dientamoeba fragilis* is a low-grade but persistent pathogen that is occasionally diagnosed in travelers.
- The individual pathogens are each discussed in their own sections in Chapter 5, and persistent diarrhea is discussed in Chapter 4.

Occurrence

- The most important determinant of risk is travel destination, and there are regional differences in both the risk for and etiology of diarrhea.
- The world is generally divided into three grades of risk: low, intermediate, and high.
  - ○ Low-risk countries include the United States, Canada, Australia, New Zealand, Japan, and countries in Northern and Western Europe.
  - ○ Intermediate-risk countries include those in Eastern Europe, South Africa, and some of the Caribbean islands.
  - ○ High-risk areas include most of Asia, the Middle East, Africa, Mexico, and Central and South America.

Risk for Travelers

Travelers' diarrhea occurs equally in male and female travelers and is more common in young adults than in older people. In short-term travelers, bouts of TD do not appear to protect against future attacks, and more than one episode of TD may occur during a single trip. A cohort of expatriates taking up residence in Kathmandu, Nepal, experienced an average of 3.2 episodes of TD per person in their first year. In more temperate regions, there may be seasonal variations in diarrhea risk. In South Asia, for example, during the hot months preceding the monsoon, much higher TD attack rates are commonly reported.

In environments where large numbers of people do not have access to plumbing or outhouses, the amount of stool contamination in the environment will be higher and more accessible to flies. Inadequate electrical capacity may lead to frequent blackouts or poorly functioning refrigeration, which can result in unsafe food storage and an increased risk for disease. Inadequate water supplies can lead to the absence of sinks for handwashing by restaurant staff. Poor training in handling and preparation of food may lead to cross-contamination from meat and inadequate sterilization of food preparation surfaces and utensils. In destinations in which effective food handling courses have been provided, the risk for TD has been demonstrated to decrease. It should be noted, however, that pathogens that cause TD are not unique to developing countries. The risk of TD is associated with the hygiene practices in specific destinations and the handling and preparation of food in restaurants in developed countries as well.

Clinical Presentation

- Bacterial diarrhea presents with the sudden onset of bothersome symptoms that can range from mild cramps and urgent loose stools, to severe abdominal pain, fever, vomiting, and bloody diarrhea.
- Viral enteropathogens present in a similar fashion to bacterial pathogens, although with norovirus vomiting may be more prominent.
- Protozoal diarrhea, such as that caused by *Giardia intestinalis*, or *Entamoeba histolytica*, generally has a more gradual onset of low-grade symptoms, with 2–5 loose stools per day.
- The incubation period of the pathogens can be a clue to the etiology of TD.
  - ○ Bacterial and viral pathogens have an incubation period of 6–48 hours.

○ Protozoal pathogens generally have an incubation period of 1–2 weeks and rarely present in the first few weeks of travel. An exception can be *Cyclospora cayetanensis*, which can present quickly in areas of high risk.

- Untreated bacterial diarrhea lasts 3–5 days. Viral diarrhea lasts 2–3 days. Protozoal diarrhea can persist for weeks to months without treatment.
- An acute bout of gastroenteritis can lead to persistent gastrointestinal symptoms, even in the absence of continued infection (see the Persistent Travelers' Diarrhea section in Chapter 4). Other postinfectious sequelae include reactive arthritis and Guillain–Barré syndrome.

Preventive Measures for Travelers

- For travelers to high-risk areas, several approaches may be recommended that can reduce but never completely eliminate the risk for TD. These include—
  ○ Instruction regarding food and beverage selection
  ○ Use of agents other than antimicrobial drugs for prophylaxis
  ○ Use of prophylactic antibiotics
- Carrying small containers of hand-sanitizing solutions or gels (containing at least 60% alcohol) may make it easier for travelers to clean their hands before eating.

Food and Beverage Selection

Care in selecting food and beverages for consumption might minimize the risk for acquiring TD. Travelers should be advised that foods that are freshly cooked and served piping hot are safer than foods that may have been sitting for some time in the kitchen or in a buffet. Care should be taken to avoid beverages diluted with nonpotable water (reconstituted fruit juices, ice, and milk) and foods washed in nonpotable water, such as salads. Other risky foods include raw or undercooked meat and seafood, and unpeeled raw fruits and vegetables. Safe beverages include those that are bottled and sealed, or carbonated. Boiled beverages and those appropriately treated with iodine or chlorine may also be safely consumed. Although food and water precautions continue to be recommended, travelers may not always be able to always adhere to the advice. Furthermore, many of the factors that ensure food safety, such as restaurant hygiene, are out of the traveler's control.

Nonantimicrobial Drugs for Prophylaxis

The primary agent studied for prevention of TD, other than antimicrobial drugs, is bismuth subsalicylate (BSS), which is the active ingredient in Pepto-Bismol. Studies from Mexico have shown this agent (taken daily as either 2 oz of liquid or two chewable tablets four times per day) reduces the incidence of TD from 40% to 14%. BSS commonly causes blackening of the tongue and stool and may cause nausea, constipation, and rarely tinnitus. BSS should be avoided by travelers with aspirin allergy, renal insufficiency, and gout, and by those taking anticoagulants, probenecid, or methotrexate. In travelers taking aspirin or salicylates for other reasons, the use of BSS may result in salicylate toxicity. Caution should be used in administering BSS to children with viral infections, such as varicella or influenza, because of the risk for Reye syndrome. BSS is not recommended for children <3 years of age. Studies have not established the safety of BSS use for periods >3 weeks.

The use of probiotics, such as Lactobacillus GG and *Saccharomyces boulardii*, has been studied in the prevention of TD in limited numbers of subjects. Results are inconclusive, partially because standardized preparations of these bacteria are not reliably available.

Prophylactic Antibiotics

Prophylactic antibiotics have been demonstrated to be quite effective in the prevention of TD. Controlled studies have shown that diarrhea attack rates are reduced from 40%

to 4% by the use of antibiotics. The prophylactic antibiotic of choice has changed over the past few decades as resistance patterns have evolved. Agents such as trimethoprim-sulfamethoxazole and doxycycline are no longer considered effective antimicrobial agents against enteric bacterial pathogens. The fluoroquinolones have been the most effective antibiotics for the prophylaxis and treatment of bacterial TD pathogens, but increasing resistance to these agents, mainly among *Campylobacter* species, may limit their benefit in the future. A nonabsorbable antibiotic, rifaximin, is being investigated for its potential use in TD prophylaxis. In the only study published to date, rifaximin reduced the risk for TD in travelers to Mexico by 77%. At this time, prophylactic antibiotics should not be recommended for most travelers. In addition to affording no protection against nonbacterial pathogens, the use of antibiotics may be associated with allergic or adverse reactions in a certain percentage of travelers. The use of prophylactic antibiotics should be weighed against the result of using prompt, early self-treatment with antibiotics when TD occurs, which can limit the duration of illness to 6–24 hours in most cases.

Prophylactic antibiotics may be considered for short-term travelers who are high-risk hosts (such as those who are immunosuppressed) or are taking critical trips during which even a short bout of diarrhea could impact the purpose of the trip.

Treatment

Antibiotics are the principal element in the treatment of TD. Adjunctive agents used for symptomatic control may also be recommended.

Antibiotics

As bacterial causes of TD far outnumber other microbial etiologies, empiric treatment with an antibiotic directed at enteric bacterial pathogens remains the best therapy for TD. The benefit of treatment of TD with antibiotics has been proven in numerous studies. The effectiveness of a particular antimicrobial depends on the etiologic agent and its antibiotic sensitivity. Both as empiric therapy or for treatment of a specific bacterial pathogen, first-line antibiotics include those of the fluoroquinolone class, such as ciprofloxacin or levofloxacin. Increasing microbial resistance to the fluoroquinolones, especially among *Campylobacter* isolates, may limit their usefulness in some destinations such as Thailand, where *Campylobacter* is prevalent. Isolated anecdotal case reports of resistant *Campylobacter* diarrhea occur periodically from other destinations. An alternative to the fluoroquinolones in this situation is azithromycin. Rifaximin has been approved for the treatment of TD caused by noninvasive strains of *E. coli*. However, since it is often difficult for travelers to distinguish between invasive and noninvasive diarrhea and since they would have to carry a back-up drug in the event of invasive diarrhea, the overall usefulness of rifaximin as empiric self-treatment remains to be determined.

Single-dose or 1-day therapy for TD with a fluoroquinolone is well established, both by clinical trials and clinical experience. The best regimen for azithromycin treatment is not yet established. One study used a single dose of 1,000 mg, but side effects (mainly nausea) may limit the acceptability of this large dose. Azithromycin, 500 mg per day for 1–2 days, appears to be effective in most cases of TD.

Antimotility Agents

Antimotility agents provide symptomatic relief and serve as useful adjuncts to antibiotic therapy in TD. Synthetic opiates, such as loperamide and diphenoxylate, can reduce bowel movement frequency and enable travelers to ride on an airplane or bus while awaiting the effects of antibiotics. Loperamide appears to have antisecretory properties as well. The safety of loperamide when used along with an appropriate antibiotic has been well established, even in cases of invasive pathogens. Loperamide can be used in children, and liquid formulations are available. In practice, however, these drugs are rarely given to small children.

Oral Rehydration Therapy

Fluids and electrolytes are lost in cases of TD, and replenishment is important, especially in young children or adults with chronic medical illness. In adult travelers who are otherwise healthy, severe dehydration resulting from TD is unusual unless prolonged vomiting is present. Nonetheless, replacement of fluid losses remains an important adjunct to other therapy and helps the traveler feel better more quickly. Travelers should remember to use only beverages that are sealed or carbonated, or otherwise known to be purified. For more severe fluid loss, replacement is best accomplished with oral rehydration solutions (ORS), such as the WHO ORS solutions, which are widely available at stores and pharmacies in most developing countries (see Table 2-25 for details). ORS is prepared by adding one packet to the appropriate volume of boiled or treated water. Travelers may find most ORS formulations to be relatively unpalatable, due to their saltiness. In most cases, rehydration can be maintained with any palatable liquid.

Treatment of TD Caused by Protozoa

The most common parasitic cause of TD is *Giardia intestinalis*, and treatment options include metronidazole, tinidazole, and nitazoxanide. Although cryptosporidiosis is usually a self-limited illness in immunocompetent persons, nitazoxanide can be considered as a treatment option. Cyclosporiasis is treated with trimethoprim–sulfamethoxazole. Treatment of amebiasis is with metronidazole or tinidazole, followed by treatment with a luminal agent such as paromomycin.

Treatment for Children

Children who accompany their parents on trips to high-risk destinations may be expected to have TD as well. There is no reason to withhold antibiotics from children who contract TD. In older children and teenagers, treatment recommendations for TD follow those for adults, with possible adjustments in the dose of medication. Macrolides such as azithromycin are considered first-line antibiotic therapy in children, although some experts now use short-course fluoroquinolone therapy for travelers <18 years of age. Rifaximin is approved for use starting at 12 years of age.

Infants and younger children are at higher risk for developing dehydration from TD, which is best prevented by the early use of ORS solutions. Breastfed infants should continue to nurse on demand, and bottle-fed infants can continue to drink their formula. Older infants and children may eat a regular diet, depending on the level of their appetite while they are ill. Infants in diapers are at risk for developing a painful, ecxematous rash on their buttocks in response to the liquid stool. Hydrocortisone cream will quickly improve this rash. More information about diarrhea and dehydration are discussed in the Traveling Safely with Infants and Children section in Chapter 7.

Table 2-25. Composition of WHO oral rehydration solution (ORS) for diarrheal illness

Ingredient	Amount	Measurement
Sodium chloride	3.5 g/L	½ tsp
Potassium chloride	1.5 g/L	1¼ tsp
Glucose	20.0 g/L	2 tbsp
Trisodium citrate (or sodium bicarbonate)	2.9 g/L (or 2.5 g/L)	½ tsp
Water	1,000 g	1 liter

References

1. Steffen R. Epidemiology of travellers' diarrhoea. Scand J Gastroenterol Suppl. 1983;84:5–17.

2. Black RE. Epidemiology of travelers' diarrhea and relative importance of various pathogens. Rev Infect Dis. 1990;12(Suppl 1):S73–9.

3. Adachi JA, Jiang ZD, Mathewson JJ, et al. Enteroaggregative *Escherichia coli* as a major etiologic agent in traveler's diarrhea in 3 regions of the world. Clin Infect Dis. 2001;32(12):1706–9.

4. von Sonnenburg F, Tornieporth N, Waiyaki P, et al. Risk and aetiology of diarrhoea at various tourist destinations. Lancet. 2000;356(9224):133–4.

5. Shlim DR. Update in traveler's diarrhea. Infect Dis Clin North Am. 2005;19(1):137–49.

6. DuPont HL, Ericsson CD. Prevention and treatment of traveler's diarrhea. N Engl J Med. 1993;328(25):1821–7.

7. Connor BA. Sequelae of traveler's diarrhea: focus on postinfectious irritable bowel syndrome. Clin Infect Dis. 2005;41(Suppl 8):S577–86.

8. Hoge CW, Gambel JM, Srijan A, et al. Trends in antimicrobial resistance among diarrheal pathogens isolated in Thailand over 15 years. Clin Infect Dis. 1998;26:341–5.

9. DuPont HL, Jiang ZD, Ericsson CD, et al. Rifaximin versus ciprofloxacin for the treatment of traveler's diarrhea: a randomized double blind clinical trial. Clin Infect Dis. 2001;33(11):1807–15.

Perspectives: Global Impact of Diarrheal Disease

Sean W. Pawlowski, Richard L. Guerrant

Travelers frequently acquire the enteric pathogens that are present in food and water at their destinations and develop travelers' diarrhea. Mercifully, this is usually a nonfatal nuisance for travelers from developed nations, who, due to their well-nourished state, lack of other co-morbidities, antibiotic availability, and lack of repetitive infections, recover from their illness (more often than not) with few lasting effects.

In the short term, for those living in developing countries, infections due to enteric organisms are potentially life threatening, particularly in children and when combined with other illnesses, such as measles. Oral rehydration is the mainstay of treatment, but children suffering repeated, malnourishing illnesses at weaning require critical nutrient and micronutrient therapy as well.

While those traveling to aid in humanitarian efforts, including missionaries and volunteers, may feel they are well prepared to meet the challenges they face, many may not fully understand the profound impact that the lack of availability of clean water and sanitation has on indigenous populations. Travel health advisors, as well, should understand the serious implications and consequences of the global burden of these diarrheal illnesses as their occurrence is centered in the destinations of many U.S. travelers. Recent figures estimate 1.6 million deaths per year worldwide in children <5 years of age in these areas. Fortunately, this rate is dramatically down from 4.6 million per year (estimates from 1955 to 1979), in large part due to the implementation of oral rehydration therapy. However, the morbidity rates either have not fallen or have slightly increased. In addition, as the AIDS pandemic continues to spread, complications associated with endemic enteric pathogens will likely increase both mortality and morbidity.

More difficult to quantify is the global burden of repeated or persistent diarrheal illnesses. Unfortunately, these contribute significantly to the impairment of physical and cognitive development of children and to long-term disability, which ultimately result in substantial national economic losses.

REFERENCES

1. UNICEF. The state of the world's children 2008. [cited 2008 Nov 26]. Available from: http://www.unicef.org/sowc08/.

2. Kosek M, Bern C, Guerrant R. The global burden of diarrhoeal disease, as estimated from studies published between 1992 and 2000. Bull WHO. 2003;81(3):197–204.

3. Guerrant R, Oria R, Bushen OY, et al. Global impact of diarrheal diseases that are sampled by travelers: the rest of the hippopotamus. Clin Infect Dis 2005;41(Suppl 8):S524–30.

4. Guerrant R, Kosek M, Moore S, et al. Magnitude and impact of diarrheal diseases. Arch Med Res 2002;33(4):351–5.

5. Guerrant RL, Oriá RB, Moore SR, et al. Malnutrition as an enteric infectious disease, with long-term effects on child development. Nutr Rev. 2008;66(9):487-505.

6. Checkley W, Buckley G, Gilman RH, et al. The Childhood Malnutrition and Diarrhea Network. Multi-country analysis of the effects of diarrhea on childhood stunting. Internat J Epidemiol. 2008;37(4):816-30.

ALTITUDE ILLNESS

Peter H. Hackett, David R. Shlim

Occurrence

The stresses of the high-altitude environment include cold, low humidity, increased ultraviolet (UV) radiation, and decreased air pressure, all of which can cause problems for travelers. The greatest concern, however, is hypoxia. At 10,000 ft (3,000 m), for example, the inspired PO_2 is only 69% of sea-level value. The degree of hypoxic stress depends upon altitude, rate of ascent, and duration of exposure. Sleeping at high altitude produces the greatest hypoxia; day trips to high altitude with return to low altitude are much less stressful on the body.

Acclimatization

The human body adjusts very well to moderate hypoxia, but requires time to do so (Box 2-3). The process of acute acclimatization to high altitude takes 3–5 days; therefore, acclimatizing for a few days at 8,000–9,000 ft before proceeding to higher altitude is ideal. Acclimatization prevents altitude illness, improves sleep, and increases comfort and well-being, although exercise performance will always be reduced compared with low altitude. Increase in ventilation is the most important factor in acute acclimatization; therefore, respiratory depressants must be avoided. Increased red-cell production does not play a role in acute acclimatization.

Risk for Travelers

Inadequate acclimatization may lead to altitude illness in any traveler going to 8,000 ft (2,500 m) or higher. Susceptibility and resistance to altitude illness are genetic traits, and no screening tests are available to predict risk. Risk is not affected by training or physical fitness. Children are equally susceptible as adults; persons >50 years of age have slightly lower risk. How a traveler has responded to high altitude previously is the most reliable guide for future trips but is not infallible. However, given certain baseline susceptibility, risk is greatly influenced by rate of ascent and exertion.

Box 2-3. Tips for acclimatization

The following are helpful tips for people traveling to high altitude destinations.

- Ascend gradually, if possible. Try not to go directly from low altitude to >9,000 ft (2,750 m) sleeping altitude in one day.
- Consider using acetazolamide (Diamox) to speed acclimatization if abrupt ascent is unavoidable.
- Avoid alcohol for the first 48 hours.
- Participate in only mild exercise for the first 48 hours.
- Having a high-altitude exposure at >9,000 ft (2,750 m), for 2 nights or more within 30 days prior to the trip is useful.
- Treat an altitude headache with simple analgesics.

Determining an itinerary that will avoid any occurrence of altitude illness is difficult because of variations in individual susceptibility, as well as in starting points and terrain. Itineraries with a high risk for altitude illness include flying directly to >9,000 ft or rapid hiking ascents, such as climbing Mt. Kilimanjaro. It is best to average no more than 1,000 ft (300 m) ft per day in altitude gain above 12,000 ft (3,660 m).

Examples of high-altitude cities with airports are Cuzco, Peru (11,000 ft; 3,326 m); La Paz, Bolivia (12,000 ft; 3,660 m); and Lhasa, Tibet (12,500 ft; 3,810 m). Travelers flying into these locations may require a period of acclimatization before proceeding higher, and drug prophylaxis may be indicated.

Clinical Presentation

Altitude illness is divided into three syndromes:

- Acute mountain sickness (AMS)
- High-altitude cerebral edema (HACE)
- High-altitude pulmonary edema (HAPE)

Acute Mountain Sickness (AMS)

AMS is the most common form of altitude illness, striking, for example, 25% of all visitors sleeping above 8,000 ft (2,500 m) in Colorado. Symptoms are those of an alcohol hangover: headache is the cardinal symptom, sometimes accompanied by fatigue, loss of appetite, nausea, and, occasionally, vomiting. Headache onset is usually 2–12 hours after arrival at a higher altitude, and often during or after the first night. Preverbal children may develop loss of appetite, irritability, and pallor. AMS generally resolves with 24–72 hours of acclimatization.

High-Altitude Cerebral Edema (HACE)

HACE is a severe progression of AMS and is rare; it is most often associated with pulmonary edema. In addition to AMS symptoms, lethargy becomes profound, with drowsiness, confusion, and ataxia on tandem gait test. A person with HACE requires immediate descent; death from HACE can ensue within 24 hours of developing ataxia if the person fails to descend.

High-Altitude Pulmonary Edema (HAPE)

HAPE can occur by itself or in conjunction with AMS and HACE; incidence is 1/10,000 skiers in Colorado and up to 1 of 100 climbers at >14,000 ft (4,270 m). Initial symptoms are increased breathlessness with exertion, and eventually increased breathlessness at rest, associated with weakness and cough. Oxygen or descent of 1,000 m or more is life-saving. HAPE can be more rapidly fatal than HACE.

Pre-Existing Medical Problems

- Travelers with medical conditions, such as heart failure, myocardial ischemia (angina), sickle cell disease, or any form of pulmonary insufficiency, should be advised to consult a physician familiar with high-altitude medical issues before undertaking high-altitude travel.
- The risk for new ischemic heart disease in previously healthy travelers does not appear to be increased at high altitudes.
- Diabetics can travel safely to high altitude, but they must be accustomed to exercise and carefully monitor their blood glucose. Diabetic ketoacidosis may be triggered by altitude illness and may be more difficult to treat in those on acetazolamide. Not all glucose meters may read accurately at high altitudes.
- Most people do not have visual problems at high altitude. However, at very high altitudes some persons who have had radial keratotomy may develop acute

farsightedness and be unable to climb by themselves. LASIK and other newer procedures may produce only minor visual disturbances at high altitudes.

- There are no studies or case reports of harm to a fetus if the mother travels briefly to high altitude during pregnancy. However, it may be prudent to recommend that pregnant women stay at sleeping altitudes of 12,000 ft (3,658 m) if possible. The dangers of having a pregnancy complication in remote, mountainous terrain should also be discussed.

Treatment

Acetazolamide

Acetazolamide (Diamox) prevents AMS when taken before ascent and can speed recovery if taken after symptoms have developed. The drug works by acidifying the blood, which causes an increase in respiration and thus aids acclimatization. An effective dose that minimizes the common side effects of increased urination and paresthesias of the fingers and toes is 125 mg every 12 hours, beginning the day before ascent and continuing the first 2 days at altitude, or longer if ascent continues. Allergic reactions to acetazolamide are uncommon, but the drug is related to sulfonamides and should not be used by sulfa-allergic persons with history of anaphylaxis. A trial dose taken in a safe environment before travel may be useful for those with a more mild allergic history to sulfonamides. People with history of severe penicillin allergy have occasionally had allergic reactions to acetazolamide.

Dexamethasone

Dexamethasone is very effective for prevention and treatment of AMS and HACE, and perhaps HAPE as well. Unlike acetazolamide, rebound can occur if the drug is discontinued at altitude prior to acclimatization. Acetazolamide is preferable to prevent AMS while ascending, with dexamethasone reserved for treatment during descent. Adult dosage is 4 mg every 6 hours.

HAPE is always associated with increased pulmonary artery pressure, and pulmonary vasodilators are useful for preventing and treating HAPE.

Nifedipine

Nifedipine prevents and ameliorates HAPE in persons who are particularly susceptible to the condition. The adult dosage is 20 mg of extended release every 8–12 hours. PDE-5 inhibitors can also selectively lower pulmonary artery pressure, with less effect on systemic blood pressure.

Other Medications

Tadalafil (Cialis), 10 mg twice a day, during ascent can prevent HAPE and is being studied for treatment. When taken before ascent, gingko biloba, 100–120 mg twice daily, was shown to reduce AMS in adults in some trials, but it was not effective in others, probably due to variation in ingredients. Gingko biloba has not yet been compared directly with acetazolamide.

Preventive Measures for Travelers

The main point of instructing travelers about altitude illness is not to prevent any possibility of altitude illness, but to prevent death from altitude illness. The onset of symptoms and clinical course is sufficiently slow and predictable that there is no reason for someone to die from altitude illness unless trapped by weather or geography in a situation in which descent is impossible. The three rules that travelers should be made aware of to prevent death from altitude illness are—

- Know the early symptoms of altitude illness and be willing to acknowledge when they are present.
- Never ascend to sleep at a higher altitude when experiencing symptoms of altitude illness, no matter how minor they seem.
- Descend if the symptoms become worse while resting at the same altitude.

For trekking groups and expeditions going into remote high-altitude areas, where descent to a lower altitude could be problematic, a pressurization bag (such as the Gamow bag) can prove extremely beneficial. A foot pump produces an increased pressure of 2 lbs. per in^2, mimicking a descent of 5,000–6,000 ft (1,500–1,800 m), depending on the starting altitude. The total packed weight of bag and pump is 6.5 kg.

For most travelers, the best way to avoid altitude illness is by gradual ascent, with extra rest days at intermediate altitudes every 3,000 ft (900 m) or less. If ascent must be rapid, acetazolamide may be used prophylactically, and dexamethasone and pulmonary artery pressure-lowering drugs, such as nifedipine or sildenafil, may be carried for emergencies.

References

1. Hackett PH, Roach RC. High-altitude illness. N Engl J Med. 2001;345(2):107–14.
2. Hackett PH, Roach RC. High-altitude medicine. In: Auerbach PS, editor. Wilderness medicine 5th ed. Philadelphia: Mosby Elsevier; 2007.
3. Pollard AJ, Murdoch DR. The high altitude medicine handbook. 3rd ed. Abingdon, UK: Radcliffe Medical Press; 2003.
4. Hackett PH. High altitude and common medical conditions. In: Hornbein TF, Schoene RB, editors. High altitude: an exploration of human adaptation. New York: Marcel Dekker, Inc.; 2001:839–85.
5. Strom BL, Schinnar R, Apter AJ, et al. Absence of cross-reactivity between sulfonamide antibiotics and sulfonamide nonantibiotics. N Engl J Med. 2003;349(17):1628–35.
6. Johnson TS, Rock PB, Fulco CS, et al. Prevention of acute mountain sickness by dexamethasone. N Engl J Med. 1984;310(11):683–6.
7. Maggiorini M, Brunner-La Rocca HP, Peth S, et al. Both tadalafil and dexamethasone may reduce the incidence of high-altitude pulmonary edema: a randomized trial. Ann Intern Med. 2006;145(7):497–506.

JET LAG

Emad Yanni

Description

Jet lag is a temporary disorder among air travelers who rapidly travel across three or more time zones. Jet lag results from the slow adjustment of the body clock to the destination time, so that daily rhythms and the internal drive for sleep and wakefulness are out of synchrony with the new environment.

The intrinsic body clock resides in the suprachiasmatic nuclei at the base of the hypothalamus, which contains melatonin receptors. The body clock receives information about light from the eyes and is also thought to receive input via the intergeniculate leaflet that carries information about physical activities and general excitement. Melatonin is manufactured in the pineal gland from tryptophan, and its synthesis and release are stimulated by darkness and suppressed by light; consequently, the secretion of melatonin is responsible for setting our sleep–wake cycle. The body clock is adjusted to the solar day by rhythmic cues in the environment known as zeitgebers (time-givers). The main zeitgebers are the light–dark cycle and this rhythmic secretion of melatonin. Exercise might also exert a weaker effect on the body clock than other zeitgebers. Although incompletely understood, the body clock is partly responsible for the daily rhythms in core temperature and plasma hormone concentrations as well.

Occurrence

- Eastward travel is associated with difficulty in falling asleep at the destination bedtime and difficulty arising in the morning.
- Westward travel is associated with early evening sleepiness and predawn awakening.
- Travelers flying within the same time zone typically experience the fewest problems.
- Crossing more time zones or traveling eastward generally increases the time required for adaptation.
- Jet lag lasts for several days, roughly equal to two-thirds the number of time zones crossed for eastward flights, and about half the number of time zones crossed after westward flights.

Risk for Travelers

- Individual responses to crossing time zones and the ability to adapt to new time zones vary. The intensity and duration of jet lag are related to the following:
  - Number of time zones crossed
  - Direction of travel
  - Ability to sleep while traveling
  - Availability and intensity of local circadian time cues at the destination
  - Individual differences in phase tolerance
- Although more data are needed, risk factors cited by the American Academy of Sleep Medicine include the following:
  - Older individuals tend to experience fewer jet lag symptoms than those who are younger.
  - Exposure to local (natural) light–dark cycle usually accelerates adaptation after jet travel over 2 to 10 time zones

Clinical Presentation

Signs of jet lag include the following:

- Poor sleep, including delayed sleep onset (after eastward flight), early awakening (after westward flight), and fractionated sleep (after flights in either direction).
- Poor performance in both physical and mental tasks during the new daytime.
- Negative subjective changes, such as increased fatigue, frequency of headaches and irritability, and decreased ability to concentrate.
- Gastrointestinal disturbances (indigestion, frequency of defecation, and the altered consistency of stools) and decreased interest in and enjoyment of meals.

Preventive Measures for Travelers

Prior to Travel

- Stay healthy by continuing to exercise, eating a nutritious diet, and getting plenty of rest.
- Consider timed bright light exposure prior to and during travel (although it requires high motivation and strict compliance with the prescribed light–dark schedules).
- Break up the journey with a stop-over.

Note: The use of the nutritional supplement melatonin is controversial for the prevention of jet lag. Some clinicians advocate the use of 0.5 mg to 5 mg of melatonin during the first few days of travel, and there are data to suggest its efficacy. However, the quality control of its production is not regulated by the U.S. Food and Drug Administration, and contaminants have been found in commercially available products.

Current information does not support the use of special diets to ameliorate jet lag.

During Travel

Travelers should be advised to—

- Avoid large meals, alcohol, and caffeine.
- Drink plenty of water.
- Move around on the plane to promote mental and physical acuity.
- Wear comfortable shoes and clothing.
- Sleep, if possible, during long flights.

On Arrival at the Destination

Travelers should be advised to—

- Avoid situations requiring critical decision-making, such as important meetings, on the first day after arrival.
- Adapt to the local schedule as soon as possible. However, if the travel period is 2 days or less, travelers should remain on home time.
- Optimize exposure to sunlight following arrival in either direction.
- Eat meals appropriate to the local time.

Treatment

- The 2008 American Academy of Sleep Medicine (AASD) recommendations include promoting sleep with hypnotic medication, although the effects of hypnotics on daytime symptoms of jet lag have not been well studied.
- The prescription of nonaddictive sedative hypnotics (nonbenzodiazepines), such as zolpidem, has been shown in some studies to promote longer periods of high-quality sleep. If a benzodiazepine is preferred, a short-acting one, such as temazepam, is recommended to minimize oversedation the following day.
- Because alcohol intake is often high during international travel, the risk for interaction with hypnotics should be emphasized with patients.

References

1. Waterhouse J, Reilly T, Atkinson G, et al. Jet lag: trends and coping strategies. Lancet. 2007;369(9567):1117–29.
2. Dubocovich ML, Markowska M. Functional MT1 and MT2 melatonin receptors in mammals. Endocrines. 2005;27(2):101–10.
3. Reid KJ, Chang AM, Zee PC. Circadian rhythm sleep disorders. Med Clin North Am. 2004;88(3):631–51.
4. Waterhouse J, Edward B, Nevill A. et al. Do subjective symptoms predict our perception of jet lag? Ergonomics. 2000;43(10):1514–27.
5. Sack RL, Auckley D, Auger RR, et al. Circadian rhythm sleep disorders: part 1, basic principles, shift work and jet lag disorders: An American Academy of Sleep Medicine Review. Sleep. 2007;30(11):1460–83.
6. Jamieson AO, Zammit GK, Rosenberg RS, et al. Zolpidem reduces the sleep disturbance of jet lag. Sleep Med. 2001;2(5):423–30.
7. Daurat A, Benoit O, Buguet A. Effects of zopiclone on the rest/activity rhythm after a westward flight across five time zones. Psychopharmacology. 2000;149(3):241–5.
8. Reilly T, Waterhouse J, Edwards B. Jet lag and air travel: implications for performance. Clin Sports Med. 2005;24(2):367–80.
9. Herxheimer A. Jet lag. Clin Evid. 2005;13:2178–83.

MOTION SICKNESS

I. Dale Carroll

Occurrence

Motion sickness is the result of a conflict between the various senses in regard to motion. The semicircular canals and otoliths in the inner ear sense angular and vertical motion, while the eyes and the proprioceptors determine the body's position in space. When signals received by the eyes or the proprioceptors do not match those being transmitted by the inner ear, motion sickness occurs. It can occur in either the presence or absence of actual motion, such as when viewing a slide through a microscope. Symptoms include nausea, vomiting, pallor, sweating, and often a sense of impending doom. Motion sickness is likely to occur when there is movement simultaneously in multiple planes, such as on amusement rides, on board ships, or during air travel.

Risk for Travelers

- All individuals, given sufficient stimulus, will develop motion sickness.
- Children 2–12 years of age are especially susceptible, while infants and toddlers seem relatively immune.
- Women, especially when pregnant, menstruating, or on hormones, are more likely to have motion sickness.
- Persons with migraine are more prone to either migraine or motion sickness at the same time as the other malady.
- Those who expect to be sick are more apt to experience symptoms.

Treatment

There are both nonpharmacologic and pharmacologic interventions for the prevention or management of motion sickness. None are ideal, and the medications typically cause drowsiness or similar adverse effects. Some feel that permitting continued exposure to motions that induce motion sickness will decondition the response and diminish the symptoms; however, most persons traveling for a limited time will understandably not be willing to endure the symptoms in the hope of deconditioning and will instead want to avail themselves of some of the suggestions that follow or the medications listed in Table 2-26.

Medications

- Antihistamines are the most commonly used and available medications, although nonsedating ones appear to be the least effective.
- Pyridoxine hydrochloride (vitamin B_6) plus doxylamine succinate (an antihistamine) is prescribed under the brand name of Diclectin in Canada and often recommended in their separate forms by clinicians in the United States.
- Sedation is the primary side effect of all the efficacious drugs.
  - Sedation is problematic when treating patients who perform essential tasks such as flying a plane or acting as crew on a ship, or in travelers who wish to participate in activities such as scuba diving or hang gliding.
- Some common prescription medications used by travelers may aggravate the nausea of motion sickness (see Table 2-27).

Medications in Children

- For symptomatic treatment of children 2–12 years of age, dimenhydrinate, 1–1.5 mg/kg per dose, or diphenhydramine, 0.5–1 mg/kg per dose up to 25 mg, can be given 1 hour before travel and every 6 hours during the trip.
- Because some children have paradoxical agitation with these medicines, a test dose should be given at home before departure.
- Scopalamine causes potentially dangerous adverse effects in children and should not be used; prochlorperazine and metoclopramide should be used with caution in children.
- Antihistamines are not FDA approved for use for the prevention or treatment of motion sickness in children. Caregivers should be reminded to always ask a

Table 2-26. Pharmacologic interventions for motion sickness (adult dosing)

Medication	Dose	Caution/Safety Information	Adverse Effects	Drug Interactions
Vitamin supplements Vitamin B$_6$	Various			
Pyridoxine–doxylamine (Example of brand: Diclectin)	Fixed combination available by Rx. in Canada. Sold separately in U.S.	More than 200,000 participants in controlled studies of nausea in pregnancy		
Anticholinergic Scopolamine (Examples of brands: Scopace, Transderm-scop)	Patch: 1.5 mg q 3 days, apply behind ear at least 4 hrs before travel Oral: 0.4–0.8 mg q 8 hrs beginning 1 hr before travel	Contraindicated in narrow-angle glaucoma, urinary retention, GI obstruction, myasthenia gravis. Wash hands after patch application to prevent transfer to eyes. Caution in hot environment or with thyroid, cardiopulmonary, GE reflux, liver, or kidney disease, seizure or psychotic disorder	*Common:* dry mouth/ nose/throat, blurred vision, drowsiness *Less common:* palpitations, urinary retention, bloating, constipation, headache, confusion, hyperexcitability, insomnia, toxic psychosis	Additive effects with alcohol and other CNS depressants. Antacids impair absorption of oral scopolamine. May impair GI motility when used with antidiarrheal drugs. May impair absorption of oral medications
Antihistamines Dimenhydrinate (Examples of brands: Calm X, Dramamine, Triptone)	Tablets 50 mg, syrup 12.5 mg/5 mL. Take 30 min before travel. Adults 50–100 mg q 4–6 hours	Caution in glaucoma, urinary retention, GI obstruction, liver or kidney disease, chronic obstructive pulmonary disease (COPD), seizure disorder. Should not be used in children <2 yrs. Take with food or milk to reduce nausea.	*Common:* drowsiness, anticholinergic symptoms (dry mouth/nose/throat, blurred vision, urinary retention), thick respiratory secretions *Less common:* dizziness, weakness, hypotension or hypertension, cardiac arrhythmia, wheezing, sweating, nausea, vomiting, bloating, diarrhea, constipation, jaundice, anorexia, headache, confusion, tinnitus, paradoxical hyperexcitability, seizures, psychosis, acute dystonic reaction, paresthesias, photosensitivity, anaphylaxis	Additive effects with alcohol and other CNS depressants. Antihistamine effects may be potentiated by monamine oxidase inhibitors. Antacids may impair absorption.
Diphenhydramine (Brands: multiple)	Available in oral capsules and tablets (25 mg, 50 mg),	As above	As above	As above

(Continued)

Table 2-26. Pharmacologic interventions for motion sickness (adult dosing) *(Continued)*

Medication	Dose	Caution/Safety Information	Adverse Effects	Drug Interactions
Diphenhydramine *(Continued)*	elixir (12.5 mg/5 mL). Adults 10–50 mg q 4–6 hours 12.5 mg, 25 mg, 50 mg			
Meclizine (Brands: Antivert [Rx], Bonine [OTC], Dramamine II [OTC], Meclicot [Rx], Medivert [Rx])	Adult dose 25–50 mg q 24 hours	As above	As above	As above
Cyclizine (Brand: Marezine [OTC])	50 mg tablets. Adult dose 50 mg q 4–6 hrs	As above	As above	As above
Antidopaminergic Promethazine (Brands: Phenergan, Promacot)	Available in oral tablets (12.5 mg, 25 mg, 50 mg), syrup (6.25 mg/5 mL, 25 mg/5 mL), rectal suppositories, and intramuscular injection. Adults: 25 mg every 8–12 hrs 5 mg and 10 mg tablets	Caution in sulfite allergy (some formulations contain sulfite), cardiovascular disease, peptic ulcer disease	Pronounced sedation, postural hypotension, skin rash, body temperature dysregulation, extrapyramidal symptoms, delirium, neuroleptic malignant syndrome	May interact with other neurologic drugs
Metoclopramide (Brands: Reglan)	Adults: 10–15 mg q 6 hrs	Unproven benefit as antinausea agent with motion sickness, but may help by hastening gastric emptying	Sedation, insomnia, extrapyramidal symptoms	May decrease absorption of medications from stomach while increasing absorption from intestine. May necessitate change in insulin dose or timing in diabetics
Sympathomimetics Pseudoephedrine	Adults: 60 mg q 6 hours	Sometimes used to counteract sedating effect of other medications	Difficult urination, dry mouth, restlessness, headache	
Benzodiazepines Diazepam (Brand: Valium)	2 mg, 5 mg and 10 mg tablets. Adult dose 2–10 mg q 6 hrs	Very sedating; perhaps of value when added to other medications		
Other antiemetics Prochlorperazine (Brand: Compazine)	5 mg and 10 mg tablets. Adult dose 5–10 mg q 6 hrs	Effective against nausea but not specific for motion sickness.	May cause photosensitization, extrapyramidal symptoms	

(Continued)

Table 2-26. Pharmacologic interventions for motion sickness (adult dosing) *(Continued)*

Medication	Dose	Caution/Safety Information	Adverse Effects	Drug Interactions
Ondansetron (Brand: Zofran)	4 mg and 8 mg tablets; Adult dose 4–8 mg q 8–12 hrs	Orally disintegrating tablets contain phenylalanine	Contraindicated with apomorphine. Effect may be decreased with some anticonvulsants (carbamazepine, phenytoin) and rifamycin (rifampin, rifabutin)	

Table 2-27. Medications that may increase nausea

Medication Class	Examples
Antibiotics	Azithromycin, metronidazole, erythromycin, trimethoprim-sulfamethoxazole
Antiparasitics	Albendazole, thiabendazole, iodoquinol, chloroquine, mefloquine
Estrogens	Oral contraceptives, estradiol
Cardiovascular	Digoxin, levodopa
Narcotic analgesics	Codeine, morphine, meperidine
Nonsteroidal analgesics	Ibuprophen, naproxen, indomethacin
Antidepressants	Fluoxetine, paroxitene, sertraline
Asthma medication	Aminophylline
Bisphosphonates	Alendronate sodium, ibandronate sodium, risedronate sodium

physician, pharmacist, or other health-care professional if they have any questions about how to use or dose antihistamines in children before they administer the medication. Oversedation of young children with antihistamines can lead to life-threatening side effects.

Medications in Pregnancy
- Drugs with the most safety data regarding the treatment of the nausea of pregnancy would seem to be the logical first choice.
- Letter scoring of the safety of medications in pregnancy may not be helpful, and practitioners should review the actual safety data or call the patient's obstetrical provider for suggestions.
- Web-based information may be found at www.Motherisk.org and www.Reprotox.org.

Preventive Measures for Travelers

Nonpharmacologic interventions include—
- Being aware of those situations which tend to trigger symptoms.
- **Optimizing positioning**—Driving a vehicle instead of riding in it, as well as sitting in the front seat of a car or bus, sitting over the wing of an aircraft or being in the central cabin on a ship can help reduce symptoms.
- **Eating or drinking**—Eating before the onset of symptoms may hasten gastric emptying, but in some individuals, can aggravate motion sickness. Drinking caffeinated beverages along with taking one of the medications suggested can help manage motion sickness.

- **Reducing sensory input**—The reduction of aggravating stimuli (e.g., lying prone, looking at the horizon, or shutting eyes) can help alleviate symptoms.
- **Adding distractions**—Aromatherapy using mint, lavender, or ginger (oral) helps some; flavored lozenges may help as well. They may function as placebos or, in the case of oral ginger, may hasten gastric emptying.
- **Using acupressure or magnets**—Advocated by some to prevent or treat nausea (not specifically for motion sickness), although scientific data are lacking.

References

1. Priesol AJ. Motion Sickness. In: Rose BD, editor. Waltham MA: UpToDate, 2008.
2. Takeda N, Morita M, Horii A, et al. Neural mechanisms of motion sickness. J Med Invest. 2001;48(1–2):44–59.
3. Benline TA, French J, Poole E. Anti-emetic drug effects on pilot performance: granisetron vs. ondansetron. Aviat Space Environ Med 1997; 68(11):998–1005.
4. FDA. Pregnancy and lactation labeling. 2008 [cited 2008 Oct 8]. Available from: www.fda.gov/cder/regulatory/pregnancy_labeling.

RESPIRATORY INFECTIONS

Regina C. LaRocque, Edward T. Ryan

Respiratory infections are an underappreciated risk for travel. Respiratory infection is a leading cause of seeking medical care in returning travelers and has been reported to occur in up to 20% of all travelers. Thus, respiratory infections may be almost as common as travelers' diarrhea. Upper respiratory infection is more common than lower respiratory infection. In general, the types of respiratory infections that affect travelers are similar to those in nontravelers, and exotic causes are rare. Travelers may be exposed to respiratory tract pathogens while in transit, while in close contact with other individuals, and while at their final destination.

Infectious Agent

- Viral pathogens are the most common cause of respiratory infection in travelers; causative agents include coronavirus, adenovirus, rhinovirus, influenza virus, parainfluenza virus, human metapneumovirus, and respiratory syncytial virus.
- Bacterial pathogens are less common but include *Streptococcus pneumoniae*, *Mycoplasma pneumoniae*, *Haemophilus influenzae*, *Chlamydophila pneumoniae*, and *Legionella* species. Viral pathogens may set the stage for subsequent bacterial sinusitis or bronchitis.

Occurrence

- Outbreaks are usually associated with common exposure in hotels and cruise ships or among tour groups.
- A few specific pathogens have been associated with outbreaks in travelers, including influenza, *Legionella pneumophila*, severe acute respiratory syndrome (SARS), and histoplasmosis.
- The peak influenza season in the temperate northern hemisphere is December through February. In the temperate southern hemisphere, the peak influenza season is June through August. Travelers to tropical zones are at risk year round.
- Exposure to an infected individual from another hemisphere, such as on a cruise ship or package tour, can lead to an outbreak of influenza at any time or place.

Risk for Travelers

Factors contributing to respiratory infection in travelers include—

- Air-pressure changes during ascent and descent of aircraft. These baropressure changes can facilitate the development of sinusitis and otitis media.
- Intermingling of large numbers of people in airports, travel hubs, transport vehicles, cruise ships, and hotels can facilitate transmission.
- Direct air-borne transmission of respiratory tract pathogens aboard aircraft is unusual because of frequent air recirculation and filtration, although sporadic cases of SARS, influenza, tuberculosis, and other agents have occurred in modern aircraft. Transmission of infection may occur between passengers who are seated in proximity to one another, usually through direct contact or droplets.
- Air quality at many travel destinations may not be optimal, and exposure to sulfur dioxide, nitrogen dioxide, carbon monoxide, ozone, and particulate matter in air is associated with a number of health risks, including increased risk for respiratory tract inflammation, exacerbations of asthma and chronic obstructive pulmonary disease, and increased risks of bronchitis and pneumonia.
- Certain epidemiologic characteristics of travelers that have been associated with a higher risk for respiratory tract infection include children, the elderly, and individuals with co-morbid pulmonary conditions, such as asthma and chronic obstructive pulmonary disease.
- The risk for tuberculosis among travelers is very low (see the Tuberculosis section in Chapter 5).

Clinical Presentation

- Most respiratory tract infections, especially those of the upper respiratory tract, are mild and not incapacitating.
- Lower respiratory tract infections, particularly pneumonia, can be more severe.
- Individuals with influenza commonly have acute onset of fever, myalgia, headache, and cough.
- Travelers with a viral upper respiratory infection may have persistent symptoms and should consider the possibility of subsequent bacterial sinusitis or bronchitis with symptoms that worsen after one week.

Diagnosis

- Identifying a specific etiologic agent, especially in the absence of pneumonia, is often difficult and not clinically necessary.
- If indicated, the following methods of diagnosis can be used:
  - Molecular methods are available for the diagnosis of a number of respiratory viruses, including influenza virus, parainfluenza virus, adenovirus, human metapneumovirus, and respiratory syncytial virus, and for certain nonviral pathogens such as *Legionella pneumophila*.
  - Rapid tests are also available for detecting group A streptococcal pharyngitis.
  - Microbiologic culturing of sputum and blood, although insensitive, can assist in identifying a causative respiratory pathogen in persons with pneumonia.

Treatment

- Affected travelers are usually managed similarly to nontravelers, although travelers with progressive or severe illness should be evaluated for illnesses specific to their travel destinations and exposure history.
- Most respiratory infections of travelers are due to viruses, are mild, and do not

require specific treatment or antibiotics. No systematic study of self-treatment of travelers with respiratory infections has been reported.

- Self-treatment usually involves supportive measures and may include the use of analgesics, decongestants, increased fluid intake, and inhaled moisture.
- Self-treatment with antibiotics can be considered for upper respiratory infections that are worsening after 7 days of symptoms, particularly if specific symptoms of sinusitis or bronchitis are present. A respiratory-spectrum fluoroquinolone such as levofloxacin or a macrolide such as azithromycin may be prescribed to the traveler for this purpose prior to travel.
- The rate of influenza infection among travelers is not known. The difficulty in self-diagnosing influenza makes it problematic to decide whether to provide travelers with a self-treatment dose of a neuraminidase inhibitor. This practice should probably be limited to travelers with a specific underlying condition that may predispose them to severe influenza.

Medical Interventions

Specific situations that may require medical intervention include—

- Pharyngitis without rhinorrhea, cough, or other symptoms that may indicate infection with group A streptococcus.
- Sudden onset of cough, chest pain, and fever that may indicate pneumonia, resulting in a situation where the traveler may be sick enough to seek medical care right away.
- Travelers with underlying medical conditions, such as asthma, pulmonary disease, or heart disease, who may need to seek medical care earlier than otherwise healthy travelers.

Preventive Measures for Travelers

- Vaccines are available for the prevention of a number of respiratory tract pathogens, including influenza, *S. pneumoniae*, *H. influenzae* type B (in young children), pertussis, diphtheria, varicella, and measles. Unless contraindicated, travelers should be vaccinated against influenza.
- The prevention of respiratory illness while traveling may not be possible, but common-sense preventive measures include—
  - Trying to minimize close contact with persons who are coughing and sneezing
  - Frequent handwashing, either with soap and water or alcohol-based hand sanitizers (containing at least 60% alcohol)
  - Using a vasoconstricting nasal spray immediately prior to air travel, if the traveler has a pre-existing eustachean tube dysfunction.

References

1. Ansart S, Pajot O, Grivois JP, et al. Pneumonia among travelers returning from abroad. J Travel Med. 2004;11(2):87–91.
2. Leder K, Sundararajan V, Weld L, et al. Respiratory tract infections in travelers: a review of the GeoSentinel surveillance network. Clin Infect Dis. 2003;36(4):399–406.
3. Freedman DO, Weld LH, Kozarsky PE, et al. Spectrum of disease and relation to place of exposure among ill returned travelers. N Engl J Med 2006;354(2):119–30.
4. Miller JM, Tam TW, Maloney S, et al. Cruise ships: high-risk passengers and the global spread of new influenza viruses. Clin Infect Dis. 2000;31(2):433–8.
5. Weitzel EK, McMains KC, Rajapaksa S, et al. Aerosinusitis: pathophysiology, prophylaxis, and management in passengers and aircrew. Aviat Space Environ Med. 2008;79(1):50–3.
6. Zitter JN, Mazonson PD, Miller DP, et al. Aircraft cabin air recirculation and symptoms of the common cold. JAMA. 2002;288(4):483–6.
7. Schwela D. Air pollution and health in urban areas. Rev Environ Health. 2000;15(1–2):13–42.
8. Luna LK, Panning M, Grywna K, et al. Spectrum of viruses and atypical bacteria in intercontinental air travelers with symptoms of acute respiratory infection. J Infect Dis. 2007;195(5):675–9.

9. Camps M, Vilella A, Marcos MA, et al. Incidence of respiratory viruses among travelers with a febrile syndrome returning from tropical and subtropical areas. J Med Virol. 2008;80(4):711–5.

10. Redman CA, Maclennan A, Wilson E, et al. Diarrhea and respiratory symptoms among travelers to Asia, Africa, and South and Central America from Scotland. J Travel Med. 2006;13(4):203–11.

11. Rack J, Wichmann O, Kamara B, et al. Risk and spectrum of diseases in travelers to popular tourist destinations. J Travel Med. 2005;12(5):248–53.

12. Morgan J, Cano MV, Feikin DR, et al. A large outbreak of histoplasmosis among American travelers associated with a hotel in Acapulco, Mexico, spring 2001. Am J Trop Med Hyg. 2003;69(6):663–9.

13. Leder K, Newman D. Respiratory infections during air travel. Intern Med J. 2005;35(1):50–5.

14. Medina-Ramon M, Zanobetti A, Schwartz J. The effect of ozone and PM10 on hospital admissions for pneumonia and chronic obstructive pulmonary disease: a national multicity study. Am J Epidemiol. 2006;163(6):579–88.

15. Farhat SC, Paulo RL, Shimoda TM, et al. Effect of air pollution on pediatric respiratory emergency room visits and hospital admissions. Braz J Med Biol Res. 2005;38(2):227–35.

16. Leder K, Tong S, Weld L, et al. Illness in travelers visiting friends and relatives: a review of the GeoSentinel Surveillance Network. Clin Infect Dis. 2006;43(9):1185–93.

17. Cobelens FG, van Deutekom H, Draayer-Jansen IW, et al. Risk of infection with *Mycobacterium tuberculosis* in travellers to areas of high tuberculosis endemicity. Lancet. 2000;356(9228):461–5.

OCCUPATIONAL EXPOSURE TO HIV

Eli W. Warnock III, L. Casey Chosewood

Risk for Health-Care Workers in International Locations

The safety practices and facility standards in health-care settings of developing countries may be less stringent than those in developed settings. The health-care resources and training of health-care workers in these settings may also be limited. These conditions have the potential to increase the risk for occupational HIV exposure to visiting health-care workers in developing countries. Lack of access to personal protective equipment may also increase risk.

Additionally, the prevalence of HIV infection in some developing countries is higher than that in the United States. Due to limited access to adequate treatment, infected source material in some developing countries may have higher viral loads than source material in the United States. Occupational exposure to source material with higher viral loads increases the risk for acquiring HIV occupationally.

Infectious Agent

Human immunodeficiency virus (HIV) is one of the pathogens, along with hepatitis C virus (HCV) and hepatitis B virus (HBV), that may be transmitted occupationally to health-care workers.

Mode of Transmission

Occupational transmission of HIV and transmission of other blood-borne pathogens typically occur via percutaneous exposure to contaminated sharps, including needles, lancets, scalpels, and broken glass. It can also occur when mucous membranes or nonintact skin comes into contact with infected blood or other body fluids.

Occurrence

- The estimated annual number of health-care workers worldwide exposed to sharps injuries contaminated with HIV was 327,000 in 2005.

- The risk of HIV infection following percutaneous exposure with a contaminated sharp is estimated to be 0.3%, or approximately 3 infections per 1,000 exposures.
- Worldwide, the total number of HIV infections attributable to sharps injuries has been estimated to be 1,000 (range 200–5,000).
- A 2005 study estimated that these infections would result in the worldwide premature deaths of 736 (range 129–3,578) health-care workers during the years 2000 to 2030.

Preventive Measures for Travelers

Health-care providers working internationally who will be engaging in high-risk occupational activities, such as drawing blood or the other use of sharps during patient care, should—

- Consistently follow standard precautions to reduce the risk of occupational exposure to HIV and other blood-borne pathogens. Standard precautions involve the use of protective barriers such as gloves, gowns, aprons, masks, or protective eyewear, which can reduce the risk of exposure of the health-care worker's skin or mucous membranes to potentially infective materials. Additional information about occupational health and safety standards for blood-borne pathogens can be found on the Occupational Safety and Health Administration (OSHA) website at www.osha.gov/pls/oshaweb/owadisp.show_document?p_table=STANDARDS&p_id=10051.
- Always be mindful of the hazards posed by sharps injuries.
- Maintain strict safety standards while working in environments that may have less stringent standards.
- Use devices with safety features and improved work practices as recommended by the National Institute for Occupational Safety and Health (NIOSH) to prevent injuries caused by needles, scalpels, and other sharp instruments or devices. Additional information about preventing needlestick injuries in health-care settings can be found on the NIOSH website: www.cdc.gov/niosh/2000-108.html#8.
- Consider bringing their own protective equipment if they are unsure of its availability at their destination.
- Consider bringing postexposure prophylaxis (PEP) for HIV with them for use in the event that they experience a sharps injury with a contaminated or potentially contaminated needle.

Postexposure Management

Health-care providers who have been occupationally exposed to HIV or have been exposed to potentially infectious material from a source person who is likely to be infected with HIV should immediately—

- Wash the exposed area with soap and water thoroughly. If mucous membrane exposure has occurred, flush the area with copious amounts of water or saline.
- Seek qualified medical evaluation as soon as possible to guide decisions on postexposure treatment and testing.
- Contact the National Clinicians' Postexposure Prophylaxis Hotline (PEPline) at 1-888-448-4911 (24 hours/7 days a week) for assistance in assessing risk and advice on managing occupational exposures to HIV, hepatitis, and other blood-borne pathogens. Additional information about PEPline can be found on the National HIV/AIDS Clinicians' Consultation Center website at www.ucsf.edu/hivcntr/Hotlines/PEPline.html.
- Consider beginning postexposure prophylaxis (PEP) for HIV.

Postexposure Prophylaxis

- A number of medication combinations are available for PEP.

- Refer to MMWR's Updated U.S. Public Health Service Guidelines for the Management of Occupational Exposures to HIV, Recommendations for Postexposure Prophylaxis, Updated Information Regarding Antiretroviral Agents Used as HIV Postexposure Prophylaxis for Occupational HIV Exposures (www.aidsinfo.nih.gov/Guidelines/GuidelineDetail.aspx?MenuItem=Guidelines&Search=Off&GuidelineID=10&ClassID=3) and the PEPline for more information about PEP recommendations.
- Specific regimens should be individually determined for those travelers at risk by health-care providers familiar with the medications and the traveler's medical history.
- If the exposed person chooses to initiate PEP, they must do so within hours, as delays lead to a significant decline in PEP effectiveness.
- If indicated, arrange for procurement or shipment of additional postexposure prophylaxis from a credible source to complete the recommended 4-week course of treatment.
- Consider other potential infectious disease exposures from the source material as well, to include HBV or HCV, and manage if appropriate.

Postexposure Testing

- Persons with occupational exposure to HIV should receive baseline postexposure HIV-antibody testing by enzyme immunoassay, postexposure counseling, and medical evaluation, whether or not they receive PEP. In addition to baseline HIV-antibody testing, persons occupationally exposed should receive follow-up HIV-antibody testing by enzyme immunoassay for 6 months following exposure, at 6 weeks, 12 weeks, and 6 months (aidsinfo.nih.gov/contentfiles/HealthCareOccupExpoGL.pdf).
- The U.S. Public Health Service also recommends that health-care workers occupationally exposed to a source co-infected with HIV and HCV and who acquire HCV infection receive extended HIV postexposure surveillance for up to 12 months following exposure.
- Exposed health-care providers should be advised to use precautions (e.g., avoid blood or tissue donations, breastfeeding, or pregnancy) to prevent secondary transmission, especially during the first 6–12 weeks postexposure.
- For exposures for which PEP is prescribed, health-care providers should be informed about—
  - possible drug toxicities and the need for monitoring
  - possible drug interactions
  - the need for adherence to PEP regimens
- Consider re-evaluation of exposed health-care providers, if possible, 72 hours postexposure, especially after additional information about the exposure or source person becomes available and when adverse events of any medication can be assessed.

References

1. OSHA. Regulations (Standards—29 CFR): Bloodborne pathogens—1910.1030. [cited 2008 Apr 1]. Available from: http://www.osha.gov/pls/oshaweb/owadisp.show_document?p_table=STANDARDS&p_id=10051.

2. CDC. Preventing needlestick injuries in health care settings. [cited 2008 Apr 10]. Available from: http://www.cdc.gov/niosh/2000-108.html#8.

3. National Clinicians' Post-Exposure Prophylaxis Hotline (PEPline). [cited 2007 Dec 20]. Available from: http://www.ucsf.edu/hivcntr/PEPline/index.html.

4. Sepkowitz KA. Occupationally acquired infections in health care workers. Part II. Ann Intern Med. 1996;125(11):917–28.

5. Romea S, Alkiza ME, Ramon JM, et al. Risk of occupational transmission of HIV infection among health care workers. Study in a Spanish hospital. Eur J Epidemiol. 1995;11(2):225–9.

6. EPINet—Exposure Prevention Information Network. Uniform needle stick and sharp object injury report. International Health Care Worker Safety Center, University of Virginia, USA. 1998. [2008 Nov 26]. Available from: http://www.healthsystem.virginia.edu/internet/epinet/home.cfm

7. Canadian Center for Occupational Health and Safety. Needlestick injuries. 2000. [cited 2007 Dec]. Available from: http://www.ccohs.ca/oshanswers/diseases/needlestick_injuries.html.

8. Puro V, De Carli G, Petrosillo N, et al. Risk of exposure to blood borne infection for Italian healthcare workers, by job category and work area. Studio Italiano Rischio Occupazionale da HIV Group. Infect Control Hosp Epidemiol. 2001;22(4):206–10.

9. Prüss-Üstün A, Rapiti E, Hutin Y. Estimation of the global burden of disease attributable to contaminated sharps injuries among health-care workers. Am J Industr Med. 2005;48(6):482–90.

10. Bell DM. Occupational risk of human immunodeficiency virus infection in health care workers: an overview. Am J Med. 1997;102(5B):9–15.

11. Sagoe-Moses C, Pearson RD, Perry J, et al. Risks to health care workers in developing countries. N Engl J Med. 2001;345(7):538–41.

12. Panlilio AL, Cardo DM, Grohskopf LA, et al. Updated U.S. Public Health Service guidelines for the management of occupational exposures to HIV and recommendations for Postexposure Prophylaxis. MMWR Recomm Rep. 2005;54(RR-9):1–17.

13. CDC. Updated information regarding antiretroviral agents used as HIV postexposure prophylaxis for occupational HIV exposures. MMWR Morb Mortal Wkly Rep. 2007;56(49):1291–2.

14. Uslan DZ, Verk A. Postexposure chemoprophylaxis for occupational exposure to Human Immunodeficiency Virus in traveling health care workers. J Travel Med. 2005;12(1):14–8.

15. CDC. Updated U.S. Public Health Service guidelines for the management of occupational exposures to HBV, HCV, and HIV and recommendations for postexposure prophylaxis. MMWR Recomm Rep. 2001;50(RR-11):1–42.

Counseling and Advice for Travelers

PROTECTION AGAINST MOSQUITOES, TICKS, AND OTHER INSECTS AND ARTHROPODS

Emily Zielinski-Gutierrez, Robert A. Wirtz, Roger S. Nasci

Although vaccines or chemoprophylactic drugs are available to protect against some important vector-borne diseases such as yellow fever and malaria, travelers still should be advised to use repellents and other general protective measures against biting arthropods. The effectiveness of malaria chemoprophylaxis is variable, depending on patterns of drug resistance, bio-availability, and compliance with medication, and no similar preventive measures exist for other mosquito-borne diseases such as dengue or chikungunya.

CDC recommends the use of products containing active ingredients that have been registered by the U.S. Environmental Protection Agency (EPA) for use as repellents applied to skin and clothing (see below). EPA registration of active ingredients indicates the materials have been reviewed and approved for efficacy and human safety when applied according to the instructions on the label.

General Protective Measures

- **Avoid outbreaks:** To the extent possible, travelers should avoid known foci of epidemic disease transmission. The CDC Travelers' Health webpage provides alerts and information on regional disease transmission patterns and outbreak alerts (www.cdc.gov/travel).
- **Be aware of peak exposure times and places:** Exposure to arthropod bites may be reduced if travelers modify their patterns of activity or behavior. Although mosquitoes may bite at any time of day, peak biting activity for vectors of some

diseases (e.g., dengue, chikungunya) is during daylight hours. Vectors of other diseases (e.g., malaria) are most active in twilight periods (i.e., dawn and dusk) or in the evening after dark. Avoiding the outdoors or focusing preventive actions during peak hours may reduce risk. Place also matters; ticks are often found in grasses and other vegetated areas. Local health officials or guides may be able to point out areas with greater arthropod activity.

- **Wear appropriate clothing:** Travelers can minimize areas of exposed skin by wearing long-sleeved shirts, long pants, boots, and hats. Tucking in shirts and wearing socks and closed shoes instead of sandals may reduce risk. Repellents or insecticides such as permethrin can be applied to clothing and gear for added protection; this measure is discussed in detail below.
- **Check for ticks:** Travelers should be advised to inspect themselves and their clothing for ticks during outdoor activity and at the end of the day. Prompt removal of attached ticks can prevent some infections.
- **Bed nets:** When accommodations are not adequately screened or air conditioned, bed nets are essential to provide protection and to reduce discomfort caused by biting insects. If bed nets do not reach the floor, they should be tucked under mattresses. Bed nets are most effective when they are treated with an insecticide or repellent such as permethrin. Pretreated, long-lasting bed nets can be purchased prior to traveling, or nets can be treated after purchase. The permethrin will be effective for several months if the bed net is not washed. (Long-lasting pretreated nets may be effective for much longer.)
- **Insecticides:** Aerosol insecticides, vaporizing mats and mosquito coils can help to clear rooms or areas of mosquitoes; however, some products available internationally may contain pesticides that are not registered in the United States. Insecticides should always be used with caution, avoiding direct inhalation of spray or smoke.

Optimum protection can be provided by applying the repellents described in the following sections to clothing and to exposed skin.

Repellents for Use on Skin and Clothing

CDC has evaluated information published in peer-reviewed scientific literature and data available from EPA to identify several EPA-registered products that provide repellent activity sufficient to help people avoid the bites of disease-carrying mosquitoes. Products containing the following active ingredients typically provide reasonably long-lasting protection:

- **DEET** (chemical name: *N,N*-diethyl-*m*-toluamide or *N,N*-diethly-3-methyl-benzamide). Products containing DEET include but are not limited to Off!, Cutter, Sawyer, and Ultrathon.
- **Picaridin** (KBR 3023, aka Bayrepel, and icaridin outside the United States; chemical name 2-(2-hydroxyethyl)-1-piperidinecarboxylic acid 1-methylpropyl ester). Products containing picaridin include but are not limited to Cutter Advanced, Skin So Soft Bug Guard Plus and Autan (outside the United States).
- **Oil of lemon eucalyptus*** or **PMD** (chemical name: *para*-menthane-3,8-diol) the synthesized version of oil of lemon eucalyptus. Products containing OLE and PMD include but are not limited to Repel.
- **IR3535** (chemical name: 3-[*N*-butyl-*N*-acetyl]-aminopropionic acid, ethyl ester) Products containing IR3535 include but are not limited to Skin so Soft Bug Guard Plus Expedition.

*Note: This recommendation refers to EPA-registered repellent products containing the active ingredient oil of lemon eucalyptus (or PMD). "Pure" oil of lemon eucalyptus (e.g., essential oil) is not the same product and has not received similar, validated testing for safety and efficacy, is not registered with EPA as an insect repellent, and is not covered by this recommendation.

EPA characterizes the active ingredients DEET and picaridin as "conventional repellents" and oil of lemon eucalyptus, PMD, and IR3535 as "biopesticide repellents," which are derived from natural materials.

Repellent Efficacy

- Published data indicate that repellent efficacy and duration of protection vary considerably among products and among mosquito species.
- Product efficacy and duration of protection are also markedly affected by ambient temperature, amount of perspiration, exposure to water, abrasive removal, and other factors.
- In general, **higher concentrations of active ingredient provide longer duration of protection**, regardless of the active ingredient. Products with ≤10% active ingredient may offer only limited protection, often from 1–2 hours.
- Products that offer **sustained release or controlled release (i.e., micro-encapsulated) formulations, even with lower active ingredient concentrations, may provide longer protection times.**
- Studies suggest that concentrations of DEET above ~50% do not offer a marked increase in protection time against mosquitoes (i.e., DEET efficacy tends to plateau at around 50%).
- Regardless of what product is used, if travelers start to get mosquito bites they should reapply the repellent according to the label instructions or leave the area with biting insects if possible.

Repellents should be purchased before traveling and can be found in hardware stores, drug stores and supermarkets. A wider variety of repellents can be found in camping, sporting goods, and military surplus stores. When purchasing repellents overseas, look for the EPA-registered active ingredients on the product labels; some names of products available internationally have been specified above.

Repellents and Sunscreen

Repellents that are applied according to label instructions may be used with sunscreen with no reduction in repellent activity. Products that combine sunscreen and repellent are not recommended, because sunscreen may need to be reapplied with greater frequency and in greater amounts than are needed to provide protection from biting insects. **In general, the recommendation is to apply sunscreen first, before applying the repellent.**

Repellents/Insecticides for Use On Clothing

- **Clothing, shoes, bed nets, mesh jackets, and camping gear can be treated with permethrin for added protection.**
- Products such as Permanone and Sawyer permethrin are registered with EPA specifically for this use.
- Permethrin is a highly effective insecticide and repellent. Permethrin-treated clothing repels and kills ticks, mosquitoes, and other arthropods. Clothing and other items must be treated several days in advance of travel to allow them to dry. As with all pesticides, follow the label instructions when using permethrin clothing treatments. Alternatively, clothing pretreated with permethrin is commercially available (e.g., products from Buzz Off/Insect Shield).
- Permethrin-treated materials retain repellency/insecticidal activity after repeated laundering but should be retreated as described on the product label to provide continued protection. Clothing treated with the other repellent products described above (e.g., DEET) provides protection from biting arthropods but will not last through washing and will require more frequent reapplications.

Precautions when Using Insect Repellents

- Apply repellents only to exposed skin and/or clothing, as directed on the product label. Do not use repellents under clothing.
- Never use repellents over cuts, wounds or irritated skin.
- Do not apply repellents to eyes or mouth, and apply sparingly around ears. When using sprays, do not spray directly on face-spray on hands first and then apply to face. Wash hands after application to avoid accidental exposure to eyes.
- Do not allow children to handle repellents. When using on children, adults should apply repellents to their hands first, and then put it on the child. It may be advisable to avoid applying to children's hands.
- Use just enough repellent to cover exposed skin and/or clothing. Heavy application and saturation are generally unnecessary for effectiveness. If biting insects do not respond to a thin film of repellent, apply a bit more.
- After returning indoors, wash treated skin with soap and water or bathe. This is particularly important when repellents are used repeatedly in a day or on consecutive days. Also, wash treated clothing before wearing it again. (This precaution may vary with different repellents—check the product label.)
- If anyone experiences a rash or other bad reaction from an insect repellent, the repellent use should be discontinued, the repellent should be washed off with mild soap and water, and a local poison control center should be called for further guidance. If seeking health care because of the repellent, take the repellent to the doctor's office and show the doctor.
- Permethrin should never be applied to skin, but only to clothing, bed nets, or other fabrics as directed on the product label.

Children

- Most repellents can be used on children >2 months of age.
- Protect infants <2 months of age from biting mosquitoes by using an infant carrier draped with mosquito netting with an elastic edge for a tight fit.
- Products containing oil of lemon eucalyptus specify that they should not be used on children <3 years of age.
- Other than the safety tips listed above, EPA does not recommend any additional precautions for using registered repellents on children or on pregnant or lactating women.

Useful Links

- U.S. Environmental Protection Agency. How to Use Insect Repellents Safely; [updated 2007 July 5; cited 2008 Nov 29]. Available from: www.epa.gov/pesticides/health/mosquitoes/insectrp.htm.
- Centers for Disease Control and Prevention. Insect Repellent Use and Safety; [updated 2008 May 14; cited 2008 Nov 29]. Available from: www.cdc.gov/ncidod/dvbid/westnile/qa/insect_repellent.htm.
- Health Canada's Pest Management Regulatory Agency. Safety Tips on Using Personal Insect Repellents; [updated 2004 September 17; cited 2008 Nov 29]. Available from: www.pmra-arla.gc.ca/english/consum/insectrepellents-e.html.

References

1. Barnard DR, Xue RD. Laboratory evaluation of mosquito repellents against *Aedes albopictus, Culex nigripalpus,* and *Ochlerotatus triseriatus* (Diptera: Culicidae). J Med Entomol. 2004;41(4):726–30.

2. Barnard DR, Bernier UR, Posey KH, et al. Repellency of IR3535, KBR3023, *para*-menthane-3,8-diol, and deet to Black Salt Marsh mosquitoes (Diptera: Culicidae) in the Everglades National Park. J Med Entomol. 2002;39(6):895–9.

3. Fradin MS, Day JF. Comparative efficacy of insect repellents against mosquito bites. N Engl J Med. 2002;347(1):13–8.
4. Murphy ME, Montemarano AD, Debboun M, et al. The effect of sunscreen on the efficacy of insect repellent: a clinical trial. J Am Acad Dermatol. 2000;43(2 Pt 1):219–22.
5. Thavara U, Tawatsin A, Chompoosri J, et al. Laboratory and field evaluations of the insect repellent 3535 (ethyl butylacetylaminopropionate) and deet against mosquito vectors in Thailand. J Am Mosq Control Assoc. 2001;17(3):190–5.

WATER DISINFECTION FOR TRAVELERS

Howard D. Backer

Risk for Travelers

Waterborne disease is a risk for international travelers who visit countries that have poor hygiene and inadequate sanitation, and for wilderness users relying on surface water in any country, including the United States. Worldwide, more than one billion people have no access to potable water and 2.4 billion do not have adequate sanitation. In developing countries, the influence of high-density population and rampant pollution, along with absent, overwhelmed, or insufficient sanitation and water treatment systems, means that surface water may be highly polluted with human waste and even urban tap water may become contaminated. Primarily humans, but also animals, are the source of microorganisms that contaminate water sources and cause intestinal infections.

The list of potential waterborne pathogens is extensive and includes bacteria, viruses, protozoa, and parasitic helminths. Most of the organisms that can cause travelers' diarrhea can be waterborne, although the majority of travelers' intestinal infections are probably transmitted by food. Microorganisms with small infectious doses can even cause illness through recreational water exposure, via inadvertent water ingestion.

Bottled water has become the convenient solution for most travelers, but in some places, it may not be superior to tap water. Moreover, the plastic bottles create a huge ecological problem, since most developing countries do not recycle plastic bottles. All international travelers, especially long-term travelers or expatriates, should become familiar with and utilize simple methods to ensure safe drinking water. Disinfection, the desired result of field water treatment, means the removal or destruction of harmful microorganisms. The goal of disinfection is to reduce the risk of gastrointestinal infection and diarrheal illness. Table 2-28 compares benefits and limitations of different methods.

Field Techniques for Water Treatment

Heat

Common intestinal pathogens are readily inactivated by heat. Microorganisms are killed in a shorter time at higher temperatures, whereas temperatures as low as 140° F (60° C) are effective with a longer contact time. Pasteurization uses this principle to kill food-borne enteric pathogens and spoiling organisms at temperatures between 140° F (60° C) and 158° F (70° C), well below the boiling point of water (212° F; 100° C).

Although attaining boiling temperature is not necessary for inactivation of common intestinal pathogens, it is the only easily recognizable endpoint without using a thermometer. Microorganisms begin to die as water is heated on a stove or fire from 150° F (65° C) to boiling. All organisms except bacterial spores, which are not usually waterborne enteric pathogens, are killed within seconds at boiling temperature. Therefore, any water brought to a boil should be adequately disinfected. CDC and the Environmental Protection Agency recommend boiling for 1 minute to allow for a margin of safety and so users are clear that the water is truly boiling. Because the boiling

Table 2-28. Comparison of water disinfection techniques

Technique	Advantages	Disadvantages
Heat	• Does not impart additional taste or color • Single step that inactivates all enteric pathogens • Efficacy is not compromised by contaminants or particles in the water as for halogenation and filtration	• Does not improve taste, smell or appearance of poor quality water • Fuel sources may be scarce, expensive or unavailable • Does not prevent recontamination during storage
Filtration	• Simple to operate • Requires no holding time for treatment • Large choice of commercial products • Adds no unpleasant taste and often improves taste and appearance of water • Rationally combined with halogens for removal or destruction of all pathogenic waterborne microbes	• Adds bulk and weight to baggage • Many are not reliable for removal of viruses • Channeling of water or high pressure can force microorganisms through the filter • Relatively expensive, compared to chemical treatment • Eventually clogs from suspended particulate matter and may require some maintenance or repair in the field
Halogens	• Inexpensive and widely available in liquid or tablet forms • Taste can be removed by several techniques • Flexible dosing • Equally easy to treat large and small volumes	• Corrosive and stains clothing • Imparts taste and odor to water • Flexibility requires understanding of principles • Iodine is physiologically active, with potential adverse effects • Not readily effective against *Cryptosporidium* oocysts • Efficacy decreases with low water temperature and decreasing water clarity
Chlorine Dioxide	• Low doses have no taste or color • Simple to use and available in liquid or tablet form • More potent than equivalent doses of chlorine • Effective against all waterborne pathogens	• Volatile and sensitive to sunlight: do not expose tablets to air and use generated solutions rapidly • No persistent residual, so does not prevent recontamination during storage
Ultraviolet	• Imparts no taste • Portable devices now available • Effective against all waterborne pathogens	• Requires clear water • Does not improve taste or appearance of water • Relatively expensive • Requires batteries or power source • Difficult to know if devices are delivering required UV doses

point decreases with increasing altitude, CDC advises boiling water for 3 minutes at altitudes greater than 6,562 feet (>2000 m).

If no other means of water treatment is available, a potential alternative to boiling is to use tap water that is too hot to touch, which is probably at a temperature between 131° F (55° C) and 140° F (60° C). This temperature may be adequate to kill pathogens if the water has been kept hot in the tank for some time. However, because one cannot know for certain that this temperature has been maintained for long enough to kill all waterborne pathogens, boiling is still advisable if possible. Travelers with access to electricity can bring a small electric heating coil or a lightweight beverage warmer to boil water.

Filtration

Filter pore size is the primary determinant of a filter's effectiveness, but microorganisms also adhere to filter media by electrochemical reactions. Microfilters with "absolute" pore sizes of 0.1–0.4 μm are usually effective for removal of cysts and bacteria but may not adequately remove viruses, which are a major concern in water with high levels of fecal contamination (Table 2-29). Environmental Protection Agency (EPA) designation of water "purifier" indicates that company-sponsored testing has substantiated claims for removing 10^4 (9,999 of 10,000) viruses although EPA does not independently test the validity of these claims.

Reverse osmosis filtration can both remove microbiologic contamination and desalinate water. The high price and slow output of small hand-pump reverse-osmosis units currently prohibit use by land-based travelers; however, they are important survival aids for ocean voyagers.

If the water supply is suspected of being heavily contaminated with biologic wastes and additional assurance is needed, then a second step with chemical treatment of the water before filtration can kill viruses. Many filters contain a charcoal stage that will remove the taste of added chlorine or iodine.

Chemical Disinfection

The most common chemical water disinfectants are chlorine and iodine (halogens). Worldwide, chemical disinfection with chlorine is the most commonly used method for improving and maintaining microbiologic quality of drinking water. Sodium hypochlorite, common household bleach, is the primary disinfectant promoted by CDC and the WHO Safe Water System for individual household use in the developing world.

Primary factors that determine the rate and proportion of microorganisms killed are the concentration of halogen (measured in mg/L or parts per million) and the length of time microorganisms are exposed to the halogen (contact time, measured in minutes). Given adequate concentrations and contact times, both chlorine and iodine have similar activity and are effective against many bacteria. Due to many uncontrolled factors in the field, extending the contact time adds a margin of safety. Cloudy water contains material that will use added disinfectant so it will require higher concentrations or contact times. However, some common waterborne parasites such as *Cryptosporidium*, are poorly inactivated by halogen disinfection, even at practical extended contact times. Therefore, chemical disinfection should be supplemented with adequate filtration to remove these disease-causing microorganisms from drinking water.

Both chlorine and iodine are available in liquid and tablet form (Table 2-30). Iodine has physiologic activity (it is used by the thyroid), so WHO recommends limiting iodine water disinfection to a few weeks of emergency use. It is not recommended in persons with unstable thyroid disease, known iodine allergy, or pregnancy (because of the potential effect on the fetal thyroid).

The taste of halogens in water can be improved by several means:

- Reduce concentration and increase contact time.
- Use a filter that contains activated carbon after contact time.
- Add a tiny pinch of ascorbic acid (vitamin C, available in powder or crystal form and an ingredient in most flavored drink mixes) after the required contact time to remove the taste of halogens. (This works by converting iodine to iodide or chlorine to chloride, which have no taste or color.)

Table 2-29. Microorganism size and susceptibility to filtration

Organism	Average Size (μm)	Maximum recommended filter rating (μm Absolute)[1]
Viruses	0.03	Not specified
Enteric bacteria (*E. coli*)	0.5 × 3.0–8.0	0.2–0.4
Cryptosporidium oocyst	4–6	1
Giardia cyst	6.0–10.0 × 8.0–15.0	3.0–5.0

1 NSF 53 rating on a filter certifies for cyst/oocyst removal.

Table 2-30. Iodine and chlorine formulations and doses

Iodination Techniques added to 1 liter or quart of water	Yield 4 mg/L Contact (Wait) Time 45 min at 30° C 180 min at 5° C[1]	Yield 8 mg/L Contact (Wait) Time 15 min at 30° C 60 min at 5° C[1]
Iodine tablets (tetraglycine hydroperiodide) (e.g., Potable Aqua, Globaline)	½ tablet	1 tablet
2% iodine solution (tincture)	0.2 mL 5 gtts[2]	0.4 mL 10 gtts[2]
Saturated solution: iodine crystals in water (e.g., Polar Pure)	13.0 mL	26.0 mL
Chlorination techniques	**Yield 5 mg/L**	**Yield 10 mg/L**
Sodium hypochlorite Household bleach 5%	0.1 mL 2 drops	0.2 mL 4 drops
Sodium dichloroisocyanurate (e.g., AquaClear)		1 tablet
Chlorine plus flocculating agent (e.g., Chlor-floc)		1 tablet

1 Very cold water requires prolonged contact time with iodine or chlorine to kill *Giardia* cysts. These contact times have been extended from the usual recommendations in cold water to account for this and for the uncertainty of residual concentration.
2 Drops per minute.

Iodine Resins

Iodine resins transfer iodine to microorganisms that come into contact with the resin, but leave little iodine dissolved in the water. The resins have been incorporated into many different filter designs available for field use. Most contain a 1-µm cyst filter, which should effectively remove protozoan cysts (it should say 1-µm or 1 micron "absolute"). Few models are sold in the United States because of inconsistent test results, but some models are still available for international use.

Salt (Sodium Chloride) Electrolysis

Passing a current through a simple brine salt solution generates mixed oxidants, primarily chlorine, which can be used for disinfection of microbes. See the discussion on chlorine above. The process was recently designed in a pocket-sized instrument that uses salt, water and electrical current generated from camera batteries to produce a disinfectant solution that is added to water.

Chlorine Dioxide

Chlorine dioxide (ClO_2) is capable of inactivating most water-borne pathogens, including *Cryptosporidium* oocysts, at practical doses and contact times. There are several new chemical methods for generating chlorine dioxide in the field for small-quantity water treatment.

Ultraviolet (UV) Light

UV light can be used as a pathogen reduction method against microorganisms. The technology requires effective pre-filtering due to its dependence on low water turbidity (cloudiness), the correct power delivery, and correct contact times to achieve maximum pathogen reduction. UV might be an effective method in pathogen reduction in backcountry water. However, there is a lack of independent testing data available on specific systems.

Solar Irradiation and Heating

UV irradiation by sunlight in the UVA range can substantially improve the microbiologic quality of water. Recent work has confirmed the efficacy and optimal procedures of the solar disinfection (SODIS) technique. Transparent bottles (e.g., clear plastic beverage bottles), preferably lying on a dark surface, are exposed to sunlight for a minimum of 4 hours. UV and thermal inactivation are synergistic for solar disinfection of drinking water. Use of a simple reflector or solar cooker can achieve temperatures of 149° F (65° C), which will pasteurize the water after 4 hours. In emergency situations such as refugee camps and disaster areas, where strong sunshine is available, solar disinfection of drinking water can improve water quality.

Silver and Other Products

Silver ion has bactericidal effects in low doses and some attractive features, including absence of color, taste, and odor. The use of silver as a drinking water disinfectant is popular in Europe, but it is not approved for this purpose in the United States because silver concentration in water is strongly affected by adsorption onto the surface of the container and there has been limited testing on viruses and cysts.

Several other common products have known antibacterial effects in water and are marketed in commercial products for travelers, including hydrogen peroxide, citrus juice, and potassium permanganate. None have sufficient data to recommend them for water disinfection in the field.

Granular activated carbon (GAC) removes organic and inorganic chemicals (including chemical disinfectants) through adsorption onto carbon particles, thereby improving odor and taste. GAC may trap but does not kill microorganisms. GAC is a common component of field filters.

Coagulation–flocculation (CF) removes suspended particles that cause a cloudy appearance and bad taste and do not settle by gravity; this process removes many but not all microorganisms. Alum, or one of several other substances, is added to the water, stirred well, allowed to settle, then poured through a simple coffee filter or fine cloth to remove the sediment. CF is an ancient technique that is still used routinely in municipal water treatment in conjunction with other treatment methods, such as disinfection, filtration, UV radiation, and ozonation.

The Preferred Technique

The optimal technique for an individual or group depends on personal preference, size of the group, water source, and the style of travel. Boiling is most effective but may not be practical in all situations. Unfortunately, alternative treatment may require a two-step process of 1) coagulation–flocculation and/or filtration and 2) halogenation. It is best to filter first and then add the halogen. On long-distance, oceangoing boats where water must be desalinated during the voyage, only reverse-osmosis membrane filters are adequate.

When the water will be stored for a period of time, such as on a boat, motor home, or a home with rainwater collection, halogens should be used to prevent the water from becoming recontaminated. A tightly sealed container is best to decrease risk of contamination. A minimum residual of 3–4 mg/L of hypochlorite should be maintained in the stored water. For short-term home storage, narrow-mouth jars or containers with water spigots prevent contamination from repeated contact with hands or utensils.

References

1. Backer HD. Field water disinfection. In: Auerbach PS, editor. Wilderness medicine. 5th ed. Philadelphia: Mosby; 2007. p. 1368–417.
2. Backer H, Hollowell J. Use of iodine for water disinfection: iodine toxicity and maximum recommended dose. Environ Health Perspect. 2000;108(8):679–84.
3. Groh CD, MacPherson DW, Groves DJ. Effect of heat on the sterilization of artificially contaminated water. J Travel Med. 1996;3(1):11–3.

4. Joyce TM, McGuigan KG, Elmore-Meegan M, et al. Inactivation of fecal bacteria in drinking water by solar heating. Appl Environ Microbiol. 1996;62(2):399–402.

5. Korich DG, Mead JR, Madore MS, et al. Effects of ozone, chlorine dioxide, chlorine, and monochloramine on *Cryptosporidium parvum* oocyst viability. Appl Environ Microbiol 1990;56(5):1423–8.

6. McGuigan KG, Joyce TM, Conroy RM, et al. Solar disinfection of drinking water contained in transparent plastic bottles: characterizing the bacterial inactivation process. J Appl Microbiol. 1998;84(6):1138–48.

7. Marchin GL, Fina LR. Contact and demand-release disinfectants. Crit Rev Environ Contr. 1989;19(4):227–90.

8. Sobsey MD. Managing water in the home: accelerated health gains from improved water supply. Geneva: World Health Organization, 2002. [cited 6 Feb 2007]. Available from: http://www.who.int/water_sanitation_health/dwq/wsh0207/en/index.html.

9. World Health Organization and United Nations Children's Fund. The global water supply and sanitation assessment 2000 report. 2000. [cited 6 Feb 2007]. Available from: http://www.who.int/water_sanitation_health/monitoring/globalassess/en/.

SUNBURN

Vernon E. Ansdell

Description

- Travelers to the tropics and subtropics are at increased risk of overexposure to the sun. Important consequences include sunburn, premature aging of the skin, wrinkling, and skin cancer, including melanoma.
- Sunlight consists of ultraviolet (UV) rays (i.e., UVA, UVB, and UVC).
  - UVA rays are present throughout the day and are the most important cause of premature aging of the skin. In addition, UVA rays are responsible for photosensitivity reactions and also contribute to skin cancer.
  - UVB rays are intense from 10 am to 4 pm and are most responsible for sunburn and skin cancer development.
  - UVC rays are filtered by the ozone layer and do not reach the earth's surface.
- The benefits of UV radiation include vitamin D protection, which is important for calcium absorption.

Occurrence and Risk For Travelers

Increased exposure to UV radiation occurs nearer the equator, during summer months, at higher elevation and between 10 am and 4 pm. Reflection from the snow, sand, and water increases exposure, a particularly important consideration for beach activities, skiing, swimming, and sailing.

Commonly Used Medications that May Cause Photosensitivity Reactions

Antimicrobials

Fluoroquinolones, sulfonamides, and tetracyclines (especially demeclocycline); less frequently, doxycycline, oxytetracycline, and tetracycline; rarely, minocycline.

Antimalarials

Doxycycline.

Others

Nonsteroidal anti-inflammatory drugs, thiazide diuretics, furosemide, amiodarone, sulfonylureas, acetazolamide (Diamox), phenothiazines.

Clinical Presentation

- Symptoms from sunburn appear 3–5 hours after overexposure, worsen over the next 24–36 hours, and resolve in 3–5 days.
- Serious burns are painful, and the skin may be tender, swollen and blistered. There may be fever, headache, itching, and malaise. Skin peeling occurs 3–8 days after excessive sun exposure.
- Overexposure to the sun over several years leads to premature aging of the skin, wrinkling, age spots, and an increased risk for skin cancer, including melanoma.
- Overexposure to the sun can cause red, dry painful eyes. Repeated exposure to sunlight results in pterygium formation and important causes of blindness such as cataracts and macular degeneration.

Preventive Measures for Travelers

Sun Protection Factor (SPF)

SPF defines the extra protection against UVB rays that an individual will get by using a sunscreen. For example, if a person using SPF 15 sunscreen normally acquires a sunburn within 20 minutes without protection, the benefit will be 20 × 15 minutes extra protection with sunscreen (i.e., 300 minutes = 5 hours). SPF does not refer to protection against UVA rays. Products containing Mexoryl, Parsol 1789, titanium dioxide, zinc oxide, or avobenzone block UVA rays.

UV Index

The UV index provides travelers with an indication of the risk of UV radiation. Information is often available on the Internet or in local newspapers. The UV index ranges from 1 (low) to 11 or higher (extremely high).

Sun Avoidance

Staying indoors or seeking shade between 10 am and 4 pm is very important in limiting exposure to UV rays, particularly UVB rays. Be aware that sunburn and sun damage can occur even on cloudy days.

Protective Clothing

- Wide-brimmed hats and long sleeves and pants provide important protection against UV rays.
- Tightly woven clothing and darker fabrics provide additional protection.
- High SPF sun-protective clothing is recommended for those at increased risk of sunburn or with a history of skin cancer. This type of clothing contains colorless compounds, fluorescent brighteners, or specifically treated resins that absorb UV rays and often provides an SPF of 30 or higher.
- Sunglasses that provide 100% protection against UV radiation are strongly recommended.

Sunscreens

Sunscreens protect the skin by absorbing or reflecting UV radiation.

Physical Sunscreens contain large particulate substances such as titanium dioxide and zinc oxide, which act to reflect and scatter both visible and UV light. They are effective sunscreens but are less popular because of aesthetically unappealing characteristics such as opaqueness and tendency to stain clothing. They are recommended for those who burn easily or who take medications that may cause photosensitivity reactions.

Chemical Sunscreens absorb rather than reflect UV radiation. A combination of agents is recommended to provide broad-spectrum protection against UVA and UVB rays.

Key Points Regarding Sunscreens

- Choose a sunscreen with at least 15 SPF.
- Select a water- and sweat-resistant product that provides protection against both UVA and UVB rays.
- Look for a sunscreen with at least three different active ingredients to provide broad-spectrum UVA and UVB ray protection. These ingredients generally include PABA derivatives, salicylates (homosalate, octyl salicylate), or cinnamates (octyll methoxycinnamate and cinoxate) for UVB ray absorption; benzophenones (oxybenzone, dioxybenzone, sulisobenzone) for shorter-wavelength UVA ray protection; and avobenzone (Parsol1789), ecamsule (Mexoryl), titanium dioxide, or zinc oxide for the remaining UVA spectrum.
- Apply 30 minutes before exposure to the sun.
- At least 1 oz of sunscreen is needed for total body application (i.e., quarter of a 4-oz bottle).
- Apply to all exposed areas, especially the ears, scalp, lips, back of the neck, tops of the feet, and backs of the hands.
- Reapply after 1–2 hours and after sweating, swimming, or toweling (even on cloudy days).
- Many sunscreens lose potency after 1–2 years.
- Sunscreens should be applied to the skin before insect repellents.
- Avoid products that contain sunscreens and insect repellents. (DEET-containing insect repellents may decrease the effectiveness of sunscreens and may increase absorption of DEET through the skin.)

Treatment

- Hydration and staying in a cool, shaded, or indoor environment
- Topical and oral nonsteroidal anti-inflammatory drugs decrease erythema if used before or soon after exposure to UVB rays and may relieve symptoms such as headache, fever, and local pain. Topical steroids are of limited benefit, and systemic steroids appear to be ineffective.
- Moisturizing creams, aloe vera, and diphenhydramine may help to relieve symptoms.
- In severe cases, narcotic analgesics may be indicated to relieve pain.

References

1. Kaplan LA, Exposure to radiation from the sun. In: Auerbach PS, editor. Wilderness medicine. 5th ed. Philadelphia: Mosby; 2007. p. 351–71.
2. McClean DI, Gallagher R. Sunscreens. Use and misuse. Dermatol Clin. 1998;16(2):219–26.
3. Diffey BL, Grice J. The influence of sunscreen type on photoprotection. Br J Dermatol. 1997;137(1):103–5.
4. Murphy ME, Montemarano AD, Debboun M, et al. The effect of sunscreen on the efficacy of insect repellent: a chemical trial. J Am Acad Dermatol. 2000;43:219–22.
5. Gu X, Wang T, Collins DM, et al. In vitro evaluation of concurrent use of commercially available insect repellent and sunscreen preparations. Br J Dermatol. 2005;152(6):1263–7.
6. Han A, Maibach HI. Management of acute sunburn. Am J Clin Dermatol. 2004;5(1):39–47.

PROBLEMS WITH HEAT AND COLD

Howard D. Backer, David R. Shlim

Background

Foreign travel involves heading into new environments, and climate is one of the most important factors to consider. Travelers may encounter temperature and weather extremes that are either much hotter or colder than they are used to, and either extreme can have health consequences.

Travelers should try to determine the likely climate extremes that they will face during their journey and to prepare with proper clothing, knowledge, and equipment. This section gives a brief overview of the topic.

Problems Associated with a Hot Climate

Risk for Travelers

Many of the most popular travel destinations are tropical or desert areas. Travelers who sit on the beach or by the pool and do only short walking tours incur minimal risk of heat illness. Those who do strenuous hiking or biking in the heat may have significant risk, especially travelers coming from cool or temperate climates who are not in good physical condition and unacclimatized to the heat.

Clinical Presentations

Physiology of Heat Injuries

Tolerance to heat depends primarily on physiologic factors, unlike cold environments where adaptive behaviors are more important. The major means of heat dissipation are radiation at rest and evaporation of sweat during exercise, both of which become minimal with air temperatures above 95° F (35° C) and high humidity.

The major organs involved in temperature regulation are the skin, where sweating and heat exchange take place, and the cardiovascular system, which must greatly increase blood flow to shunt heat from the core to the surface while meeting the metabolic demands of exercise. Cardiovascular status and conditioning are the major physiologic variables affecting the response to heat stress at all ages. Dehydration is the most important predisposing factor in heat illness; temperature and heart rate increase in direct proportion to the level of dehydration. Sweat is a hypotonic fluid containing sodium and chloride. Sweat rates commonly reach 1–2 L/hr, which may result in significant fluid and sodium loss.

Minor Heat Disorders

Heat cramps are painful muscle contractions following exercise in heat. They begin an hour or more after stopping exercise, most often involving heavily used muscles in the calves, thighs, and abdomen. If rest and passive stretching of the muscle do not resolve cramps, an oral salt solution, as in rehydration solutions, will rapidly relieve symptoms.

Heat syncope is sudden fainting in heat that occurs in unacclimatized people while standing or after 15–20 minutes of exercise. Consciousness rapidly returns to normal when the patient is supine. Rest, relief from heat, and oral fluids are sufficient treatments.

Heat edema is mild swelling of the hands and feet, which is more frequent in women during the first few days of heat exposure. It resolves spontaneously and should not be treated with diuretics, which may delay acclimatization and cause dehydration.

Prickly heat (e.g., miliaria, heat rash) manifests as small, red, pruritic lesions on the skin caused by obstruction of the sweat ducts. It is best prevented by wearing light, loose clothing and avoiding heavy, continuous sweating.

Major Heat Disorders

Heat Exhaustion

- Most people who experience acute collapse or other symptoms associated with exercise in the heat are suffering from heat exhaustion, simply defined as the inability to continue exertion in the heat.
- The presumed cause of heat exhaustion is loss of fluid and electrolytes, but there are no objective markers to define the syndrome, which is a spectrum ranging from minor complaints to a vague boundary shared with heat stroke.

- Transient mental changes, such as irritability, confusion, or irrational behavior, may be present, but neurologic signs, such as seizures or coma, would indicate heat stroke or hyponatremia.
- Body temperature may be normal or elevated.
- Most cases can be treated with supine rest in a cool place and oral water or fluids containing glucose and salt. Spontaneous cooling occurs, and patients recover within hours, preventing progression to more serious illness. An oral solution for treating minor heat disorders or for fluid and electrolyte replacement can be made by adding ¼ teaspoon or two 1-gm salt tablets to 1 liter of water, plus 4–8 tsp of sugar if desired for taste.
- Subacute heat exhaustion may develop over several days and is often misdiagnosed as "summer flu" because of findings of weakness, fatigue, headache, dizziness, anorexia, nausea, vomiting, and diarrhea. Treatment is as described for acute heat exhaustion.

Exercise-Induced Hyponatremia

- Some travelers are so concerned about preventing heat illness and dehydration that they adopt the attitude that "you can't drink too much." Sadly, this attitude can lead to tragic outcomes.
- Hyponatremia due to excessive water intake occurs in both endurance athletes and recreational hikers, particularly if the person is replacing sodium loss through sweating with plain water.
- In the field setting, altered mental status with normal body temperature and a history of large volumes of water intake are highly suggestive of hyponatremia. The vague and nonspecific symptoms are the same as those described for hyponatremia in other settings (e.g., anorexia, nausea, emesis, headache, muscle weakness, lethargy, confusion, and seizures).
- Until clinically apparent alterations in mental status appear, heat exhaustion is difficult to distinguish from early hyponatremia.
- A delay before onset of major symptoms or deterioration after cessation of exercise and heat exposure are unique aspects of hyponatremia.
- Prevention includes sodium supplementation with prolonged exercise or heat exposure. For hikers and wilderness users, food is the most efficient vehicle for salt replacement. Trail snacks should include salty foods (e.g., trail mix, crackers, pretzels, jerky), and not just sweets.

Heat Stroke

- Heat stroke is an extreme medical emergency requiring aggressive cooling measures and hospitalization for support.
- Heat stroke is the only form of heat illness in which the mechanisms for thermal homeostasis have failed. As a result of uncontrolled fever and circulatory collapse, organ damage can occur in the brain, liver, kidneys, and heart.
- The onset of heat stroke may be acute (exertional heat stroke) or gradual (nonexertional heat stroke, also referred to as classic or epidemic).
- A presumptive diagnosis of heatstroke is made when patients have hyperpyrexia and marked alteration of mental status.
- Body temperatures in excess of 106° F (41° C) can be observed; even without a thermometer, these patients will feel hot to touch. If a thermometer is available, a rectal temperature is the safest and most reliable way to check the temperature in someone who may have heatstroke.
- In the field, institute evaporative cooling by maximizing skin exposure, spraying tepid water on the skin, and maintaining air movement over the body by fans. If ice is available, apply cold packs to the neck, axillas, and groin and massage the skin with ice. Immersion in a nearby pool or natural body of water can initiate cooling.
- Unless the recovery is very rapid, the person should be evacuated to a hospital. If that is not possible, encourage rehydration, if the person is able to take oral fluids, and monitor closely for several hours.

Prevention of Heat Disorders

Heat Acclimatization

Heat acclimatization is a process of physiologic adaptation to a hot environment that occurs in both residents and visitors. The result of acclimatization is an increase in sweating, and decreased energy expenditure with lower rise in body temperature for a given workload. Only partial adaptation occurs by passive exposure to heat. Full acclimatization, especially cardiovascular response, requires 1–2 hours of exercise in the heat each day. Most acclimatization changes occur within 10 days, provided a suitable amount of exercise is taken each day in the heat. After this time, only increased physical fitness will result in further exercise tolerance. Decay of acclimatization occurs within days to weeks if there is no heat exposure.

Physical Conditioning and Acclimatization

Higher levels of physical fitness improve exercise tolerance and capacity in heat, but not as much as acclimatization. If possible, travelers should acclimatize before leaving by exercising at least 1 hour daily in the heat. If this is not possible before departing, exercise in heat during the first week of travel should be limited in intensity and duration (30- to 90-minute periods) with rest in between. It is a good idea to conform to the local practice in most hot regions and avoid strenuous activity during the hottest part of the day.

Clothing

Clothing should be lightweight, loose, and light-colored to allow maximum air circulation for evaporation yet give protection from the sun. A wide-brimmed hat markedly reduces radiant heat exposure.

Fluid and Electrolyte Replacement

During exertion, fluid intake improves performance and decreases the likelihood of illness. Reliance on thirst alone is not sufficient to prevent significant dehydration. During mild to moderate exertion, electrolyte replacement offers no advantage over plain water. However, for those exercising many hours in heat, a weak solution similar to commercial electrolyte drinks is recommended. Salty snacks or light salting of mealtime food or fluids is the most efficient way to replace salt losses. Salt tablets, when swallowed whole, may cause gastrointestinal irritation and vomiting, but two tablets can be dissolved in one liter of water. Urine volume and color are a readily available means to monitor fluid needs.

Problems Associated with a Cold Climate

Risk for Travelers

Travelers do not have to be in an arctic or high-altitude environment to encounter problems with the cold. Humidity, rain, and wind can produce hypothermia even with temperatures around 50° F (12° C–14° C). Reports of severe hypothermia in international travelers are rare. Many high-altitude destinations are not wilderness areas, and villages offer an escape from extreme weather. In Nepal, trekkers almost never experience hypothermia except in the rare instance in which they may get lost in a storm. Even in a temperate climate, the traveler in a small boat that overturns in very cold water can rapidly become hypothermic.

Clinical Presentations

Hypothermia

Hypothermia can be defined, in general terms, as having a core body temperature of <95° F (35° C). When persons are faced with an environment in which they cannot keep warm, they first feel chilled, then begin to shiver, and eventually stop shivering as their metabolic reserves are exhausted. At that point, body temperature continues to decrease, dependent upon the ambient temperatures. As the core temperature falls, neurologic functioning decreases until almost all hypothermic people with a core temperature of ≤86° F (30° C) are comatose. The record low core body temperature in an adult who survived is 56° F (13° C). Travelers headed to a cold climate should be encouraged to ask questions and research appropriate clothing and equipment.

Travelers who will be recreating or working around cold water face a different sort of risk. Immersion hypothermia can render a person unable to swim or keep floating within 30–60 minutes. In these cases, a personal flotation device is critical, as is knowledge about self-rescue and righting a capsized boat.

The other medical conditions associated with cold affect mainly the skin and the extremities. These can be divided into nonfreezing cold injuries and freezing injuries (frostbite).

Nonfreezing Cold Injury

The nonfreezing cold injuries are—

- **Trench foot** (immersion foot): This condition is caused by prolonged immersion of the feet in cold water (32° F–59° F, 0° C–15° C). The damage is mainly to nerves and blood vessels, and the result is pain that is aggravated by heat and a dependent position of the limb. Severe cases can take months to resolve. Unlike the treatment for frostbite, immersion foot should not be rapidly rewarmed, which can make the damage much worse.
- **Pernio** (chilblains): Pernio are localized, inflammatory lesions that occur mainly on the hands of susceptible individuals. They can occur with exposure to only moderately cold weather. The bluish-red lesions are thought to be caused by prolonged, cold-induced vasoconstriction. As with trench foot, rapid rewarming should be avoided, as it makes the pain worse. Nifedipine may be an effective treatment.
- **Cold urticaria**: This condition involves the formation of localized or general wheals and itching after exposure to cold. It is not the absolute temperature that induces this form of urticara, but the rate of change of temperature in the skin.

Freezing Cold Injury

Categories of Frostbite

- Frostbite is the term that is used to describe tissue damage from direct freezing of the skin.
- Modern equipment and clothing have greatly decreased the risk of frostbite in most adventurous tourist destinations, and frostbite occurs mainly during an accident, severe unexpected weather, or as a result of poor planning.
- Once frostbite injury has occurred, little can be done to reverse the changes. Therefore, taking great care to prevent frostbite is crucial.
- Frostbite is usually graded like burns.
  - First-degree frostbite involves reddening of the skin without deeper damage. The prognosis for complete healing is virtually 100%.
  - Second-degree frostbite involves blister formation. Blisters filled with clear fluid have a better prognosis than blood-tinged blisters.
  - Third-degree frostbite represents full-thickness injury to the skin, and possibly the underlying tissues. No blister forms, the skin darkens over time and may turn black, and if the tissue is completely devascularized, amputation will be necessary.

Management of Frostbite

Frostbitten skin is numb and appears whitish or waxy. The generally accepted method for treating a frozen digit or limb is through rapid rewarming in water heated to 104° F–108° F (40° C–42° C). The frozen area should be completely immersed in the warm water. A thermometer is needed to maintain the water at the correct temperature. Rewarming can be associated with severe pain, and analgesics can be given if needed. Once the area is rewarmed, it must be safeguarded against freezing again. It is thought to be better to keep digits frozen a little longer and rapidly rewarm them, than to allow them to thaw out slowly or to thaw and refreeze. A cycle of freeze–thaw–refreeze is devastating to tissue and leads more directly to the need for amputation.

Once the area has rewarmed, it can be examined. If blisters are present, it is important to note whether they extend to the end of the digit. Proximal blisters usually mean that the tissue distal to the blister has suffered full-thickness damage. Treatment consists of avoiding further mechanical trauma to the area and preventing infection. Reasonable field treatment consists of washing the area thoroughly with a disinfectant such as povidone–iodine, putting dressings between the toes or fingers to prevent maceration, using fluffs (expanded gauze sponges) for padding, and covering with a roller gauze bandage. These dressings can safely be left on for up to 3 days at a time. By leaving the dressings on longer, the traveler can preserve what may be limited supplies of bandages. Prophylactic antibiotics are not needed in most situations.

Once the patient has reached a definitive medical setting, there should be no rush to do surgery. The usual time from injury to surgery is 4–5 weeks. By that time the dead tissue has begun to separate from viable tissue, and the surgeon can plan surgery that maximizes the remaining digits.

References

1. Moran DS, Gaffin SL. Clinical management of heat-related illnesses. In: Auerbach PS, editor. Wilderness medicine. 5th ed. Philadelphia: Mosby; 2007.
2. Epstein Y, Moran DS. Extremes of temperature and hydration. In: Keystone JS, Kozarsky PE, Freedman DO, Nothdurft HD, Connor BA, editors. Travel medicine. 2nd ed. Philadelphia: Mosby; 2008. p. 413–22.
3. Noakes TD. The hyponatremia of exercise. Int J Sport Nutr. 1992;2(3):205–28.
4. Backer HD, Shopes E, Collins SL, et al. Exertional heat illness and hyponatremia in hikers. Am J Emerg Med. 1999;17(6):532–9.
5. McCauley RL, Killyon GW, Smith DJ Jr, et al. Frostbite. In: Auerbach PS, editor. Wilderness medicine. 5th ed. Philadelphia: Mosby; 2007.

FOOD POISONING FROM MARINE TOXINS

Vernon E. Ansdell

Description

- Seafood poisoning from marine toxins is an underrecognized hazard for travelers, particularly in the tropics and subtropics. Furthermore, the risk is increasing as a result of multiple factors such as global warming, coral reef damage, and spread of toxic algal blooms.
- **Ciguatera fish poisoning** and shellfish poisoning are caused by potent toxins that originate in small marine organisms (dinoflagellates and diatoms).
- **Scombroid** poisoning is caused by eating improperly chilled fish that contains large quantities of histamine.

Ciguatera Fish Poisoning

Ciguatera fish poisoning occurs after eating reef fish contaminated with toxins such as ciguatoxin or maitotoxin. These potent toxins originate from small marine organisms (dinoflagellates) that grow on and around coral reefs. Dinoflagellates are ingested by herbivorous fish, and the toxins are concentrated as they pass up the food chain to large (usually >6 pounds) carnivorous fish and finally to humans. Toxin in fish is concentrated in the liver, intestinal tract, roe, and head.

Gambierdiscus toxicus, which produces ciguatoxin, tends to proliferate on dead coral reefs. The risk of ciguatera is likely to increase as more coral reefs die as a result of factors such as global warming, construction, and nutrient runoff.

Risk for Travelers

- Over 50,000 cases of ciguatera poisoning occur every year.
- The incidence in travelers to endemic areas has been estimated as high as 3/100.
- Ciguatera is widespread in tropical and subtropical waters, usually between the latitudes of 35 degrees north and 35 degrees south; it is particularly common in the Pacific and Indian Oceans and the Caribbean Sea.
- Fish that are most likely to cause ciguatera poisoning are carnivorous reef fish, including barracuda, grouper, moray eel, amberjack, sea bass, or sturgeon. Omnivorous and herbivorous fish such as parrot fish, surgeon fish, and red snapper can also be a risk.

Clinical Presentation

- Typical ciguatera poisoning results in a gastrointestinal illness, followed by neurologic symptoms and, very rarely, cardiovascular collapse.
- The first symptoms usually appear 1–3 hours after eating contaminated fish and include nausea, vomiting, diarrhea, and abdominal pain.
- Neurologic symptoms appear 3–72 hours after the meal and include paresthesias, pain in the teeth or the sensation that the teeth are loose, itching, metallic taste, blurred vision, or even transient blindness. Temperature reversal (hot objects feel cold and cold objects feel hot) is very characteristic. Neurologic symptoms usually last a few days to several weeks.
- Chronic neuropsychiatric symptoms resembling chronic fatigue syndrome may be very disabling, last several months, and include malaise, depression, headaches, myalgias, and fatigue. Cardiac manifestations include bradycardia, other arrythmias, and hypotension.
- Overall mortality from ciguatera poisoning is about 0.1% but varies due to the toxin dose absorbed and availability of adequate medical care to deal with serious complications such as cardiovascular collapse or respiratory failure.
- The diagnosis of ciguatera poisoning is based on the clinical signs and symptoms and a history of eating fish that are known to carry ciguatera toxin. Commercial kits are available to test for ciguatera in fish, but there is no test for ciguatera in humans.

Preventive Measures for Travelers

- Avoid or limit consumption of the reef fish listed above, particularly when the individual fish weighs 6 pounds or more.
- Never eat high-risk fish such as barracuda or moray eel.
- Avoid the parts of the fish that concentrate ciguatera toxin, such as liver, intestines, roe, and head.
- Remember that ciguatera toxins do not affect the texture, taste or smell of fish, and they are not destroyed by gastric acid, cooking, smoking, freezing, canning, salting, or pickling.
- Commercial kits (if available) can be used to check if the fish is safe to eat.

Treatment

- There is no specific antidote for ciguatoxin or maitotoxin.

- Treatment is generally symptomatic and supportive.
- Intravenous mannitol has been reported to reduce the severity and duration of neurologic symptoms, particularly if given early.

Scombroid

Scombroid, one of the commonest fish poisonings, occurs worldwide in both temperate and tropical waters. The illness occurs after eating improperly refrigerated or preserved fish containing high levels of histamine and often resembles a moderate to severe IgE-mediated allergic reaction.

Fish that cause scombroid have naturally high levels of histidine in the flesh and include tuna, mackerel, mahimahi (dolphin fish), sardine, anchovy, herring, bluefish, amberjack, and marlin. Histidine is converted to histamine by bacterial overgrowth in fish that has been improperly stored (over 20° C) after capture. Histamine and other scombrotoxins are resistant to cooking, smoking, canning, or freezing.

Scombroid fish poisoning occurs worldwide in both temperate and tropical waters.

Clinical Presentation

- Symptoms of scombroid poisoning resemble an acute allergic reaction and usually appear 10–60 minutes after eating contaminated fish. They include flushing of the face and upper body (resembling sunburn), severe headache, palpitations, itching, blurred vision, abdominal cramps, and diarrhea.
- Untreated, symptoms usually resolve within 12 hours. Rarely, there may be respiratory compromise, malignant arrythmias, and hypotension requiring hospitalization.
- Diagnosis is usually clinical. A clustering of cases helps to exclude the possibility of fish allergy.

Preventive Measures for Travelers

- Fish contaminated with histamine may have a peppery, sharp, salty, or bubbly taste, but may also look, smell, and taste normal.
- The key to prevention is to make sure that the fish is promptly chilled (below 15° C–20° C) after capture.
- Cooking, smoking, canning, or freezing will not destroy histamine in contaminated fish.

Treatment

- Scombroid poisoning usually responds well to H1 antihistamines.
- H2 antihistamines may also be of benefit.

Shellfish Poisoning

There are several forms of shellfish poisoning. All occur after ingesting filter-feeding bivalve mollusks, such as mussels, oysters, clams, scallops, and cockles containing potent toxins. The toxins originate in small marine organisms (dinoflagellates or diatoms) that are ingested and concentrated by shellfish.

Risk for Travelers

Contaminated shellfish may be found in temperate and tropical waters, typically during or after dinoflagellate blooms or "red tides."

Clinical Presentation

Poisoning results in gastrointestinal and neurologic illness of varying severity. Symptoms typically appear 30–60 minutes after ingesting toxic shellfish but can be delayed for several hours. Diagnosis is usually made clinically together with a history of recent shellfish ingestion.

Paralytic Shellfish Poisoning

This is the most common and most severe form of shellfish poisoning. Symptoms usually appear 30–60 minutes after eating toxic shellfish and include numbness and tingling of the face, lips, tongue, arms, and legs. There may be headache, nausea, vomiting, and diarrhea. Severe cases are associated with ingestion of large doses of toxin and clinical features such as ataxia, dysphagia, mental status changes, flaccid paralysis, and respiratory failure. The case–fatality rate averages 6% and may be particularly high in children.

Neurotoxic Shellfish Poisoning

Usually presents as gastroenteritis accompanied by minor neurologic symptoms, resembling mild ciguatera poisoning or mild paralytic shellfish poisoning. Inhalation of aerosolized toxin in the sea spray associated with a red tide may cause an acute respiratory illness, rhinorrhea, and bronchoconstriction.

Diarrheic Shellfish Poisoning

This produces chills, nausea, vomiting, abdominal cramps, and diarrhea. No fatalities have been reported.

Amnesic Shellfish Poisoning

This is a rare form of shellfish poisoning that produces a gastroenteritis that may be accompanied by headache, confusion, and permanent short-term memory loss. In severe cases, seizures, paralysis, and death may occur.

Preventive Measures for Travelers

- Shellfish poisoning can be prevented by avoiding potentially contaminated bivalve molluscs. This is particularly important in areas during or shortly after "red tides."
- Travelers to developing countries should avoid eating all shellfish, because they carry a high risk of viral and bacterial infections.
- Marine shellfish toxins cannot be destroyed by cooking or freezing.

Treatment

- Treatment is symptomatic and supportive.
- Severe cases of paralytic shellfish poisoning may require mechanical ventilation.

References

1. Ansdell V. Food-borne illness. In: Keystone JS, Kozarsky PE, Freedman DO, Nothdurft HD, Connor BA, editors. Travel medicine. 2nd ed. Philadelphia: Mosby; 2008. p. 475–84.
2. Isbister GK, Kiernan MC. Neurotoxic marine poisoning. Lancet Neurol. 2005;4(4):219–28.
3. Sobel J, Painter J. Illnesses caused by marine toxins. Clin Infect Dis. 2005;41(9):1290–6.
4. Palafox NA, Jain LG, Pinano AZ, et al. Successful treatment of ciguatera fish poisoning with intravenous mannitol. JAMA. 1988;259(18):2740–2.
5. Schnorf H, Taurarii M, Cundy T. Ciguatera fish poisoning: a double-blind randomized trial of mannitol therapy. Neurology. 2002;58(6):873–80.

ANIMAL-ASSOCIATED HAZARDS

Nina Marano, G. Gale Galland

Human Interaction with Animals: A Risk Factor for Injury

Animals in general tend to avoid human beings, but they can attack if they perceive threat, are protecting their young or territory, or are injured or ill. Although attacks by wild animals are more dramatic, attacks by domestic animals are far more common. Animals cause injury through bites, kicks, or blunt trauma, or by the use of horns or claws. Further damage can occur if injuries become secondarily infected, as these infections may result in serious systemic disease. In addition, animals can transmit zoonotic infections such as rabies. A recent 10-year retrospective review of dog bites in Austria showed that 75% of the bites were preventable because the person intentionally interacted with the dog.

Bite Wounds

Prevention

- Before departure, travelers should have a current tetanus vaccination or should have documentation of receiving a booster vaccination within the prior 5–10 years. An assessment of the traveler's need for pre-exposure rabies immunization should be made according to guidelines in Table 2-17.
- During travel, travelers should never try to pet, handle, or feed unfamiliar animals, domestic or wild, particularly in areas of endemic rabies. Young children are more likely to be bitten by animals and sustain more severe injuries from animal bites.

Management

- All wounds should receive prompt local treatment by thorough cleansing and debridement of the wound if necrotic tissue or dirt is present to prevent infection and illness, especially tetanus or rabies-prone wounds (see the Rabies and Tetanus sections earlier in this chapter).
- Any animal bite should be evaluated by a health-care provider as soon as possible, after cleaning the wound. Travelers who might have been exposed to rabies should contact a reliable health practitioner for advice about rabies postexposure prophylaxis (see the Rabies section earlier in this chapter). Since rabies immune globulin or rabies vaccine may not be available in the destination country, travelers should have a strategy in place prior to travel as to how to respond to a possible rabies exposure. This strategy may require the traveler to fly to a different country to obtain the appropriate treatment.
  - Travelers who have purchased medical evacuation insurance should contact their insurance provider for guidance on seeking medical care.
  - U.S. citizens can contact the local U.S. Embassy or Consulate in the country they are visiting for assistance in locating a health-care professional at their destination. Consular personnel at U.S. Embassies and Consulates abroad and in the United States are available 24 hours a day, 7 days a week, to provide emergency assistance to U.S. citizens. To contact the U.S. Department of State's Overseas Citizens Services:
    - Dial: 888-407-4747 if calling from the U.S. or Canada
    - Dial: 202-501-4444 if calling from overseas
- Travelers who received their most recent tetanus toxoid-containing vaccine >5 years previously or who have not received at least three doses of tetanus toxoid-

containing vaccines may require a dose of tetanus toxoid-containing vaccine (Tdap, Td, or DTaP), according to the guidelines in Table 2-21.

A wide variety of animals and insects can cause illness and injury to travelers; a short synopsis of risks by species is provided below.

Monkeys

- Macaques, a type of monkey, pose a threat for rabies and herpes B virus. Macaques are native to Asia and Northern Africa. They are also housed in research facilities, zoos, wildlife or amusement parks, and are kept as pets in private homes throughout the world. Monkey bites occasionally occur in certain urban sites, such as temples in Nepal or India.
- Herpes B virus is related to the herpes simplex viruses, which cause oral and genital ulcers. Herpes B virus was discovered in 1933, and since that time approximately 50 cases have been reported in humans, with an 80% mortality rate. Herpes B infection is rare in humans, and most documented cases have resulted from occupational exposures. No cases of herpes B infection have been reported in travelers or others exposed to monkeys in the wild. However, travelers to areas where free-ranging macaques exist should be aware of the potential risk. An infected monkey may appear completely healthy.
- Documented routes of human infection include animal bites and scratches, exposure to infected tissue or body fluids from splashes, and, in one instance, human-to-human spread. Even minor scratches or bites should be considered potential exposures as, experimentally, herpes B virus has been isolated from surfaces for up to 2 weeks after it was applied (unpublished data, National Institutes of Health B Virus Reference Laboratory).
- The incubation period for herpes B may be less than 1 week to a month or longer.
- Neurologic symptoms develop as the virus infects the central nervous system and may lead to ascending paralysis and respiratory failure.
- Increased public and physician awareness about the risks associated with an injury from a macaque, improved first aid postexposure, the availability of better diagnostic tests, and improved anti-viral therapeutics have decreased the mortality rate to 20% in treated individuals. As a result, from 1987 to 2004 there have been only five fatal infections.

Prevention

Travelers should never attempt to feed, pet, or otherwise handle any monkeys.

Management

- Travelers should seek first aid immediately after being bitten or scratched by a monkey. The wound should be thoroughly cleaned, and travelers should seek health care immediately.
- If the history is strongly suggestive of exposure to herpes B through contact with monkeys, there are published guidelines for the prevention of herpes B infection after exposure and for the treatment of established infection. These guidelines have recommendations for serologic tests and postexposure prophylaxis. When potentially exposed travelers return home, they should follow up with their health-care providers for care. Additional information and photos of macaques can be found at the website for the National B Virus Resource Center at the Georgia State University Viral Immunology Center: www2.gsu.edu/~wwwvir/.

Snakes

- Poisonous snakes are hazards in many locations, although deaths from snakebites are rare. Snakebites usually occur in areas where dense human populations coexist with dense snake populations (e.g., Southeast Asia, sub-Saharan Africa, and tropical America).

- Common sense is the best precaution. Most snakebites are the direct result of startling, handling, or harassing snakes. Therefore, all snakes should be left alone. Travelers should maintain awareness of their surroundings, especially at night and during warm weather when snakes tend to be more active. For extra precaution, when practical, travelers should wear heavy, ankle high or higher boots, and long pants when walking outdoors at night in areas possibly inhabited by venomous snakes.

Management

- Travelers should be advised to seek immediate medical attention any time a bite wound breaks the skin, or when snake venom is ejected into their eyes or mucous membranes.
- Immobilization of the affected limb and application of a pressure bandage that does not restrict blood flow are recommended first-aid measures while the victim is moved as quickly as possible to a medical facility.
- Incision of the bite site and tourniquets that restrict blood flow to the affected limb are not recommended.
- Specific therapy for snakebites is controversial and should be left to the judgment of local emergency medical personnel. Specific antivenins are available for some snakes in some areas, so trying to ascertain the species of snake that bit the victim may be critical.

Insects

Bites and stings from insects such as spiders and scorpions can be painful and can result in significant morbidity and mortality, particularly among infants and children. Many insects can transmit communicable diseases, even without the traveler's awareness of the bite. This is particularly true when camping or staying in rustic accommodations.

Prevention

Exposure to insect bites and scorpion envenomations can be avoided by wearing long sleeves and pants while hiking, sleeping under mosquito nets, and shaking clothing and shoes before putting them on.

Management

Travelers should be advised to seek medical attention if an insect bite or sting causes redness, swelling, bruising, or persistent pain. Those who have a history of severe allergic reactions to insect bites or stings should also ask their physician to evaluate them for the need to carry an epinephrine autoinjector (EpiPen) to use in case of recurrence (both in general and especially while traveling).

Bats

- Bats can be found almost anywhere in the world except the polar regions and extreme deserts. Bats are reservoir hosts for viruses that can cross species barriers to infect humans and other domestic and wild mammals. Viruses such as rabies virus can be transmitted directly from bats to people.
- It is not possible to tell if a bat has rabies; however, any bat that is active by day, is found in a place where bats are not usually seen (for example, indoors or outdoors in areas in close proximity to humans), or is unable to fly is far more likely than others to be rabid.

- Human exposure to bats can occur during adventure activities such as caving. Exposure can include bites, scratches, and mucosal or cutaneous exposure to bat saliva. Like any other wild animal, any bat, whether it is sick or healthy, will bite in self-defense if handled.

Prevention

Bats should never be handled. Travelers should be discouraged from going into caves that have a large bat infestation. Depending on the country being visited, pre-exposure rabies vaccination may be recommended for persons engaged in outdoor activities such as caving and spelunking.

Management

- If a bite occurs or if infectious material (such as saliva) from a bat gets into the eyes, nose, mouth, or a wound, the traveler should wash the affected area thoroughly and get medical advice immediately. Any suspected or documented bite or scratch from a bat should be grounds for seeking postexposure rabies immunoprophylaxis.
- People usually know when they have been bitten by a bat. However, bats have tiny teeth and not all wounds may be apparent. There are situations in which travelers should seek medical advice even in the absence of an obvious bite wound, such as upon awakening and finding a bat in the room or seeing a bat in the room of a child.

Marine Animals

- Venomous injuries from marine fish and invertebrates are increasing with the popularity of surfing, scuba diving, and snorkeling. The majority of species responsible for human injuries and envenomation reside in tropical coastal waters and include stingrays, jellyfish, stonefish, and scorpionfish.
- Travelers should be advised to use protective footwear and maintain vigilance while engaging in recreational water activities. Traumatic injury, envenomation and wound infection are common sequelae. Identification of the species involved is helpful in determining the best course of treatment.

Birds

- When traveling in an area that is experiencing an outbreak of avian influenza (www.cdc.gov/flu/avian/outbreaks/current.htm), travelers should avoid all contact with poultry (e.g., chickens, ducks, geese, pigeons, turkeys, and quail) or any wild birds, and avoid settings where H5N1-infected poultry may be present, such as commercial or backyard poultry farms and live poultry markets.
- Travelers should not eat uncooked or undercooked poultry or poultry products, including dishes made with uncooked poultry blood.

References

1. Callahan M. Bites, stings, and envenoming injuries. In: Keystone JS, Kozarsky PE, Freedman DO, Nothdurft HD, Connor BA, editors. Travel medicine. 2nd ed. Philadelphia: Mosby; 2008. p. 463–74.

2. Anonymous. Rabies. In: Acha PN, Szyfres B. editors. Zoonoses and communicable diseases common to man and animals. 3rd ed. Vol. 2, Chlamydioses, rickettsioses, and viruses. Washington (DC): PAHO; 2003. p. 246–76.

3. Schalamon J, Ainoedhofer H, Singer G, et al. Analysis of dog bites in children who are younger than 17 years. Pediatrics. 2006;117(3):e374–9.

4. Huff JL, Barry PA. B-virus (Cercopithecine herpesvirus 1) infection in humans and macaques: potential for zoonotic disease. Emerg Infect Dis. 2003;9(2):246–50.

5. Cohen JI, Davenport DS, Stewart JA, et al.; B Virus Working Group. Recommendations

for prevention of and therapy for exposure to B virus (Cercopithecine Herpesvirus 1). Clin Infect Dis. 2002;35(10):1191–203.

6. Gold BS, Dart RC, Barish RA. Bites of venomous snakes. N Engl J Med. 2002;347(5):347–56.

7. Warrell DA. Treatment of bites by adders and exotic venomous snakes. BMJ. 2005;331(7527):1244–7.

8. CDC. Nonfatal dog bite-related injuries treated in hospital emergency departments—United States, 2001. MMWR Morb Mortal Wkly Rep. 2003;52(26):605–10.

9. Löe J, Röskaft E. Large carnivores and human safety: a review. Ambio. 2004;33(6):283–8.

10. Schalamon J, Ainoedhofer H, Singer G, et al. Analysis of dog bites in children who are younger than 17 years. Pediatrics. 2006;117(3):e374–9.

11. Feldman KA, Trent R, Jay MT. Epidemiology of hospitalizations resulting from dog bites in California, 1991–1998. Am J Public Health. 2004;94(11):1940–1.

12. CDC. Dog-bite-related fatalities—United States, 1995–1996. MMWR Morb Mortal Wkly Rep. 1997;46(21):463–7.

13. Diaz JH. The global epidemiology, syndromic classification, management, and prevention of spider bites. Am J Trop Med Hyg. 2004;71(2):239–50.

14. Gibbons RV. Cryptogenic rabies, bats, and the question of aerosol transmission. Ann Emerg Med. 2002;39(5):528–36.

DEEP VEIN THROMBOSIS AND PULMONARY EMBOLISM

Deborah Nicolls Barbeau

Background

Venous thromboembolism (VTE) consists of two related conditions: 1) deep vein thrombosis (DVT) and 2) pulmonary embolism (PE). DVT occurs when there is a partial or complete blockage of a deep vein by a blood clot, most commonly in the legs. The clot may break off and travel to the vessels in the lung, causing a life-threatening PE.

VTE associated with air travel was first described in the early 1950s. Previous studies have shown a two- to four-fold increased risk of VTE following air travel. In 2001, the World Health Organization set up the WHO Research into Global Hazards of Travel (WRIGHT) Project, a large collaborative research study to confirm the association between VTE and air travel. The goals of this project are to determine the magnitude of the risk of VTE due to air travel, to determine the effect of other factors on the association, and to study the effect of preventive measures on risk. The results of Phase I of the project were published recently. Phase II will address the effect of preventive measures.

Risk for Travelers

Several factors have been associated with an increased risk for developing VTE (Box 2-4).

Combined effects have been observed between these established risk factors and different forms of travel. A population-based case–control study of adults receiving treatment for their first VTE found that long-distance travel (≥4 hours) doubled the risk of VTE. The effect was greatest in the first week after travel but remained elevated for 2 months. Travel by air increased the risk to the same extent as travel by bus, train, or car, suggesting that the increased risk of air travel is due primarily to prolonged immobility. Synergistic effects were noted with factor V Leiden mutations, women who used oral contraceptives, BMI >30 kg/m^2, and height >1.9 m (approximately 6 ft 3 in). Some of these effects were greatest following air travel. Furthermore, people shorter than 1.6 m (approximately 5 ft 3 in) had an increased risk of VTE only after prolonged air travel. These findings suggest that additional factors related to air travel may be involved in the increased risk for VTE.

Box 2-4. Risk factors for venous thromboembolism (VTE)

Risk factors for developing VTE include:

- Recent major surgery[1]
- Paralytic spinal cord injury
- Multiple trauma
- Malignancy
- Congestive heart failure or respiratory failure
- Hormone replacement therapy, oral contraceptive
- Previous venous thromboembolism

- Inherited hypercoagulable condition
- Acquired hypercoagulable condition
- Pregnancy
- Age >40 years
- Obesity
- Immobility
- Male

[1]Especially cardiothoracic, abdominal, major orthopedic surgery.
Adapted from Anderson FA Jr, Spencer FA. Risk factors for venous thromboembolism. Circulation. 2003;107(23 Suppl 1):I9–I16.

Occurrence

Two recent retrospective cohort studies address the issue of air travel-associated VTE incidence. The first was a cohort of 2,499 healthy Dutch commercial pilots. The incidence of VTE in this group was 0.3 per 1,000 person-years. When the data were adjusted for age and sex, the rate was not different from that in the general Dutch population. There was no association between the number of hours flown.

The second study was among 8,755 employees of several international organizations. The overall incidence of VTE following flights >4 hours was 1.4 per 1,000 person-years. The absolute risk of VTE was 1 per 4,656 flights. The rates of VTE were higher in women, especially those using oral contraceptives. Incidence was also higher in employees with a BMI >25 kg/m^2 and those with height <1.65 m (5 ft 5 in) or >1.85 m (6 ft 1 in). The risk of VTE increased with flight duration and with the number of times the employee flew during an 8-week period; the risk of VTE tripled in employees who went on five or more long-haul (≥4 hours) flights. Each extra flight increased the risk of VTE 1.4-fold. The risk of VTE was highest in the first 2 weeks after a long-haul flight and gradually decreased to baseline after 8 weeks.

Both these studies were performed among populations that are younger (mean age 35–40 years) and healthier than the general population and are not, therefore, generalizable to a higher-risk population.

Clinical Presentation

Symptoms of DVT include swelling, redness, pain, or tenderness, and increased warmth over the skin. It may be difficult to distinguish from muscle strain, injury, or skin infection.

Symptoms of PE range from mild and nonspecific to acute, resembling heart attack or stroke. Once a clot has traveled to the lungs, common symptoms of PE are chest pain and shortness of breath. Other symptoms include dizziness, fainting, anxiety, and malaise. PE can occur in the absence of overt signs of DVT.

Diagnosis

Specialized imaging tests (e.g., duplex venous ultrasound, venography, computed tomography (CT) scans, and magnetic resonance imaging) are needed to make a definitive diagnosis of DVT. Helical CT or ventilation–perfusion scans are commonly used to diagnose PE.

Preventive Measures for Travelers

Several randomized, controlled trials have been performed to assess the effect of prophylactic measures on VTE risk after air travel. All studies examined the risk of asymptomatic DVT in travelers making flights ≥7 hours. All travelers were encouraged to do regular exercises and to drink nonalcoholic beverages during the flight. DVT was diagnosed by venous ultrasound from 90 minutes to 48 hours after the flight. Interventions that were studied include compression stockings, aspirin, low-molecular weight heparin, and various natural extracts with anticoagulant properties. No significant effect was seen in any of the pharmacologic interventions. Compression stockings (10–20 mm Hg and 20–30 mm Hg) were shown to significantly reduce the risk of asymptomatic DVT; however, four travelers wearing compression stockings in one study developed superficial thrombophlebitis. Symptomatic DVT and PE were not observed in any of the travelers enrolled in the studies.

All travelers should keep hydrated, wear loose-fitting clothing, and make efforts to walk and stretch at regular intervals during long-distance travel. Compression stockings may be beneficial to travelers with other risk factors for VTE. Currently no convincing data suggest that pharmacologic interventions reduce the risk of significant VTE during travel.

The American College of Chest Physicians published the 8th edition of their Antithrombotic and Thrombolytic Therapy Evidence-Based Clinical Practice Guidelines in a June 2008 Supplement to Chest. Recommendations for long-distance travel associated VTE are the following:

- For travelers who are taking flights >8 hours, the following general measures are recommended: avoidance of constrictive clothing around the lower extremities or waist, maintenance of adequate hydration, and frequent calf muscle contraction (Grade 1C).
- For long-distance travelers with additional risk factors for VTE, we recommend the general measures listed above. If active thromboprophylaxis is considered because of a perceived high risk of VTE, we suggest the use of properly fitted, below-knee graduated compression stockings (GCS), providing 15–30 mm Hg of pressure at the ankle (Grade 2C), or a single prophylactic dose of low-molecular-weight heparin (LMWH), injected prior to departure (Grade 2C).
- For long-distance travelers, we recommend against the use of aspirin for VTE prevention (Grade 1B).

References

1. Anderson FA Jr, Spencer FA. Risk factors for venous thromboembolism. Circulation. 2003;107(23 Suppl 1):I9–16.
2. World Health Organization. WHO Research into Global Hazards of Travel (WRIGHT) project: Final Report of Phase I. Geneva (Switzerland): World Health Organization; 2007 [cited 2008 May 30]. Available from: http://www.who.int/cardiovascular_diseases/wright_project/en.
3. Kuipers S, Cannegieter SC, Middeldorp S, et al. The absolute risk of venous thrombosis after air travel: a cohort study of 8,755 employees of international organisations. PLoS Med. 2007;4(9):e290.
4. Goodacre S, Sutton AJ, Sampson FC. Meta-analysis: the value of clinical assessment in the diagnosis of deep venous thrombosis. Ann Intern Med. 2005;143(2):129–39.
5. Kuipers S, Schreijer AJ, Cannegieter SC, et al. Travel and venous thrombosis: a systematic review. J Intern Med. 2007;262(6):615–34.
6. Geerts WH, Bergqvist D, Pineo GF, et al.; American College of Chest Physicians. Prevention of venous thromboembolism: American College of Chest Physicians Evidence-Based Clinical Practice Guidelines (8th Edition). Chest. 2008;133(6 Suppl):381S–453S.

INJURIES AND SAFETY

David A. Sleet, L.J. David Wallace, David R. Shlim

Overview

According to the World Health Organization, injuries are among the leading causes of death and disability in the world, and they are the leading cause of preventable death in travelers. Of the approximately five million people killed due to injuries in the world, approximately 1.2 million people died of road traffic incidents, 815,000 from suicide and 520,000 from homicides. In addition to the considerable number of deaths, millions more are wounded or suffer other nonfatal health consequences. Worldwide, among persons aged 5–44 years, injuries account for 6 of the 15 leading causes of death.

In 2007, just over 64 million Americans traveled outside the United States. The vast majority of these trips occurred without any serious health problems, but fatal and serious injuries occur to Americans every year while traveling internationally. Among travelers abroad, injuries are one of the leading causes of death. Compared with injuries, infectious diseases, for example, only account for a small proportion (2%) of deaths to overseas travelers.

The U.S. Department of State collects data on U.S. citizens who die in a foreign country from non-natural causes for the most recent 3-year period and makes these data available on the Department of State website. These deaths are categorized by location where the death occurred, date of death, and cause of death. These deaths should be considered a conservative estimate of the true number of U.S. citizens who die in foreign countries, as some deaths may not be reported to the Department of State. We analyzed these data and found that from 2003 to 2005 an estimated 2,276 U.S. citizens died from injuries and violence while in foreign countries (excluding deaths occurring in Iraq and Afghanistan). Road traffic crashes headed the list of causes (34%), followed by homicide (17%), and drowning (13%) (Figure 2-3). By comparison to U.S. injury fatalities in 2003, road traffic crashes accounted for 27%, homicide 11%, and drowning 2% of all injury deaths.

Depending on travel destination, duration, and planned activities, other common injury and safety concerns include natural hazards and disasters, civil unrest, terrorism, hate crimes against Americans, falls, burns, poisoning, drug-related overdose, and suicide. If seriously injured, emergency care may not be available or acceptable by U.S. standards. Trauma centers which are capable of providing optimal trauma care are uncommon outside urban areas.

Males, compared with females, are more likely to die from injury causes while traveling internationally. Acquaintance rape and sexual assault are among the important risks to women travelers. Travelers should be aware of the increased risk of certain injuries while traveling abroad, particularly in low-income countries, and be prepared to take preventive steps to avoid them.

Road Traffic Injuries

Road traffic injuries are the leading cause of injury-related deaths worldwide. An estimated 3,000 people are killed each day around the world in road traffic crashes involving cars, buses, motorcycles, bicycles, trucks, or pedestrians. Each year another 20 to 50 million are seriously injured. In response to this crisis, in 2008 the United Nations General Assembly, passed resolution 62/244 'Improving global road safety" to strength international cooperation to develop policies and practices to reduce crash risks around the world.

According to U.S. Department of State data, road traffic crashes are also the leading cause of injury death to U.S. citizens while traveling internationally (see Figure 2-3). An estimated 768 Americans were killed in road traffic crashes in the period from 2003 to 2005. Approximately 13% of these road traffic deaths involved motorcycles and 7% were pedestrians. A study from Bermuda reported that tourists sustain a much higher rate of motorbike injuries than the local population, with the highest rate in persons aged 50–59 years. Loss of vehicular control, unfamiliar equipment, and inexperience with motorized two-wheelers contributed to crashes and injuries, even when traveling at speeds less than 30 mph. Road traffic crashes are also a leading cause of nonfatal injury among U.S. citizens requiring emergency transport back to the United States.

Road traffic crashes are common in foreign tourists for a number of reasons: lack of familiarity with the roads, driving on the opposite side of the road than in one's home country, poorly made or maintained vehicles, travel fatigue, poor road surfaces without shoulders, unprotected curves and cliffs, and poor visibility due to lack of adequate lighting, both on the road and on the vehicle. In many low-income areas of the world, unsafe roads and vehicles and an inadequate transportation infrastructure contribute to the traffic injury problem. A safety concern in low-income countries is the mixing of motor vehicles with vulnerable road users such as pedestrians, bicyclists, and motorbike users. It is common in low-income countries to have cars, buses, and large trucks all sharing the same road with pedestrians, motorbikes, bicycles, rickshaws and even animals. This mixing of road users all in the same travel lane increases the risk for crashes and injuries.

Sometimes travelers have few options in getting to remote areas, but if there are choices, they should look for better-maintained vehicles, daytime travel, seatbelts and a trained and licensed or hired driver.

Prevention of Road Traffic Injuries

Health advisors should counsel the traveler to:

- Use safety belts and child safety seats whenever possible. Safety belts reduce the risk of death in a crash by 45%–60%, child safety seats by 54% and infant seats by 70%. When traveling, rent newer vehicles with safety belts and airbags and bring a child safety seat from home.
- Rent larger vehicles if possible, because they provide more protection in a crash.
- Try to ride only in taxis with functional safety belts and ride in the rear seat.
- Wear helmets when riding motorcycles, motorbikes, and bicycles. If helmets are likely to be unavailable at the destination, they should be brought from home.
- Avoid drinking alcohol and driving or biking. U.S. data show that an alcohol-impaired driver has a 17 times greater risk of being involved in a fatal crash.
- Visit the websites of the Association for International Road Travel (ASIRT) (www.asirt.org) and Make Roads Safe (www.makeroadssafe.org), both NGOs, which have useful safety tips for international travelers, including road safety checklists and country specific driving risks.
- Check the safety and security information from the U.S. Department of State (www.travel.state.gov).
- Consider hiring a driver familiar with the destination, the language and an expert in maneuvering through local traffic.
- Avoid riding on overcrowded, overweight, top heavy busses, or minivans, or riding with any driver who has consumed alcohol.
- Be aware of pedestrians and be aware as a pedestrian of the dangers. Walk with a friend, rather than alone, as this helps with safety.

Water Injuries

Drowning accounts for 13% of deaths of Americans abroad. The risk factors have not been clearly defined, but are suspected to be related to unfamiliarity with local water currents and water conditions. Drowning was the leading cause of injury death to Americans visiting countries where exposure to water recreation was a major activity such as Fiji, Dutch Antilles, Aruba, and Costa Rica. Studies have found that young men are particularly at risk of head and spinal cord injuries from diving into shallow water, with alcohol a factor in some cases. In 2000, approximately 449,000 people drowned worldwide; the exact number of travelers who suffer from nonfatal drowning is not precisely known.

Alcohol is also a suspected contributing factor to both drowning and boating mishaps.

Scuba diving is a frequent pursuit of travelers in ocean destinations. Travelers should either be experienced divers, or dive with a reliable dive shop and instructors. They should be reminded not to dive on the same day they arrive by airplane. The fatality rate among all divers, worldwide, is thought to be 15 to 20 deaths per 100,000 divers per year.

Other Unintentional Injuries

From 2003 to 2005, other than drowning, airplane crashes, natural disasters, and other unintentional injuries accounted for over a third of all injury deaths to Americans in foreign countries (see Figure 2-3). Fires can be a substantial risk in low-income countries where building codes are not present or enforced, where there's an absence of smoke alarms, where there is no emergency access to 9-1-1 services, and where the fire department focus is on putting out fires rather than on fire prevention or victim rescue.

Preventing Other Unintentional Injuries

Health advisors should counsel the traveler on the following:

- Travelers should consider purchasing special health and evacuation insurance if their destinations include countries where there may not be access to good medical care.
- Because trauma care is poor in many countries, victims of injuries can die before ever reaching a hospital, and there may be no coordinated ambulance services. In remote areas, medical assistance, drugs and medicines may be unavailable and travel can take a long time to the nearest medical facility.
- Where possible avoid using local unscheduled small aircraft. If available choose larger aircraft (greater than 30 seats) as they have undergone more strict and regular safety inspections. Larger aircraft also provide more protection in the event of a crash. From 2003 to 2005 an estimated 83 Americans were killed in airplane crashes in foreign countries (see Figure 2-3). For country-specific airline crash events, see www.airsafe.com.
- To prevent fire-related injuries, select accommodations on the 6th floor or below (fire ladders generally cannot reach above the 6th). If possible, stay in hotels with smoke alarms and preferably sprinkler systems. Be alert for improperly vented heating devices which may cause poisoning from carbon monoxide (CO), a colorless odorless gas and by-product of all fossil fuel combustions. Some travelers choose to carry a personal CO detector. Travelers should identify two escape routes from buildings and remember to escape a fire by crawling low under smoke and by covering one's mouth with a wet cloth.

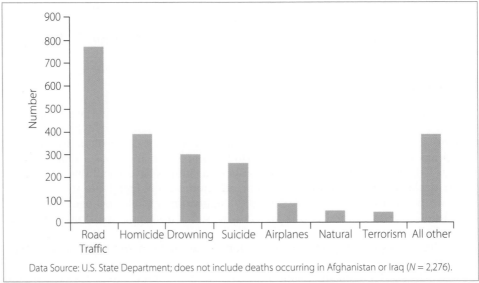

Data Source: U.S. State Department; does not include deaths occurring in Afghanistan or Iraq (*N* = 2,276).

Figure 2-3. Leading causes of injury death of U.S. citizens in foreign countries, 2003–2005.

(From U.S. Department of State. U.S. citizen deaths from non-natural causes. Washington D.C.: U.S. Department of State. Available from: http://travel.state.gov/law/family_issues/death/death_600.html.)

Violence-Related Injuries

Violence is a leading worldwide public health problem and a growing concern of travelers. In 2000, about 1.6 million persons lost their lives to violence and only one-fifth were casualties of armed conflicts. Rates of violent deaths in low- to middle-income countries are more than 3 times those in higher-income countries, although there are great variations within countries, depending on regional demographic differences.

Homicide was the second leading cause of injury death among American travelers in foreign countries accounting for almost 400 deaths from 2003 to 2005 (see Figure 2-3). For some low-income countries such as Honduras, Colombia, Guatemala, and Haiti homicide was the leading cause of injury death for Americans accounting for 43%–65% of all injury deaths.

Terrorism-related deaths among Americans in foreign countries, while alarming, are still relatively rare events and accounted for only 2% of all injury deaths (see Figure 2-3). The vast majority of terrorism deaths among Americans occurred in countries of the Middle East. According to data from the State Department, 2003–2005, 82% of the injury deaths among Americans in Saudi Arabia and 55% of injury deaths in Israel/West Bank/Gaza were from terrorism.

Suicide is the fourth leading cause of injury death to U.S. citizens traveling abroad (see Figure 2-3). Factors contributing to homicide and suicide may be different while traveling than at home. Unfamiliarity with a destination, not being vigilant to one's surroundings, and alcohol involvement may increase risk of assault and homicide. For longer-term travelers (e.g., missionaries and volunteers), social isolation and substance abuse, particularly in the face of living in areas of poverty and rigid gender roles, may increase the risk of depression and suicide.

If a traveler is the victim of a crime overseas, the nearest U.S. embassy, consulate, or consular agency for assistance should be contacted at www.travel.state.gov.

Prevention of Violence

U.S. travelers are viewed by many criminals as wealthy, naïve targets, who are inexperienced and unfamiliar with the culture and inept at seeking assistance once victimized. Traveling in high poverty areas, civil unrest, alcohol or drug use, and traveling in unfamiliar environments at night increase the likelihood that a U.S. traveler will be the victim of planned or random violence.

To avoid violence while traveling, limit travel at night, travel with a companion, and vary the routine travel habits. Travelers should wear locally available accessories that are more typical of a country-savvy expatriate community and avoid expensive or provocative clothing, or accessories. Accommodations on the ground floor of hotels or immediately next to the stairwell should be avoided. Criminals are less likely to victimize upper level floors. All doors and windows should be locked. Some carry a door intruder alarm, a smoke alarm, and a rubber door stop that can be used as a supplemental door lock. Persons unknown to the traveler should not be invited into one's accommodations as this can be misinterpreted or against local laws and customs.

The U.S. Department of State website (www.travel.state.gov) has useful information regarding safety and security.

Summary

Injuries and violence are as much a public health problem to travelers overseas as are infectious and chronic diseases—and they are in many ways more deadly. Injuries are still the most frequent cause of death abroad in developing countries. Effective prevention strategies are available, particularly for travelers who find themselves in new environments and who may be more likely to be unaware of risks or complacent in exotic surroundings. Despite greater understanding and increased research efforts in this field, data on the magnitude and severity of injuries is still incomplete or unreliable in many countries. Existing data indicate that injury and violence are among the most important causes of premature death and ill-health to U.S. travelers overseas. Travel health advisors and other health-care providers should alert the public to the known risks and especially about simple and effective preventive measures to implement during international travel.

References

1. Peden M, McGee K, Sharma G. The injury chart book: a graphical overview of the global burden of injuries [Internet]. [cited 2008 Nov 25] Geneva (Switzerland): World Health Organization; 2002. Available from: http://www.who.int/violence_injury_prevention/publications/other_injury/chartb/en/

2. U.S. Department of Commerce. The Office of Travel and Tourism Industries. 2007 United States resident travel abroad [cited 2008 Nov 25]. Available from: http://tinet.ita.doc.gov/outreachpages/outbound.general_information.outbound_overview.html.

3. McInnes RJ, Williamson LM, Morrison A. Unintentional injury during foreign travel: a review. J Travel Med. 2002;9(6):297–307.

4. U.S. Department of State. U.S. citizen deaths from non-natural causes by foreign country [cited 2006 June]. Available from: http://travel.state.gov/law/family_issues/death/death_600.html

5. CDC. Web-based Injury Statistics Query and Reporting System (WISQARS) [cited 2008 June]. Available from: www.cdc.gov/ncipc/wisqars

6. MacPherson DW, Guérillot F, Streiner DL, et al. Death and dying abroad: the Canadian experience. J Travel Med. 2000; 7(5):227–33.

7. Hargarten SW, Baker TD, Guptill K. Overseas fatalities of United States citizen travelers: an analysis of deaths related to international travel. Ann Emerg Med. 1991;20(6):622–6.

8. Peden M, Scurfield R, Sleet D, et al., editors. World report on road traffic injury prevention. Geneva (Switzerland): World Health Organization; 2004. [cited 2008 Nov 25]. Available from: http://www.who.int/violence_injury_prevention/publications/road_traffic/world_report/en/.

9. Sleet DA, Branche CM. Road safety is no accident. J Safety Res. 2004;35(2):173–4.

10. Carey MJ, Aitken ME. Motorbike injuries in Bermuda: a risk for tourists. Ann Emerg Med. 1996;28(4):424–9.

11. Hargarten SW, Bouc GT. Emergency air medical transport of U.S.-citizen tourists: 1988 to 1990. Air Med J. 1993;12(10):398–402.

12. Barss P, Smith GS, Baker SP, et al. Injury prevention: an international perspective. New York: Oxford University Press; 1998.

13. Zaza S, Sleet DA, Shults RA, et al. Reducing injuries to motor vehicle occupants. In: Zaza S, Briss P, Harris K, editors. The guide to community preventive services: what works to promote health? New York: Oxford University Press, 2005. p. 329–84.

14. The Association for International Road Travel. [cited 2008 Nov 25]. Available from: www.asirt.org

15. Commission for Global Road Safety. Make Roads Safe. [cited 2008 Nov 25] Available from: www.makeroadssafe.org

16. U.S. Department of State. Bureau of Consular Affairs [cited 2008 Nov 25]. Available from: http://travel.state.gov/travel/travel_1744.html.

17. Krug EG, Dahlberg LL, Mercy JA, et al. World report on violence and health. Geneva (Switzerland): World Health Organization; 2002. [cited 2008 Nov 25]. Available from: www.who.int/violence_injury_prevention/violence/world_report/en

18. Jeannel D, Allain-Ioos S, Bonmarin I, et al. Les décès de français lors d'un séjour à l'étranger et leurs causes. Bull Epid Heb. 2006(23–4):166–8.

19. Ball DJ, Machin N. Foreign travel and the risk of harm. Int J Inj Contr Saf Promot. 2006; 13(2):107–15.

20. Cortés LM, Hargarten SW, Hennes HM. Recommendations for water safety and drowning prevention for travelers. J Travel Med. 2006;13(1):21–34.

21. United Nations General Assembly. Resolution A/RES/62/244 Improving global road safety. Sixty-second session, agenda item 46. 87th Plenary meeting, 2008 March 31. Passed 2008 April.

NATURAL DISASTERS AND ENVIRONMENTAL HAZARDS

Josephine Malilay, Dahna Batts, Armin Ansari, Charles W. Miller, Clive M. Brown

Natural Disasters

Travelers should be aware of the potential for natural phenomena such as hurricanes, tornadoes, or earthquakes. Natural disasters can contribute to the transmission of some diseases, especially since water supplies and sewage systems may be disrupted, sanitation and hygiene compromised by population displacement and overcrowding, and normal public health services interrupted.

Disease Risks

- The risk for infectious diseases is minimal unless a disease is endemic in an area prior to the disaster event, since transmission cannot take place unless the causative agent is present.
  - Although typhoid can be endemic in developing countries, natural disasters have seldom led to epidemic levels of disease.
  - Floods have been known to prompt outbreaks of leptospirosis in areas where the organism is found in water sources (see the Leptospirosis section in Chapter 5).
- When water and sewage systems have been disrupted, safe water and food supplies are of great importance in preventing enteric disease transmission. If contamination is suspected, water should be boiled and appropriately disinfected (see the Water Disinfection for Travelers section earlier in this chapter).
- Travelers who are injured during a natural disaster should have a medical evaluation to determine what additional care may be required for wounds potentially contaminated with feces, soil, or saliva or that have been exposed to fresh or sea water that may contain parasites or bacteria.
- Tetanus booster status should always be kept current.

Injuries

- When arriving at a destination, travelers should be familiar with local risks for seismic, flood-related, landslide-related, tsunami-related, and other hazards, as well as warning systems, evacuation routes, and shelters in areas of high risk.
- After natural disasters, deaths are rarely due to infectious diseases but most often to blunt trauma, crush-related injuries, or drowning. Travelers should thus be aware of the risks for injury before, during, and after a natural disaster.
- In floods, people should avoid driving through swiftly moving water.
- Travelers should exercise caution during clean-up, particularly when encountering downed power lines, water-affected electrical outlets, interrupted gas lines, and stray or frightened animals.
- During natural disasters, technological malfunctions may release hazardous materials (e.g., release of toxic chemicals from a point source displaced by strong winds, seismic motion, or rapidly moving water).

Environmental Risks

- Natural disasters often lead to wide-ranging air pollution in large cities. Uncontrolled forest fires have caused widespread pollution over vast expanses of the world.
- Natural or manmade disasters resulting in massive structural collapse or dust clouds can cause the release of chemical or biologic contaminants (e.g., asbestos or the arthrospores that lead to coccidioidomycosis).
- Health risks associated with these environmental occurrences have not been fully studied.
- Travelers with chronic pulmonary disease may be more susceptible to adverse effects from these exposures.

Event-Specific Information

Typically, following natural disasters of a magnitude that may impact travelers, current information about the disaster, as well as travel health information specific to those needing entry into such regions, is provided on the CDC Travelers' Health website (www.cdc.gov/travel). Recommendations may include specific immunizations or cautions regarding unique hazards in the affected area.

Environmental Hazards

Air

- Air pollution may be found in large cities throughout the world; its sources are often attributed to automobile exhaust and industrial emissions and may be aggravated by climate and geography.
- The harmful effects of air pollution are difficult to avoid when visiting some cities; limiting strenuous activity and not smoking can help.
- Any risk to healthy short-term travelers to such areas is probably small, but persons with pre-existing health conditions (e.g., asthma or chronic obstructive pulmonary disease) could be more susceptible.
- Avoidance of dust clouds and areas of heavy dust or haze may be wise.

Water

- Rivers, lakes, and the ocean may be contaminated with—
  o organic or inorganic chemical compounds (e.g., heavy metals or other toxins);
  o harmful algal blooms (i.e., cyanobacteria) that can be toxic both to fish and to people who eat the fish or who swim or bathe in the water; and
  o pathogens from human and animal waste that may cause disease in swimmers.
- Such hazards may not be immediately apparent in a body of water.
- Extensive water damage after major hurricanes and floods increases the likelihood of mold contamination in buildings. U.S. residents may visit flooded areas overseas as part of emergency, medical, or humanitarian missions. Mold is a greater hazard for persons with conditions such as impaired host defenses or mold allergies. To prevent exposure that could result in adverse health effects from disturbed mold, persons should—
  o Avoid areas where mold contamination is obvious.
  o Use personal protective equipment (PPE) (e.g. gloves, goggles, tight-fitting NIOSH-approved N-95 respirator). Travelers should take sufficient PPE with them, as these may be scarce in the countries visited.
  o Keep hands, skin, and clothing clean and free from mold-contaminated dust.
  o The CDC MMWR guidance, "Mold Prevention Strategies and Possible Health Effects in the Aftermath of Hurricanes and Major Floods," provides recommendations for dealing with mold in these settings.

Radiation

- Natural background radiation levels can vary substantially from region to region, but these natural variations are not a health concern for either the traveler or resident population.
- Travelers should be aware of regions known to have been contaminated with radioactive materials, such as the area surrounding the Chernobyl nuclear power station, 100 km (62 miles) northwest of Kiev, Ukraine. This unprecedented radiation emergency and subsequent contamination primarily affected regions in three republics—Ukraine, Belarus, and Russia—with the highest radioactive ground contamination within 30 km (19 miles) of Chernobyl.
- In most countries, known areas of radioactive contamination are fenced or marked with signs. These areas should not be trespassed.
- Any traveler seeking long-term (more than a few months) residence near a known or suspected contaminated area should consult with staff of the nearest U.S. Embassy and inquire about any applicable advisories in that area regarding

drinking water quality or purchase of meat, fruit, and vegetables from local farmers.

- Radiation emergencies are rare events. In case of such an emergency, however, travelers should:
  - Follow instructions provided by local emergency and public health authorities.
  - If such information is not forthcoming, U.S. travelers should immediately seek advice from the nearest U.S. embassy.
- Natural disasters (such as floods) may also result in displacement of industrial or clinical radioactive sources. In all circumstances, travelers should exercise caution when they encounter unknown objects or equipment, especially if they bear the radioactive symbol. If a questionable object is encountered, appropriate authorities should be notified.

References

1. Pan American Health Organization. Natural disasters: protecting the public's health. Washington (DC): Pan American Health Organization; 2000 [cited 2006 Jun 21]. Available from: http://www.paho.org/English/dd/ped/SP575.htm

2. Watson JT, Gayer M, Connolly MA. Epidemics after natural disasters. Emerg Infect Dis. 2007;13(1):1–5.

3. Noji EK, editor. The public health consequences of disasters. New York: Oxford University Press; 1997.

4. Young S, Balluz L, Malilay J. Natural and technologic hazardous material releases during and after natural disasters: a review. Sci Total Environ. 2004;322(1–3):3–20.

5. Nukushina J. Japanese earthquake victims are being exposed to high density of asbestos. We need protective masks desperately. Epidemiol Prev. 1995;19(63):226–7.

6. Schneider E, Hajjeh RA, Spiegel RA, et al. A coccidioidomycosis outbreak following the Northridge, Calif, earthquake. JAMA. 1997;277(11):904–8.

7. Brant M, Brown C, Burkhart J; CDC. Mold prevention strategies and possible health effects in the aftermath of hurricanes and major floods. MMWR Recomm Rep. 2006;55(RR-8):1–27.

8. National Council on Radiation Protection and Measurements. Exposure of the population in the United States and Canada from natural background radiation. Report No 94. Bethesda (Md); 1987.

9. Eisenbud M, Gessel T. Environmental radioactivity from natural, industrial, and military sources. 4th ed. San Diego: Academic Press; 1997.

10. United Nations Scientific Committee on the Effects of Atomic Radiation. Annex J: Exposures and effects of the Chernobyl accident. In: Sources and effects of ionizing radiation; United Nations Scientific Committee on the Effects of Atomic Radiation. UNSCEAR 2000 Report to the General Assembly with Scientific Annexes. Volume II: Effects. New York: United Nations; 2000. p. 451–556.

11. U.S. Food and Drug Administration, Center for Devices and Radiological Health. Accidental radioactive contamination of human food and animal feeds: recommendations for state and local agencies. Rockville (MD): U.S. Food and Drug Administration; 1998 [cited 2006 Jun 22]. Available from: http://www.fda.gov/cdrh/dmqrp/84.html.

SCUBA DIVING

Daniel A. Nord

Scuba diving can present a variety of unique medical challenges for the traveling diver. Because diving injuries are generally rare, few health-care providers are trained in their diagnosis and treatment. Thus, the recreational diver must be able to recognize the signs of injury and ensure the availability of dive medicine help when needed.

Fitness to Dive

Planning for dive-related travel should take into account any changes in health status, recent injuries, or surgery. In general, respiratory disorders, as well as any disorders affecting higher function and consciousness (e.g., diabetes mellitus or seizures), respiratory function (e.g., asthma), psychological problems (e.g., anxiety), and pregnancy raise special concerns about diving fitness.

Diving Disorders

Barotrauma

Ear and Sinus

Ear barotrauma is the most common injury in divers. On descent, failure to equalize pressure changes within the middle ear space creates a pressure gradient across the eardrum, which can cause bleeding or fluid accumulation in the middle ear, as well as stretching or rupture of the eardrum and the membranes covering the windows of the inner ear. Symptoms can include—

- pain
- tinnitus (ringing in the ears)
- vertigo (dizziness or sensation of spinning)
- sensation of fullness
- effusion (fluid accumulation in the ear)
- decreased hearing

Paranasal sinuses, because of their relatively narrow connecting passageways, are uniquely susceptible to barotraumas, generally on descent. With small changes in pressure (depth), symptoms are usually mild and short lived, but can be exacerbated by continued diving. Larger pressure changes, especially with forceful attempts at equilibration (e.g., valsalva maneuver), can be more injurious. Additional risk factors for ear and sinus barotrauma include—

- earplugs
- medications
- ear and/or sinus surgery
- nasal deformity
- disease

A diver who may have sustained ear or sinus barotrauma should discontinue diving and seek medical attention.

Pulmonary

It is critical for a scuba diver to exhale (or breathe normally) while ascending slowly. Overinflation of the lungs, which usually happens when a novice diver panics, can result as a scuba diver ascends toward the surface without exhaling. During ascent, compressed gas trapped in the lung increases in volume until the expansion exceeds the elastic limit of lung tissue, causing damage and allowing gas bubbles to escape into one or more of three possible locations, as follows:

- Gas entering the pleural space can cause lung collapse or pneumothorax.
- Gas entering the mediastinum (space around the heart, trachea and esophagus) causes mediastinal emphysema and frequently tracks under the skin (subcutaneous emphysema) or into the tissue around the larynx, sometimes precipitating a change in the voice characteristics.
- Gas rupturing the alveolar walls can dissect into the pulmonary capillaries and pass via the pulmonary veins to the left side of the heart, where it is distributed according to relative blood flow, resulting in arterial gas embolism (AGE).

While mediastinal or subcutaneous emphysema usually resolves spontaneously, pneumothorax generally requires specific treatment to remove the air and reinflate the lung. AGE is a medical emergency requiring appropriate intervention, which includes recompression treatment with hyperbaric oxygen.

Lung overinflation injuries from scuba diving can range from dramatic and life threatening to mild symptoms of chest pain and dyspnea. Although pulmonary barotrauma is relatively uncommon in divers, prompt medical evaluation is necessary, and evidence for this condition should always be considered in the presence of respiratory or neurologic symptoms following a dive.

Decompression Illness

Decompression illness (DCI) is an all-inclusive term that describes the dysbaric injuries, AGE, and decompression sickness (DCS). Because the two diseases are considered to result from separate causes, they are described here separately. However, from a clinical and practical standpoint, distinguishing between them in the field may be impossible—and unnecessary, since the initial treatment is the same for both. DCI can occur even in divers who have carefully followed the standard decompression tables and the principles of safe diving.

Arterial Gas Embolism (AGE)

Gas entering the arterial blood through ruptured pulmonary vessels can distribute bubbles into the body tissues, including the heart and brain, where they disrupt circulation. AGE may cause minimal neurologic symptoms or dramatic symptoms that require immediate attention. These signs and symptoms include—

- numbness
- weakness
- tingling
- dizziness
- visual blurring
- chest pain
- personality change
- paralysis or seizures
- loss of consciousness
- death

In general, any scuba diver who surfaces unconscious or loses consciousness within 10 minutes after surfacing should be assumed to have AGE. Intervention with basic life support is indicated, including the administration of 100% oxygen, followed by rapid evacuation to a hyperbaric oxygen treatment facility.

Decompression Sickness

Breathing air under pressure causes excess inert gas (usually nitrogen) to dissolve in body tissues. The amount dissolved is proportional to and increases with depth and time. As the diver ascends to the surface, the excess dissolved gas must be cleared through respiration via the bloodstream. Depending on the amount dissolved and the rate of ascent, some gas can supersaturate tissues, where it separates from solution to form bubbles, interfering with blood flow and tissue oxygenation and causing signs and symptoms of decompression sickness. These symptoms include—

- joint aches or pain
- numbness and/or tingling
- mottling or marbling of skin
- coughing spasms or shortness of breath
- itching
- unusual fatigue
- dizziness
- weakness
- personality changes
- loss of bowel or bladder function

- staggering, loss of coordination, and/or tremors
- paralysis
- collapse or unconsciousness

Serious permanent injury may result from either AGE or DCS.

Flying after Diving

The risk of developing decompression sickness is increased when divers are exposed to increased altitude too soon following a dive. The cabin pressure of commercial aircraft may be the equivalent of 8,000 ft (2,438 m). Thus, divers should avoid flying or an altitude exposure >2,000 ft (610 m) for—

- a minimum of 12 hours after surfacing from a single no-decompression dive, or
- after repetitive dives and/or multiple days of diving, wait a minimum of 18 hours before ascending to altitude, to reduce the risk of decompression sickness.

These recommended preflight surface intervals do not guarantee avoidance of DCS. Longer surface intervals will further reduce DCS risk.

Prevention of Diving Disorders

Recreational divers should dive conservatively and well within the limits of their dive tables or computers. Risk factors for DCI are primarily dive depth and bottom time; however, factors such as rapid ascent, repetitive dives, strenuous exercise, dives >60 feet, altitude exposure soon after a dive, and physiological variability also increase risk. Divers should be cautioned to stay well hydrated and rested, dive within the limits of their training, and follow established guidelines for dives unique to their travel destination. Diving is a skill that requires appropriate training and certification and should be done with a companion.

Treatment of Diving Disorders

Definitive treatment of DCI begins with early recognition of symptoms, followed by recompression with hyperbaric oxygen. A high concentration (100%) of supplemental oxygen is considered effective first aid in relieving the signs and symptoms of decompression illness and should be administered as soon as possible. Divers are often dehydrated, either because of incidental causes, immersion, or DCI itself, which can cause a capillary leak. Administration of isotonic glucose-free intravenous fluid is recommended in most cases. Oral rehydration fluids may also be helpful, provided they can be safely administered (e.g., if the diver is conscious). The definitive treatment of DCI is recompression and oxygen administration in a hyperbaric chamber.

The Divers Alert Network (DAN) maintains a 24-hour emergency consultation and evacuation assistance at 919-684-8111 or 919-684-4326 (collect calls are accepted). DAN will provide assistance with management of the injured diver, help in deciding if recompression is needed, the location of the closest recompression facility, and assistance in arranging patient transport. DAN can also be contacted for routine nonemergency consultation by telephone at 919-684-2948, ext. 222, or by accessing the website www.diversalertnetwork.org.

Travelers who plan to scuba dive may want to ascertain whether there are recompression facilities at their destination prior to embarking on their trip.

References

1. Brubakk AO, Neuman TS, editors. Bennett and Elliot's physiology and medicine of diving. 5th ed. London: Saunders Ltd.; 2003.

2. Moon RE. Treatment of decompression illness. In: Bove AA, Davis J, editors. Diving medicine. 4th ed. London: Saunders; 2004. p. 195–223.

3. Sheffield PJ, Vann RD. Flying after recreational diving: workshop proceedings. Divers Alert Network. 2004 [cited 2008 Nov 25]. Available from: http://www.diversalertnetwork.org/research/projects/fad/workshop/.

4. Thalmann ED. DAN dive and travel medical guide. rev. ed. 2003. Durham, NC: Divers Alert Network.

MEDICAL TOURISM

Christie M. Reed

Introduction

Travel for the purpose of obtaining health care abroad has received a great deal of attention in the popular media recently—even Wikipedia has recently devoted a section to the practice (http://en.wikipedia.org/wiki/Medical_tourism). However, it is not the only form of "medical tourism." The term has also been applied to travel by health-care professionals for the purpose of providing health care. The extent of either form of travel is not well characterized, but the overarching issues for both types of travelers, their primary health-care providers, and travel medicine providers are outlined below.

Travel to Obtain Care

Data from the annual U.S. Department of Commerce in-flight survey during 2003–2006 show an overall annual increase in the number of trips taken by U.S. residents for which at least one purpose was health care. In 2006, there were approximately half a million overseas trips in which health treatment was at least one purpose of travel. Common cited procedures include:

- Dentistry
- Reproductive procedures
- Surgeries (cosmetic, joint replacement, and cardiac)

Lower cost is often mentioned as the motivation for this type of medical tourism, and an entire industry has grown up around this phenomenon. One can search for a provider and research accreditation status of the facility online, opt for an online concierge service that will make all the arrangements or, more recently, find that health insurance coverage may include the option of "outsourced" health care.

The dynamic nature of the field was described in a recent roundtable discussion in Merrell et al.,

> In recent years, standards have been rising in other parts of the world even faster than prices have surged in the U.S. Many physicians abroad trained in the U.S. and the Joint Commission International (JCI) applies strict standards to accreditation of offshore facilities. Those facilities use the same implants, supplies, and drugs as their U.S. counterparts. However, a heart bypass in Thailand costs $11,000 compared to as much as $130,000 in the U.S. Spinal fusion surgery in India at $5,500 compares to over $60,000 in the U.S.

However, the quality of facilities, assistance services, and care is neither uniform nor regulated; thus, in most instances, responsibility for assessing suitability of an individual program or facility lies solely with the traveler.

Guidelines for Travelers Seeking Care Abroad

Potential patients should consider that, whatever procedure is being contemplated, travelers undergoing medical treatment outside their accustomed environment are almost always at a disadvantage, particularly if there are complications. Concerns are—

- Resolution of financial issues if costs escalate, such as in the case of complications.
- Language and cultural differences may impede accurate interpretation of both verbal and nonverbal communication.
- Religious and ethical differences may be encountered over issues such as heroic efforts to preserve life or limb or in care of the terminally ill.
- Lack of familiarity with the local medical system, limited access to past medical history, unfamiliar drugs and medicines.
- Legal recourse may be fairly limited, difficult to obtain, or nonexistent.
- Follow-up care back in the United States may be more difficult to arrange and may be fraught with problems, should there be complications.

Potential patients should consider the guiding principles developed by the American Medical Association for employers, insurance companies, and other entities that facilitate or offer incentives for care outside the United States, although in some circumstances it is unclear how realistic they may be (see www.ama-assn.org/ama1/pub/upload/mm/31/medicaltourism.pdf). These principles stipulate that international care must be voluntary and provided by accredited institutions; financial incentives should not inappropriately limit or restrict patient options; there should be continuity of care, including coverage of costs upon return; patients should be informed of their rights and legal recourse before travel; patients should have access to licensing, outcome, and accrediting information when seeking care; medical record transfers should comply with Health Insurance Portability and Accountability Act (HIPAA) guidelines; and patients should be informed of potential risks of combining surgical procedures with long flights and vacation activities. The American Society for Plastic Surgery emphasizes plastic surgery is "real" surgery and outlines the issues every patient undergoing surgery should consider, whether at home or abroad, on their website at www.plasticsurgery.org/patients_consumers/patient_safety/Medical-Tourism.cfm. Several clusters of mycobacterial wound infections in travelers returning from cosmetic procedures abroad have been published. Similarly, the American Dental Association provides informational documents, including: "Traveler's Guide to Safe Dental Care" through the Global Dental Safety Organization for Safety and Asepsis Procedures at www.osap.org and "Dental Care Away from Home" at www.ada.org/public/manage/care/index.asp.

Individuals researching accreditation status should note that, although facilities may be part of a chain, they are surveyed and accredited individually. They should also check the duration of the accreditation and validate that the information is current by consulting the public portion of the appropriate accrediting agency website (see references below).

Pre-Travel Advice for the Medical Tourist

As discussed in the Planning for Healthy Travel section in Chapter 1, patients who do elect to travel should consult a travel health-care practitioner for advice tailored to individual health needs, preferably at least 4–6 weeks in advance of travel. This is particularly true for patients considering invasive procedures, who should consult as soon as travel is considered to allow for assessment of hepatitis B vaccination status (see the Hepatitis B section earlier in this chapter). Hepatitis B and C viruses and HIV are examples of blood-borne infections that can be transmitted via contaminated equipment, from infected health-care providers during invasive procedures, via transfusion of blood or blood products, or through transplantation of tissue or organs that have not been properly screened. Prevalence rates of these viruses vary considerably around the world and are generally higher in developing parts of the world than in the United States. U.S. policies address hepatitis B vaccination status of health-care workers, but these policies are not uniform worldwide and there are no currently licensed vaccines for hepatitis C and HIV. Blood transfusion programs in the United States and other developed areas rely on voluntary, nonremunerated donors; screen the donated blood for a variety of potentially blood-borne pathogens; and are closely regulated. Standards in other parts of the world vary. Based on data from 2000–2001, the latest available on the WHO Global Database on Blood Safety (www.who.int/bloodsafety/global_database/en/), 70 countries did not test all donated blood for the three major blood-borne viruses, HIV and hepatitis B and C.

Organ Transplantation

Organ transplantation in the United States is also a voluntary, closely monitored process coordinated by the United Network for Organ Sharing (www.optn.org). The need for transplantable organs, however, far exceeds the available supply worldwide. Travel to a country with less rigorous methods of distribution for the purpose of obtaining a transplant has been termed "transplant tourism" or "organ trafficking." Recently, there have been reports in the media of investigations and arrests associated with "rings" that use unscrupulous methods to obtain organs. In 2004, the World Health Assembly Resolution 57.18 encouraged member countries to protect vulnerable populations. Some countries have begun experimenting with controlled programs to relieve the shortage, support the health of the donor, and remove incentives for clandestine operations. A revised set of eleven WHO Guiding Principles on Human Cell, Tissue and Organ Transplantation will be presented to the World Health Assembly in 2009 (www.who.int/transplantation/).

Travel for the Purpose of Delivering Health Care

There are many structured opportunities for health-care professionals, students, or trainees to participate in established programs in developing areas of the world that are mutually beneficial to both the local population and the traveler. Travel by health-care workers in their professional capacity should be governed by the principle of *Primum non nocere*, or "first, do no harm." The traveling health-care worker should have sufficient experience or be at a stage in training to be able to contribute labor, knowledge, and skills to the host community. Benefits to the traveling health-care worker include exposure to patients with tropical diseases and conditions that are not commonly seen or are at a more advanced stage than in the country of residence; local diagnostic skills which are often less dependent on technology; and new cultures and new ways of thinking, in addition to any personal gratification. Many medical schools and universities have established reciprocal relationships with institutions in developing areas in which there is an exchange of students and faculty. A variety of organizations match volunteers with local needs for skills-building or to address specific problems. Doctors Without Borders/Médecins Sans Frontières (MSF), which received the Nobel Peace Prize in 1999 for humanitarian efforts around the world, requires a minimum 6-month commitment from physicians and a shorter commitment for surgeons. Interventional programs such as dentistry or surgery simultaneously provide reparative or reconstructive services to the population and train local staff to perform the procedures and provide follow-up care, often donating excess supplies. Other ongoing volunteer relationships exist between faith-based or service organizations and local communities. The involvement of the local health establishment is key to determining needs and maximizing benefit to the local population, as well as educating the visitors on local customs and medical issues and providing translation, if needed, to adequately assess the patients, obtain consent, and advise on postprocedure care.

These forms of international capacity-building should be differentiated from—

- medicine that is practiced on local populations ad hoc by independent travelers to areas that seem to have no system of health care,
- the development of adventure holidays sold to groups of doctors specifically for the purposes of research or providing health care in the absence of prior consultation, and
- students or trainees who travel to "gain practical experience" beyond their training with minimal supervision or absence of structured learning, or practitioners performing outside the area of their expertise.

The acts performed in a life-threatening emergency are justified, but if a local health-care system exists there should still be follow-up with the nearest local provider. Health-care professionals contemplating an international clinical experience should also consult the Humanitarian Aid Workers section in Chapter 8 for a discussion of emotional and physical fitness to participate, preparation, and after-care issues.

The Primary Health-Care Provider

Primary health-care providers play a crucial role in several aspects of medical tourism. For un- or under-insured patients who cannot afford their prescribed course of treatment, the primary care provider may be asked to provide counsel regarding international treatment options, assist with vetting available options, optimize patient status prior to travel, or coordinate care on return. Each provider will need to assess individually his or her ability to address travel health issues or refer to a travel medicine provider.

Clinicians who care for immigrant populations should also be aware that the majority of health-seeking travelers in 2004 were current U.S. citizens born outside the United States, followed by non-U.S. citizens. Health-care needs, such as dentistry, are often included in visits home, due to familiarity with care in the country of origin, the high cost of health care in the United States, and lack of insurance coverage in these populations. There are also recent reports that patients on transplant waiting lists may also travel abroad for the procedure and return to the developed country of residence for continued care, often requiring immediate hospitalization and intense initial management with little documentation. Options for dialysis care are also increasing in developing areas; thus patients requiring this level of care may return home for visits and obtain local care. Acute hepatitis B infections have been diagnosed in patients returning to developed countries from both scenarios. Clinicians providing care to immigrant populations should consider routinely inquiring about future or recent travel home to visit friends and relatives, whether health care will be sought or occurred during travel and advise accordingly (see the VFR section in Chapter 8).

Travel Medicine Providers

Patients who plan to seek medical care abroad may not divulge this activity during the consultation. The desire for anonymity may be a reason for seeking procedures, such as cosmetic surgery or sex-change operations, abroad. As previously mentioned, cost is often an issue, and patients may be uncomfortable self-disclosing. Clinicians may find that routine discussion of hepatitis B vaccination with all patients in the context of risk due to tattoo, sex, emergency medical care, and invasive procedures offers an environment for patients to initiate further discussion.

Health-care providers may also find that the medical industry and associated resources that are rapidly expanding in the developing world related to medical tourism intersect directly with the medical care options for patients with pre-existing illness who travel, emergency care for travelers, and health-care options for expatriates (see the Obtaining Health Care Abroad for the Ill Traveler section later in this chapter).

Additional Resources for Medical Tourism and Accredidation

- Joint Commission International (jointcommissioninternational.org/)
- Trent International Accreditation Scheme (trentaccreditationscheme.org/)
- Australian Council for Healthcare Standards International (www.achs.org.au/ACHSI/)
- Canadian Council on Health Services (www.cchsa.ca/)
- International Society of Plastic Surgery also certifies international surgeons who meet U.S. standards (www.isaps.org)

References

1. U.S. Department of Commerce. Office of Travel and Tourism Industries survey of international air travelers US to overseas and Mexico 2006 report, 2006 January–December. 2007.

2. U.S. Department of Commerce. Office of Travel and Tourism Industries survey of international air travelers US to overseas and Mexico by birth and citizenship. 2004 report, 2004 January–December. 2005.

3. U.S. Department of Commerce. Office of Travel and Tourism Industries survey of international air travelers US to overseas and Mexico 2005 report, 2005 January–December. 2006.

4. U.S. Department of Commerce. Office of Travel and Tourism Industries survey of international air travelers US to overseas and Mexico by birth and citizenship. 2003 report, 2003 January–December. 2005.

5. Reed CM. The health-seeking traveler. In: Keystone JS, Kozarsky PE, Freedman DO, Nothdurft HD, Connor BA, editors. Travel medicine. 2nd ed. Philadelphia: Mosby; 2008. p. 343–50.

6. Merrell RC, Boucher D, Carabello L, et al. Medical tourism. Telemed J E Health. 2008;14(1):14–20.

7. Wapner J. American Medical Association provides guidance on medical tourism. BMJ. 2008;337:a575.

8. Furuya EY, Paez A, Srinivasan A, et al. Outbreak of *Mycobacterium abscessus* wound infections among "lipotourists" from the United States who underwent abdominoplasty in the Dominican Republic. Clin Infect Dis. 2008;46(8):1181–8.

9. Oleksyn V. Top transplant surgeons involved in organ trafficking, expert says. The Associated Press [updated 2008 Feb 14]. Available from: http://www.bookrags.com/news/top-transplant-surgeons-involved-in-moc/

10. U.S. Health Resources and Services Administration, Healthcare Systems Bureau, Division of Transplantation. 2007 Annual Report of the U.S. Organ Procurement and Transplantation Network and the Scientific Registry of Transplant Recipients: Transplant Data 1997–2006. Rockville (MD): 2007. [cited 2008 Jul 22]. Available from: http://www.ustransplant.org/annual_reports/current/

11. Bishop R, Litch JA. Medical tourism can do harm. BMJ. 2000;320(7240):1017.

12. O'Leary A. Working vacation. Yale Alumni Magazine. 2008;71(5) [cited 2008 Oct 13]. Available from: http://www.yalealumnimagazine.com/issues/2008_05/ notebook.html.

13. U.S. Department of Commerce. Office of Travel and Tourism Industries survey of international air travelers US to overseas and Mexico by birth and citizenship. 2004 report, 2004 January–December. 2005.

14. Merion RM, Barnes AD, Lin M, et al. Transplants in foreign countries among patients removed from the US transplant waiting list. Am J Transplant. 2008;8(4 Pt 2):988–96.

15. Harling R, Turbitt D, Millar M, et al. Passage from India: an outbreak of hepatitis B linked to a patient who acquired infection from health care overseas. Public Health. 2007;121(10):734–41.

Perspectives: Counterfeit Drugs

Michael D. Green

GENERAL INFORMATION

Counterfeit and substandard drugs are an international problem contributing to morbidity, mortality, toxicity, and drug resistance. A counterfeit medicine is a compound that is not made by an authorized manufacturer but is presented to the consumer as if it were. Overall, global estimates of drug counterfeiting are somewhat ambiguous, depending on geographic region, but proportions range from 1% of sales in developed countries to >10% in developing countries. In specific regions in Africa, Asia, and Latin America, chances of purchasing a counterfeit drug may be higher than 30%. Although the availability of fake drugs is a worldwide occurrence, developing countries lacking adequate resources to effectively monitor and maintain good drug quality are most susceptible. These conditions allow for the proliferation of counterfeit as well as substandard medicines.

Since counterfeit drugs are not made by the legitimate manufacturer and are produced under unlawful circumstances, contaminants or lack of proper ingredients may result in serious harm to one's health. For example, the active pharmaceutical ingredient (API) may be completely lacking, present in small quantities, or substituted by another less-effective compound. In addition, the wrong inactive ingredients (excipients) can contribute to poor drug dissolution and bioavailability. As a result, a patient may not respond to treatment, or they may exhibit adverse reactions to unknown substituted ingredients.

Prior to international departure, travel clinics should alert travelers of the dangers of counterfeit and substandard drugs and provide suggestions on how to avoid them. Listed are main points of which to be aware.

HOW TO AVOID COUNTERFEIT DRUGS WHEN TRAVELING

The best way to avoid counterfeit drugs is to reduce the need to purchase medications abroad. Anticipated amounts of medications for chronic conditions such as hypertension, sinusitis, arthritis, hay fever, etc., medications for gastroenteritis (travelers' diarrhea), and prophylactic medications for infectious diseases such as malaria (depending on the destinations) should all be purchased at home prior to traveling.

To do before you leave:

- **Make sure you have all your vaccinations before embarking.** Immunizations provide the best protection against many serious diseases.
- **Purchase in advance, in your home country, all the medicines you will need for the entire trip.** Prescriptions from your doctor usually cannot be filled overseas, and over-the-counter medicines may not be available in many foreign countries. Checked baggage can get lost; therefore pack as much as possible in a carry-on bag. Bring along extra in case of travel delays.
- **Make sure your medicines are in their original containers.** If the drug is a prescription, make sure your name and dosage requirements are on the container.
- **Bring your "Patient Prescription Information" sheet.** This sheet provides information on common generic and brand names, usage, side effects, precautions, and drug interactions.

What to do if you run out and require additional medications:

- **Purchase medicines from a legitimate pharmacy.** In some places, it is difficult to know if a pharmacy has a genuine license. Your chances of receiving a counterfeit drug are less if you avoid buying from open markets, street vendors, or suspicious-looking pharmacies. Request a receipt when making the purchase. The U.S. Embassy may be able to assist you in finding a legitimate pharmacy in the area.
- **Do not buy medicines that are significantly cheaper than the typical price.** Although generics are usually less expensive, many counterfeited brand names are sold at prices significantly below the normal price for that particular brand.
- **Make sure the medicines you purchase are in their original packages or containers.** Many times medicines are sold to the pharmacy in bulk and the pharmacist will dispense the required amount of medicine into another container. If you receive medicines as loose tablets or capsules supplied in a plastic bag or envelope, ask the pharmacist to see the container from which it was originally dispensed. Record the brand, batch number, and expiration date. Sometimes a wary consumer will prompt the seller into making sure he or she supplies you with quality medicine.
- **Be familiar with your medications.** The size, shape, color, and taste of counterfeit medicines may be different from the authentic. Discoloration, splits, cracks, spots, and stickiness of the tablets or capsules are indications of a possible counterfeit. Keep examples of authentic medications available for comparison if you purchase the same brand.
- **Be familiar with the packaging.** Different color inks, poor-quality print or packaging material, and misspelled words are clues to counterfeit material. Also, keep an example of packaging for comparison. Observe the expiration date to make sure the medicine has not expired and the package contains the drug insert.

USEFUL WEBSITES ON COUNTERFEITS

- General Information:
  - CDC:
    - wwwn.cdc.gov/travel/contentCounterfeitDrugs.aspx
    - www.cdc.gov/malaria/travel/counterfeit_drugs.htm
  - World Health Organization: who.int/mediacentre/factsheets/fs275/en

- U.S. Food and Drug Administration: www.fda.gov/counterfeit/
- U.S. Pharmacopeia: www.usp.org/worldwide/dqi/drugQuality.html
- Warnings and alerts: www.safemedicines.org/in_the_news/drug_alerts.php
- What can you pack in your luggage (for travelers with disabilities and medical conditions):
  - Transportation Security Administration: www.tsa.gov/travelers/airtravel/specialneeds/editorial_1059.shtm
- What can you bring back:
  - U.S. Customs and Border Protection: www.cbp.gov/xp/cgov/travel/clearing/restricted/medication_drugs.xml
- Reporting counterfeit cases: www.who.int/medicines/services/counterfeit/report/en/

REFERENCES

1. Newton PN, Green MD, Fernández FM, et al. Counterfeit anti-infective drugs. Lancet Infect Dis. 2006;6(9):602–13.

2. World Health Organization. Counterfeit medicines. Fact sheet no. 275. Nov. 2006 [updated 2006 Nov 14; cited 2008 Jun 6]. Available from: http://who.int/mediacentre/factsheets/fs275/en.

3. Newton PN, Fernandez FM, Green MD. Counterfeit and substandard antimalarial drugs. In: Schlagenhauf-Lawlor P, editor. Travelers' malaria. 2nd ed. Hamilton (Canada): BC Decker, Inc.: 2008. p. 331–42.

DRUG–VACCINE AND DRUG–DRUG INTERACTIONS

Elizabeth D. Barnett

The pre-travel travel medicine visit potentially exposes people to a number of different vaccines, prophylactic medications, and therapeutic drugs. In addition, the traveler may already be taking one or more medications on a regular basis. Travel medicine practitioners need to think about the possible interactions between all these products. Although a comprehensive list of interactions is beyond the scope of this section, some of the more significant interactions of commonly used vaccines and medications are discussed here.

Interactions between Travel Vaccines and Drugs

Oral Typhoid Vaccine

There is a concern that antibiotics or anti-malarials with antibiotic activity should not be taken at the same time as the oral typhoid vaccine (a live-bacteria vaccine) as they may be active against the vaccine strain and prevent an adequate immune response to the vaccine. These issues should be addressed separately.

Sulfonamides and antibiotics taken orally should not be taken at the same time as oral typhoid vaccine. Parenteral typhoid vaccine is a more appropriate choice for individuals taking antibiotics.

The current mefloquine (Lariam) product insert recommends vaccinations with attenuated live bacteria be completed at least 3 days before the first dose of Lariam. However, one study in humans failed to show any decrease in immunogenicity when the vaccine was given to those on mefloquine prophylaxis. Mefloquine can be given concurrently with the oral typhoid vaccine. Although the antibody response to oral typhoid vaccine was reduced by higher dose proguanil in one study examining the effects of concomitant use of oral typhoid vaccine and chloroquine, mefloquine, and proguanil, a second study using approved prophylaxis doses of atovaquone–proguanil showed no decrease in immunogenicity. Atovaquone–proguanil at prophylaxis doses can be given concurrently with the oral typhoid vaccine. However, since the oral typhoid vaccine should be completed 14 days prior to traveling, there should be no opportunity for concomitant administration with atovaquone/proguanil in most travelers. This same study also showed no decrease in immunogenicity with chloroquine. Chloroquine can be given concurrently with the oral typhoid vaccine.

Doxycycline is an antibiotic with both antibacterial and antimalarial activity. Thus it should not be given concurrently with oral typhoid vaccine. However, since the oral typhoid vaccine should be completed 14 days prior to traveling, there should be no opportunity for interaction with doxycycline in most travelers.

Rabies Vaccine

Concomitant use of chloroquine may reduce antibody response to intradermal rabies vaccine administered for pre-exposure prophylaxis. The intramuscular route should be used for persons taking chloroquine concurrently (the intradermal route is currently not approved for use in the United States); ideally, the rabies pre-exposure prophylaxis series should be completed before beginning chloroquine.

Corticosteroids and other immunosuppressive agents may interfere with response to rabies immunization; when these are used concurrently with rabies vaccine for postexposure prophylaxis, testing should be done to ensure adequate antibody response.

Interactions between Antimalarials and Other Drugs

Mefloquine

Mefloquine may interact with several categories of drugs, including other antimalarials, drugs that alter cardiac conduction, and anticonvulsants. Although the antimalarial halofantrine is not available in the United States, potentially fatal prolongation of the QTc interval of the electrocardiogram may occur if halofantrine is given after mefloquine. Halofantrine should not be given with or after mefloquine. If halofantrine is given for treatment of malaria, mefloquine for prophylaxis should not be resumed until at least 12 hours after the last halofantrine dose. However, no conclusive data are available with regard to coadministration of mefloquine and other drugs that may theoretically have an impact on cardiac conduction. These include anti-arrhythmic or beta-blocking agents, calcium-channel blockers, antihistamines, H1-blocking agents, tricyclic antidepressant, or phenothiazines. Use of these drugs along with mefloquine should be avoided, if possible.

Mefloquine used with the anticonvulsants valproic acid, carbamazepine, phenobarbital, or phenytoin may lower anticonvulsant plasma levels, thus lowering seizure threshold. Monitoring anticonvulsant levels would be appropriate in persons for whom mefloquine must be used concomitantly with these drugs.

Chloroquine

Chloroquine absorption may be reduced by antacids or kaolin; at least 4 hours should elapse between doses of these medications. Concomitant use of cimetidine and chloroquine should be avoided, as cimetidine can inhibit the metabolism of chloroquine and may increase drug levels. Chloroquine inhibits bioavailability of ampicillin; 2 hours should elapse between doses.

Atovaquone–Proguanil

Tetracycline, rifampin, and rifabutin may reduce plasma concentrations of atovaquone and should not be used concurrently with atovaquone–proguanil. Metaclopramide may reduce bioavailability of atovaquone; unless no other antiemetics are available, this antiemetic should not be used for treatment of the vomiting that may accompany use of atovaquone at treatment doses. Atovaquone–proguanil should not be used with other proguanil-containing medications. Patients on anticoagulants may need to reduce their anticoagulant doses or more closely monitor their prothrombin time while taking atovaquone proguanil.

Doxycycline

Doxycycline use theoretically may lead to decreased efficacy of oral contraceptives, although it has been difficult to quantify this effect in a way that is useful for counseling travelers. Changes in hormone levels in women taking oral contraceptives concurrently with doxycycline have not been demonstrated. Phenytoin, carbamazepine, and barbiturates may decrease the half-life of doxycycline. Patients on anticoagulants may need to reduce their anticoagulant doses while taking doxycycline because of its ability to depress plasma prothrombin activity. Absorption of tetracyclines may be impaired by bismuth subsalicyclate, iron-containing preparations, and antacids containing calcium, magnesium, or aluminum; these preparations should not be taken within 1–3 hours of doxycycline. Doxycycline absorption is not markedly affected by food or milk taken concurrently. Doxycyline may interfere with the bactericidal activity of penicillin, and these drugs should not be taken concurrently.

Interactions with Antidiarrheal Drugs

Fluoroquinolones

Increase in the international normalized ratio (INR) has been reported when levofloxacin and warfarin are used concurrently. Concurrent administration of ciprofloxacin and magnesium or aluminum hydroxide containing antacids may reduce bioavailability of ciprofloxacin significantly. Ciprofloxacin decreases clearance of theophylline and caffeine; theophylline levels should be monitored when ciprofloxacin is used concurrently. Ciprofloxacin should not be used with tazanidine.

Azithromycin

Close monitoring for side effects of azithromycin is recommended when azithromycin is used with nelfinavir. Increased anticoagulant effects have been noted when azithromycin is used with warfarin; monitoring of prothrombin time is recommended for such individuals.

Rifaximin

No clinically significant drug interactions have been reported to date with rifaximin. Although the drug induces cytochrome P450 3A4 (CYP3A4), studies of concurrent administration of rifaximin with midazolam and with a single dose of the oral contraceptive ethinyl etradiol and norestironate did not show changes in the pharmacokinetics of these drugs.

Interactions with Drugs Used for Travel to High Altitude

Acetazolamide

Acetazolamide produces alkaline urine that can increase the rate of excretion of barbiturates and salicylates and may potentiate salicylate toxicity. Decreased excretion of dextroamphetamine, anticholinergics, mecamylamine, ephedrine, mexiletine, or quinide may also occur. Hypokalemia caused by corticosteroids may be potentiated by concurrent use of acetazolamide.

Dexamethasone

Dexamethasone interacts with multiple classes of drugs. Use of this drug for treatment of altitude illness may, however, be lifesaving. Interactions may occur with the following drugs and drug classes: macrolide antibiotics, anticholinesterases, anticoagulants, hypoglycemic agents, isoniazid, digitalis preparations, oral contraceptives, and phenytoin.

References

1. Kollaritsch H, Que JU, Kunz C, et al. Safety and immunogenicity of live oral cholera and typhoid vaccines administered alone or in combination with antimalarial drugs, oral polio vaccine, or yellow fever vaccine. J Infect Dis. 1997;175(4):871–5.

2. Horowitz H, Carbonaro CA. Inhibition of the Salmonella Typhi oral vaccine strain, Ty21a, by mefloquine and chloroquine. J Infect Dis. 1992;166(6):1462–4.

3. Brachman PS Jr, Metchock B, Kozarsky PE. Effects of antimalarial chemoprophylactic agents on the viability of the Ty21a vaccine strain. Clin Infect Dis. 1992;15(6):1057–8.

4. Pappaioanou M, Fishbein DB, Dreesen DW, et al. Antibody response to preexposure human diploid-cell rabies vaccine given concurrently with chloroquine. N Engl J Med. 1986;314(5):280–4.

5. Matson PA, Luby SP, Redd SC, et al. Cardiac effects of standard-dose halofantrine therapy. Am J Trop Med Hyg. 1996;54(3):229–31.

6. CDC. Sudden death in a traveler following halofantrine administration—Togo, 2000. MMWR Morb Mortal Wkly Rep. 2001;50(9):169–70, 179.

7. Neely JL, Abate M, Swinker M, et al. The effect of doxycycline on serum levels of ethinyl estradiol, norethindrone, and endogenous progesterone. Obstet Gynecol. 1991;77(3):416–20.

Perspectives: PPD Testing of Travelers

Philip LoBue

Screening travelers for asymptomatic tuberculosis (TB) infections should only be carried out among travelers who will be at significant risk of acquiring TB (see the TB section in Chapter 5). Screening with a tuberculin skin test (TST) in a very low-risk population may result in a false-positive test, leading to unnecessary further screening or unnecessary therapeutic treatment. Using even highly sensitive and specific tests in very low-prevalence populations will produce more false positives than true positives.

Therefore, the TST should be considered only for travelers anticipating an extended stay over a period of years in a country with a high risk of TB or for those who could be expected to come in contact routinely with hospital, prison, or homeless shelter populations. The general recommendation is that persons at low risk for TB, which includes the vast majority of travelers, do not need to be screened before or after travel.

For travelers who anticipate a long stay or contact with a high-risk population, careful pre-travel screening should be carried out. The two-step TST is recommended in this population, for the following reasons:

■ The use of two-step testing can reduce the number of positive TSTs that would otherwise be misclassified as recent skin test conversions during future periodic screenings.

■ Certain persons who were infected with *Mycobacterium tuberculosis* years earlier exhibit waning delayed-type hypersensitivity to tuberculin. When they are skin tested years after infection, they might have a false-negative TST result (even though they are truly infected). However, this first skin test years after the infection might stimulate the ability to react to subsequent tests, resulting in a "booster" reaction. When the test is repeated, the reaction might be misinterpreted as a new infection (recent conversion) rather than a boosted reaction.

■ For two-step testing, persons whose baseline TSTs yield a negative result are retested 1–3 weeks after the initial test. If the second test result is negative, they are considered not infected. If the second test result is positive, they are classified as having had previous TB infection.

■ Two-step testing should be considered for the baseline testing of persons who report no history of a recent TST and who will receive repeated TSTs as part of an ongoing monitoring of whether they have been exposed to TB.

- If the two-step TST result is negative, the traveler should have a repeat TST 8–10 weeks after returning from their trip, or as part of a periodic screening examination for those who remain at high risk.

Two-step testing is particularly important for travelers who will have potential prolonged TB exposure; it is particularly important among those going to areas where drug resistance is very high. Two-step testing prior to travel will detect boosting and potentially prevent "false conversions"-positive TST results that appear to be indicative of infection acquired during travel, but which are really the result of previous TB infection. This is particularly important if the traveler is going to a country where XDR TB is rampant. It would be critical to know whether the person's skin test had actually been positive before the travel.

Persons having repeat TSTs must be tested with the same commercial antigen, as switching antigens can also lead to false TST conversions.

An alternative to two-step TST is a single FDA-approved interferon-gamma release assay (IGRA), such as the QuantiFERON TB test (Gold or Gold In-Tube versions). IGRAs are about equally specific as TST in non-BCG-vaccinated populations and much more specific in BCG-vaccinated populations. For a traveler whose time before departure is short, a single-step TST would be an acceptable alternative if there were insufficient time for the two-step TST and the IGRA were not available.

In general it is best not to mix tests. There is about 15% discordance between TST and IGRA, usually with the TST positive and the IGRA negative. There are multiple reasons for the discordance, and in any individual it is often difficult to be confident about the reason for discordance. However, if the health-care provider decides to mix tests, it is better to go from TST to IGRA than the other way around, because the likelihood of having a discordant result, with the TST negative and the IGRA positive, is much lower. Such discordant results may become unavoidable as more medical establishments switch from TSTs to IGRAs.

The use of TST among those visiting friends and relatives in TB-endemic areas should take into account the high rate of TST positivity in this population. In a study among 53,000 adults in Tennessee, the prevalence of a positive TST among the foreign born was 10 times that of the U.S. born (34.2% vs. 3.2%). Confirming TST status prior to travel would prevent the conclusion that a positive TST after travel was due to recent conversion.

REFERENCES

1. Leder K, Tong S, Weld L, et al. Illness in travelers visiting friends and relatives: a review of the GeoSentinel Surveillance Network. Clin Infect Dis. 2006;43(9):1185–93.

2. Jung P, Banks RH. Tuberculosis risk in US Peace Corps volunteers, 1996 to 2005. J Travel Med. 2008;15(2):87–94.

3. Cobelens FG, van Deutekom H, Draayer-Jansen IW, et al. Risk of infection with Mycobacterium tuberculosis in travellers to areas of high tuberculosis endemicity. Lancet 2000;356(9228):461–5.

4. Haley CA, Cain KP, Yu C, et al. Risk-based screening for latent tuberculosis infection. South Med J. 2008;101(2):142–9.

5. Al-Jahdali H, Memish ZA, Menzies D. Tuberculosis in association with travel. Int J Antimicrob Agents. 2003;21(2):125–30.

6. Johnston VJ, Grant AD. Tuberculosis in travellers. Travel Med Infect Dis. 2003;1(4):205–12.

TRAVEL HEALTH KITS

Amanda D. Whatley, Deborah Nicolls Barbeau

The purpose of packing a travel health jit is to ensure travelers have supplies they need to—

- manage pre-existing medical conditions and treat any exacerbations of these conditions,

- prevent illness related to traveling, and
- take care of minor health problems as they occur.

Traveling with Medications

When medications are necessary for travel, it is important to remember the following:

- **Original containers:** All medications should be carried in their original containers with clear labels, so the contents are easily identified. Although many travelers like placing medications into small containers or packing them in the daily-dose containers, officials at ports of entry may require proper identification of medications.
- **Prescriptions:** Travelers should carry copies of all prescriptions, including their generic names.
- **Physician notes:** For controlled substances and injectable medications, travelers are advised to carry a note from the prescribing physician on letterhead stationery.
- **Restricted medications:** Travelers should be aware that certain medications are not permitted in certain countries. If there is a question about these restrictions, particularly with controlled substances, travelers are recommended to contact the embassy or consulate of the destination country.
- **Availability:** A travel health kit is useful only when it is available. It should be carried with the traveler at all times (e.g., in a carry-on bag). Due to airline security rules, sharp objects and some liquids and gels must remain in checked luggage.

Pre-Existing Medical Condition Supplies

Travelers with pre-existing medical conditions are advised to carry enough medication for the duration of their trip and an extra supply, in case the trip is extended for any reason. If additional supplies or medications are needed for the management of exacerbations of existing medical conditions, these should be carried as well. The health-care provider managing a traveler's pre-existing medical conditions should be consulted for the best plan of action (see the section Traveling with Chronic Medical Illnesses in Chapter 8).

Persons with pre-existing conditions, such as diabetes or allergies to envenomations or medications, should consider wearing an alert bracelet and making sure this information is on a card in their wallet and with their other travel documents.

General Travel Health Kit Supplies

A variety of health kits is available commercially and may even be purchased over the Internet (see below); however, similar kits can be assembled at home, often at lower cost. The specific contents of the health kit are based on destination, duration of travel, type of travel, and the traveler's pre-existing medical conditions.

Although this is not a comprehensive list, basic items that should be considered are listed below. See Chapters 7 and 8 for additional suggestions that may be useful in planning the contents of a kit for travelers with specific needs.

Medications

- Destination-related, if applicable:
  - Antimalarial medications
  - Medication to prevent or treat high-altitude illness
- Pain or fever (one or more of the following, or an alternative):
  - Acetaminophen
  - Aspirin
  - Ibuprofen
- Stomach upset or diarrhea:
  - Over-the-counter antidiarrheal medication (such as loperamide or bismuth subsalicylate)

- ○ Antibiotic for self-treatment of moderate to severe diarrhea
- ○ Oral rehydration solution packets
- ○ Mild laxative
- ○ Antacid
- Items to treat throat and respiratory symptoms:
  - ○ Antihistamine
  - ○ Decongestant, alone or in combination with antihistamine
  - ○ Cough suppressant/expectorant
  - ○ Throat lozenges
- Anti-motion sickness medication.
- Epinephrine auto-injector (such as an EpiPen), especially if history of severe allergic reaction. Smaller-dose packages are available for children.
- Any medications, prescription or over the counter, taken on a regular basis at home.

Basic First Aid

- Disposable gloves (at least two pairs)
- Adhesive bandages, multiple sizes
- Gauze
- Adhesive tape
- Elastic bandage wrap for sprains and strains
- Antiseptic
- Cotton swabs
- Tweezers*
- Scissors*
- Antifungal and antibacterial ointments or creams
- 1% hydrocortisone cream
- Anti-itch gel or cream for insect bites and stings
- Aloe gel for sunburns
- Moleskin or molefoam for blisters
- Digital thermometer
- Saline eye drops
- First-aid quick reference card

Other Important Items

- Insect repellent
- Sunscreen (SPF 15 or greater)
- Antibacterial hand wipes or an alcohol-based hand sanitizer containing at least 60% alcohol
- Useful items in certain circumstances:
  - ○ Extra pair of contacts or prescription glasses, or both, for people who wear corrective lenses
  - ○ Mild sedative (such as zolpidem), other sleep aid, or anti-anxiety medication
  - ○ Latex condoms
  - ○ Water purification tablets
  - ○ Commercial suture/syringe kits to be used by a local health-care provider. (These items will also require a letter from the prescribing physician on letterhead stationery.)

*Note: Pack these items in checked baggage, since they may be considered sharp objects and confiscated by airport or airline security if packed in carry-on bags.

Contact Card

It is also important for travelers to locate and record important contact information, in case it is needed during their trip. Often this information is needed quickly; having a contact card with the following items will help save time in these urgent situations.

Items to include on a contact card should be the address and phone numbers of the following:

- Family member or close contact still in the United States
- Health-care provider at home
- Area hospitals or clinics
- U.S. Embassy or Consulate in the destination country or countries

See the next section in this chapter, Obtaining Health Care Abroad for the Ill Traveler, for information about how to locate local health care and embassy/consulate contacts.

Commercial Medical Kits

Commercial medical kits are available for a wide range of circumstances, from basic first aid to advanced emergency life support. Many pharmacy, grocery, retail, and outdoor sporting goods stores sell their own basic first-aid kits. Travelers who choose to purchase a health kit rather than assemble their own should be certain to review the contents of the kit carefully to ensure that it has everything needed; additional items may be necessary.

For more adventurous travelers, a number of companies produce advanced medical kits and will even customize kits based on specific travel needs.

In addition, specialty kits are available for managing diabetes, dealing with dental emergencies, and handling aquatic environments.

Below is a list of websites supplying a wide range of medical kits. There are many suppliers, and this list is not meant to be all-inclusive.

- American Red Cross: www.redcrossstore.org
- Adventure Medical Kits: www.adventuremedicalkits.com
- Chinook Medical Gear: www.chinookmed.com
- Travel Medicine, Inc.: www.travmed.com
- Wilderness Medicine Outfitters: www.wildernessmedicine.com

References

1. Weiss EA, Franco-Paredes C. Travel health and medical kits. In: Keystone JS, Kozarsky PE, Freedman DO, Nothdurft HD, Connor BA, editors. Travel medicine. 2nd ed. Philadelphia: Mosby; 2008. p. 69–74.

2. Reynolds SA, Levy F, Walker ES. Hand sanitizer alert. Emerg Infect Dis. 2006;12(3):527–9.

OBTAINING HEALTH CARE ABROAD FOR THE ILL TRAVELER

Theresa Sommers, Gary W. Brunette

An important aspect of preparing for a trip abroad is to consider the possibility of becoming sick or injured during travel. The following resources and information will be useful to travelers, should they require medical assistance abroad.

Traveling While Ill

Health-care providers should advise their patients about the possible need to avoid traveling if they become ill during their trip. Those with certain health conditions may need to postpone their travel arrangements, including air and public ground transportation. In general, travelers who are ill with a communicable disease that is spread easily to other people should discuss the need for rescheduling travel with their provider.

Travelers should be aware that some airlines check for visibly sick passengers in the waiting area and during boarding. If a waiting passenger looks visibly ill, the airline may prohibit that person from getting on the airplane.

Locating a Health-Care Provider

Several resources are available to American citizens who require medical attention during their travels. The following resources can assist travelers in finding adequate care:

- The U.S. Department of State:
  - A U.S. consular officer can assist in locating appropriate medical services, as well as in notifying friends, family, or employer of an emergency.
  - For more information, see http://travel.state.gov/travel/tips/brochures/brochures_1215.html.
- The International Society of Travel Medicine (ISTM):
  - ISTM maintains a directory of health-care professionals with expertise in travel medicine in almost 50 countries worldwide.
  - To access the directory, see www.istm.org.
- The American Society of Tropical Medicine and Hygiene (ASTMH):
  - ASTMH maintains a worldwide directory of providers specializing in tropical medicine, medical parasitology, and travelers' health.
  - To access the directory, see www.astmh.org.
- International Association for Medical Assistance to Travelers (IAMAT):
  - IAMAT maintains an international network of physicians, hospitals, and clinics who have agreed to treat IAMAT members in need of medical care while abroad.
  - Membership is free, although a donation to support IAMAT efforts is suggested. Members receive a directory of participating physicians and medical centers and have access to a variety of travel-related informational brochures.
  - For more information, see www.iamat.org.
- Travel Health Online:
  - This resource maintains a list of travel medicine providers worldwide. Information is obtained from a variety of sources, so the quality of services and the expertise of the providers cannot be guaranteed.
  - For more information, see https://www.tripprep.com.

Travelers may also get information about local health care from embassies and consulates of other countries, hotel doctors, credit card companies, and multinational corporations, which may offer health-care services for their employees. In addition, travelers who obtain evacuation insurance before travel will have access to a 24-hour hotline for help in any medical emergency.

Accreditation of International Health-Care Facilities

The quality of health care from foreign medical centers can be variable, particularly in developing countries. To ensure a higher quality of care abroad, Joint Commission International attempts to continuously improve the safety and quality of care in the international community through the provision of education and consultation services and international accreditation.

A list of accredited international health-care facilities is available at the Joint Commission International website (www.jointcommissioninternational.org).

Drugs/Pharmaceuticals Abroad

The quality of drugs and medical products abroad cannot be guaranteed, as they may not meet U.S. standards or could be counterfeit (see *Perspectives:* Counterfeit Drugs earlier in this chapter). Travelers are advised to—

- Bring with them all the drugs and medicines that they think they will need, including pain relievers, antidiarrheal medication, and, if applicable, antimalarials.
- Exercise caution when buying medications (especially those that do not require a prescription). In many developing countries, virtually any drug can be purchased without prescription.
- Travelers who may require an injection(s) abroad should bring their own injection supplies (see the Travel Health Kits section earlier in this chapter).
- Travelers who do not have their own injection supplies yet require an injection should ask if the equipment is disposable and insist that a new needle and syringe be used.

Emergency Care Abroad

The quality and availability of proper emergency medical care abroad may be variable and, in situations requiring a blood transfusion, the safety of blood products often cannot be guaranteed.

- Not all countries have accurate, reliable, and systematic screening of blood donations for infectious agents, which increases the risk of transfusion-related transmission of disease.
- The 2001–2002 WHO Global Database on Blood Safety report supports this view:
  - 40 countries reported they did not test all donated blood for HIV, hepatitis B and C viruses, and syphilis.
  - 39 countries reported that, due to unavailable testing supplies, blood was released for clinical use without testing for transfusion-transmissible infections.
- Due to this increased risk, travelers in developing countries should only receive a blood transfusion in life-and-death situations for which there may be no other options.
- When a situation requires blood transfusion, travelers should make every effort to ensure that the blood has been screened for transmissible diseases, including HIV.
- All travelers should consider being immunized against hepatitis B virus before their trip, especially—
  - Those who travel frequently to developing countries
  - Travelers whose itinerary indicate spending a prolonged period of time in developing countries
  - Travelers whose activities put them at higher risk for serious injury (e.g., adventure travel).
- There are no medical indications for travelers to take blood with them from their home countries.
- The limited storage period of blood and the need for special equipment negate the feasibility of independent blood banking for individual travelers or small groups. The international shipment of blood for transfusion is practical only when handled by agreement between two responsible organizations, such as national blood transfusion services. This mechanism is not useful for the emergency needs of individual travelers and should not be attempted by private travelers or organizations not operating recognized blood programs.

References

1. World Health Organization. Global database on blood safety report 2001–2002. Available from: http://www.who.int/bloodsafety/GDBS_Report_2001-2002.pdf. Geneva: World Health Organization [cited 2008 Jun 30].
2. Kolars JC. Rules of the road: a consumer's guide for travelers seeking health care in foreign lands. J Travel Med. 2002;9(4):198–201.
3. Joint Commission International. c2002–08 [cited 2008 Jun 30]. Available from: http://www.jointcommissioninternational.org.

TRAVEL INSURANCE AND EVACUATION INSURANCE

Theresa Sommers, Gary W. Brunette

It is important for travelers to consider the financial consequences of a severe illness or injury abroad. A growing number of people do not have health insurance at home. Those who do need to check their policies to determine if their care abroad will be covered and what limitations may apply. Those who have adequate health insurance may not be covered for medical evacuation from a resource-poor area to a hospital where definitive care can be obtained. Even if they have a policy that would reimburse evacuation costs, the health insurance company may not have the resources to help organize the evacuation. Evacuation-only policies are available to fill this gap. Evacuation by air ambulance can cost $50,000 to $100,000 and must be paid in advance by those who do not have insurance.

Paying for Health Services Abroad

Travelers who receive medical care in other countries will usually be required to pay in cash or with a credit card at the point of service, even if they have insurance coverage abroad. This could result in a large out-of-pocket expenditure of perhaps thousands of dollars for medical care.

- Travelers with health insurance coverage should be sure to obtain copies of all bills and receipts from overseas medical care.
- The U.S. consular office can assist travelers who are U.S. citizens with transferring funds from the United States.
- In extreme circumstances, the U.S. consular office may be able to approve small government loans until private funds are available.
- Medical evacuation insurance may only cover the cost to the nearest destination where definitive care can be obtained. Some policies will cover eventual repatriation to one's home country. The traveler should be sure to understand what coverage is purchased.

Health Insurance Abroad

- Some health insurance carriers in the United States may provide coverage for emergencies that occur while traveling.
- The first step for travelers is to examine their present coverage and planned itinerary. Determine exactly which medical services will be covered abroad and what supplemental insurance you will need. Things to look for include—
  - Exclusions for treatment of exacerbations of pre-existing medical conditions
  - The company's policy for "out-of-network" services
  - Coverage for complications of pregnancy
  - Exclusions for high-risk activities such as skydiving, scuba diving, and mountain climbing
  - Exclusions regarding psychiatric emergencies or injuries related to terrorist attacks or acts of war
  - Whether pre-authorization is needed for treatment, hospital admission, or other services
  - Whether a second opinion is required before obtaining emergency treatment
- Medicare and Medicaid will not cover services outside the United States, except in very limited circumstances.

Travel Health and Medical Evacuation Insurance

Travelers need to evaluate their existing health insurance policies to see whether they already have adequate coverage. Short-term supplemental policies that cover health-care costs on a trip can be purchased. Evacuation coverage can be sold separately or in conjunction with overseas health insurance. Evacuation companies often have better resources and experience in some parts of the world than others. Travelers may want to check with them about their resources in a given area before making a purchase. In general, travelers should purchase a policy that provides the following:

- Arrangements with hospitals to guarantee payments directly. Travelers may want to check on this possibility for the planned itinerary.
- Assistance via a 24-hour physician-backed support center. This is critical if the traveler is going to pay for evacuation insurance.
- Emergency medical transport, including repatriation. Medical evacuation can be costly, ranging from a few thousand dollars to over $100,000.

While travel health and medical evacuation insurance is a consideration for all travelers, it is particularly important for travelers who—

- Will be outside the United States for an extended period of time.
- Have underlying illnesses. These travelers should make certain that complications of the underlying condition will be covered by the chosen policy.
- Participate in activities involving greater risk for injury.

Finding a Travel Health and Medical Evacuation Insurance Provider

The following list, while not all-inclusive, gives a sample of resources for travelers seeking to purchase travel health and medical evacuation insurance:

- U.S. Department of State (www.travel.state.gov)
- International SOS (www.internationalsos.com)
- MEDEX (www.medexassist.com)
- International Association for Medical Assistance to Travelers (www.iamat.org)

Special Considerations for Travelers with Underlying Medical Conditions

Travelers with underlying medical conditions may want to take extra precautions in preparing for travel.

- Travelers should choose a medical assistance company that allows customers to store their medical history before departure, so it can be accessed from anywhere in the world, if needed.
- Travelers should carry a letter from their physician listing underlying medical conditions and all current medications (including their generic names).
- If possible, travelers may want to carry with them the name of their medical condition and medications written in the local language(s) of the areas they plan to visit.

Special Considerations for Medicare/Medicaid Beneficiaries

- The Social Security Medicare program does not provide coverage for medical costs outside the United States, except under very limited circumstances.

- Medicare beneficiaries can purchase supplemental travel health insurance to cover medical expenses outside of the United States.
- Some Medigap plans available to people enrolled in the original Medicare plan provide limited coverage for emergency care abroad.
- As with all travelers, Medicare beneficiaries should examine their present coverage carefully to know exactly what will be covered abroad and supplement with additional travel health insurance as appropriate.

References

1. U.S. Department of State. Medical information for Americans abroad. [cited 2008 Jun 30] Available from: http://travel.state.gov/travel/tips/brochures/brochures_1215.html.
2. Centers for Medicare and Medicaid Services.

Medicare coverage outside the United States. [cited 2008 Jun 30] Available from: http://www.medicare.gov/Publications/Pubs/pdf/11037.pdf.

MENTAL HEALTH AND TRAVEL

Victor Balaban

Description

Travel is undertaken for a number of reasons, such as adventure, pleasure, business, or personal growth. While most travelers complete their journeys with a manageable amount of stress, foreign travel can produce a wide range of psychiatric, behavioral, and neurologic issues in travelers. Any journey can produce challenges, but longer journeys to more remote and strange environments can increase the psychological stresses for travelers.

Risk Factors

Risk factors that have been identified for developing psychiatric and neurologic problems during and after travel include—

- Pre-existing psychiatric issues: Stress can trigger or exacerbate psychiatric reactions in travelers with pre-existing psychiatric or behavioral conditions.
- Side effects of mefloquine or other drugs:
  - People with underlying psychiatric disorders should not receive the antimalarial medication mefloquine. The neuropsychiatric side effects associated with mefloquine may become pronounced in these patients.
  - The neuropsychiatric side effects associated with mefloquine may also be compounded when administered concurrently with the antiretroviral medication efavirenz, which also carries the risk of neurologic toxicity.
  - Elderly travelers and travelers with memory or cognitive deficits may be more prone to develop delirium in flight, particularly when combined with dehydration, alcohol, or the use of sleep aids such as zolpidem.
  - The use of recreational drugs has also been found to be a trigger for psychiatric symptoms in travelers.
- Stressful events during travel, such as loneliness, a feeling of loss of control, financial difficulties, or a traumatic event such as a serious illness or viewing disturbing sights, can have behavioral and psychosocial consequences for travelers.

Occurrence and Risk for Travelers

Data are limited on the prevalence of travel-related psychiatric and neurologic disorders:

- A study of Israeli long-term travelers to Southeast Asia found that 11.3% reported psychiatric or neurologic symptoms during travel. The most common symptoms were sleep disturbances, fatigue, and dizziness. The majority of symptoms were short-lived and transient, but 2.5% of travelers reported severe psychiatric or neurologic symptoms, and 1.2% had symptoms lasting more than 2 months.
- A study of urgent repatriation of British diplomats found that 41% of evacuations for nonphysical causes were due to depression.
- Adventure travelers in extreme settings, such as polar expeditions, have been found to undergo psychiatric changes, including disturbed sleep, impaired cognitive ability, negative affect, and interpersonal tension and conflict; approximately 5% have been found to meet the Diagnostic and Statistical Manual of Mental Disorders (DSM-IV) or the International Classification of Diseases (ICD) criteria for psychiatric disorders (including substance-related and sleep disorders).

Pre-Travel Mental Health Evaluation

Pre-travel screening should assess risk factors that might indicate a need for a traveler to be referred to a mental health professional for evaluation, especially prior to travel that is likely to be stressful. Factors that should be assessed include—

- pre-existing psychiatric diagnoses, such as depression or anxiety disorders
- history of psychosis in the traveler or a close family member
- history of suicide attempts
- evidence of depressed mood at assessment
- exposure to prior traumas (e.g., disasters, severe injury, abuse, assault, etc.), particularly prior to travel that could involve re-exposure to traumatic events or situations
- recent major life stressors or emotional strain
- use of medications that may have psychiatric or neurologic side effects
- pre-travel anxieties and phobias that are severe enough to interfere with a patients' ability to function or to prepare for and enjoy their travel.

Long-term travelers, aid workers, military personnel and other travelers likely to be exposed to stressful situations should be advised that the stresses and challenges they may face, particularly if combined with long hours of work, lack of sleep, or fatigue, can contribute to stress and anxiety. Long-term travelers should be encouraged to—

- learn how to recognize signs of stress, exhaustion, depression, and anxiety in themselves;
- take care of themselves physically by eating and exercising regularly; and
- use their full allotment of time off or annual leave, particularly if they recognize signs of stress or exhaustion in themselves.

During Travel

Severe mental illness occurring abroad can be extremely stressful for travelers, their families, and those who try to care for them. Acute psychosis leading to disruptive behavior can land a traveler in jail in a developing country. Inpatient psychiatric facilities may be either nonexistent or completely inadequate for a foreigner. It can be very difficult to repatriate a psychotic person until the symptoms have been brought under control with medication. Someone will most often have to accompany the person home. Many evacuation insurance plans specifically exclude psychiatric illness from their coverage.

Post-Travel Mental Health Evaluation

Returning travelers may have experienced physical illnesses, personal difficulties, or traumas that could result in psychiatric reactions. Travel-related injuries and diseases that affect quality of life can also have profound and long-term psychiatric impacts. Even in the absence of trauma, some returning long-term travelers report experiencing "reverse culture shock" after their return, characterized by feelings of disorientation, unfamiliarity, and loss of confidence. Approximately 36% of aid workers report depression shortly after returning home, and as many as 60% of returned aid workers have reported feeling predominantly negative emotions on returning home, even though many reported that their time overseas was positive and fulfilling.

Post-travel evaluations should assess—

- Behavioral and psychiatric symptoms, including:
  - Experiences during or soon after travel, which have been painful, hard to reconcile or which still cause distress, anxiety, or avoidance.
  - Persistent sleep disturbance or unusual fatigue.
  - Excessive use of alcohol or drugs.
  - Behavioral or interpersonal difficulties in home, school, work, in friendships or relationships.
- Somatic symptoms that can also be indications of distress, including:
  - Unexplained somatic symptoms, such as headaches, backaches, or abdominal pain; and somatic disorders such as fibromyalgia, chronic fatigue syndrome, temporomandibular disorder, and irritable bowel syndrome.
  - Rashes, itching, and skin diseases, such as psoriasis, atopic dermatitis, and urticaria, which can be exacerbated by stress.

Clinicians should be aware that some travelers may be reluctant to acknowledge psychiatric symptoms or distress. For example, many cultures have stigmas associated with experiencing or disclosing behaviors associated with mental illness, as well as different culturally appropriate ways of expressing grief, pain, and loss. In addition, some travelers may fear being penalized or stigmatized at work if they have psychiatric diagnoses noted on their medical records.

Regardless of the type or duration of travel, and whether or not travelers appear to meet criteria for a psychiatric diagnosis, returned travelers who are having difficulties functioning or who appear to be unduly depressed or distressed should be encouraged to seek appropriate treatment or counseling.

References

1. Lankester T. Health care of the long-term traveler. Travel Med Infect Dis. 2005;3(3):143–55.
2. Beny A, Paz A, Potasman I. Psychiatric problems in returning travelers: features and associations. J Travel Med. 2001;8(5):243–6.
3. Bhadelia N, Klotman M, Caplivski D. The HIV-positive traveler. Am J Med. 2007;120(7):574–80.
4. Reed CM. Travel recommendations for older adults. Clin Geriatr Med. 2007;23(3):687–713, ix.
5. Potasman I, Beny A, Seligmann H. Neuropsychiatric problems in 2,500 long-term young travelers to the tropics. J Travel Med. 2000;7(1):5–9.
6. Patel D, Easmon C, Dow C, et al. Medical repatriation of British diplomats resident overseas. J Travel Med. 2000;7(2):64–9.
7. Palinkas LA, Suedfeld P. Psychological effects of polar expeditions. Lancet. 2008;371(9607):153–63.
8. Espino CM, Sundstrom SM, Frick HL, et al. International business travel: impact on families and travellers. Occup Environ Med. 2002;59(5):309–22.
9. Bor R. Psychological factors in airline passenger and crew behaviour: a clinical overview. Travel Med Infect Dis. 2007;5(4):207–16.
10. Balaban V. Psychological assessment of children in disasters and emergencies: a review. Disasters. 2006;30(2):178–98.
11. Hochedez P, Vinsentini P, Ansart S, et al. Changes in the pattern of health disorders diagnosed among two cohorts of French travelers to Nepal, 17 years apart. J Travel Med. 2004;11(6):341–6.
12. Rolfe M, Tang CM, Sabally S, et al. Psychosis and cannabis abuse in The Gambia. A case–control study. Br J Psychiatry. 1993;163:798–801.
13. Crofford LJ. Violence, stress, and somatic syndromes. Trauma Violence Abuse. 2007;8(3):299–313.
14. Urpe M, Buggiani G, Lotti T. Stress and psychoneuroimmunologic factors in dermatology. Dermatol Clin. 2005;23(4):609–17.

3

Select Destinations and Travel Itineraries

RATIONALE FOR SELECT DESTINATIONS

David R. Shlim

We are all aware that the quality of our travel health advice is improved if we know something about the destination—where people go, how they travel, and what hidden joys and difficulties might be associated with that locale. A person living in or traveling frequently to a destination is often best able to reveal the answers to questions that are more difficult to ascertain from afar. These destination sections are a completely new feature. We invited authors who were familiar with particular destinations to convey their experience with insights that would be helpful to providers who have not traveled to that area. These sections are therefore personal points of view or editorial pieces, similar to the *Perspectives* boxes scattered throughout the text. Please consult the appropriate sections in Chapter 2 for CDC prevention recommendations for specific diseases and destinations.

The risks for certain diseases may be geographically specific within a country, but this level of detail is often unavailable in general references. In addition, the approach to prevention of certain diseases may vary according to the philosophy of the experts involved. It is a common experience for travelers from different continents to meet at an exotic location and, in comparing their respective preparations for their trips, to find that they received sometimes different medications, vaccinations and advice by providers in their home countries. Travel health providers need to be able to account for these disparities when discussing these issues with their patients. The earlier section *Perspectives:* Why Guidelines Differ in Chapter 1 makes some attempt to discuss the range of approaches, from the conservative to the more permissive. These sections will highlight some of these approaches in the context of specific destinations. The travel medicine practitioner and the traveler will then be able to weigh these approaches and come to a decision which reflects their perception and tolerance of risk.

The destinations were selected because of a consensus that these locales were commonly visited, and that there was a broad range of styles in preparing travelers for these trips. As travel medicine practitioners, we have found preparing a traveler for a destination with which we are familiar is an easier experience. The goal of these sections is to allow more of us to feel comfortable giving advice about specific destinations that we may never have visited ourselves.

CUZCO–MACHU PICCHU, PERU

Alan J. Magill

Destination Background

Peru is about twice the size of the state of Texas, with a population of almost 30 million people. Thousands of tourists are drawn to Peru every year to enjoy the magnificent geographic, biologic, and cultural diversity. The primary destination for most travelers is the remarkable Incan ruins of Machu Picchu, recently named as one of the modern Seven Wonders of the World and a United Nations Educational, Scientific, and Cultural Organization (UNESCO) World Heritage site. Machu Picchu stands in the middle of a tropical mountain forest, in an extraordinarily beautiful setting. It was probably the most amazing urban creation of the Inca Empire at its height; its giant walls, terraces, and ramps seem as if they have been cut naturally in the continuous rock escarpments. The natural setting, on the eastern slopes of the Andes, is in the upper Amazon Basin, with its rich diversity of flora and fauna.

A typical visit to Peru includes arrival at the capital city of Lima, a large megacity the size of the state of Rhode Island, with about a third of Peru's population. Interestingly, many persons think Lima is a high-altitude Incan city, but it is actually located on the Pacific coast at sea level. After a few days in Lima, one takes an hour-long flight to Cuzco, the gateway to Machu Picchu and a worthwhile destination of its own. Tourists can visit multiple Inca-era ruins and Peruvian mountain villages and markets in the Vallee Sagrado before taking the train to Machu Picchu. Many individuals also wish to add a tropical rainforest experience to their Cuzco trip and take the 30-minute flight from Cuzco to Puerto Maldonado, 55 km west of the Bolivian border, on the confluence of the Rio Tambopata with the Madre de Dios River, a major tributary of the Amazon River. The majority of travelers take a boat up the Rio Tambopata to one of several rustic lodges. Visitors wanting to see the Amazon rainforest also may go to Manu National Park in the south, also reached via Cuzco, or the northern Amazon rainforest by visiting lodges around Iquitos or by the increasingly popular Amazon river cruises that go both up- and downstream from Iquitos. Ecotourism is a growing activity in Peru, as elsewhere. Peru is also home to the Cordillera Blanca, a several hundred-mile range of spectacular snow covered peaks that form the backbone of the Andes Mountains in Peru.

Health Issues

Important pre-travel information for Peru includes advice on preventing high-altitude illness, the risk for cutaneous leishmaniasis, appropriate use of yellow fever vaccine, and the risk for malaria for travelers visiting popular jungle lodges.

Altitude and Acute Mountain Sickness (AMS)

All travelers to Machu Picchu will arrive and transit through Cuzco, 3,395 m (11,203 ft) above sea level. Many arriving travelers will find the near 3,500 m elevation leads to some degree of AMS, with the initial symptoms of headache, nausea, and loss of appetite beginning 4–8 hours after arrival. The hypoxemia of high altitude can also dramatically affect the quality of sleep in the first few nights in Cuzco, with restless sleep, frequent awakening, and Cheyne–Stokes breathing (periodic breathing), even in those who appear to be doing well during the day. A minority of travelers may progress to severe forms of altitude illness, to include high-altitude pulmonary edema and high-altitude cerebral edema. The symptoms of AMS can markedly impair the traveler and prevent enjoyment of the sights of Cuzco.

Surveys have shown that most travelers arrive in Cuzco with limited or no knowledge of AMS and its prevention with the prophylactic use of acetazolamide. **Every traveler to Cuzco should be counseled about AMS pre-travel and be prepared to prevent or self-treat AMS.** The use of acetazolamide (Diamox) can minimize or eliminate the symptoms of AMS. (More information about prevention and treatment of altitude illness can be found in the Altitude Illness section in Chapter 2.) Locals refer to AMS as "soroche" and will almost always offer the new arrival a cup of hot coca tea (mate de coca) when checking in to the hotel. Although many believe mate de coca can prevent and treat soroche, no data support its use in the prevention or treatment of AMS. Perhaps of concern to some who may experience random drug screening as a condition of employment, individuals who drink a single cup of coca tea will test positive for cocaine metabolites in standard drug toxicology screens for several days. However, sitting quietly and resting while enjoying a cup of tea is a most civilized activity and a pleasant memory.

New arrivals may also find it helpful to transit directly to the Valle Sagrado (~2,800–3,000 m; 9,500 ft) of the Rio Urubamba to spend the first few days and nights at this somewhat lower altitude. One can board the train to Machu Picchu in Ollantaytambo, at the south end of the Valle Sagrado, and the not-to-be-missed visit to Cuzco can be made on return from Machu Picchu, when people are better acclimatized. The train follows the Rio Urubamba north (downstream) to Aguas Calientes (2,000 m; 6,600 ft). Machu Picchu (2,430 m; 7,970 ft) is located on a ridge above the town.

Cutaneous Leishmaniasis (CL)

Many areas in the Pacific valleys of the Andes and the Amazon tropical rainforest are endemic for CL, a parasitic infection transmitted by bites of sand flies (see the Leishmaniasis, Cutaneous section in Chapter 5). While this disease is widespread in southeastern Peru, the highest risk for travelers seems to be the Manu Park area in Madre de Dios. In Manu, CL is most often caused by *Leishmania braziliensis,* and there is a risk of both simple CL and mucosal leishmaniasis. There is no visceral leishmaniasis in Peru. Travelers should be counseled to be meticulous about vector precautions, as there is no vaccine or chemoprophylaxis to prevent leishmaniasis. Any person with a skin lesion persisting more than a few weeks should be evaluated for CL.

Yellow Fever (YF)

Proof of YF vaccination is not required for entry into Peru. Travelers who are limiting travel to the cities of Lima, Cuzco, and Machu Picchu do not need YF vaccination. Peru recommends vaccination for those who intend to visit any jungle areas of the country <2,300 m (<7,546 ft).

Malaria

In general, the risk of malaria in travelers visiting Peru is relatively low. There are, on average, 5 cases reported in the United States each year that were acquired in Peru. Both *Plasmodium vivax* malaria and *P. falciparum* malaria are found in the Peruvian Amazon.

There is no malaria risk for travelers visiting only Lima and vicinity, coastal areas south of Lima, or the popular highland tourist areas (Cuzco, Machu Picchu, and Lake Titicaca).

The malaria risk areas for most tourists are the neotropical rainforests of the Amazon. There are two major destinations. The city of Iquitos in the northern rainforest is a frequent arrival destination for those traveling to jungle lodges around the city or for

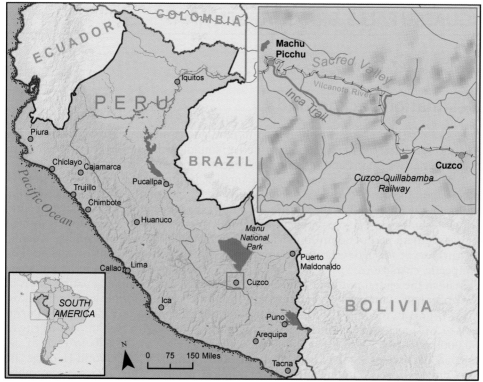

Map 3-1. Destination map of Peru.

boarding river cruise boats for rainforest travel. Malaria transmission occurs in the areas in and around Iquitos. Chemoprophylaxis is recommended for most travelers.

The city of Puerto Maldonado is a thirty minute flight from Cuzco and a popular arrival destination for those visiting the rainforest lodges on the Rio Tambopata. Newly arrived travelers usually transit directly from the airport to the boats that take them up the river to numerous lodges. Peruvian Ministry of Health data document that malaria transmission occurs in Puerto Maldonado. Most cases reported in the region occur in local loggers and gold miners in the forests. It is the opinion of this author that travelers transiting Puerto Maldonado for a short 2–3 day visit to lodges on the Rio Tambopata may not need chemoprophylaxis.

Risk for the traveler varies with itinerary, style of travel and location of accommodations. Malaria in the Peruvian Amazon is unpredictable from season to season, with *P. falciparum* epidemics occasionally occurring. When making a decision on whether to recommend chemoprophylaxis or simply mosquito precautions, all of these factors and data need to be taken into consideration.

References

1. Merritt AL, Camerlengo A, Meyer C, Mull JD. Mountain sickness knowledge among foreign travelers in Cuzco, Peru. Wilderness Environ Med. 2007;18(1):26–9.

2. Mazor SS, Mycyk MB, Wills BK, et al. Coca tea consumption causes positive urine cocaine assay. Eur J Emerg Med. 2006;13(6):340–1.

3. Cabada MM, Maldonado F, Quispe W, et al. Pretravel health advice among international travelers visiting Cuzco, Peru. J Travel Med. 2005;12(2):61–5.

4. Behrens RH, Carroll B, Beran J, et al.; TropNetEurop. The low and declining risk of malaria in travellers to Latin America: is there still an indication for chemoprophylaxis? Malar J. 2007;6:114.

IGUASSU FALLS, BRAZIL/ARGENTINA

David O. Freedman

Destination Background

Iguassu Falls (Iguazú in Spanish; Iguaçu in Portuguese, the language of Brazil) in the Atlantic rainforest region of South America straddles the border of the southern Brazilian state of Paraná and the northern Argentine province of Misiones.

Brazil, occupying most of eastern South America, is immense and varies from tropical plains and jungle at the equator to cooler uplands in the south. Brazil is a developing nation in the lower half of the world's economies, but the highly industrialized south, which includes São Paulo, is affluent with modern infrastructure. Argentina is located in the southern part of South America, between the Andes Mountains and the Atlantic Ocean. Except for a tiny northernmost fringe, which is tropical, all of Argentina is temperate, characterized by a cool, very dry climate in the south and a more moderate climate in the central portion of the country. Argentina is a developing nation but is in the upper half of the world's economies. In addition, Paraguay is only a few miles away. Most visitors to the falls stay in either the city of Foz do Iguaçu, Paraná, or in Puerto Iguazú, Misiones, each about 12 miles from the falls and each a well developed city of 60,000 people. However, there is one sizeable hotel right at the falls in each of the separate national parks on either side of the border. This UNESCO World Heritage site also protects an astounding diversity of tropical wildlife. There are airports called Iguassu Falls in both countries, but travelers can fly to the Brazilian airport (IGU) only from Brazil and to the Argentinean airport (IGR) only from Argentina.

Higher than Niagara Falls, Iguassu is rivaled only by Southern Africa's Victoria Falls, which are higher but narrower. Iguassu Falls is a waterfall system consisting of 275 falls along 1.67 miles of the Iguassu River, varying from 210 to 270 ft in height. The main feature, the Devil's Throat, is a U-shaped cliff, 490 by 2,300 ft , that marks the border between Argentina and Brazil. Two-thirds of the falls are on the Argentine side of the gorge, giving the Brazilian side the best view. However, one cannot directly approach the falls from the Brazilian side. Travelers visiting the Argentine side are able to pass over and under the actual falls on a series of catwalks and trails. The bridge connecting the two sides of the river is a number of miles away and crosses the Brazil–Argentina border.

U.S. travelers require a visa, which must be obtained in advance, to enter Brazil. Many organized day trips simply do not stop at the Brazilian immigration post, and this seems to be tolerated. However, a U.S. citizen in Brazil without a visa in his/her passport may face arrest or imprisonment if stopped for any reason by authorities during the short visit. U.S. travelers staying on the Brazilian side on a single-entry Brazilian visa are now able to re-enter Brazil after a day trip to Argentina. No visa is required to enter Argentina from Brazil. Ideally, one really should visit both sides, but most people do not because their stay is too short to deal with the somewhat complicated logistical issues.

Health Issues

The infrastructure in tourist accommodation around Iguassu Falls is good, and most travelers are tourists staying only for a short time. Travelers utilizing usual accommodation and dining facilities are at modest risk for enterically transmitted diseases. Travelers should carry an antibiotic for self-treatment of travelers' diarrhea. Hepatitis A vaccine is recommended for all travelers and typhoid vaccine only for those with adventurous dietary habits or eating away from usual tourist locations.

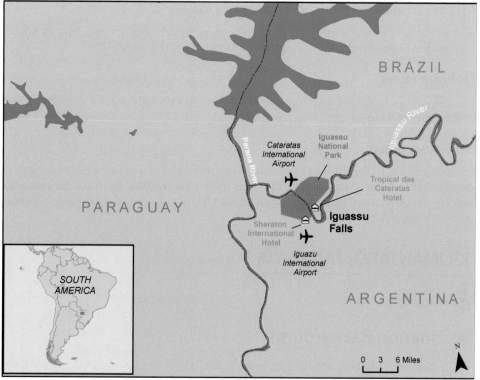

Map 3-2. Destination map of Iguassu Falls.

Yellow Fever

Yellow fever virus currently circulates in monkeys in the forested regions along the Iguassu and Paraná rivers. All travelers, even those on a typical 1- to 2-day itinerary, should be vaccinated. Although requirements may change from time to time, at present neither Brazil nor Argentina requires an International Certificate of Vaccination or prophylaxis for yellow fever for any traveler.

Malaria

Some transmission of *Plasmodium vivax* does occur at the falls and in surrounding areas. In making a decision on whether to recommend chemoprophylaxis or simply mosquito precautions, the itinerary, style of travel, and location of accommodations all need to be taken into consideration. Typical 1- to 2-night travelers on assuredly fixed itineraries and staying at the hotels at the falls or in upscale accommodation in the adjacent towns may well decide on insect precautions only. Other types of travelers to the area may be at increased risk and may decide to use chemoprophylaxis in consultation with their provider.

Rabies

Both canine and bat rabies are risks in parts of Brazil, but no cases in animals or humans have been reported from around Iguassu Falls. Pre-exposure vaccine is not necessary for typical travelers, but travelers should be educated about seeking adequate medical care for any bite injuries or bat exposures that do occur.

Leishmaniasis

This protozoan disease, transmitted by sandflies, occurs in Brazil and is most common in the Amazonian and northeast regions but is present in Paraná. Cases have not been described in visitors to Iguassu Falls.

Chagas Disease (American Trypanosomiasis)

Risk to travelers is unknown but is thought to be negligible. Few travelers stay in houses constructed of mud, adobe brick, or palm thatch where the vectors live.

Dengue Fever

Dengue occurs in urban and rural areas in the Iguassu Falls region. Daytime insect precautions will reduce risk.

Schistosomiasis

Schistosomiasis, transmitted in freshwater lakes and rivers, is a public health problem in many states in Brazil. Historically, rare cases have been reported from the Iguassu area, but no recent data are available. Cautious travelers should avoid freshwater exposure while visiting the area.

KILIMANJARO, TANZANIA

Kevin C. Kain

Destination Background

As the highest mountain in Africa and one of the largest freestanding volcanoes in the world, Kilimanjaro remains a revered and classic image of east Africa. Its snowcapped peak rising (19,344 ft; 5,896 m) above the tropical African savanna is an irresistible draw for trekkers, particularly since no technical climbing is required to reach the summit. Kilimanjaro is one of the "seven summits" representing the highest peaks on each continent. However, because it does not involve technical climbing, the difficulties are often misjudged. Climbing Kilimanjaro is a serious undertaking requiring serious preparation. Despite being higher than classic trekking destinations in Nepal such as Kalar Pattar (18,450 ft; 5,625 m) or Everest base camp (17,500 ft; 5,335 m), typical ascent rates on Kilimanjaro are considerably faster (4–6 days vs. 8–12 days).

The classic route up Kilimanjaro is the Marangu route (64 km) usually sold as a "5 day/4 night" trip. Marangu is frequently nicknamed the "Coca Cola" route, since accommodation and food are provided in bunkhouses and the trail is wide and relatively easy compared to other routes. There are at least nine other alternative routes, including the stunningly beautiful Machame route (the so-called "Whiskey" route, since the days are generally longer, with tougher climbs). This author can vouch for the dramatic rugged beauty of this hike. Machame and other routes involve camping but are usually sold as 6- to 9-day packages, providing more opportunity to acclimatize and greater chances to successfully summit. Kilimanjaro can be climbed throughout the year (March–April is often the wettest), but the weather is unpredictable and the climber must be prepared for extreme weather and rain at any time of the year.

Health Issues

The main travel medicine-related issues for those attempting Kilimanjaro include the prevention and treatment of altitude illness and the potential for drug interactions between medications used for altitude illness and antimalarial or antidiarrheal agents commonly used by travelers to Tanzania.

Altitude and Acute Mountain Sickness (AMS)

- Altitude illness is a significant problem on Kilimanjaro and a major contributor to

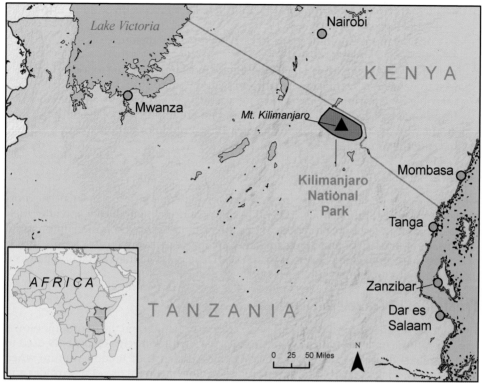

Map 3-3. Destination map of Tanzania.

why only 50% of those attempting the standard Marangu route reach the crater rim, known as Gillman's Point (18,600 ft; 5,680 m), and only 10% reach the summit, known as Uhuru (Freedom) Peak (19,344 ft; 5,896 m). *Every hiker on Kilimanjaro should receive pre-travel advice on AMS, be able to recognize symptoms, and know how to prevent and treat it.*

- Individuals with certain underlying medical conditions, including pregnancy, cardiac and lung disease, and ocular and neurologic conditions, may be more susceptible to altitude-associated problems or may be taking medications that may interact with altitude medications and should consult a health provider with knowledge of altitude illness before travel.
- Enjoying the experience and successfully reaching the summit can be significantly enhanced by allowing more time to acclimatize. For example—
  - If Ngorongoro crater is part of the planned combined itinerary, try to end the safari with a few nights here, because its elevation (7,500 ft; 2,286 m) will aid acclimatization for the Kilimanjaro trek.
  - It is strongly encouraged to add at least an extra day or two to the ascent of Kilimanjaro regardless of the route, but especially on routes normally promoted as 4- to 6-day routes.
  - If possible before attempting Kilimanjaro, acclimatize by hiking nearby Mt. Meru (14,976 ft; 4,566 m) or Mt. Kenya (to Point Lenana, 16,055 ft; 4,895 m). A number of combined climbing trips for Mt. Kenya and Kilimanjaro are now offered commercially.
- For those with a past history of susceptibility to AMS and for those in whom adequate acclimatization is not possible (most "Kili" clients), the use of medications such as acetazolamide to prevent altitude illness is recommended.
  - Acetazolamide accelerates acclimatization and is effective in preventing (beginning the day before ascent) and treating AMS and is safe in children.
  - For those who are intolerant or allergic to acetazolamide, dexamethasone is an

alternative for prevention of AMS, but there are cautions involved in using dexamethasone for ascent.

  ○ Consideration should be given to carrying a treatment course of dexamethasone for HACE.

- Individuals with symptoms of altitude illness must not continue to ascend and need to descend if symptoms are worsening at the same altitude.
- A flexible itinerary and having an extra guide that can accompany any member of the group who becomes ill down the mountain are important considerations.
- See the Altitude Illness section in Chapter 2 for more information about prevention and treatment of altitude illness.

Malaria

Kilimanjaro is unique in that its tropical malaria-endemic location means that most trekkers will be on antimalarials and will need to continue them during and after their climb. Fortunately, there are no reported drug interactions between common antimalarial prophylaxis agents (atovaquone/proguanil, doxycycline, or mefloquine) and acetozolamide or dexamethasone used to prevent or treat AMS. There is a potential interaction between mefloquine and nifedipine, used for HAPE.

Treatment of Travelers' Diarrhea

There are no reported drug interactions between acetozolamide and the fluoroquinolones (e.g., ciprofloxacin, levofloxacin) or macrolides (e.g., azithromycin) commonly used to treat travelers' diarrhea. There is a potential increased risk of tendon rupture when dexamethasone is used with fluoroquinolones. Avoid concurrent use of macrolides and nifedipine.

Remote Travel

Treks on Kilimanjaro are physically demanding and require a good level of fitness and preparation for the elements. Kilimanjaro weather is characterized by extremes: be prepared for tropical heat, heavy rains, and bitter cold. Ensure one's gear is kept in waterproof bags, especially one's sleeping bag. Travelers should have adequate health insurance, including medical evacuation.

Carry a first-aid kit that includes bandages, tape, blister kit, antibacterial and antifungal cream, antibiotics for travelers' diarrhea, antimalarials, antiemetics, antihistamines, analgesics, cold and flu medications, throat lozenges, and altitude meds.

Conclusion

Climbing Kilimanjaro is a dream for many who visit Africa. However, a large number of travelers are ill-prepared, ascend too quickly, and consequently fail to summit. With due preparation and more reasonable ascent rates, climbing "Kili" is an aspiration that can be successfully and safely accomplished by many.

References

1. Hackett PH, Roach RC. High-altitude illness. N Engl J Med. 2001;345(2):107–14.
2. Barry PW, Pollard AJ. Altitude illness. BMJ. 2003;326(7395):915–9.
3. Luks AM, Swenson ER. Medication and dosage considerations in the prophylaxis and treatment of high-altitude illness. Chest. 2008;133(3):744–55.
4. Luks AM, Swenson ER.Travel to high altitude with pre-existing lung disease. Eur Respir J. 2007;29(4):770–92.
5. Jean D, Leal C Kriemler S, et al. Medical recommendations for women going to altitude. High Alt Med Biol. 2005;6(1):22–31.
6. Baumgartner RW, Siegel AM, Hackett PH. Going high with preexisting neurological disorders. High Alt Med Biol. 2007;8(2):108–16.
7. Mader TH, Tabin G. Going to high altitude with preexisting ocular conditions. High Alt Med Biol. 2003; 4(4):419–30.

8. Basnyat B, Gertsch JH, Holck PS, et al. Acetazolamide 125 mg BD is not significantly different from 375 mg BD in the prevention of acute mountain sickness: the prophylactic acetazolamide dosage comparison for efficacy (PACE) trial. High Alt Med Biol. 2006;7(1):17–27.

9. Bärtsch P, Gibbs JS. The effect of altitude on the heart and lungs. Circulation. 2007;116(19):2191–2202.

10. Strom BL, Schinnar R, Apter AJ, et al. Absence of cross-reactivity of sulfonamide antibiotics with sulfonamide nonantibiotics. N Engl J Med. 2003;349(17):1628–35.

SAFARIS IN EAST AND SOUTHERN AFRICA

Jay S. Keystone

Destination Background

East and Southern Africa remain among the last regions of the world where visitors can experience spectacular wide expanses and free-roaming animals in their natural state. The African Safari has long been the dream vacation for many Westerners. Individuals and families are now choosing safari vacations in lieu of the more traditional sightseeing tours of Europe's capitals. The typical quest to observe the Big Five (lion, leopard, rhino, Cape buffalo, and elephant), the striking birds and reptiles, and the extraordinary plant life draws many to African lands. Most of these safaris are planned through tour operators, who offer travelers both the adventure and thrill of the wilderness and the luxury of modern accommodations. These tour operators offer an innumerable variety of scheduled and customized safari options.

East African safaris are typically undertaken in the major game parks in Kenya and Tanzania. Kenya has many game reserves, most notably the Masai Mara, which hosts the start of the annual migration of over one million wildebeest and 200,000 zebras. Tanzania also possesses some of the most famous safari destinations, such as two UNESCO World Heritage Sites—Serengeti National Park and the Ngorongoro Conservation Area—which includes the Ngorongoro Crater, Ruaha National Park, and Selous Game Reserve, and in the north, Tarangire National Park. East African safaris are typically undertaken during the drier months, from mid-December through January or from June to August. Temperatures in the daytime usually range between 70° F–80° F, while mornings and evenings may be quite chilly. Itineraries within these countries may include exotic destinations on the coast, such as Zanzibar in Tanzania and the Kenyan coastal areas around Mombasa and Lamu, or visits to mountainous areas, such as the Usambara Mountains and Mount Kilimanjaro.

In the south of the continent, large game reserves are located in South Africa, Botswana, and Namibia. The Southern African parks can be enjoyed year round, but travelers may prefer the dry season, as during the drier months of April through October daytime temperatures are mild with little humidity and nights are crisp and cool. During this time, game viewing is usually better, because of sparser vegetation. Northwest of Botswana lies the huge expanse of the Okavango Delta and the nearby Chobe National Park. Water activities and more rare types of animals make exploring the Okavango Delta particularly exciting. In Namibia, the Etosha National Park partly comprises a wide salt pan formed 1,000 million years ago. Etosha's wildlife features the black-faced impala and endangered black rhino, as well as flamingo and pelicans. The South African game reserves are spread around the country. To the east of Johannesburg is the famous Kruger National Park (larger in size than Israel) and satellite reserves in the surrounding area. Many of these safaris include exquisite cuisine and luxurious lodging. In Kwa-Zulu Natal is the Hluhluwe-Umfolozi Game Reserve, the oldest reserve in Africa. This game reserve is famous for being the home of both black and white rhino and many other endangered species. On the southern coast are the Shamwari Game Reserve and the Addo Elephant Park. The private Shamwari Game Reserve supports five ecosystems and for multiple years has been named the World's Leading Conservation Company and Game Reserve.

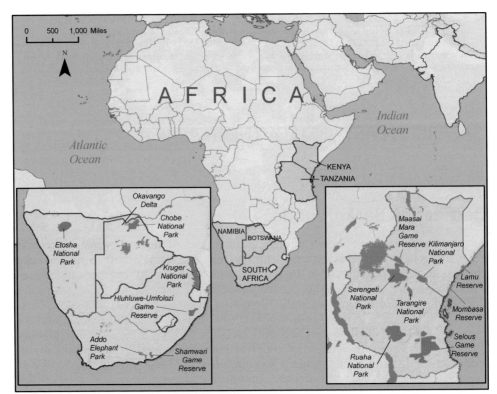

Map 3-4. Destination map of East and Southern Africa.

Health Issues

For most travelers, the African safari is a relatively low risk undertaking. The actual risk depends on the specific destination, duration of visit, and style of travel. Most of safaris are usually short-term (<2 weeks), guided by experts, and often in a style comparable to western standards. However, accommodations can vary, and the health advisor will need to know if the traveler will be in luxury tented camps and lodges or in more rustic surroundings.

As for travel in any developing country, travelers' diarrhea remains a major cause of illness. Food and water precautions are important, despite the fact that the traveler may be part of a luxury tour. Other illnesses that are common are minor skin infections, insect bites, suprainfection of bites, and minor respiratory illnesses.

The major risks to the safari-goer are vector-borne diseases, such as malaria and African tick-borne fever. Rarely, African trypanosomiasis has been reported.

Vector-Borne Diseases

Malaria

- Malaria transmission occurs in these areas (except for the southern coastal region of South Africa), and most infections are due to *Plasmodium falciparum* (see the Malaria section in Chapter 2).
- Chloroquine-resistant *P. falciparum* is universal.
- Personal protection measures are an important adjunct to malaria chemoprophylaxis. Bed nets are usually supplied at high-end lodges. Permethrin-impregnated bed nets may be required for "do-it-yourself" and budget safaris.

Yellow Fever

The country in which the safari is being taken determines whether yellow fever is a risk and whether the vaccine is recommended (see the table Yellow Fever Vaccine Requirements and Recommendations, by Country in Chapter 2).

African Tick-Borne Fever

Rickettsial infection (*Rickettsia africae*) is transmitted in rural areas by ticks, primarily in southern Africa. Typhus illness is characterized by fever, sometimes along with localized lymphadenopathy, rash, and presence of an eschar. In addition to using repellents, prevention includes tucking pant legs into socks and doing "tick checks" daily.

African Trypanosomiasis

African trypanosomiasis is transmitted by day-biting tsetse flies (*Glossina*), which are attracted to movement and dark colors. Rarely, cases occur in travelers on safari. Flies may bite through clothing and are often not discouraged by insect repellents. Light-colored clothing is recommended.

Ectoparasites

Myiasis (Tumbu Fly)

Myiasis is caused by fly larvae penetrating the skin and causing a boil-like lesion with a central aperture. Eggs are usually laid on clothing left to dry out of doors and enter skin when clothing is put on. Clothing should not be placed on the ground out of doors or should be ironed before wearing.

Tungiasis

Tungiasis is caused by direct penetration of skin by a sand flea (*Tunga penetrans*) that causes a small, painful or pruritic nodule on the foot, often adjacent to a toenail. Wearing closed-toed footwear and avoiding walking barefoot help to prevent this problem.

Waterborne Disease

Schistosomiaisis (Bilharzia)

Infection is widespread throughout Africa. Exposure to freshwater ponds, lakes or rivers, no matter how enticing, should be avoided (see the Schistosomiasis section in Chapter 5).

Other Health and Safety Risks

Although the above issues are the most important, travelers should be aware of other risks. Rare deaths and severe injuries have been the result of attacks by game animals, especially lions, buffalo, elephants, rhinoceros, snakes, and crocodiles. Prevention includes common-sense behavior, such as remaining inside of game park vehicles unless otherwise directed, avoiding close contact with animals, using flashlights at night, being cautious when exiting accommodations after dark, and not dangling arms and legs in the water while boating.

Robbery and personal injury from crimes are rare occurrences to those on safari because of increased law enforcement practices. However, in some major urban centers, notably Johannesburg, Nairobi, and Mombasa, street muggings during both the day and the night are common. The rates of motor vehicle accidents are among the highest in the world. Within game parks, for the most part, low rates of speed and poor quality roads (in some parks) ensure that high-speed, severe motor vehicle accidents are rare. However, high risk occurs during travel in rural areas between parks, especially after dark.

References

1. Durrheim DN, Braack L, Grobler D, et al. Safety of travel in South Africa: The Kruger National Park. J Travel Med. 2001;8(4):176–91.

2. Reyburn H, Mbatia R, Drakeley C, et al. Overdiagnosis of malaria in patients with severe febrile illness in Tanzania: a prospective study. BMJ. 2004;329(7476):1212.

3. Sinha A, Grace C, Alston WK, et al. African trypanosomiasis in two travelers from the United States. Clin Infect Dis. 1999;29(4):840–4.

4. Leggat PA, Durrheim DN, Apps PJ. Occupational risks posed by wild mammals in South African wildlife reserves. J Occup Health Saf Aust NZ. 2000;16:47–54.

5. Moore DA, Edwards M, Escombe R, et al. African trypanosomiasis in travelers returning to the United Kingdom. Emerg Infect Dis. 2002;8(1):74–6.
6. United Nations Office at Nairobi. Security Advice for United Nations visitors to Kenya [Internet]. [cited 2008 Jun 30]. Available from: http://www.unon.org/unoncomplex/security_advice.php.
7. Peden M, Scurfield R, Sleet D, Mohan D, Hyder AA, Jarawan E, Mathers C, editors. World Report on Road Traffic Injury Prevention. Geneva: WHO; 2004.

ANGKOR WAT, CAMBODIA

Kathrine R. Tan

Destination Background

Angkor, located in the province of Siem Reap in Cambodia, is the capital of the ancient Khmer empire. Located in dense jungle 20 miles from Lake Tonle Sap, Angkor contains hundreds of ancient temples built during the 9th to the 15th centuries. The most famous of these temples is Angkor Wat, the world's largest religious building. Ideal months for travel are November through January with cooler temperatures and little rain. Starting in February, temperatures start rising to peaks as high as 104° F (40° C) in April. While the monsoon season in May through October brings afternoon rains that can turn the roads to outlying temples into quagmires of mud, intrepid tourists this time of year are rewarded by views of Angkor framed by verdant, lush foliage.

Since there are no accommodations in Angkor, most tourists stay in Siem Reap and take local transportation for the 20-minute ride to Angkor. From Siem Reap, there are several options to get to Angkor. Tuk-tuks, or motorcycle taxis, are the most popular mode of transportation. There are also tour buses and cars for hire. Because of Angkor's size, most travelers hire transportation for the whole day to get to various parts of the temple complex. The temples of Angkor cover an area of 400 km², so travelers would do best to plan their itinerary carefully, taking into consideration accessibility of sites by road. Angkor Wat, the largest temple, is by the ancient city of Angkor Thom and is the most easily accessible area. Other groups of temples include sites east and north to Angkor Thom (Le Petit Circuit and Le Grand Circuit), the Roluos group located 15 km east of Siem Reap, and other outlying temples that are located more than 20 km from Angkor Wat.

Lighting at sunrise and sunset makes for the most dramatic viewing of the temples, and these are therefore popular times to visit. Visitors are suggested to wear long pants or long skirts and covered shoulders as a sign of respect, because Angkor is considered a holy site. A typical itinerary starts early at the northern reflecting pool to watch the sun rise behind Angkor Wat. The day can then be spent taking a tour of the archaeological wonders of Angkor Wat and Angkor Thom. While being surrounded by ancient relics, visitors are reminded of the present day by hawkers of food, drink, and souvenirs in front of many of the temples. At the end of the day, visitors climb up the steep steps of Phnom Bakheng to watch the sun set over Angkor.

Health Issues

Immunizations

Hepatitis A Vaccine

Hepatitis A is highly endemic in Cambodia. All travelers should be protected against hepatitis A.

Typhoid Vaccine

All travelers should be protected against typhoid. Although the vaccine provides good

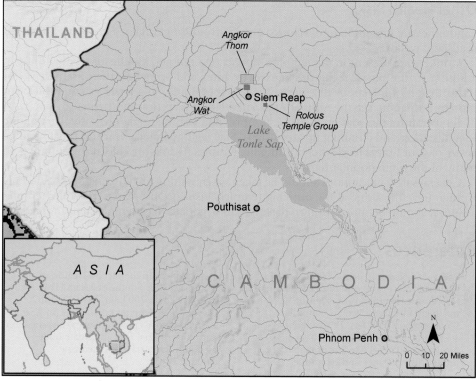

Map 3-5. Destination map of Cambodia.

protection against typhoid infection, no vaccine is 100% effective, so precautions should still be taken in selecting food and drinks.

Japanese Encephalitis (JE) Vaccine

JE is endemic countrywide with transmission season extending from May through October. Vaccination is recommended only for travelers who will be visiting rural areas of Cambodia during the transmission season with extensive outdoor exposure (see the JE section in Chapter 2). Most visitors to Angkor who are planning on a typical tour of the temples will not need JE vaccination.

Rabies Vaccine

Visitors to Angkor should avoid contact with animals, such as stray dogs in Siem Reap city and monkeys in the Angkor temple complex. Do not pet or feed animals. If bitten, seek medical attention.

Malaria

Angkor is often visited at sunrise and sunset when mosquitoes are likely to bite, putting travelers at risk for mosquito-borne diseases such as malaria and dengue. Malaria chemoprophylaxis and mosquito avoidance are both recommended.

Atovaquone/proguanil or doxycycline should be taken to prevent malaria. Chloroquine and mefloquine are not recommended because *P. falciparum* may be resistant to these drugs in this area. Purchase malaria prophylaxis drugs in the United States before travel, because counterfeit malaria drugs have been found in Southeast Asia.

Avoid mosquito bites by using a recommended repellent, sleeping under a mosquito net if not in an air conditioned room, and wearing protective clothing. Mosquito bites can transmit not only malaria but other diseases such as dengue and Japanese encephalitis.

Other Health Risks

Landmines are present in undeveloped areas surrounding Angkor. Stay on well-traveled roads and walkways.

Monkeys are present in the temple complex. Do not pet, handle, or feed wildlife. In addition to the physical injuries caused by bites and scratches, there is the risk for transmission of infectious diseases such as herpes B and, to a lesser extent, rabies. For more information, see the Animal-Associated Hazards section in Chapter 2.

Temperatures can soar up to 40° C in April, and visiting Angkor will involve walking long distances and climbing up steep steps. Stay well-hydrated, wear sun block, and be aware of your fitness level when touring the temples. Drinks are sold at the entrances to many of the more popular temples.

General safety precautions should be taken when visiting Angkor after dark, especially women traveling alone at the outlying temples. Visitors who plan to view the temples at sunset should be sure to bring a flashlight to negotiate steep temple steps in the dark.

References

1. Reynes JM, Soares JL, Keo C, et al. Characterization and observation of animals responsible for rabies post-exposure treatment in Phnom Penh, Cambodia. Onderstepoort J Vet Res. 1999;66(2):129–33.
2. Socheat D, Denis MB, Fandeur T, et al., Meekong Malaria II. Update of malaria, multi-drug resistance and economic development in the Mekong region of Southeast Asia. Southeast Asian J Trop Med Public Health. 2003;34(Suppl 4):1–102.
3. Newton PN, Fernandez FM, Plancon A, et al. A collaborative epidemiological investigation into the criminal fake artesunate trade in South East Asia. PloS Medicine. 2008;5(2):e32.

INDIA

Phyllis E. Kozarsky

Destination Background

India is about one-third the size of the United States, with a population of over 1 billion people—the seventh largest country and the second most populous. Rich in history, vibrant culture, and diversity, it is home to the origin of four world religions: Hinduism, Buddhism, Jainism, and Sikhism. Despite the growth of megacities such as Mumbai (14 million) and Delhi (12 million), 70% of the population still resides in rural areas and 60% work in agriculture. Although India is one of the fastest-growing economies, the literacy rate is still only 60%, with a high level of poverty. The topography is varied, ranging from tropical beaches to foothills, deserts, and the Himalayan Mountains. The north sees a more temperate climate, while the south is more tropical year round. Many travelers prefer India during the winter—November through March, when the temperatures are more agreeable, although some, particularly families with children, must travel during the summer vacation time.

India is becoming more popular for U.S. travelers, and rates of travel from the United States are increasing. International businesses are flourishing in India; tourists are flocking to the temples, beaches, and the Taj Mahal; and for some new U.S. residents, India remains their homeland, with frequent visits to family and friends.

Just as one could not visit all the tourist sites in the United States during a 2-week holiday, tourists usually select a part of India for any given trip. A typical itinerary in the north of India includes Delhi, Agra, and cities in Rajasthan. Agra is the home of the Taj Mahal, a breathtaking monument to lost love. Along the northern travel circle, one can stop to enjoy the magnificent bird sanctuary at Keoladeo Ghana and the tiger reserve at

Ran Thambore. Another frequent stop is Goa and its beaches on the western coast. Swaying coconut palms form the backdrop for great parties and old-time hippies. Mumbai, another common entry point to India, hosts Bollywood, the largest film industry in the world. Kolkata is considered the cultural capital of the country. Bengaluru (Bangalore) in the south central region has become a worldwide information technology center and has managed to meld the very old and traditional India with a new image of a modern hub. Despite the many and varied itineraries, most health recommendations for travelers to India are similar. The incidences of some illnesses, such as those transmitted by mosquitoes, increase during the monsoon season with the high temperatures, heavy rains, and the risk of flooding.

Some of the most important health considerations of travel to India are those for travelers who are visiting friends and relatives (VFRs). These individuals often travel without seeking pre-travel health advice, since they are returning to their land of origin. Such travelers may stay in rural areas often not visited by tourists or business people, live in homes, and eat and drink with their families and thus are at greater risk of many travel-related illnesses.

Health Issues

Immunizations

Hepatitis A Vaccine

All travelers to India should be protected against hepatitis A. Although some assume that those born in India would have been exposed to hepatitis A in childhood and thus be immune, this may no longer be true, particularly for younger people. Serology for hepatitis A IgG should be checked in these VFR travelers, or they should be immunized.

Typhoid Vaccine

The incidence of typhoid in U.S. citizens traveling to the Indian subcontinent has been reported to be at least 18 times higher than from any other geographic region. It is the country from which most travel-related typhoid is imported, and thus, even for short-term travel, one of the typhoid vaccines should be recommended. More compelling for those who are hesitant is the fact that typhoid fever acquired in India is becoming increasingly resistant to quinolone antibiotics, often requiring parenteral therapy.

Japanese Encephalitis (JE) Vaccine

Although there has been an absence of reported cases in travelers, there is a risk for JE, particularly during the monsoon season from May to October. In the south, some areas experience cases year round. Vaccination is not recommended for the typical tourist unless they will be traveling for extended periods during the monsoon season or will be out of doors and exposed in rice-growing areas (see the JE section in Chapter 2). Publicized outbreaks in recent years have not been in typical tourist destinations. The cost–benefit of the vaccine needs consideration, especially for travelers on a budget.

Rabies Vaccine

India has one of the highest incidences of rabies in the world, with estimates of 30,000–50,000 human cases per year. Dogs roam in packs in all areas of the country. Unfortunately, human rabies immune globulin is not readily available in India, so that if someone does not have pre-exposure rabies vaccination, a bite may result in the traveler having to leave the country for postexposure prophylaxis. Even so, a pre-exposure series is not recommended for all travelers to India. Cost is a consideration for many. Long-term travelers, expatriates, missionaries, and volunteers may want to ensure their children receive a pre-exposure series. Travelers may want to check to see if medical evacuation policies purchased prior to leaving home will cover travel for recommended rabies postexposure prophylaxis.

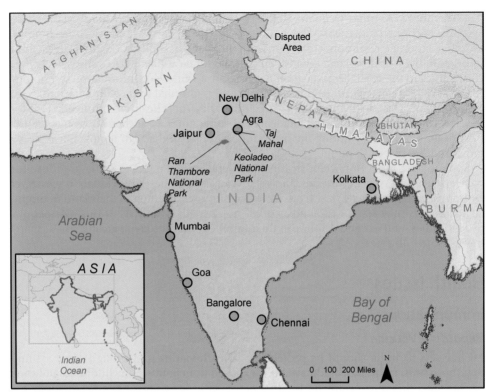

Map 3-6. Destination map of India.

Malaria

Although the intensity of malaria may be related to the season, unlike other countries in Asia, malaria is holoendemic in India and occurs in both rural and urban areas. Rates of *Plasmodium falciparum* have increased over the last two decades, and thus chemoprophylaxis is recommended for all destinations. For very short-term travelers spending 1–2 days in Delhi, a major city, in the winter, insect precautions alone may be sufficient for malaria prevention.

Other Infections

Dengue

Large outbreaks have occurred in India, particularly in the north, and particularly at the end of the monsoon season (September–October).

Hepatitis E

This illness is being recognized with greater frequency in travelers to India. A traveler who develops symptomatic hepatitis despite being immunized against hepatitis A will likely have hepatitis E.

Animal Bites and Wounds

Aside from rabies, other diseases can be transmitted by animal bites and wounds. Cellulitis, fasciitis, and wound infections may result from scratches or bites of any animal. Herpes B virus is carried by Old World monkeys and may be transmitted by active macaques that are kept as pets, inhabit many of the temples, and scatter themselves in many tourist gathering places. Monkeys can be very aggressive and often approach travelers because they are commonly fed. It is important to stress to travelers that monkeys and other animals should not be handled at all and bites can be dangerous. First aid should include vigorous washing with soap and water until medical assistance is accessed.

Travelers' Diarrhea (TD)

The risk for TD is moderate to high in India, with an estimated 30%–50% risk during a 2-week journey. Travelers should carry an antibiotic for empiric self-treatment of TD.

Miscellaneous

Arrival in India for the first time may be shocking to travelers who have never ventured into the developing world. The crowds, the intense colors, heat, and smells are striking and invade all the senses at once. It is difficult to enjoy the beauty without being touched by the enormity of the poverty. The close juxtaposition of the old and new is noteworthy. At times this can be overwhelming for travelers. Health care is quite variable in India and very dependent on the location.

Transportation in India remains problematic. While traveling through India, travelers should be advised to carry food and beverages with them in the event of delays, almost inevitable no matter the mode of transport. Traveling by train system is exciting, and negotiating a busy railway station is an experience. Roadways are some of the most hazardous in the world. Animals, rickshaws, motor scooters, people, bicycles, trucks, and overcrowded buses compete for space in an unregulated free-for-all. Rural, nighttime driving should be discouraged, even when a paid driver has been hired.

In general, travelers feel safe while in India. Peddlers and promoters are aggressive with tourists, however, and may require a firm "no" to leave tourists alone. It is always wise to pay attention to U.S. Department of States advisories in case of issues that arise at some borders or occasional increases in religious tensions.

References

1. Bacaner N, Stauffer B, Boulware DR, et al. Travel medicine considerations for North American immigrants visiting friends and relatives. JAMA. 2004;291(23):2856–64.

2. Chatterjee S. Compliance of malaria chemoprophylaxis among travelers to India. J Travel Med. 1999;6(1):7–11.

3. Leder K, Tong S, Weld L, et al.; GeoSentinel Surveillance Network. Illness in travelers visiting friends and relatives: a review of the GeoSentinel Surveillance Network. Clin Infect Dis. 2006;43(9):1185–93.

4. Connor B, Schwartz E. Typhoid and paratyphoid fever in travellers. Lancet Infect Dis. 2005;5(10):623–8.

5. Steinberg EB, Bishop R, Haber P, et al. Typhoid fever in travelers: who should be targeted for prevention? Clin Infect Dis. 2004;39(2):186–91.

6. Das K, Jain A, Gupta S, et al. The changing epidemiological pattern of hepatitis A in an urban population of India: emergence of a trend similar to the European countries. Eur J Epidemiol. 2000;16(6):507–10.

CHINA

Sarah T. Borwein

Destination Background

China, with more than 1.3 billion people, is the most populous country in the world, and the fourth largest geographically, behind Russia, Canada, and the United States. It shares a border with 14 other countries. China is divided into 23 provinces, five autonomous regions, and four municipalities.

This large landmass is home to diverse climates, topography, languages, and customs. China has one of the world's oldest continuous civilizations, dating back more than 5,000 years. It has the world's longest continuously used written language system and is the source of many major inventions, including the "four great inventions of Ancient

China": paper, the compass, gunpowder, and printing. Today, China is considerably more advanced (with the ability to put men in space, for example) and wealthier than many other developing countries, yet rural poverty and underdevelopment are still significant problems, particularly in the western part of the country.

About 800 million Chinese live in rural areas. Urban areas are growing rapidly, however, and China is now home to many of the world's largest megacities. Shanghai and Beijing each have close to 20 million inhabitants, and Chongqing, with a population exceeding 30 million, is the fastest-growing urban center in the world. Rivers play a central role in China's economy, history, and culture. The Yangtze River basin, stretching 4,000 miles from the Tibetan plateau to the East China Sea near Shanghai, is home to approximately 10% of the world's population.

In 2006, about 50 million tourists visited China, and by 2020, China is widely predicted to be both the largest tourist destination and the largest source for tourists to other countries. China's 5,000 years of continuous civilization and varied natural beauty can be traced in its 37 UNESCO World Heritage Sites, from the imperial grandeur of the Forbidden City and the Temple of Heaven to the marvel of the Great Wall, the Terracotta Warriors in Xi'an, and the spectacular mountainous sanctuaries of the west. Popular itineraries often include Beijing and the Great Wall, Xi'an, and the Yangtze River. Other important tourist destinations include—

- Shanghai and Hong Kong, with their futuristic architecture and East-meets-West mystique
- Lijiang and Yunnan, home to many of China's ethnic minorities, as well as its iconic symbol, the panda
- Guilin, famous for its uniquely shaped limestone Karst mountains that are so often featured in Chinese paintings
- Tibet, accessible now by the world's highest railroad directly to Lhasa, with a maximum altitude of 16,640 ft (5,072 m)

Specialized itineraries are increasingly being offered, including hiking, mountain climbing, village tours, the Silk Road, and other more remote regions. Aside from tourism, increasing numbers of people travel to China to visit friends and relatives, to study, or to adopt children. These groups may be at particularly high risk of illness because they underestimate their risks, are less likely to seek pre-travel advice, and stay in more local or rural accommodations. People traveling to China to adopt children often worry about the health of the child but neglect their own travel health safety.

Health Issues

Although China is now the world's third-largest economy, in per capita terms it is still a low-income country, with wide disparity in income and development between rural and urban and east and west. Health risks vary accordingly.

Immunizations

Routine vaccinations should be up-to-date, including tetanus/diphtheria, measles, rubella, varicella, influenza, and pneumococcal vaccines, as indicated. In addition, hepatitis A, hepatitis B, and typhoid vaccinations are usually recommended. Measles immunity is particularly important, as China reports upwards of 100,000 measles cases annually. A few travelers have made news headlines by triggering outbreaks in their own countries on return from trips to China.

Rabies Vaccine

Rabies is a serious problem in China, as in much of Asia, with more than 3,000 human deaths per year reported in recent years. This mortality rate has made rabies, at least officially, the most important infectious disease killer of humans in China. Animal bites in any area of China, including urban areas, must be considered high risk for

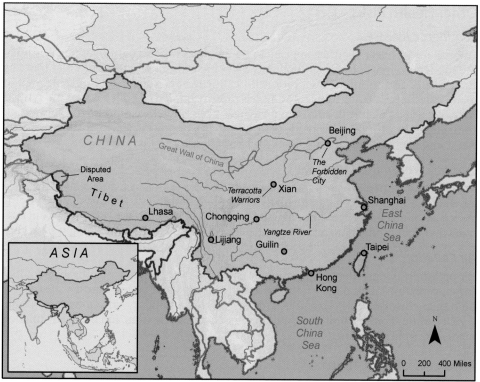

Map 3-7. Destination map of China.

rabies. As international standard rabies immune globulin is generally unavailable, animal bites are often trip-enders, requiring evacuation to Hong Kong or home for postexposure prophylaxis. Bites are surprisingly common in tourists; dog bites were the most common dermatologic problem seen after China travel in a recent analysis of data from the GeoSentinel Network. Rabies risk and prevention should be discussed in pre-travel consultations, and a strategy for dealing with a possible exposure should be developed.

Japanese Encephalitis Vaccine

Japanese encephalitis (JE) occurs in all regions except Qinghai, Xinjiang, and Xizang (Tibet). Although the JE season varies by region, most human cases are reported from April to October. The risk of JE for most travelers to China is very low but varies based on season, destination, duration, and activities. Risk is highest among travelers to rural areas during the transmission season. JE vaccine is only recommended for travelers who plan to spend a month or longer in endemic areas or shorter-term travelers who plan to spend significant time in rural areas or doing outdoor activities. However, rare sporadic cases have occurred on an unpredictable basis in short-term travelers, including those on Yangtze River cruises or in peri-urban Beijing.

Malaria

Malaria is very rarely a consideration for travelers to China, with the exception of those visiting rural parts of Anhui, Yunnan, or Hainan Island. For these areas, chemoprophylaxis should be considered; for travelers to other regions, the risk is too low to warrant it. Rare cases occur in other rural parts of the country below 1,500 m (4,921 ft) between May and December, and only insect precautions are recommended.

Other Health Risks

Foodborne Illnesses

The risk for travelers' diarrhea appears to be low in deluxe accommodations in China, but moderate elsewhere. Usual food and water precautions should apply, and travelers should carry an antibiotic for empiric self-treatment. Tap water is not drinkable even in major cities, except Hong Kong. Most hotels provide bottled or boiled water, and bottled water is easily available. In addition, there have been several well-publicized episodes of contamination of food with pesticides and other substances. Travelers should strictly avoid undercooked fish and shellfish, and unpasteurized milk.

Sexually Transmitted Diseases

Sexually transmitted diseases, including syphilis, HIV, gonorrhea, and chlamydia, are a growing problem in China, particularly along the booming eastern seaboard. Travel is associated with loosened inhibitions and increased casual sexual liaisons. Aside from risk-reduction counseling, remember hepatitis B vaccination for those who might be at risk.

Air Pollution

Air pollution is a problem in most major cities in China. There is significant potential for exacerbation of respiratory conditions, including asthma and chronic obstructive pulmonary disease (COPD), and heightened risk for respiratory infections. Susceptible travelers should receive influenza and pneumococcal vaccination and bring any inhaled medications they may use.

Medical Care in China

Western-style medical facilities that meet international standards are available in Beijing, Shanghai, and Hong Kong. Some hospitals in other cities have "VIP wards" (*gaogan bingfang*), which may have English-speaking staff. The standard of care in such facilities is somewhat unpredictable, and cultural and regulatory differences can cause difficulties for travelers. In rural areas, only rudimentary medical care may be available. Hepatitis B transmission from poorly sterilized medical equipment remains a risk outside major centers.

Pharmacies often sell prescription medications over the counter. Such medications have sometimes been counterfeit, substandard, or even contaminated. Travelers should carry all their regular medications in sufficient quantity; if more or other medications are required, it is advisable to visit a reputable clinic or hospital.

Some travelers wish to try traditional Chinese medicine and acupuncture. While most do so uneventfully, there is potential risk from nonsterile acupuncture needles and contamination of traditional medicine products with heavy metals or pharmaceutical agents. Acupressure may be preferable to acupuncture.

Language and Culture

Finally, language will be a problem for many travelers to China. Outside major tourist destinations, English speakers may be rare, and most signage will be in Chinese characters. In general, people are helpful and friendly to tourists, and personal safety is rarely an issue. Cultural sensitivity is essential, however. Chinese will often ask near strangers about their weight, their age, and their income, subjects that are taboo in many Western cultures. Travelers should try to avoid taking offense. In turn, Westerners may offend Chinese by raising their voice, losing their temper, or otherwise bringing conflict into the open. Whatever the problem, patience, firmness, and sensitivity to "face" will almost always work better in China than open confrontation.

References

1. Measles among adults associated with adoption of children in China—California, Missouri and Washington, July–August 2006. MMWR Morb Mortal Wkly Rep 2007;56(7):144–6.

2. Zhang YZ, Xiong CL, Xiao DL, et al. Human rabies in China [letter]. Emerg Infect Dis. 2005;11(12):1983–4.
3. Tang X, Luo M, Zhang S, et al. Pivotal role of dogs in rabies transmission, China. Emerg Infect Dis. 2005;11(12):1970–2.
4. Davis XM, MacDonald S, Borwein S, et al. Health risks in travelers to China: the GeoSentinel experience and implications for the 2008 Beijing Olympics. Am J Trop Med Hyg. 2008;79(1):4–8.
5. Shaw MT, Leggat PA, Borwein S. Traveling to China for the Beijing 2008 Olympic and Paralympic Games. Travel Med Infect Dis. 2007:5(6):365–73.
6. Cutfield J, Anderson NE, Brickell K, et al. Japanese encephalitis acquired during travel in China. Intern Med J. 2005;35(8):497–8.
7. Shlim DR, Solomon T. Japanese encephalitis: Exploring the limits of risk. Clin Infect Dis. 2002;35(2):183–8.
8. Chen XS, Gong XD, Liang GJ, et al. Epidemiologic trends of sexually transmitted diseases in China. Sex Transm Dis. 2000; 27(3):138–42.

COSTA RICA

Christie M. Reed

Destination Background

What better name than "rich coast" to describe this 19,730-mi^2 (51,000-km^2) country with only 0.03% of the world's landmass, but a total of 802 miles of coastline (132 miles on the Caribbean and 631 miles on the Pacific) and 5% of the world's biodiversity? Exotic birds, butterflies, howler monkeys, and sloths put the country first on the list of destinations for an increasing number of U.S. travelers.

About the same size as West Virginia or Vermont and New Hampshire combined, Costa Rica is often compared to the former for the many rivers that make whitewater rafting and kayaking popular. One-fourth of the land is protected in a series of reserves, such as the Cloud Forests of Monteverde (private) and Santa Elena (public), which straddle the Continental Divide running from Nicaragua in the north to Panama in the south–southeast. The mountain range contains Cerro Chirripo, at 12,532 ft the fifth highest peak in Central America, and active volcanoes, such as Arenal, with the Smithsonian Institution Observatory Lodge on its flank and Costa Rica's largest lake, Lake Arenal, nearby. In addition to picturesque beaches, several islands are also contained within Costa Rica's 589,000 km^2 of territorial waters. Calero is the largest at 151.6 km^2 (58.5 mi^2), but the farthest from shore is Cocos, only 24 km^2 (9.25 mi^2) but 300 miles (480 km) from Puntarenas in the Pacific. Puntarenas is only a 3-hour car ride (284 km) from Limon City on the Caribbean coast.

Tourism has replaced bananas and coffee as the major source of foreign exchange. If growth continues as it has for the past few years, more than 2 million visitors are expected to visit in 2008, up from 1,725,000 in 2006, attracted by the physical beauty and the opportunities for adventure- and eco-tourism.

Approximately half the visitors are from the United States and Canada, arriving almost equally by air and water; Costa Rican ports on both coasts are included on many of the cruises that traverse the canal in adjoining Panama. About 30,000–50,000 U.S. citizens, including many retirees, reside in the country.

The military was abolished over 50 years ago in favor of social programs such as health care and education, resulting in a literacy rate of 96%. However, about 16% of the population live below the poverty line and inflation is high. There is an extensive tourism infrastructure and a well-developed ecotourism industry that does conduct inspections, but the standards may not be the same as in the United States. Resources to maintain or modify facilities unfortunately may not be able to keep pace with utilization by rapidly increasing numbers of tourists. However, Costa Rica intends to be the first carbon-neutral country by 2021.

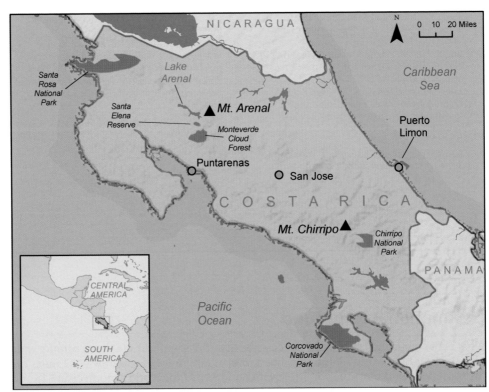

Map 3-8. Destination map of Costa Rica.

Health Issues

Physical Concerns for the Traveler

Crime

The U.S. Department of State considers the crime rate to be high. Tourists are frequently targeted for scams, including a series of robberies at gunpoint of cars leaving the Juan Santa Maria Airport after 10:30 pm in 2006. These events ceased with police intervention, but the U.S. Embassy in the capitol, San Jose has received more reports of lost passports as of April 2008 than any Embassy in the world, frequently because of thefts of belongings in rental cars.

Traffic

Speed, aggressive driving, and alcohol are universal contributors to road fatalities, but here the features that may make the countryside picturesque, such as narrow gorges, animals, and lack of signs, or even the presence of other tourists as cyclists, may also play a role in accidents, which are common (see the Injuries and Safety section in Chapter 2). Rules of the road may not be observed, and pedestrians are not given the right of way. During the rainy season (May to November), mudslides, road washouts, and the resultant potholes are a concern. Weather may vary throughout the country's microclimates, but flooding can occur in low-lying areas year round.

Natural Disasters

In countries on the Pacific Rim or "ring of fire," earthquakes are not uncommon, and Costa Rica is home to seven active volcanoes. The last earthquake to cause significant damage occurred in 1991, was 7.6 on the Richter scale, and killed 47 people. The last major volcanic eruption was in 1963. Special building codes are reported to be strictly followed in high-population areas like the capital city of San Jose, and long-term residents are encouraged to have an earthquake emergency plan.

Beaches

Beaches are one of the main attractions, with over 50 named tourist resorts, the vast majority of which are on the west coast. Just as on other beaches along the Pacific and Caribbean coasts, currents can be swift and dangerous with riptides or sudden drop-offs from shallow water. Travelers should be vigilant. The absence of warning signs and lifeguard stations, for example, on public beaches does not represent an absence of risk. The U.S. Department of State reports that 8–12 American citizens drown in Costa Rica each year.

Infectious Disease Concerns

Travelers should observe basic food and water precautions and consult with their travel medicine clinician regarding self-treatment for travelers' diarrhea and vaccination for hepatitis A. Those who will be staying or living in more rural areas or who will be staying in Costa Rica long-term should consider typhoid vaccination.

Vector-Borne Diseases

The distribution and extent of vector-borne infections are not static. The exact parameters are not well understood, but alterations in climactic conditions, such as rainfall and temperature, interventions such as control measures, alteration in habitat or host, or spillover from a nearby area can affect the temporal and geographic distribution of the diseases listed below. The CDC Travelers' Health website (www.cdc.gov/travel) should be consulted for the most current information. For more details on the individual infectious agents, please see the relevant sections in Chapters 2 and 5.

Leishmaniasis

Cutaneous leishmaniasis (CL) is considered one of the main emergent diseases in the Americas. An interplay of environmental factors, climate cycles (such as those associated with El Niño), social factors, and deforestation, are thought to play a role in explaining variations in disease risk. *Leishmania* spp. are endemic in most parts of Costa Rica, and the CDC's Division of Parasitic Diseases has noted increasing numbers of inquiries/consults about diagnosis and treatment of CL in travelers returning from vacation, sometimes involving more than one person in a group of travelers. *Leishmania* spp. are transmitted by the bite of an infected sandfly. Sandflies typically feed, like the anopheline mosquitoes which transmit malaria, from dusk to dawn, thus travelers are most at risk at twilight or while they sleep. Travelers to areas that are not considered to be at risk of malaria may not appreciate the need for insect repellent and barrier precautions such as bed nets. Travelers who engage in water sports, such as rafting and whitewater kayaking, or adventure sports may not recognize the need to reapply insect repellent after excessive sweating or emerging from water. Their activities may also disturb resting sandflies, prompting them to bite during the day. Clinicians should therefore advise travelers of preventive measures, have a high degree of suspicion for CL in the differential diagnosis of skin lesions in returning travelers, and, if needed, consult the CDC's Division of Parasitic Diseases for assistance with diagnosis and management (see the Cutaneous Leishmaniasis section in Chapter 5 for contact information).

Malaria

Malaria transmission occurs principally in Limon province, but not in Limon City, the port of entry to the country from the Caribbean. Longer term travelers may prefer to use chloroquine for malaria prevention when traveling here. Because this is an area with mostly *P. vivax*, shorter term travelers (with normal G6PD activity) may prefer to use primaquine. Rare cases occur in Puntarenas, Alajuela, Guanacaste, and Heredia Provinces as well, but mosquito avoidance measures only are recommended for travelers to these areas.

Cutaneous Larva Migrans (CLM)

CLM is a common linear, parasitic skin infestation which results from the direct exposure of skin to infected sand that has been contaminated with cat or dog hookworm larvae.

It can be prevented by maintaining a barrier, such as a towel or shoes, between the traveler's skin and beaches that have been contaminated by animal feces.

Myiasis

Infestation with the larval form of the bot fly (*Dermatobium hominis*) can result in a painful skin lesion. The larvae often gain access to the skin from contact with eggs laid on clothes left outside to dry. The heat from ironing clothes is usually effective in preventing infestation if the clothes cannot be hung inside to dry.

Dengue

Autochthonous cases of dengue reappeared in Costa Rica in 1993, associated with reinfestation of *Aedes aegypti* after a 30-year absence. Over 25,000 cases were reported in 2007, and all four serotypes have been detected. Travelers should be advised to observe mosquito precautions at all times.

Summary

Most of the health risks described above are avoidable with a bit of planning. Travelers should be reminded that the environmental factors that contribute to a varied, lush ecosystem also provide suitable environments for vectors capable of transmitting disease. Awareness of the potential for exposure can allow use of barrier and insect avoidance measures or prompt diagnosis and treatment. Avoidance of the physical hazards primarily involves the application of common sense. The diversity, proximity, and stability of Costa Rica are appealing to many types of U.S. travelers, including families, adventure tourists, and expatriates, who reside or have retired there. Costa Rica's proximity and diversity make it an ideal locale that demands fewer preventive interventions than perhaps many other "exotic" destinations.

References

1. World Resources Institute. Earthtrends: Energy and resources country profiles, Costa Rica. [cited 2008 Nov 29]. Available from: http://earthtrends.wri.org/country_profiles/index.php?theme=6.
2. United Nations World Tourism Organization. International Tourist Arrivals by Country of Destination [Table]. World Tourism Barometer. 2008;6(2):30. [cited 2008 Oct 16]. Available from: http://www.tourismroi.com/Content_Attachments/27670/File_633513750035785076.pdf.
3. Overseas Security Advisory Council. Costa Rica 2008 Crime and Safety Report. Washington D.C.: U.S. Department of State; 2008. [cited 2008 Apr 11]. Available from: https://www.osac.gov/Reports/report.cfm?contentID=81286.
4. U.S. Department of State. Background Note: Costa Rica. [2008 Oct 8]. Available from: http://www.state.gov/r/pa/ei/bgn/2019.htm.
5. Chaves LF, Cohen JM, Pascual M, Wilson ML. Social exclusion modifies climate and deforestation impacts of a vector-borne disease. PLoS Negl Trop Dis. 2008;2(2):e176.
6. Saenz R, Bissel RA, Paniagua F. Post disaster malaria in Costa Rica. Prehospital Diaster Med. 1995;10(3):154–60.
7. Troyo A, Porcelain S, Calderon-Arguedas O, et al. Dengue in Costa Rica: the gap in local scientific research. Rev Panam Salud Publica. 2006;20(5):350–60.

NEPAL

David R. Shlim

Destination Background

Nepal is a country of over 27 million people that stretches for 500 miles (805 km) along the Himalayan mountains that form the border of Nepal and Tibet. The topography rises from low plains with an altitude of 200 ft (70 m) to the highest point in the world at 29,135 ft (8,848 m), the peak of Mt. Everest. About 25% of tourists come to Nepal to trek into the mountains, while others come to experience the culture and stunning natural beauty. Kathmandu is the capital city, with a population of over 1 million people. It sits in a lush valley at 4,300 ft in altitude (1,300 m). Nepal's latitude of 28° north (the same as Florida) means that the nonmountainous areas are temperate year round. Most of the annual rainfall comes during the monsoon season (June through September). The main tourist seasons are in the spring (March to May) and fall (October and November). The winter months, December through February, are pleasant in the lowlands, but can be too cold to make trekking enjoyable in the high mountains.

There are three main trekking areas: the Mt. Everest region east of Kathmandu, the Annapurna region to the west, and the Langtang region north of Kathmandu. Trekkers into the Mt. Everest region routinely sleep at altitudes of over 14,000–16,000 ft (4,200–4,900 m) and hike to altitudes over 18,000 ft (5,500 m). This prolonged exposure to very high altitudes means that tourists must be knowledgeable about the risks of high-altitude illness and may need to carry specific medications to prevent and treat the problem (see the Altitude Illness section in Chapter 2). The majority of trekkers into the Mt. Everest region arrive there by flying to a tiny airstrip at Lukla at 9,000 ft (2,700 m). The following day they reach Namche Bazaar at 11,300 ft (3,500 m). Acetazolamide prophylaxis can greatly decrease the chances of developing acute mountain sickness in Namche.

In the Annapurna region, short-term trekkers may choose to hike to viewpoints in the foothills without reaching any high altitudes. Others may undertake the 15- to 20-day trek around the Annapurna massif, going over a 17,700-ft (5400-m) pass. The total exposure to high altitude is less in this region than in the Everest region. The Langtang region has a high point of 14,000 ft (4,200 m).

In addition to trekking, Nepal has some of the best rafting and kayaking rivers in the world. Jungle lodges in Chitwan National Park allow tourists to view a wide range of wildlife, including tigers, rhinocerous, bears, and crocodiles. It is also possible to travel by road to comfortable lodges in the foothills that afford panoramic views of the Himalayas.

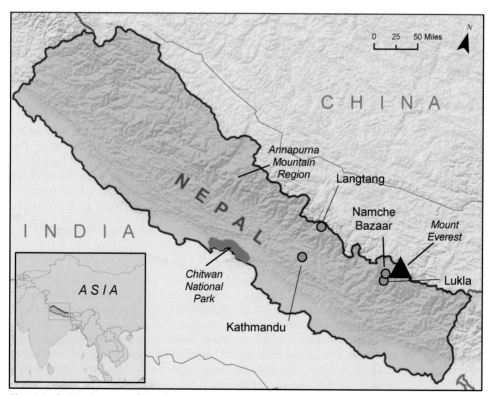

Map 3-9. Destination map of Nepal.

Health Issues

Nepal has a high risk for enterically transmitted diseases. Hepatitis A vaccine and typhoid vaccine are the two most important immunizations. The risk for typhoid fever among travelers to Nepal is one of the highest in the world.

Japanese encephalitis (JE) is endemic in Nepal, mainly in the Terai region during and immediately after the monsoon season, which usually runs from mid-June to mid-September. JE has been detected in local people living in the Kathamandu Valley (outside the city), but there have been no reported cases of JE in a tourist or expatriate in Nepal. The vaccine is not recommended for usual tourists or trekkers unless they will be spending time living in rural low-altitude areas during the season of risk. However, in recent years, expatriates living in Nepal are usually immunized against JE because they may frequently take side trips outside Kathmandu (see the JE section in Chapter 2).

Malaria is not a risk for the vast majority of travelers to Nepal. There is no risk for malaria in Kathmandu or Pokhara, the two main cities in Nepal. All the main trekking routes in Nepal are free of malaria risk. Chitwan National Park is a popular tourist destination for wildlife viewing in the Terai. While it is noted that the Nepalese Ministry of Health and other regional organizations regard the Terai to be a malaria transmission area, this author, in 25 years of treating travelers in Nepal, has not seen a single case of malaria in a traveler to Chitwan, and therefore considers the risk within Chitwan National Park for malaria to be low.

Cyclospora cayetanensis is an intestinal protozoal pathogen that is highly endemic in Nepal. The risk for infection is distinctly seasonal: transmission occurs almost exclusively from May to October, with a peak in June and July. Because this is outside the main tourist seasons, the primary impact is on expatriates who stay through the monsoon. Profound anorexia and fatigue are the hallmark symptoms of *Cyclospora* infection. The treatment of choice is trimethoprim–sulfamethoxazole; no highly effective alternatives have been identified.

Hepatitis E virus is endemic in Nepal, and several cases each year are diagnosed in tourists or expatriates. There is no vaccine commercially available against hepatitis E.

The Kathmandu Valley often has air pollution. People with asthma or even just a history of asthma may suffer exacerbations in Kathmandu, particularly after a viral upper respiratory infection. Asthma has not been a significant problem in tourists outside Kathmandu.

Rabies is highly endemic among dogs in Nepal, but in recent years there are fewer stray dogs in Kathmandu. Half of all tourist exposures (caused by bites or scratches from dogs and monkeys) that lead to postexposure rabies immunoprophylaxis occur near Swayambunath, a beautiful hilltop shrine also known as the monkey temple, so tourists should be advised to be extra cautious with both dogs and monkeys in this area. The monkeys can be aggressive if approached and can jump on a person's back if they smell food in a backpack. Clinics that specialize in the care of foreigners almost always have complete postexposure rabies immunoprophylaxis, including human rabies immune globulin. Trekkers who are bitten in the mountains are able to return to Kathmandu within an average of 5 days.

Empiric Medications

Since many tourists are heading to remote areas that do not have medical care available, they should be provided with medications for self-treatment. Travelers' diarrhea is a significant risk, and the risk in the spring trekking season (March to May) is double that in the fall trekking season (October and November). All trekkers should have an antibiotic such as ciprofloxacin for empiric treatment of bacterial diarrhea. *Campylobacter* accounts for as much as 20% of the etiology of bacterial diarrhea in Nepal, and up to 70% of the *Campylobacter* isolates are resistant to fluoroquinolones. Although ciprofloxacin remains an excellent choice for empiric treatment of bacterial diarrhea, azithromycin is an excellent alternative and should be used if there is no response to ciprofloxacin.

Viral upper respiratory infections (URI) are extremely common, and the percentage of these that lead to bacterial sinusitis or bronchitis is high. Trekkers may wish to carry an antibiotic, such as azithromycin, for empiric treatment of a prolonged URI that results in bronchitis or sinusitis. It is possible that more treks have been ruined by respiratory infection than by gastrointestinal illness.

Evacuation

Helicopter evacuation from most areas is readily available. Communication has improved from remote areas because of satellite and cell phones, and private helicopter companies accept credit cards and are eager to perform evacuations for profit. Evacuation can sometimes take place on the same day as the request, if weather permits. Helicopter rescue is usually limited to morning hours due to afternoon winds in the mountains. The cost of helicopter evacuation ranges from $3000 to $5000.

Two main clinics in Kathmandu specialize in the care of foreigners in Nepal. Contact information is available on the International Society of Travel Medicine website (www.istm.org). Hospital facilities have improved steadily over the years, and emergency general or orthopedic surgery is reliable and available in Kathmandu. The closest evacuation point for definitive care is Bangkok.

References

1. Schwartz E, Shlim DR, Eaton M, et al. The effect of oral and parenteral typhoid vaccination on the rate of infection with Salmonella Typhi and Salmonella Paratyphi A among foreigners in Nepal. Arch Intern Med. 1990;150(2):349–51.
2. Cave W, Pandey P, Osrin D, Shlim DR. Chemoprophylaxis use and the risk of malaria in travelers to Nepal. J Travel Med. 2003;10(2):100–5.
3. Hoge CW, Shlim DR, Echeverria P, et al. Epidemiology of diarrhea among expatriate residents living in a highly endemic environment. JAMA. 1996;275(7):533–8.

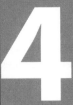

4

The Post-Travel Consultation

GENERAL APPROACH TO THE RETURNED TRAVELER

Carlos Franco-Paredes

Risk of Illness in Travelers

- An estimated 15%–70% of international travelers returning to the United States have a travel-related illness. The likelihood of developing a medical condition during travel relates to an individual's past medical history, travel destination, duration of travel, level of accommodation, pre-travel immunization history, adherence to prescribed malaria chemoprophylaxis regimens, activities during travel, and especially to his or her history of exposure to infectious agents prior to and during travel.
- While some illnesses that occur in returned travelers may begin during the travel period, others may occur weeks, months, or even years after return. In many cases, travelers may be harboring a pathogen in its incubation phase that becomes clinically evident in the immediate post-travel period. In terms of clinical severity, most travel-related illnesses are mild, but 1%–5% of travelers become sick enough to seek medical care either during or after travel. Thus, a history of travel, particularly within the previous 6 months, should be part of the routine medical history for every ill patient, especially those with a febrile illness.
- Particular groups of travelers are considered at higher risk of developing illness after returning to their place of residence. Travelers visiting friends and relatives are often less likely to seek pre-travel advice, obtain vaccinations, or take antimalarial prophylaxis. Adventure travelers and persons visiting friends and relatives overseas are at greater risk for becoming ill, in part because of increased exposure to pathogens.

Types of Illnesses

- The most frequent health problems in ill returned travelers are persistent gastrointestinal illness (10%), skin lesions or rashes (8%), respiratory infections (5%–13%, depending on season of travel), and fever (up to 3%).
- Although gastrointestinal upset is the most frequent problem, febrile illnesses represent the most serious of the spectrum of illnesses in travelers. Infections such

as malaria may be life threatening, and others may pose a serious public health hazard (e.g., tuberculosis, measles, viral hemorrhagic fever).

- A recent analysis of the GeoSentinel Surveillance Network, a partnership of the International Society of Travel Medicine (www.istm.org) and CDC that gathers data from more than 30 travel and tropical medical clinics worldwide, has shown substantial regional differences in the morbidity of various syndromic categories in relation to place of exposure among ill returned travelers. For example, dermatologic problems were among the most frequent diagnoses among travelers returning from the Caribbean or Central or South America, while the diagnosis of acute diarrhea was more common for travelers returning from South Central Asia. Malaria was identified as one of the three most frequent causes of systemic febrile illness among travelers from any region. Other than malaria, travelers returning from sub-Saharan Africa were diagnosed most often with rickettsial infections, as well as typhoid and dengue.

- Fever is a frequently reported complaint among returned travelers. Recently, the GeoSentinel Surveillance Network reviewed its data on 24,920 travelers. This global surveillance system reported that 28% (6,957) of returned travelers seen at GeoSentinel clinics from March 1997 through March 2006 had fever as their chief reason for seeking medical care.

- Fever was a marker of a potentially serious illness in up to 26% of these travelers and often resulted in hospitalization. The most frequent "tropical" causes of fever in the returned traveler are malaria, dengue, invasive bacterial diarrhea, hepatitis A, typhoid, and rickettsial infections. However, nontropical entities such as respiratory or urinary tract infections account for a large proportion of febrile illnesses in returned travelers.

- In terms of gastrointestinal illnesses, acute bacterial gastroenteritis or parasitic diarrhea caused mostly by *Giardia* represents the most common conditions reported by travelers. Parasitic diarrhea may often present as intermittent diarrhea, nausea, headache, and fatigue, but may also present with postprandial rapid expulsions of loose stool. Rarely, postinfectious celiac sprue or postinfectious inflammatory bowel disease may occur after travelers have been ill with travelers' diarrhea. More frequently, causes of persistent gastrointestinal illness are postinfectious irritable bowel syndrome and postinfectious lactose intolerance after an episode of travelers' diarrhea.

- Although infections such as giardiasis or cyclosporiasis are often treated on the basis of clinical findings (without the benefit of laboratory confirmation), intestinal parasitic infections are uncommon causes of persistent diarrhea.

- Most post-travel skin ailments reported are insect bites, pyoderma, scabies, and cutaneous larva migrans.

- A number of diseases may occur months to years after return. The risk is related to the degree of exposure, the duration and season of travel, and the underlying health of the traveler. Some of these late-appearing illnesses include chronic forms of Chagas disease, cutaneous and mucocutaneous leishmaniasis, chronic forms of brucellosis, reactivation of tuberculosis from travel-acquired latent tuberculosis infection, malaria, sequelae of schistosomiasis, and reactivation of chronic systemic mycoses, such as paracoccidioidomycosis or coccidioidomycosis.

Clinical Presentations

- Most travelers infected abroad become ill within 12 weeks after returning to the United States. However, some diseases, such as malaria, may not cause symptoms for as long as 6–12 months or more after exposure (Table 4-1).

- If travelers become ill after they return home, even many months after travel, they should be advised to tell their physician where they have traveled. In particular, fever in a traveler returned from a malarious area should be considered a medical emergency.

- The possibility of malaria as a cause of the fever should be evaluated urgently by appropriate laboratory tests and qualified personnel, and testing should be

Table 4-1. Incubation periods of frequent febrile syndromes in returned travelers

Incubation Period	Syndromes	Etiologies
<2 weeks	Fever with initial nonspecific signs and symptoms	Malaria, dengue, scrub typhus, spotted group rickettsiae, acute HIV, acute hepatitis C, *Campylobacter*, salmonellosis, shigellosis, African trypanosomiasis, leptospirosis, relapsing fever
	Fever and coagulopathy	Meningococcemia, leptospirosis, and other bacterial pathogens associated with coagulopathy, malaria, viral hemorrhagic fevers
	Fever and central nervous system involvement	Malaria, typhoid fever, rickettsial typhus (epidemic caused by *Rickettsia prowazecki*), meningococcal meningitis, rabies, arboviral encephalitis, African trypanosomiasis, encephalitis or meningitis due to worldwide distributed known pathogens, angiostrongyloidiasis, rabies
	Fever and pulmonary involvement	Influenza, pneumonia due to typical pathogens, *Legionella* pneumonia, acute histoplasmosis, acute coccidioidomycosis, Q fever, SARS, malaria
	Fever and skin rash	Viral exanthems (rubella, varicella, mumps, herpes simplex-6), dengue, spotted or typhus group rickettsiosis, typhoid fever, parvovirus B19
2–6 weeks	Various syndromes (fever with pulmonary, dermatologic, central nervous system, or involvement of other sites)	Malaria, tuberculosis, hepatitis A, hepatitis B, hepatitis E, visceral leishmaniasis, acute schistosomiasis, amebic liver abscess, leptospirosis, African trypanosomiasis, viral hemorrhagic fevers, Q fever, acute American trypanosomiasis (Chagas disease)
>6 weeks	Various syndromes (fever with pulmonary, dermatologic, central nervous system, or involvement of other sites)	Malaria, tuberculosis, hepatitis B, hepatitis E, visceral leishmaniasis, filariasis, onchocerciasis, schistosomiasis, amebic liver abscess, chronic mycoses, African trypanosomiasis, rabies, typhoid fever

repeated if the initial result is negative. In this regard, primary care physicians, general medicine practitioners, pediatricians, emergency medicine physicians, and every health-care worker dealing with a febrile returned traveler from a malaria-endemic area should take steps to ensure the patient has serial blood smears evaluated on the day of presentation and consider hospitalization if there is any need for observation.

- In evaluating patients seeking medical care, it is essential to obtain a detailed history of exposures, such as: insect bites; swimming in freshwater; animal bites; sexual contacts; and eating raw meat, seafood, or unpasteurized dairy products.
- Answers to these questions may provide important clues for diagnosis of a particular illness or syndrome in returned travelers. In addition, when an infectious disease is suspected, calculating an approximate incubation period is a useful step in ruling out possible etiologies. For example, fever beginning 3 weeks or longer after return greatly reduces the probability of dengue, rickettsial infections, and viral hemorrhagic fevers in the differential diagnosis.
- This important step helps focus the differential diagnosis on probable causative agents and eliminates unlikely considerations. As indicated by exposure history, time course of illness, and associated signs and symptoms, initial investigations for febrile travelers may include: prompt evaluation of peripheral blood for *Plasmodium* species; a complete blood cell count with differential; liver enzymes; urinalysis; culture of blood, stool, and urine; and chest radiography. More specific diagnostic assays may be useful initially for diseases such as leptospirosis (serology) and acute HIV infection (RNA viral load). However, sometimes acute- and convalescent-phase serologies are required to confirm a particular diagnosis, such as many rickettsial infections.

- Since most primary care physicians have little expertise in tropical diseases, a newly returned, ill international traveler should be preferentially evaluated by an infectious disease or tropical medicine practitioner. For assistance in finding a provider who practices clinical tropical medicine, access the American Society of Tropical Medicine and Hygiene website for a listing by state at www.astmh.org or the International Society of Travel Medicine at www.istm.org.

References

1. Hill DR. Health problems in a large cohort of Americans traveling to developing countries. J Travel Med. 2000;7(5):259–66.

2. Hill DR. The burden of illness in international travelers. N Engl J Med. 2006;354(2):115–7.

3. Ryan ET, Wilson ME, Kain KC. Illness after international travel. N Engl J Med. 2002;347(7):505–16.

4. O'Brien D, Tobin S, Brown GV, Torresi J. Fever in returned travelers: review of hospital admissions for a 3-year period. Clin Infect Dis. 2001;33(5):603–9.

5. Franco-Paredes C, Keystone J. Fever in the returned traveler. Antimicrobial Therapy and Vaccines. Empiric Section. [cited 2008 Jun 1]. Available from: http://www.antimicrobe.org.

6. Wilson ME, Weld LH, Boggild A, et al. Fever in returned travelers: results from the GeoSentinel Surveillance Network. Clin Infect Dis. 2007;44(12):1560–8.

7. Freedman DO, Weld LH, Kozarsky PE, et al; GeoSentinel Surveillance Network. Spectrum of disease and relation to place of exposure among ill returned travelers. N Engl J Med. 2006;354(2):119–30.

8. Steffen R, Rickenbach M, Wilhelm U, et al. Health problems after travel to developing countries. J Infect Dis. 1987;156(1):84–91.

9. Angell SY, Behrens RH. Risk assessment and disease prevention in travelers visiting friends and relatives. Infect Dis Clin North Am. 2005;19(1):49–65.

10. Bacaner N, Stauffer B, Boulware DR, et al. Travel medicine considerations for North American immigrants visiting friends and relatives. JAMA. 2004;291(23):2856–64.

11. Leder K, Tong S, Weld L, et al.; GeoSentinel Surveillance Network. Illness in travelers visiting friends and relatives: a review of the GeoSentinel Surveillance Network. Clin Infect Dis. 2006;43(9):1185–93.

12. Mutsch MM, Spicher VM, Gut C, Steffen R. Hepatitis A virus infections in travelers, 1988–2004. Clin Infect Dis. 2006;42(4):490–7.

13. Jensenius M, Fournier PE, Raoult D. Rickettsioses and the international traveler. Clin Infect Dis. 2004;39(10):1493–9.

14. Basnyat B, Maskey AP, Zimmerman MD, Murdoch DR. Enteric (typhoid) fever in travelers. Clin Infect Dis. 2005;41(10):1467–72.

15. Freedman DO, Leder K. Influenza: changing approaches to prevention and treatment in travelers. J Travel Med. 2005;12(1):36–44.

16. Mutsch M, Tavernini M, Marx A, et al. Influenza virus infection in travelers to tropical and subtropical countries. Clin Infect Dis. 2005;40(9):1282–7.

17. Leder K, Sundararajan V, Weld L, et al.; GeoSentinel Surveillance Group. Respiratory tract infections in travelers: a review of the GeoSentinel surveillance network. Clin Infect Dis. 2003;36(4):399–406.

18. Connor BA. Sequelae of traveler's diarrhea: focus on postinfectious irritable bowel syndrome. Clin Infect Dis. 2005;41(Suppl 8):S577–86.

19. Wilson ME, Chen LH. Dermatologic infectious diseases in international travelers. Curr Infect Dis Rep. 2004;6(1):54–62.

20. Schwartz E, Kozarsky P, Wilson M, Cetron M. Schistosome infection among river rafters on Omo River, Ethiopia. J Travel Med. 2005;12(1):3–8.

ASYMPTOMATIC SCREENING

Carlos Franco-Paredes

There are no official CDC guidelines or recommendations for screening of asymptomatic international travelers, except in special populations such as refugees at the time of their initial domestic evaluation. Cost-effectiveness studies of routine screening in asymptomatic international travelers have not shown a significant benefit to this approach on a population basis. Therefore, a clinic visit or any nonfocused laboratory screening for the majority of travelers is not indicated. Exceptions would be for those with known high-risk exposures that are linked to the transmission of certain agents.

The decision to screen for particular pathogens will depend on the type of travel, itinerary, and exposure history.

- Travelers who have engaged in casual unprotected sex or have received an injection, a body piercing, or a tattoo may be screened for HIV, hepatitis B and C, and potentially transmitted sexually transmitted diseases (such as gonorrhea) with nucleic acid hybridization tests in urine, and for *Chlamydia* infections with nucleic acid amplification tests in urine. Sometimes testing for hepatitis B DNA or hepatitis C RNA viral load and HIV RNA viral load is recommended for travelers with high-risk factors presenting with a febrile illness, in order to rule out the possibility of acute hepatitis B or C or an acute HIV syndrome, respectively.
- Travelers who have been exposed to freshwater in areas endemic for schistosomiasis should be screened for this infection by serology and stool or urine tests, or both. Travelers exposed to soil should be screened for strongyloidiasis and possibly other intestinal parasites. Eosinophilia in a returned traveler suggests the possibility of a helminth infection, of which the most important is strongyloidiasis. If left untreated, this infection may last for the lifetime of the host, and in an immunocompromised person it has the potential to disseminate.
- Travelers who resided in poorly constructed dwellings in highly endemic areas for American trypanosomiasis (Chagas disease) should be serologically screened for latent *Trypanosoma cruzi* infection.
- Asymptomatic international travelers who have been abroad for many months or longer, particularly in resource-limited settings, should be screened for certain diseases, using tests such as hepatitis B serology, HIV serology, syphilis serology, Mantoux intradermal skin test for latent tuberculosis infection (pre-departure baseline skin testing is recommended in long-term travelers visiting resource-limited settings), stool examination for ova and parasites, and complete blood count, including a peripheral eosinophil count and red blood cell parameters.

Asymptomatic screening is encouraged in special populations such as refugees or international adoptees.

- Some of the frequently recommended tests to conduct in these patient groups include—
  - Hepatitis B serologic panel
  - HIV serology
  - Syphilis serology
  - Complete blood count, including a peripheral eosinophil count and red blood cell parameters
- Screening for latent tuberculosis infection can be performed by using one of two modalities: the Mantoux tuberculin skin test (TST) or a blood assay for *Mycobacterium tuberculosis* infection. Currently, the QuantiFERON-TB Gold In-tube Test (QFT-G) is approved for such purposes in the United States in adults. Chest radiograph and sputum studies for mycobacterial staining should be performed for those with positive screening results.

CDC has published guidelines for evaluating refugees for intestinal parasites and tissue-invading parasites during domestic medical evaluations. Screening modalities vary according to predeparture presumptive parasitic therapy:

- Screening for parasitic infection among asymptomatic refugees who had no documented predeparture presumptive antiparasitic therapy should include two morning stool samples for ova and parasite examination by the concentration method.
- Screening for parasitic infection among asymptomatic refugees who received single-dose predeparture treatment with albendazole should include the following:
  - An eosinophil count should be performed in every refugee.
  - Those from Sub-Saharan Africa with persistent eosinophilia should undergo serologic testing for strongyloidiasis and schistosomiasis.
- Screening for parasitic infection among asymptomatic refugees who received high-dose predeparture albendazole (7-day therapy) or ivermectin, with or without

praziquantel should include a follow-up eosinophil count 3–6 months after antiparasitic treatment is suggested for those identified with residual eosinophilia at the initial evaluation.

Further screening and testing guidelines are expected to be issued by the CDC in the near future that will make screening for refugees more uniform and help tailor evaluations to specific populations. These guidelines will be accessible on the CDC website at www.cdc.gov/yellowbook/RefugeeGuidelines.

References

1. Carroll B, Dow C, Snashall D, et al. Post-tropical screening: how useful is it? BMJ. 1993;307(6903):541.
2. Stauffer WM, Kamat D, Walker PF. Screening of international immigrants, refugees, and adoptees. Prim Care. 2002;29(4):879–905.
3. CDC. Refugee health guidelines: domestic guidelines. Guidelines for evaluation of refugees for intestinal and tissue-invasive parasitic infections during domestic medical evaluation. Division of Global Migration and Quarantine, CDC Atlanta, 2008. [cited 2008 Nov 26]. Available from: http://www.cdc.gov/ncidod/dq/refugee/rh_guide/index.htm.

SKIN AND SOFT TISSUE INFECTIONS IN RETURNED TRAVELERS

Jay S. Keystone

Description

Next to fever and diarrheal illness, skin problems are the third most frequent medical problem in returned travelers reported to travel and tropical medicine clinics. The largest case series of dermatologic problems in returned travelers from the GeoSentinel surveillance network showed that cutaneous larva migrans, insect bites, and bacterial infections were the most frequent skin problems in returned travelers, making up 30% of the 4,742 diagnoses (Table 4-2). In another recent review of 165 travelers who returned to France with skin problems, cellulitis, scabies, and pyoderma led the list of skin conditions. These data carry an inherent bias in that they do not include skin problems that were diagnosed and, in many cases, easily managed overseas or that were self-limited.

Skin problems generally fall into one of the following two categories: those associated with fever, usually a rash or secondary bacterial infection (cellulitis, lymphangitis, bacteremia, toxin-mediated), and those not associated with fever. Most skin problems are minor and are not accompanied by fever.

The approach to the diagnosis of skin problems in returned travelers is based on the following:

- Pattern recognition of the lesions (e.g., maculopapular, linear, nodular)
- The location of the lesions (e.g., exposed or unexposed skin surfaces)
- Exposure history (e.g., freshwater, insects, animals, or human contact)
- Associated symptoms (e.g., fever, pain, pruritus)

It is important to remember that skin conditions in returned travelers may not have a travel-related cause.

Papular Lesions

Insect bites, the most common cause of papular lesions, are frequently associated with secondary infection, or hypersensitivity reactions. Bed bugs and fleas can produce

Table 4-2. **Skin lesions in returned travelers, by type of lesion**

Skin Lesion	Percentage (n = 4,742)
Cutaneous larvae migrans	9.8
Insect bite	8.2
Skin abscess	7.7
Superinfected insect bite	6.8
Allergic rash	5.5
Rash, unknown etiology	5.5
Dog bite	4.3
Superficial fungal infection	4.0
Dengue	3.4
Leishmaniasis	3.3
Myiasis	2.7
Spotted fever group rickettsiae	1.5
Scabies	1.5

Modified from Lederman ER, Weld LH, Elyazar IR, et al. Dermatologic conditions of the ill returned traveler: an analysis from the GeoSentinel Surveillance Network. Int J Infect Dis. 2008;12(6):593–602.

papules in groups of three ("breakfast, lunch, and dinner"). Scabies is a mite that frequently presents with a generalized pruritic, papular rash. Very pruritic, excoriated papules may present in a short linear fashion on the skin.

Onchocerciasis, also known as river blindness, is caused by the filarial nematode *Onchocerca volvulus* (see the Onchocerciasis section in Chapter 5). Skin lesions can present with generalized pruritus, often associated with a papular rash. The filariae are transmitted by day-biting black fly bites. The main risk occurs in long-stay travelers living in rural sub-Saharan Africa, and rarely, Latin America.

Nodular/Subcutaneous Lesions, Including Bacterial Skin Infections

Bacterial skin infections may occur more frequently following bites and other wounds in the tropics, particularly when good hygiene cannot be maintained. Organisms responsible are commonly *Staphylococcus aureus* or *Streptococcus pyogenes*. The presentations can include abscess formation, cellulitis, lymphangitis, or ulceration. Furunculosis, or recurrent pyoderma, is the result of colonization of the skin and nasal mucosa with *Staphylococcus aureus*. Boils may continue to occur weeks or months after a traveler returns.

In addition to pyodermas, cellulitis, or erysipelas may complicate excoriated insect bites or any trauma to the skin. Cellulitis and erysipelas manifest as areas of skin erythema, edema, and warmth in the absence of an underlying suppurative focus; unlike cellulitis, erysipelas lesions are raised, there is a clear line of demarcation at the edge of the lesion, and the lesions are more likely to be associated with fever. Cellulitis, on the other hand, is more likely to be associated with lymphangitis. Cellulitis and erysipelas are usually caused by beta-hemolytic steptococci; *Staphylococcus aureus* (including methicillin-resistant staphylococcus, MRSA) and gram-negative aerobic bacteria may also cause cellulitis.

Emerging antibiotic resistance among staphylococci and *Streptococcus pyogenes* (erythromycin resistance) is problematic because antimicrobial treatment may be more difficult. After return from travel, antibiotic choice will be determined by the presentation and extent of illness. If such a skin problem occurs during travel, the antibiotic choice may depend on whether medical care and follow up are available, as well as which medications are available. Some travelers may benefit from carrying an antibiotic for self-treatment in these circumstances. Choices are difficult, but include trimethoprim/sulfamethoxazole and extended penicillin, a cephalosporin, or a broad-spectrum quinolone. None of these is ideal.

Another common bacterial skin infection in the tropics, due to *S. aureus* and/or *Str. pyogenes*, is impetigo, especially in children. Impetigo is a highly contagious superficial skin infection that generally appears on the arms, legs, or face as "honey-colored" scabs formed from dried serum. The treatment of choice is a topical antibiotic such as mupirocin.

Myiaisis presents as a painful, boil-like lesion. It is caused by an infection with the larval stage of the Tumbu *(Cordylobia anthropophaga)* or bot fly *(Dermatobium hominis)*. The larvae are frequently acquired in Africa and Latin America. The lesions reveal the presence of a small, central punctum that allows the larvae to breathe. There are several described techniques for removal of the larvae.

Tungiasis is a sand flea *(Tunga penetrans)*. The female burrows into the skin, usually the foot, and produces a nodular, subcutaneous lesion with a central dark spot. The lesion expands as the female produces eggs in her uterus. The flea must be extracted surgically.

Loa Loa filariasis can rarely occur in long-stay travelers living in rural sub-Saharan Africa. It is transmitted by day-biting deer flies. The traveler may present with transient, migratory, subcutaneous, painful, or pruritic swelling produced by the adult nematode migration. Rarely, the worm can be visualized crossing the conjunctiva of the eye or eyelid. Eosinophilia is common. It can be diagnosed by finding the larval stages (microfilaria) in blood collected during the day. Serologic tests are also available, but usually not in commercial laboratories. Infection can be prevented by taking 200 mg of diethylcarbmazine once a week while at risk.

Gnathostomiasis is a nematode infection found primarily in Southeast Asia and less commonly in Africa and Latin America. Infection results from eating undercooked or raw freshwater fish. The traveler experiences transient, migratory, subcutaneous, pruritic, or painful swellings that may occur weeks or even years after exposure. The symptoms are due to a single worm migrating throughout the body, including the central nervous system. Eosinophilia is common, and the diagnosis can be made by serology.

Macular Lesions

By far the most frequent macular lesions seen in returned travelers living in warm climates are superficial mycoses such as tinea versicolor and tinea corporis.

Tinea versicolor, which is due to *Malassezia furfura* (previously *Pityrosporum ovale)*, is characterized by asymptomatic hypo- or hyperpigmented oval, slightly scaley patches measuring 1–3 cm, found on the upper chest, neck, and back. Diagnosis is by Wood's lamp or by placing a drop of methylene blue on a slide onto which clear cellulose acetate tape is placed sticky side down, after it has been touched briefly to the skin lesions to pick up superficial scales. Hyphae ("spaghetti") and spores ("meatballs") are readily visible. Treatment with topical or systemic azoles (ketoconazole, fluconazole), or terbenifine is recommended.

Tinea corporis (ringworm) is caused by a number of different superficial fungi. The lesion is often a single lesion, with an expanding red, raised ring, with a central area of clearing in the middle. Treatment is several weeks' application of a topical antifungal agent.

Lyme disease, a tick-borne infection with *Borrelia burgdorferi*, is common in North America, Europe, and Russia (see the Lyme Disease section in Chapter 5). The traveler presents with one or more large erythematous patches, with or without central clearing, surrounding a prior tickbite. The patient may not have noted the tick bite.

Linear Lesions

Cutaneous larva migrans is the result of infection of the skin with a larva from a dog or cat hookworm *(Ancylostoma brasiliensis)* (see the Cutaneous Larva Migrans section in Chapter 5). Dogs and cats that defecate on beaches appear to be one of the main risks for travelers. Lesions appear on the feet or buttocks most commonly. The traveler presents with an extremely pruritic, serpiginous, linear lesion that migrates within the skin at the rate of 2–4 cm per day. Treatment is with oral albendazole or ivermectin, but a topical cream of 10% thiabendazole is also effective.

Phytophotodermatitis results from spilling lime juice onto the skin in a sunny climate. The result is exaggerated sunburn that gives rise to a linear, asymptomatic lesion that later develops hyperpigmentation. The hyperpigmentation may take weeks or months to resolve.

Lymphocuticular spread of infection occurs when organisms spread along superficial cutaneous lymphatics, producing a raised, linear cord-like lesion along which nodules or ulcers may be found. Examples are sporotrichosis, *Mycobacterium marinum* (associated with exposure to water), bartonellosis (cat-scratch disease), tularemia, and blastomycosis.

Skin Ulcers

Ulcerated skin lesions may result from *Staphyloccus* infections or may be the direct result of an unseen spider bite. Often the etiology of such an ulcer is not clear. Of particular concern is the ulcer caused by **cutaneous leishmaniasis**, which results from the bite of a sand fly. The main areas of risk are Latin America, the Mediterranean, Middle East, and Asia. The lesion is a chronic, usually painless ulcer with heaped-up margins on exposed skin surfaces. Special diagnostic techniques are necessary to confirm the diagnosis, and treatment is problematic. If cutaneous leishmaniasis is suspected, contact the CDC for further advice (see the Leishmaniasis, Cutaneous section in Chapter 5 for contact information).

Miscellaneous Skin Infections

Skin Infections Associated with Water

Soft tissue infections can occur after both freshwater and saltwater exposure, particularly if there is associated trauma. Puncture wounds due to fishhooks and fish spines, lacerations due to inanimate objects during wading and swimming, and bites from fish or other sea creatures may be the source of the trauma leading to waterborne infections. The most common soft tissue infections associated with exposure to water or water-related animals include *Mycobacterium marinum*, *Aeromonas* species, *Edwardsiella tarda*, *Erysipelothrix rhusiopathiae*, and *Vibrio vulnificus*. A variety of skin and soft tissue manifestations may occur in association with these infections, including cellulitis, abscess formation, ecthyma gangrenosum, and necrotizing fasciitis. The majority of *Vibrio* infections occur in men; *Vibrio vunificus* may be especially severe in those with underlying liver disease. *M. marinum* lesions usually appear as solitary nodules or papules on an extremity, especially on the dorsum of feet and hands that subsequently progress to shallow ulceration and scar formation. Occasionally "sporotrichoid" spread may occur as the lesions spread proximally along superficial lymphatics.

"Hot tub folliculitis" due to *Pseudomonas aeruginosa* may result from the use of spa pools or whirlpools, or exposure to inadequately chlorinated swimming pools and hot tubs. Folliculitis typically develops 8–48 hours after exposure in contaminated water and consists of tender, pruritic papules, papulopustules, or nodules. Most patients have malaise and some have low grade fever. The condition is self-limited in 2–12 days; no antibiotic therapy is typically required.

Skin Infections Associated with Bites

Wound infections following dog and cat bites are caused by a variety of microorganisms. *Staphylococcus aureus*, alpha-, beta-, and gamma-hemolytic streptococci, several genera of gram-negative organisms, and a number of anaerobic microorganisms have all been isolated. The prevalence of *Pasteurella multocida* isolates from dog bite wounds is 20%–50% and is the major pathogen in cat bite wound infections. Management of dog and cat bites includes consideration of rabies prophylaxis, tetanus immunization, and antibiotic prophylaxis. Primary closure of puncture wounds and dog bites to the hand should be avoided. Antibiotic prophylaxis for dog bites is controversial, but because *Pasteurella multocida* is a common accompaniment of cat bites, prophylaxis with amoxicillin–clavulanate or a fluoroquinolone for 3–5 days should be considered.

Fever and Rash

Fever and rash in returned travelers are most often due to a viral infection, with dengue being the most frequent and perhaps most easily recognizable example.

Dengue fever is caused by one of four strains of dengue viruses (see the Dengue Fever section in Chapter 5). The disease is transmitted by a day-biting *Aedes* mosquito often found in urban areas. The disease is characterized by the abrupt onset of high fever, frontal headache (often accompanied by retro-orbital pain), myalgia, and a faint macular rash that becomes evident on the second to fourth day of illness. The rash may become visible only after one presses on the skin, and an area of blanching persists for several seconds.

Chikungunya fever, a virus transmitted by a day-biting *Aedes* mosquito, has recently caused major outbreaks of illness in Southeast Africa and South Asia (see the Chikungunya Fever section in Chapter 5). Chikungunya fever is similar to dengue clinically, including the rash. The major distinguishing feature is that arthritis is common with chikungunya fever and may persist for months. Treatment of the arthritis is with nonsteroidal anti-inflammatory drugs (NSAIDS). Aspirin should be avoided in dengue fever. Serologic tests are available for the diagnosis of both chikungunya and dengue, but often require a convalescent-phase serum to confirm.

South African tick typhus, or African tick bite fever (*Rickettsia africae*) is the most frequent cause of fever and rash in Southern Africa. Transmitted by ticks, the disease is characterized by fever and a papular or vesicular rash associated with localized lymphadenopathy and the presence of an eschar, a mildly painful 1–2-cm black necrotic lesion with an erythematous margin. Diagnosis can be suspected clinically and confirmed by serology. Treatment is with doxycycline.

The category of fever with rash is large, and travel medicine physicians should also consider the following diagnoses: enteroviruses, such as echovirus and coxsackie virus, hepatitis B virus, measles, Epstein–Barr virus, cytomegalovirus, typhus, leptospirosis, and HIV.

References

1. Freedman DO, Weld LH, Kozarsky PE, et al.; GeoSentinel Surveillance Network. Spectrum of disease and relation to place of exposure among ill returned travelers. N Engl J Med. 2006;354(2):119–30.

2. Lederman ER, Weld LH, Elyazar IR, et al. Dermatologic conditions of the ill returned traveler: an analysis from the GeoSentinel Surveillance Network. Int J Infect Dis. 2008;12(6):593–602.

3. Ansart S, Perez L, Jaureguiberry S, et al. Spectrum of dermatoses in 165 travelers returning from the tropics with skin diseases. Am J Trop Med Hyg. 2007;76(1):184–6.

4. Ménard A, Dos Santos G, Dekumyoy P, et al. Imported cutaneous gnathostomiasis: report of five cases. Trans R Soc Trop Med Hyg. 2003;97(2):200–2.

5. Bowers AG. Phytophotodermatitis. Am J Contact Dermat. 1999;10(2):89–93.

6. Magill AJ. Cutaneous leishmaniasis in the returning traveler. Infect Dis Clin North Am. 2005;19(1):241–66.

7. Hochedez P, Canestri A, Guihot A, et al. Management of travelers with fever and exanthema, notably dengue and chikungunya infections. Am J Trop Med Hyg. 2008;78(5):710–3.

8. Oostvogel PM, van Doornum GJ, Ferreira R, et al. African tickbite fever in travelers, Swaziland. Emerg Infect Dis. 2007;13(2):353–5.

9. Wilson ME, Chen LH. Dermatologic Infectious Diseases in International Travelers. Curr Infect Dis Rep.2004;6(1):54–62.

10. Diaz JH. The epidemiology, diagnosis, management, and prevention of ectoparasitic diseases in travelers. J Travel Med. 2006;13(2):100–11.

11. Chosidow O. Clinical practices. Scabies. N Engl J Med. 2006;354(16):1718–27.

12. Klion AD.Filarial infections in travelers and immigrants. Curr Infect Dis Rep. 2008;10(1):50–7.

13. Tristan A, Bes M, Meugnier H, et al.Global distribution of Panton–Valentine leukocidin-positive methicillin-resistant *Staphylococcus aureus*, 2006. Emerg Infect Dis. 2007;13(4):594–600.

14. Bernard P.Management of common bacterial infections of the skin. Curr Opin Infect Dis. 2008;21(2):122–8.

15. Nutman TB, Miller KD, Mulligan M, et al. Diethylcarbamazine prophylaxis for human loiasis. Results of a double-blind study. N Engl J Med. 1988;319(12):752–6.

16. Nontasut P, Bussaratid V, Chullawichit S, et al. Comparison of ivermectin and albendazole treatment for gnathostomiasis. Southeast Asian J Trop Med Public Health. 2000;31(2):374–7.

17. Huang DB, Ostrosky-Zeichner L, Wu JJ, et al. Therapy of common superficial fungal infections. Dermatol Ther. 2004;17(6):517–22

18. Heukelbach J, Feldmeier H. Epidemiological and clinical characteristics of hookworm-related cutaneous larva migrans. Lancet Infect Dis. 2008;8(5):302–9.

19. Lupi O, Tyring SK. Tropical dermatology: viral tropical diseases. J Am Acad Dermatol. 2003;49(6):979–1000.

20. Kain KC.Skin lesions in returned travelers. Med Clin North Am. 1999;83(4):1077–102.

PERSISTENT TRAVELERS' DIARRHEA

Bradley A. Connor

Although most cases of travelers' diarrhea are acute and self-limited (see the Travelers' Diarrhea section in Chapter 2), a certain percentage of travelers will develop persistent gastrointestinal symptoms.

The pathogenesis of persistent travelers' diarrhea generally falls into one of three broad categories: persistent infection or co-infection, chronic underlying gastrointestinal illness unmasked by the enteric infection, or a postinfectious process. The contribution of each of these to the total number of persistent travelers' diarrhea patients is often related to the duration of symptoms following the acute episode of diarrhea.

Persistent Infection

Most cases of travelers' diarrhea are the result of infection with bacteria. Persistent symptoms, however, suggest protozoan parasites as the etiology. Parasites as a group are the pathogens most likely to be isolated from patients with persistent diarrhea, and their probability relative to bacterial infections increases with increasing duration of symptoms. Parasites may also be the cause of persistent diarrhea in those already appropriately treated for a bacterial pathogen.

Giardia is by far the most likely persistent pathogen to be encountered in these patients. Suspicion for giardiasis should be particularly high when upper gastrointestinal symptoms predominate. Untreated, symptoms may last for months even in the immunocompetent host. The diagnosis can often be made through stool microscopy. However, as *Giardia* infects the proximal small bowel, even multiple stool specimens may fail to detect it, and a duodenal aspirate may be necessary for definitive diagnosis. Given the high prevalence of *Giardia* in persistent travelers' diarrhea, empiric therapy is a reasonable option in the appropriate clinical setting after negative stool microscopy and in lieu of duodenal sampling.

Other intestinal parasites that may cause persistent symptoms include *Cryptosporidium parvum*, *Entamoeba histolytica*, *Isospora belli*, *Microsporidia*, and *Dientamoeba fragilis*, as well as *Cyclospora cayetanensis*.

Bacteria in general rarely cause persistence of symptoms, although there are reports of persistent diarrhea in children infected with enteroadherent *Escherichia coli*. A notable exception to this self-limited nature of bacterial diarrhea is seen with *Clostridium difficile*. *C. difficile*-associated diarrhea may follow treatment of a bacterial pathogen with a fluoroquinolone or other antibiotic or may even follow malaria chemoprophylaxis. It is especially important to consider in the patient with persistent travelers' diarrhea that seems refractory to multiple courses of empiric antibiotic therapy. The initial work-up of persistent travelers' diarrhea should always include a *C. difficile* stool toxin assay. Treatment is with metronidazole or oral vancomycin, although increasing reports of resistance have been noted.

Other causes of persistent travelers' diarrhea associated with microbial pathogens include tropical sprue and Brainerd diarrhea. In each case, the offending microbial pathogen has not been identified, but there is an abundance of evidence that all these are infectious diseases. Tropical sprue is a syndrome of persistent travelers' diarrhea associated with malabsorption, fatigue, and deficiencies of vitamins absorbed in both the proximal and distal small bowel. It most commonly affects longer-term travelers, but even short-term visitors to the tropics have been afflicted. The epidemiology of tropical sprue has changed in the past few decades, insofar as there now seem to be fewer cases of tropical sprue diagnosed.

Brainerd diarrhea was first described in 1983 when an epidemic of chronic diarrhea occurred in Brainerd, Minnesota, in which unpasteurized milk from a local dairy was epidemiologically identified as the source, although no specific microbial pathogen was ever identified. At least seven subsequent Brainerd epidemics have been reported since this initial description, including one on a cruise ship in the Galápagos Islands of Ecuador.

Underlying Gastrointestinal Disease

In some cases, persistence of gastrointestinal symptoms relates to chronic underlying gastrointestinal disease or susceptibility unmasked by the enteric infection. Most prominent among these is celiac sprue, a systemic disease manifesting primarily with small bowel changes. In genetically susceptible individuals, villous atrophy and crypt hyperplasia are seen in response to exposure to antigens found in wheat, leading to malabsorption. The diagnosis is made by obtaining appropriate serologic tests, including antigliadin and tissue transglutaminase antibodies. A biopsy of the small bowel showing villous atrophy confirms the diagnosis. Treatment is with a wheat (gluten)-free diet.

Idiopathic inflammatory bowel disease (IBD), both Crohns and ulcerative colitis, may be seen following acute bouts of travelers' diarrhea. A prevailing hypothesis of the pathogenesis of IBD suggests that an initiating endogenous pathogen sets in motion, in genetically susceptible individuals, the conditions for the development of disease. In cases following travelers' diarrhea, this hypothetical process appears to be greatly accelerated.

In the appropriate clinical setting and age group, it may be necessary to do a more comprehensive search for other underlying causes of chronic diarrhea. Colorectal cancer should be considered, particularly in those passing occult or gross blood per rectum or with the onset of a new iron deficiency anemia.

Postinfectious Phenomena

In a certain percentage of patients who present with persistent gastrointestinal symptoms, no specific etiology will be found. Concurrent with recognition of the importance of persistent travelers' diarrhea as a presenting complaint has been the observation that in a certain number of patients with irritable bowel syndrome, the onset of symptoms can be traced to an acute bout of gastroenteritis. Irritable bowel syndrome that develops after acute enteritis has been termed postinfectious irritable bowel syndrome (PI-IBS). In the context of travelers' diarrhea, PI-IBS has been defined as new IBS symptoms by the Rome III criteria.

- At least 3 months of symptoms, with an onset of symptoms at least 6 months previously.
- Recurrent abdominal pain or discomfort associated with two or more of the following features:
  - Improvement with defecation

Table 4-3. Treatment of common intestinal protozoan parasites

Parasite	Disease Severity or Indication	Drug of Choice	Alternative Drugs
Amebiasis (*Entamoeba histolytica*)	Asymptomatic	**Iodoquinol** Adults: 650 mg PO tid × 20d Pediatric: 30–40 mg/kg/d (max. 2g) PO in 3 doses × 20d	**Paromomycin** Adults: 25–35 mg/kg/d PO in 3 doses × 7d Pediatric: 25–35 mg/kg/d PO in 3 doses × 7d *or* **Diloxanide furoate** Adults: 500 mg PO tid × 10d Pediatric: 20 mg/kg/d PO in 3 doses × 10d
	Mild to moderate intestinal disease	*1) Initial:* **Metronidazole** Adults: 500–750 mg PO tid × 7–10d Pediatric: 35–50 mg/kg/d PO in 3 doses × 7–10d *2) Followed by:* **Iodoquinol** Adults: 650 mg PO tid × 20d Pediatric: 30–40 mg/kg/d (max. 2g) PO in 3 doses × 20d	*1) Initial:* **Tinidazole** Adults: 2 g once PO daily × 5d Pediatric >3 yrs of age: 50 mg/kg/d (max. 2g) PO in 1 dose × 3d *2) Followed by:* **Paromomycin** Adults: 25–35 mg/kg/d PO in 3 doses × 7d Pediatric: 25–35 mg/kg/d PO in 3 doses × 7d
	Severe intestinal and extraintestinal disease	*1) Initial:* **Metronidazole** Adults: 750 mg PO tid × 7–10d Pediatric: 35–50 mg/kg/d PO in 3 doses × 7–10d *2) Followed by:* **Iodoquinol** Adults: 650 mg PO tid × 20d Pediatric: 30–40 mg/kg/d (max. 2g) PO in 3 doses × 20d	*1) Initial:* **Tinidazole** Adults: 2 g once PO daily × 5d Pediatric >3 yrs of age: 50 mg/kg/d (max. 2g) PO in 1 dose × 3d *2) Followed by:* **Paromomycin** Adults: 25–35 mg/kg/d PO in 3 doses × 7d Pediatric: 25–35 mg/kg/d PO in 3 doses × 7d
Cryptosporidiosis (*Cryptosporidium*)	Non-HIV infected (Nitazoxanide has not been shown to have efficacy in immunosuppressed persons)	**Nitazoxanide** Adults: 500 mg PO bid × 3d 1–3 yrs of age: 100 mg PO bid × 3d 4–11 yrs of age: 200 mg PO bid × 3d 12–18 yrs of age: 500 mg PO q12h × 3d	
Cyclosporiasis (*Cyclospora cayetanensis*)		**Trimethoprim/ sulfamethoxazole** Adults: TMP 160 mg/SMX 800 mg (1 DS tab) PO bid × 7–10d Pediatric: TMP 5 mg/kg/SMX 25 mg/kg/d PO in 2 doses × 7–10d	

Table 4-3. Treatment of common intestinal protozoan parasites *(Continued)*

Parasite	Disease Severity or Indication	Drug of Choice	Alternative Drugs
Dientamoeba fragilis infection		**Iodoquinol** Adults: 650 mg PO tid × 20d Pediatric: 30–40 mg/kg/d (max. 2g) PO in 3 doses × 20d	**Paromomycin** Adults: 25–35 mg/kg/d PO in 3 doses × 7d Pediatric: 25–35 mg/kg/d PO in 3 doses × 7d *or* **Tetracycline** Adults: 500 mg PO qid × 10d Pediatric: 40 mg/kg/d (max. 2g) PO in 4 doses × 10d *or* **Metronidazole** Adults: 500–750 mg PO tid × 10d Pediatric: 35–50 mg/kg/d PO in 3 doses × 10d
Giardiasis (*Giardia intestinalis*)		**Metronidazole** Adults: 250 mg PO tid × 5–7d Pediatric: 15 mg/kg/d PO in 3 doses × 5–7d *or* **Tinidazole** Adults: 2 g PO once Pediatric: 50 mg/kg PO once (max. 2 g) *or* **Nitazoxanide** Adults: 500 mg PO bid × 3d 1–3 yrs of age: 100 mg PO q12h × 3d 4–11 yrs of age: 200 mg PO q12h × 3d 12–18 yrs of age: 500 mg PO q12h × 3d	**Paromomycin** Adults: 25–35 mg/kg/d PO in 3 doses × 5–10d Pediatric: 25–35 mg/kg/d PO in 3 doses × 5–10d *or* **Furazolidone** Adults: 100 mg PO qid × 7–10d Pediatric: 6 mg/kg/d PO in 4 doses × 7–10d *or* **Quinacrine** Adults: 100 mg PO tid × 5d Pediatric: 2 mg/kg/d PO in 3 doses × 5d (max 300 mg/d)
Isosporiasis (*Isospora belli*)		**Trimethoprim/ sulfamethoxazole** Adults: TMP 160 mg/SMX 800 mg (1 DS tab) PO bid × 10d Pediatric: TMP 5 mg/kg/d/ SMX 25 mg/kg/d PO in 2 doses × 10d	
Microsporidiosis	Ocular (*Encephalitozoon hellem, E. cuniculi, Vittaforma corneae* [*Nosema corneum*])	**Albendazole** Adults: 400 mg PO bid *plus* **Fumagillin**	
	Intestinal (*E. bieneusi, E.* [*Septata*] *intestinalis*)	Drug of choice for *E. bieneusi*: **Fumagillin** Adults: 20 mg PO tid × 14d Drug of choice for *E. intestinalis*: **Albendazole** Adults: 400 mg PO bid × 21d	

(Continued)

Table 4-3. **Treatment of common intestinal protozoan parasites** *(Continued)*

Parasite	Disease Severity or Indication	Drug of Choice	Alternative Drugs
Microsporidiosis *(Continued)*	Disseminated (*E. hellem, E. cuniculi, E. intestinalis, Pleistophora* sp., *Trachipleistophora* sp., and *Brachiola vesicularum*)	**Albendazole** Adults: 400 mg PO bid	

- ○ Onset associated with a change in the frequency of stool
- ○ Onset associated with a change in form (appearance) of stool
- To be labeled PI-IBS, these symptoms should follow an episode of gastroenteritis or travelers' diarrhea if the work-up for microbial pathogens and underlying gastrointestinal disease is negative.

Postinfectious IBS is most often characterized by diarrheal symptoms; however, an array of gastrointestinal symptoms is reported, including bloating, gas, and constipation. Although only recently recognized as an important diagnosis in returning travelers, the syndrome was described more than a half century ago as "postdysenteric colitis," describing continuing symptoms of diarrhea in British troops after successful treatment of amebic dysentery. A decade later, Chaudary and Truelove described 130 patients with IBS, 34 of whom dated the onset of their symptoms to an attack of bacterial dysentery. Since then, others have suggested a high incidence of IBS postgastrointestinal infection, with estimates ranging from 4% to 31%.

Studies in the past decade have elucidated some of the pathophysiology associated with the symptoms of PI-IBS. Patients appear to be unable to down-regulate intestinal inflammation. In a recent study of selected IBS patients, there was a decreased prevalence in those with anti-inflammatory cytokines, IL-10, and TGF-beta, implying more susceptibility to prolonged and severe inflammation. Markers of mucosal inflammation are consistently elevated in patients with postinfectious IBS. The inflammatory cytokine interleukin 1-beta was present in higher levels both during and 3 months after an episode of acute gastroenteritis in the rectal mucosa of eight patients who developed postinfectious IBS, compared with seven patients whose bowel habits returned to normal. Macroscopic and conventional histologic assessment of the intestinal mucosa of patients with postinfectious IBS generally appeared normal within 2 weeks of the acute infectious illness, but chronic inflammation—as revealed by quantitative histology—persists. These changes were seen even 52 weeks after the acute episode. Some evidence indicates that postinfectious IBS may be associated with small bowel bacterial overgrowth and may be effectively treated with nonabsorbable antibiotics that reduce small bowel bacterial counts.

Evaluation of the Patient with Persistent Travelers' Diarrhea

The evaluation of the patient with persistent travelers' diarrhea includes evaluations for persistent infection or co-infection, stool microscopy with at least three ova and parasite stool examinations, *Clostridium difficile* toxin assay, D-xylose test, duodenal aspirate, or empiric treatment for *Giardia*. For underlying gastrointestinal disease, an initial evaluation should include serologic tests for celiac and inflammatory bowel disease. Subsequently, gastrointestinal endoscopy with duodenal aspirate and biopsies may be considered.

References

1. Taylor DN, Connor BA, Shlim DR. Chronic diarrhea in the returned traveler. Med Clin North Am. 1999;83(4):1033–52.

2. Taylor DN, Houston R, Shlim DR, et al. Etiology of diarrhea among travelers and foreign residents in Nepal. JAMA. 1988;260(9):1245–8.

3. Norman FF, Pérez-Molina J, Pérez de Ayala A, et al. *Clostridium difficile*-associated diarrhea after antibiotic treatment for traveler's diarrhea. Clin Infect Dis. 2008;46(7):1060–3.

4. Walker MM. What is tropical sprue? J Gastroenterol Hepatol. 2003;18(8):887–90.

5. Osterholm MT, MacDonald KL, White KE, et al. An outbreak of a newly recognized chronic diarrhea syndrome associated with raw milk consumption. JAMA. 1986;256(4):484–90.

6. Green PH, Jabri B. Coeliac disease. Lancet. 2003;362(9381):383–91.

7. Porter CK, Tribble DR, Aliaga PA, et al. Infectious gastroenteritis and risk of developing inflammatory bowel disease. Gastroenterology 2008;135(3):781–6.

8. Connor BA. Sequelae of traveler's diarrhea: focus on postinfectious irritable bowel syndrome. Clin Infect Dis. 2005;41(Suppl 8):S577–86.

9. Spiller RC. Postinfectious irritable bowel syndrome. Gastroenterology. 2003;124(6):1662–71.

10. Spiller RC, Jenkins D, Thornley JP, et al. Increased rectal mucosal enteroendocrine cells, T lymphocytes and increased gut permeability following acute *Campylobacter enteritis* and in post-dysenteric irritable bowel syndrome. Gut. 2000;47(6):804–811.

FEVER IN RETURNED TRAVELERS

Mary Elizabeth Wilson

Initial Focus

Fever commonly accompanies serious illness in returned travelers. Because it can signal a rapidly progressive infection, such as malaria, the clinician must initiate early evaluation, especially in persons who have visited areas with malaria in recent months (see the Malaria section in Chapter 2). The initial focus in evaluating a febrile returned traveler should be on identifying infections that are rapidly progressive, treatable, or transmissible. In some instances, public health officials must be alerted if the traveler may have been contagious en route or infected with a pathogen of public health importance (e.g., yellow fever) at the origin or destination.

Use of History, Location of Exposure, and Incubation to Limit Differential Diagnosis

Often the list of potential diagnoses is long, but multiple recent studies help to identify more common diagnoses. A significant proportion of illnesses in returned travelers is caused by common, cosmopolitan infections (e.g., bacterial pneumonia, pyelonephritis), so these must be considered along with unusual infections. Because the geographic area of travel determines the relative likelihood of major causes of fever, it is essential to identify where the febrile patient has traveled and lived (Table 4-4). Details about activities (e.g., freshwater exposure in schistosomiasis-endemic areas, animal bites, sexual activities, local medical care with injections) and accommodations in malaria-endemic areas (e.g., use of bed nets, presence of window screens, air conditioning) during travel may provide useful clues. Preparation before travel (e.g., hepatitis A vaccine, yellow fever vaccine) will markedly reduce the likelihood of some infections, so this is a relevant part of the history. Because each infection has a characteristic incubation period (although the range is extremely wide with some infections), the time of exposures needs to be defined in different geographic areas (Table 4-5). This knowledge may allow the clinician to exclude some infections from the differential diagnosis. The majority of serious febrile infections manifest within the first month

Table 4-4. Common causes of fever, by geographic area

Geographic areas	More Common Tropical Disease Causing Fever	Other Infections Causing Outbreaks or clusters in travelers
Caribbean	Dengue, malaria	Acute histoplasmosis, leptospirosis
Central America	Dengue, malaria (primarily *vivax*)	Leptospirosis, histoplasmosis, coccidioidomycosis
South America	Dengue, malaria (predominantly *vivax*)	Bartonellosis
Sub-Saharan Africa	Malaria, primarily *falciparum*; tick-borne rickettsiae; acute schistosomiasis; filariasis	African trypanosomiasis
South Central Asia	Dengue, enteric fever, malaria (primarily non-*falciparum*)	
Southeast Asia	Dengue, malaria (primarily non-*falciparum*)	

Table 4-5. Common infections, by incubation periods

Disease	Usual Incubation Period (Range)	Distribution
Incubation <14 days		
Malaria, *falciparum*	6–30 days (weeks to years)	Tropics, subtropics
Dengue	4–8 days (3–14 days)	Topics, subtropics
Spotted fever rickettsiae	Few days to 2–3 weeks	Causative species vary by region
Leptospirosis	7–12 days (2–26 days)	Widespread; most common in tropical areas
Enteric fever	7–18 days (3–60 days)	Especially in Indian subcontinent
Malaria, *vivax*	8–30 days (often >1 month)	Widespread in tropics/subtropics
Influenza	1–3 days	Worldwide; can also be acquired en route
Acute HIV	10–28 days (10 days to 6 weeks)	Worldwide
Legionellosis	5–6 days (2–10 days)	Widespread
Encephalitis, arboviral (e.g., Japanese encephalitis, tick-borne encephalitis, West Nile virus, other)	3–14 days (1–20 days)	Specific agents vary by region
Incubation 14 days to 6 weeks		
Malaria, enteric fever, leptospirosis	See above incubation periods for relevant diseases	See above distribution for relevant diseases
Hepatitis A	28–30 days (15–50 days)	Most common in developing countries
Hepatitis E	26–42 days (2–9 weeks)	Widespread
Acute schistosomiasis (Katayama syndrome)	4–8 weeks	Most common after travel to sub-Saharan Africa
Amebic liver abscess	Weeks to months	Most common in developing countries
Incubation >6 weeks		
Malaria, amebic liver abscess, hepatitis E	See above incubation periods for relevant diseases	See above distribution for relevant diseases
Tuberculosis	Primary, weeks; reactivation, years	
Leishmaniasis, visceral	2–10 months (10 days to years)	

after return from tropical travel, yet infections related to travel exposures can occasionally occur months or even more than a year after return. In the United States, >90% of reported cases of *falciparum* malaria manifest within 30 days of return, but almost half of cases of *vivax* manifest >30 days after return. A history of prior travel and residence should be an integral part of every medical history.

Findings Requiring Urgent Attention

Presence of associated signs, symptoms, or laboratory findings can help to focus attention on specific infections (Table 4-6). Findings that should prompt urgent attention include hemorrhage, neurologic impairment, and acute respiratory distress. Even if an initial physical examination is unremarkable, it is worth repeating the examination, as new findings may appear that will help in the diagnostic process (e.g., skin lesions, tender liver). Although most febrile illnesses in returned travelers are related to infections, the clinician should bear in mind that other problems, including pulmonary emboli and drug hypersensitivity reactions, can be associated with fever. See Box 4-1 for a list of initial studies for diagnosing patients with unexplained fever.

CDC's Division of Global Migration and Quarantine is responsible for preventing the transmission of illnesses across international borders, and in particular, for preventing transmission of such illnesses into the United States. The following syndromes deserve

Table 4-6. Common clinical findings and associated infections

Common Clinical Findings	Infections to Consider after Tropical Travel
Fever and rash	Dengue, chikungunya, rickettsioses, enteric fever (skin lesions may be sparse or absent), acute HIV infection, measles
Fever and abdominal pain	Enteric fever, amebic liver abscess
Undifferentiated fever and normal or low white blood cell count	Dengue, malaria, rickettsial infection, enteric fever, chikungunya
Fever and hemorrhage	Viral hemorrhagic fevers (dengue and others), meningococcemia, leptospirosis, rickettsial infections
Fever and eosinophilia	Acute schistosomiasis; drug hypersensitivity reaction; fascioliasis and other parasitic infections (rare)
Fever and pulmonary infiltrates	Common bacterial and viral pathogens; legionellosis, acute schistosomiasis, Q fever
Mononucleosis syndrome	Epstein–Barr virus, cytomegalovirus, toxoplasmosis, acute HIV
Fever persisting >2 weeks	Malaria, enteric fever, Epstein–Barr virus, cytomegalovirus, toxoplasmosis, acute HIV, acute schistosomiasis, brucellosis, tuberculosis, Q fever, visceral leishmaniasis (rare)
Fever with onset >6 wk after travel	*Vivax* malaria, acute hepatitis, tuberculosis, amebic liver abscess

---

Box 4-1. Initial studies for diagnosis in returned travelers with unexplained fever[1]

- Complete blood count with differential and platelet estimate
- Liver function
- Blood cultures
- Thick and thin smears for malaria (supplement with rapid diagnostic tests, as available)
- Urinalysis
- Chest X-rays

---

[1]Additional tests will depend on specific findings and exposures

further scrutiny because of their potential for signaling a disease of public health importance. Fever accompanied by—

- skin rash
- difficulty breathing
- shortness of breath
- persistent cough
- decreased consciousness
- bruising or unusual bleeding (without previous injury)
- persistent diarrhea
- persistent vomiting (other than air sickness)
- jaundice
- paralysis of recent onset

Persons who travel to visit friends and relatives (VFRs) often do not seek pre-travel medical advice. Review of GeoSentinel surveillance data showed that a greater proportion of immigrant VFRs presented with serious, potentially preventable travel-related illnesses (and required hospitalization) than did tourist travelers.

Change over Time

Clinicians now have access to many resources on the Internet that can help to provide information about geographic-specific risks, current disease activity, and other useful information, such as drug-susceptibility patterns for pathogens. Infectious diseases are dynamic, as is demonstrated by a recent review of adult returned travelers with fever and rash seen during 2006–2007 at a Paris hospital. The most common diagnosis was chikungunya fever, followed by dengue and African tick bite fever. In contrast, because of the wide use of vaccine, hepatitis A infection is becoming less common in travelers.

Common infections in returned travelers may be seen at unexpected times of the year. Because influenza transmission can occur throughout the year in tropical areas and the peak season in the southern hemisphere is May to August, clinicians in the northern hemisphere must be alert to the possibility of influenza outside the usual flu season.

The tables in this section help to identify some of the more common infections by presenting findings or other characteristics by geographic area of travel and by incubation periods. These highlight only the most common infections. The listed references and websites should be consulted for more detailed information. In most studies, a specific cause for the fever is not identified in about 25% of returned travelers.

Keep in Mind

- Initial symptoms of life-threatening and self-limited infections can be identical.
- Malaria is the most common cause of acute undifferentiated fever after travel to sub-Saharan Africa and to some other tropical areas.
- Fever in returned travelers is often caused by common, cosmopolitan infections, such as pneumonia and pyelonephritis, which should not be overlooked in the search for more exotic diagnoses.
- Patients with malaria may be afebrile at the time of evaluation but typically give a history of chills.
- Malaria, especially *falciparum*, can progress rapidly. Diagnostic studies should be done promptly and treatment instituted immediately if malaria is diagnosed (see the Malaria section in Chapter 2).
- A history of taking malaria chemoprophylaxis does not exclude the possibility of malaria.
- Patients with malaria can have prominent respiratory (including adult respiratory distress syndrome), gastrointestinal, or central nervous system findings.

- Viral hemorrhagic fevers are important to identify but are rare in travelers; bacterial infections, such as leptospirosis, meningococcemia, and rickettsial infections, can also cause fever and hemorrhage and should be always be considered because of the need to institute prompt, specific treatment.
- Sexually transmitted infections, including acute HIV, can cause acute febrile infections.
- Consider infection control, public health implications and requirements for reportable diseases.

References

1. Ryan ET, Wilson MW, Kain K. Illness after international travel. N Engl J Med. 2002;347(7):505–16.

2. Wilson ME, Weld LH, Boggild B, et al.; GeoSentinel Surveillance Network. Fever in returned travelers: results from the GeoSentinel Surveillance Network. Clin Infect Dis. 2007;44(12):1560–8.

3. Bottieau E, Clerinx J, Schrooten W, et al. Etiology and outcome of fever after a stay in the tropics. Arch Intern Med. 2006;166(15):1642–8.

4. O'Brien D, Tobin S, Brown GV, Torresi J. Fever in returned travelers: review of hospital admissions for a 3-year period. Clin Infect Dis. 2001;33(5):603–9.

5. Jensenius M, Fournier PE, Raoult D. Rickettsioses and the international traveler. Clin Infect Dis. 2004;39(10):1493–9.

6. Bottieau E, Clerinx J, Van den Enden E, et al. Infectious mononucleosis-like syndromes in febrile travelers returning from the tropics. J Travel Med. 2006;13(4):191–7.

7. Freedman DO, Weld LH, Kozarsky PE, et al. Spectrum of disease and relation to place of exposure in ill returned travelers. N Engl J Med. 2006;354(2):119–30.

8. Leder K, Tong S, Weld L, et al.; GeoSentinel Surveillance Network. Illness in travelers visiting friends and relatives: a review of the GeoSentinel Surveillance Network. Clin Infect Dis. 2006;43(9):1185–93.

9. Hochedez P, Canestri A, Guihot A, et al. Management of travelers with fever and exanthema, notably dengue and chikungunya infections. Am J Trop Med Hyg. 2008;78(5):710–3.

10. Wilson ME, Freedman DO. The etiology of travel-related fever. Curr Opin Infect Dis. 2007;20(5):449–53.

5

Other Infectious Diseases Related to Travel

Sharon Roy, Barbara L. Herwaldt, Stephanie P. Johnston

Infectious Agent

Amebiasis is caused by the protozoan parasite *Entamoeba histolytica*.

Mode of Transmission

Transmission occurs via the fecal–oral route, either directly by person-to-person contact (e.g., diaper changing, sexual practices) or indirectly by eating or drinking fecally contaminated food or water.

Occurrence

- Amebiasis occurs worldwide, but it is more common in areas of poor sanitation, particularly in the tropics. Most infections, morbidity, and mortality occur in Africa, Asia, and Central and South America.
- Only an estimated 10%–20% of individuals infected with *E. histolytica* become symptomatic. Among these, approximately 50 million cases of invasive *E. histolytica* disease occur each year, with up to 100,000 deaths. Prevalence and presentation of symptomatic amebiasis vary geographically (e.g., amebic colitis may be the predominant presentation in one country, whereas amebic liver abscesses may predominate in another country).
- The prevalence of asymptomatic infection also varies geographically, ranging from 1% to 21% in persons in developing countries based on stool tests.

Risk for Travelers

- *E. histolytica* can infect persons of all ages.
- Persons at high risk for severe disease include pregnant women, immunocompromised

individuals, and patients receiving corticosteroids. Associations with diabetes and alcohol use have also been reported.

- The rate of amebic diarrhea in returning travelers varies by travel destination. One study found rates of 1.5% in travelers returning from Southeast Asia and 3.6% in those returning from Central America. The overall rate in travelers returning from all regions was 2.7%. Other studies among travelers to the tropics provided similar estimates.
- Risk of infection for both travelers and residents is highest in settings with poor sanitation where barriers between human feces and food and water (including ice) are inadequate.

Clinical Presentation

- The clinical spectrum of *E. histolytica* ranges from asymptomatic infection to amebic diarrhea and dysentery to fulminant colitis and peritonitis to extraintestinal amebiasis.
- Acute amebiasis can present as amebic dysentery, with frequent, urgent, small bloody stools.
- Chronic amebiasis can present with alternating diarrhea and constipation every few days, combined with fatigue and weight loss.
- The incubation period is commonly 2–4 weeks but ranges from a few days to years.
- Occasionally, the parasite may spread to other organs (extraintestinal amebiasis), most commonly the liver (amebic liver abscess). Amebic liver abscess presents with fever and right upper quadrant abdominal pain, usually in the absence of diarrhea.

Diagnosis

- Microscopy does not distinguish between the amebas *E. histolytica* (pathogenic) and *E. dispar* (nonpathogenic). Enzyme immunoassay (EIA) or polymerase chain reaction (PCR) is needed to confirm the diagnosis of *E. histolytica.* Contact your state health department reference laboratory for recommendations on *E. histolytica*-specific testing.
- The recognition of two identical-appearing species, one pathogenic and one not, may explain the observation that some people with apparent *E. histolytica* infection were "asymptomatic cyst passers." Based on this new knowledge, some people passing apparent *E. histolytica* cysts, but having no symptoms, may be infected with *E. dispar* and not require treatment.
- The sensitivity of serologic tests varies depending on clinical presentation (approximately 90% extraintestinal and 70% intestinal) and cannot distinguish between current and past infection.

Treatment

- Travelers with either asymptomatic *E. histolytica* infection or symptomatic *E. histolytica* disease should be treated if the organism can be proven to be *E. histolytica.* Otherwise, asymptomatic travelers do not need to be treated.
- For asymptomatic infection, iodoquinol or paromomycin are the drugs of choice.
- For symptomatic intestinal infection and extraintestinal disease, treatment with metronidazole or tinidazole should be followed by treatment with iodoquinol or paromomycin.

Preventive Measures for Travelers

No vaccine is available. Travelers to developing countries should be advised to follow food and water precautions.

References

1. Abramowicz M, editor. The Medical Letter Report on Drugs for Parasitic Infections. New Rochelle (NY): The Medical Letter; 2007.

2. Petri WA Jr, Singh U. Diagnosis and management of amoebiasis. Clin Infect Dis. 1999;29(5):1117–25.

3. Stanley SL Jr. Amoebiasis. Lancet. 2003;361(9362):1025–34.

4. Petri WA Jr, Singh U. Enteric Amoebiasis. In: Guerrant RL, Walker DH, Weller PF, editors. Tropical infectious diseases: principles, pathogens, & practice. 2nd ed. Philadelphia: Churchill Livingstone; 2006. p. 967–83.

5. Ravdin JI, Stauffer WM. *Entamoeba histolytica* (amoebiasis). In: Mandell GL, Bennett JE, Dolin R, editors. Mandell, Bennet, & Dolin: principles and practice of infectious diseases. 6th ed. Philadelphia: Churchill Livingstone; 2005. p. 3097–111.

6. Freedman DO, Weld LH, Kozarsky PE, et al. GeoSentinel Surveillance Network. Spectrum of disease and relation to place of exposure among ill returned travelers. N Engl J Med. 2006;354(2):119–30.

7. Ansart S, Perez L, Vergely O, et al. Illnesses in travelers returning from the tropics: a prospective study of 622 patients. J Travel Med. 2005;12(6):312–8.

8. Tanyuksel M, Petri WA Jr. Laboratory diagnosis of amoebiasis. Clin Microbiol Rev. 2003;16(4):713–29.

9. World Health Organization. Amoebiasis. Wkly Epidemiol Rec. 1997;72(14):97–9.

10. Stauffer W, Abd-Alla M, Ravdin JI. Prevalence and incidence of *Entamoeba histolytica* infection in South Africa and Egypt. Arch Med Res. 2006;37(2):266–9.

11. Weinke T, Friedrich-Janicke B, Hopp P, et al. Prevalence and clinical importance of *Entamoeba histolytica* in two high-risk groups: travelers returning from the tropics and male homosexuals. J Infect Dis. 1990;161(5):1029–31.

12. de Lalla F, Rinaldi E, Santoro D, et al. Outbreak of *Entamoeba histolytica* and *Giardia lamblia* infections in travellers returning from the tropics. Infection. 1992;20(2):78–82.

13. Benetton ML, Goncalves AV, Meneghini ME, et al. Risk factors for infection by *Entamoeba histolytica/E. dispar* complex: an epidemiological study conducted in outpatient clinics in the city of Manaus, Amazon Region, Brazil. Trans R Soc Trop Med Hyg. 2005;99(7):532–40.

14. Rinne S, Rodas EJ, Galer-Unti R, et al. Prevalence and risk factors for protozoan and nematode infections among children in an Ecuadorian highland community. Trans R Soc Trop Med Hyg. 2005;99(8):585–92.

15. Amoebiasis. In: Heymann DL, editor. Control of communicable diseases manual. 18th ed. Washington D.C.: American Public Health Association; 2004. p. 11–5.

ANGIOSTRONGYLIASIS (*ANGIOSTRONGYLUS CANTONENSIS* INFECTION, NEUROLOGIC ANGIOSTRONGYLIASIS)

Barbara L. Herwaldt

Infectious Agent

Angiostrongyliasis is caused by *Angiostrongylus cantonensis*, a nematode parasite that is considered the most common infectious cause of eosinophilic meningitis in humans.

Mode of Transmission

- Rats are the definitive hosts of the parasite, snails and slugs are intermediate hosts, and humans are accidental (dead-end) hosts (Box 5-1).
- Humans become infected by ingesting third-stage larvae in raw or undercooked snails or slugs. The exposure can be recognized or presumptive: snails or slugs may be consumed for cultural reasons, "on a dare," or accidentally—such as by ingesting contaminated raw produce (e.g., lettuce or vegetable juice).
- Transmission might occur through ingestion of raw or undercooked transport hosts (e.g., freshwater shrimp or prawns, crabs, and frogs). Fish are not known to transmit the parasite.

> **Box 5-1. Classification of hosts for *Angiostrongylus cantonensis* and their roles in the life cycle and transmission of the parasite**
>
> Various species of rats are the **definitive hosts** of the parasite, also known as the rat lungworm:
> • The mature (adult) form of the parasite is found only in rats, not in humans or other hosts.
> • Infected rats shed first-stage larvae in their feces, which are infective for snails and slugs but not for humans or for transport hosts.
>
> Snails and slugs serve as **intermediate hosts**:
> • Snails and slugs become infected by ingesting first-stage larvae in rat feces.
> • These immature larvae mature to third-stage larvae, which are infective for rats (in which they develop to adult worms), humans, and various other animals.
>
> Infective larvae have been found in various **transport (paratenic) hosts**, such as freshwater shrimp or prawns, crabs, and frogs:
> • The parasite does not mature in paratenic hosts, but they can "transport" infective larvae.
> • Some transport hosts (e.g., raw frogs) have been associated with human infection; however, the importance of transport hosts in transmitting the parasite is unclear.

Occurrence

- Most of the described cases have occurred in Asia and the Pacific Basin (e.g., parts of Thailand, Taiwan, mainland China, the Hawaiian Islands, and other Pacific Islands). However, cases have been reported in many areas of the world, including the Caribbean.
- Expansion of the geographic dispersal of the parasite is ongoing; it may be facilitated by infected ship-borne rats and the diversity of snail species that can serve as intermediate hosts.

Risk for Travelers

- Both individual and outbreak-associated cases have been described.
- An outbreak of *A. cantonensis*-associated eosinophilic meningitis occurred among a group of U.S. travelers exposed in Jamaica in 2000, before angiostrongyliasis was known to be endemic there. The presumptive vehicle was the lettuce in a salad.

Clinical Presentation

- Ingested larvae can migrate to the central nervous system and cause eosinophilic meningitis.
- Typically, the incubation period is ~1–3 weeks but has ranged from approximately 1 day to >6 weeks.
- Common manifestations include headache, photophobia, stiff neck, nausea, vomiting, fatigue, and body aches. Abnormal skin sensations (e.g., tingling or painful feelings) are more common than in other types of meningitis. A low-grade fever might be noted.
- The manifestations may persist for weeks or months but usually are self-limited. Severe cases can be associated with sequelae (e.g., paralysis, blindness) or death.

Diagnosis

- Typically, the diagnosis is presumptive, on the basis of clinical and epidemiologic criteria, in persons with otherwise unexplained eosinophilic meningitis.
- If lumbar punctures are done early or late in the course of infection, few, if any, eosinophils may be found in the cerebrospinal fluid. Peripheral blood eosinophilia is occasionally noted.

- Parasitologic confirmation of the diagnosis—by detecting *A. cantonensis* larvae in the cerebrospinal fluid—is unusual in most settings.
- Serologic assays and other diagnostic modalities are considered investigational but might provide supportive evidence for the diagnosis.

Treatment

- The larvae die spontaneously, and supportive care usually suffices (e.g., analgesics).
- The use of corticosteroid and/or antiparasitic therapy should be individualized, with expert consultation. The utility of such therapy may vary among *A. cantonensis*-endemic areas.

Preventive Measures for Travelers

- No vaccine is available.
- Preventive measures are aimed at reducing the risk of ingesting the parasite. In particular, travelers are advised to:
  ○ Avoid eating raw/undercooked snails, slugs, and other possible hosts (see Box 5-1)
  ○ Follow the precautions regarding raw produce (e.g., lettuce)
  ○ Wear gloves (and wash hands) if snails or slugs are handled.

Contact Information for CDC

Clinicians may consult with CDC staff about evaluation and treatment of patients (CDC Public Inquiries, 770-488-7775, parasites@cdc.gov). Additional information can be found on the Division of Parasitic Diseases' website at www.cdc.gov/ncidod/dpd/parasites/angiostrongylus/default.htm.

References

1. Slom TJ, Cortese MM, Gerber SI, et al. An outbreak of eosinophilic meningitis caused by *Angiostrongylus cantonensis* in travelers returning from the Caribbean. N Engl J Med. 2002;346(9):668–75.
2. Hochberg NS, Park SY, Blackburn BG, et al. Distribution of eosinophilic meningitis cases attributable to *Angiostrongylus cantonensis*, Hawaii. Emerg Infect Dis. 2007;13(11):1675–80.
3. Tsai HC, Lee SS, Huang CK, et al. Outbreak of eosinophilic meningitis associated with drinking raw vegetable juice in southern Taiwan. Am J Trop Med Hyg. 2004;71(2):222–6.
4. Lai CH, Yen CM, Chin C, et al. Eosinophilic meningitis caused by *Angiostrongylus cantonensis* after ingestion of raw frogs. Am J Trop Med Hyg. 2007;76(2):399–402.

ANTHRAX

Sean V. Shadomy

Infectious Agent

Anthrax is caused by aerobic, gram-positive, encapsulated, spore-forming, nonmotile, nonhemolytic, rod-shaped bacterium *Bacillus anthracis*.

Mode of Transmission

- Anthrax is primarily transmitted by direct contact with *B. anthracis*-infected animals or contact with contaminated products from infected animals, including carcasses, meat, hides, wool, or items made with those products, such as drums or wool clothing.

- Anthrax presents in three forms: cutaneous, gastrointestinal, and inhalation. Introduction of the spores through the skin can result in cutaneous anthrax; abrasion of the skin increases susceptibility. Ingestion of infected meat can result in gastrointestinal anthrax. Inhalation anthrax typically occurs by inhaling spores aerosolized by industrial processing of contaminated materials, such as hides or wool, or among persons working with contaminated animal skins or wool; it can also result from bioterrorism.
- Anthrax in humans is not generally considered to be contagious; person-to-person transmission of cutaneous anthrax has rarely been reported.

Occurrence

- Anthrax is a zoonotic disease that primarily affects herbivores such as cattle, sheep, goats, antelope, and deer, which become infected through ingestion of contaminated vegetation, water or soil; humans are generally incidental hosts.
- Anthrax is most common in agricultural regions in Central and South America, sub-Saharan Africa, Central and Southwestern Asia, and Southern and Eastern Europe. Anthrax is now rare in the United States and Canada; however, sporadic outbreaks occur every year in livestock and wild herbivores in these countries.

Risk for Travelers

- Travelers to endemic areas have acquired anthrax through either direct or indirect contact with carcasses of animals that died from anthrax. Anthrax may also be mechanically transmitted by biting flies presumed to have fed on such carcasses.
- Cases of cutaneous and inhalation anthrax have been reported among persons who have handled or played contaminated goatskin drums from Haiti or West Africa. Cases have also been reported among persons using contaminated goatskins from West Africa for drum making, as well as members of their households exposed to environments contaminated by the drum-making process.

Clinical Presentation

- Cutaneous anthrax usually develops 1–7 days after exposure. Case–fatality rates can be as high as 20% if untreated, but typically are <1% with antimicrobial therapy. Cutaneous anthrax is characterized by localized itching, followed by the development of a painless papule, which turns vesicular and enlarges, ulcerates, and develops into a depressed black eschar within 7–10 days of the initial lesion. The head, neck, forearms, and hands are the most commonly affected sites. Edema usually surrounds the lesion, sometimes with secondary vesicles, hyperemia, and regional lymphadenopathy. Patients may have associated fever, malaise, and headache.
- Gastrointestinal anthrax usually develops 1–7 days after consumption of contaminated meat and can present in either intestinal or oropharyngeal forms. Shock and death may occur within 2–5 days of onset; case–fatality estimates for gastrointestinal anthrax are >50% if untreated, but <40% with treatment.
- Inhalation anthrax usually develops within a week after exposure, but the incubation period may be prolonged (up to 2 months). Case–fatality estimates are >85%; even with aggressive treatment mortality can be 45%. Initial symptoms are nonspecific and may mimic those of influenza, including myalgia, fever, nonproductive cough, malaise, nausea and vomiting; upper respiratory tract symptoms are rare. Two to 3 days after onset, the patient's condition dramatically worsens with development of severe respiratory distress, diaphoresis, cyanosis, shock, and frequently death.

- Hemorrhagic meningitis may result from hematogenous spread and may develop with any form of anthrax. Case–fatality rates with anthrax meningitis approach 100%.

Diagnosis

- Laboratory diagnosis depends on bacterial culture and isolation of *B. anthracis* or the detection of bacterial DNA or antigens. Serologic testing of host antibody responses requires acute- and convalescent-phase sera for diagnosis. Confirmatory testing, including isolate identification, antigen detection in tissues, or quantitative serology, should be performed by the state health department or Laboratory Response Network (LRN) laboratories.
- Guidelines for collection and submission of appropriate clinical specimens for testing, and algorithms for laboratory diagnosis are at http://emergency.cdc.gov/agent/anthrax/lab-testing/. Specimens for culture should be collected prior to initiation of antimicrobial therapy.
- Diagnostic procedures for inhalation anthrax include thoracic imaging studies for detection of a widened mediastinum or pleural effusion.

Treatment

- Ciprofloxacin is the drug of choice. Because of intrinsic resistance, neither cephalosporins nor trimethoprim–sulfamethoxazole should be used.
- Localized or uncomplicated cutaneous anthrax can be treated for 7–10 days with ciprofloxacin (500 mg orally, 2 times/day) or oral doxycycline (100 mg orally, 2 times/day), except in children <2 years of age. If susceptibility testing is supportive, oral penicillin V or amoxicillin may be used to complete the regimen.
- Theraputic treatment for severe systemic or life-threatening disease, such as: inhalation anthrax; gastrointestinal anthrax; anthrax meningitis; severe cutaneous anthrax with systemic involvement, extensive edema, or head and neck lesions; treatment of children <2 years of age; or cutaneous anthrax associated with aerosol exposure. Therapeutic recommendations are found at www.cdc.gov/mmwr/preview/mmwrhtml/mm5042a1.htm.

Preventive Measures for Travelers

- Vaccination against anthrax is not recommended for travelers.
- Travelers are warned against having direct or indirect contact with carcasses of animals found in anthrax-endemic regions or consuming meat from animals that were not determined by health officials to be healthy at the time of slaughter.
- The risk of acquiring anthrax from playing with or handling an animal-skin drum is very low. In recent years there have been a few cases of anthrax among animal-skin drum makers. Some of these cases have been fatal. Travelers who wish to bring back animal hides from anthrax-endemic regions for the purpose of drum making should strongly consider the health risks before importing animal skins.
- Currently, no tests are offered or available to determine if animal products are either contaminated with or free of *B. anthracis* spores. Animal-skin drum owners or players should report any unexplained fever or new skin lesions to their health-care provider and describe their recent contact with animal-skin drums.
- The importation of goatskin souvenirs such as goatskin drums from Haiti is prohibited by the Centers for Disease Control and Prevention (see the Taking Animals Across International Borders section in Chapter 6).
- Importation of animal products, including processed and unprocessed cattle and goat hides, is currently regulated by the United States Department of Agriculture (USDA). Animal skin products, trophies, or souvenirs from anthrax-endemic regions must be accompanied by a certificate saying they are from animals that

were free of anthrax to be imported into the United States. Cattle or goat hides that have been tanned, pickled in a solution of salt and mineral acid, or treated with lime are considered to pose less of a risk for infectious diseases and may also be imported under certain conditions. For more information, consult the USDA website at www.aphis.usda.gov and www.aphis.usda.gov/import_export/animals/animal_import/animal_imports.shtml.

References

1. Bales ME, Dannenberg AL, Brachman PS, et al. Epidemiologic response to anthrax outbreaks: field investigations, 1950–2001. Emerg Infect Dis. 2002;8(10):1163–74.

2. Van den Enden E, Van Gompel A, Van Esbroeck M. Cutaneous anthrax, Belgian traveler. Emerg Infect Dis. 2006;12(3):523–5.

3. Krishna Rao NS, Mohiyudeen S. Tabanus flies as transmitters of anthrax: a field experience. Indian Vet J. 1958;35:348–53.

4. Turell M, Knudson GB. Mechanical transmission of *Bacillus anthracis* by stable flies (*Stomoxys calcitrans*) and mosquitoes (*Aedes aegypti* and *Aedes taeniorhynchus*). Infect Immun. 1987;55(8):1859–61.

5. CDC. Cutaneous anthrax acquired from imported Haitian drums—Florida. MMWR Morb Mortal Wkly Rep. 1974;23:142–7.

6. Eurosurveillance editorial team. Probable human anthrax death in Scotland. Euro Surveill. 2006;11(8):E060817.2.

7. CDC. Inhalation anthrax associated with dried animal hides—Pennsylvania and New York City, 2006. MMWR Morb Mortal Wkly Rep. 2006;55(10):280–2.

8. CDC. Cutaneous anthrax associated with drum making using goat hides from West Africa—Connecticut, 2007. MMWR Morb Mortal Wkly Rep. 2008;57(23):628–31.

9. Jernigan DB, Raghunathan PL, Bell BP, et al. Investigation of bioterrorism-related anthrax, United States, 2001: epidemiologic findings. Emerg Infect Dis. 2002;8(10):1019–28.

10. CDC. Update: investigation of bioterrorism-related anthrax and interim guidelines for exposure management and antimicrobial therapy, October 2001. MMWR Morb Mortal Wkly Rep. 2001;50(42):909–19.

11. Inglesby TV, O'Toole T, Henderson DA, et al. Anthrax as a biological weapon, 2002: updated recommendations for management. JAMA. 2002;287(17):2236–52.

12. CDC. Use of anthrax vaccine in response to terrorism: supplemental recommendations of the Advisory Committee on Immunization Practices. MMWR Morb Mortal Wkly Rep. 2002;51(45):1024–6.

BARTONELLA-ASSOCIATED INFECTIONS

Alicia Anderson, Jennifer McQuiston

Infectious Agent

At least a dozen bacterial species in the genus *Bartonella* cause several different diseases, but very few have been shown to be significant causes of human disease. Cat-scratch disease (CSD) is caused by *B. henselae*. Oroya fever results from infection with *B. bacilliformis*. Trench fever is caused by *B. quintana*. A variety of *Bartonella* species have been associated with culture-negative endocarditis.

Mode of Transmission

- CSD is contracted through scratches and bites from domestic or feral cats, particularly kittens. The disease occurs most frequently in children <10 years of age. Cats acquire the organism through infected fleas. The subsequent infected flea dirt is harbored in their claws when they scratch themselves and may then be transmitted to a person or another cat.
- Oroya fever is transmitted by sand flies (genus *Lutzomyia*) that are infected with the organism. Much is still unknown regarding the existence of other competent

arthropod vectors and the identification of a natural, nonhuman, vertebrate reservoir for Oroya fever.
- Trench fever is transmitted by the human body louse. Because of its association with body louse infestations, trench fever is most commonly associated with homeless populations or areas of high population density and poor sanitation.

Occurrence

- CSD occurs worldwide and may be present wherever cats are found. The majority of cases occur in the fall and winter.
- Oroya fever has limited geographic distribution, with cases occurring in the Andes Mountains in western South America, including Peru, Colombia, and Ecuador. Most cases are reported in Peru.
- Trench fever has a worldwide distribution, with cases reported from Europe, North America, Africa, and China.

Risk for Travelers

- There are a few case reports of Oroya fever and verruge peruana (Peruvian wart) in travelers who visit the Andean highlands in South America, but the risk is low. In 2007, a newly recognized species of *Bartonella* was identified in an ill traveler returning from Peru.
- The risk for other species of *Bartonella* occurs worldwide.

Clinical Presentation

- The symptoms of CSD include fever; enlarged, tender lymph nodes that develop 1–2 weeks after exposure, and a papule or pustule at the inoculation site. Unusual manifestations such as granulomatous conjunctivitis, neuroretinitis, atypical pneumonia, or endocarditis may occur in a small percentage of patients.
- The manifestations of Oroya fever include fever, myalgia, headache, and anemia. Mortality may exceed 40% in untreated individuals. There is also a chronic phase of the disease (verruga peruana or Peruvian wart), which is characterized by red to purple nodular skin lesions.
- The symptoms of trench fever include fever, headache, a transient rash, and bone pain, mainly in the shins, neck and back.

Diagnosis

- Diagnosis of CSD can be made by isolation of *B. henselae* by PCR or in culture of pus or lymph node aspirates by using special techniques. CSD is usually confirmed by serology.
- Oroya fever is typically diagnosed via blood culture or direct observation of the bacilli in peripheral blood smears.
- Diagnosis of trench fever can be made by isolation of *Bartonella quintana* from blood cultured on blood or chocolate agar under 5% CO_2. Microcolonies can be seen after 1–3 weeks incubation at 37° C. Trench fever can also be confirmed by serology.

Treatment

- Most cases of CSD eventually resolve without treatment; the use of antibiotics to shorten the course of disease is controversial and has not been proven.
- A wide range of antibiotics have been shown to be effective against *Bartonella*

infections including penicillins, tetracyclines, cephalosporins, aminoglycosides, and fluoroquinolones.

Preventive Measures for Travelers

- For CSD, travelers should avoid rough play with cats to prevent scratches or bites and wash hands promptly after handling cats. Provide flea control for owned cats to prevent parasitism.
- Preventive measures for Oroya fever are aimed at protection from sand flies via clothing, repellents, and reduced outdoor activities when sand flies are most active (dusk and dawn).
- Preventive measures for trench fever are aimed at avoiding exposures to human body lice.

References

1. Margileth AM. Cat scratch disease. Adv Pediatr Infect Dis. 1993;8:1–21.
2. Maguina C, Gotuzzo E. Bartonellosis. New and old. Infect Dis Clin North Am. 2000;14(1):1–22.
3. Chamberlin J, Laughlin LW, Romero S, et al. Epidemiology of endemic *Bartonella bacilliformis*: a prospective cohort study in a Peruvian mountain valley community. J Infect Dis. 2002 Oct 1;186(7):983–90.
4. CDC. Cat-scratch disease in children—Texas, September 2000—August 2001. MMWR Morb Mortal Wkly Rep. 2002;51(10):212–4.
5. Ihler, GM. *Bartonella bacilliformis*: dangerous pathogen slowly emerging from deep background. FEMS Microbiol Lett. 1996;144(1):1–11.
6. Foucault C, Brouqui P, Raoult D. *Bartonella quintana* characteristics and clinical management. Emerg Infect Dis. 2006;12(2):217–23.
7. Rolain JM, Brouqui P, Koehler JE, et al. Recommendations for treatment of human infections caused by *Bartonella* species. Antimicrob Agents Chemother. 2004;48(6):1921–33.
8. Daily JP, Waldron MA. Case records of the Massachusetts General Hospital. Weekly clinicopathological exercises. Case 22-2003. A 22-year-old man with chills and fever after a stay in South America. N Engl J Med. 2003;349(3):287–95
9. Matteelli A, Castelli F, Spinetti A, et al. Short report: verruga peruana in an Italian traveler from Peru. Am J Trop Med Hyg. 1994 Feb;50(2):143–4.
10. Eremeeva ME, Gerns HL, Lydy SL, et al. Bacteremia, fever and splenomegaly caused by a newly recognized bartonella species. N Engl J Med. 2007;356(23):2381–7.

BRUCELLOSIS

Marta A. Guerra, Barun K. De

Infectious Agent

Brucella species are facultative, intracellular, gram-negative coccobacilli. Nine species of *Brucella* are currently defined by phenotypic and antigenic differences, in addition to differential host specificity.

- Known human pathogens: *B. abortus*, *B. melitensis*, *B. suis*, and *B. canis*.
- Pathogenicity to humans of these species is not well known: *B. ovis*, *B. neotomae*, *B. ceti*, *B. pinnipedialis*, and *B. microti*.

Mode of Transmission

- Eating or drinking contaminated milk products is the most common route of infection for *Brucella* spp.

- *Brucella* can enter the body via skin wounds, mucous membranes, or inhalation.
- Person-to-person transmission is very rare.

Occurrence

- High-risk regions include the Mediterranean basin, South and Central America, Eastern Europe, Asia, Africa, and the Middle East.
- Brucellosis is primarily an occupational disease among those working with infected livestock or handling the organism in laboratory settings.
- The infection is present in animals such as goats, sheep, pigs, and cattle, and in wildlife.
- Brucellosis is common in countries that do not have a standardized public health system or brucellosis control programs for livestock.

Risk for Travelers

- Risk is mainly associated with the consumption of unpasteurized milk and other dairy products in countries where brucellosis is endemic or enzootic.
- Unpasteurized soft goat cheeses are frequently contaminated with *Brucella* and associated with the development of brucellosis.
- Individuals exposed to contaminated fluids and tissue during events surrounding parturition, during slaughter and dressing of infected animals, and during preparation of foods from infected animals are at increased risk of infection.
- Consumption of undercooked infected meat is another route of infection.

Clinical Presentation

- Incubation period is 2–4 weeks (range 5 days to 5 months).
- Initial presentation is nonspecific, such as fever, muscle aches, fatigue, headache, and night sweats.
- Fever may be continuous or intermittent (undulant).
- Systemic infection may localize in liver, spleen, bone marrow, joints, heart, or reproductive organs.
- Endocarditis is a primary cause of mortality.
- Neuropsychiatric symptoms, such as depression or sleep disturbance, are rare.
- More severe symptoms are generally associated with *B. melitensis* or *B. suis* infections than with infections from other *Brucella* spp.

Diagnosis

- Culture is the diagnostic gold standard, and blood or bone marrow culture is the method of choice for isolation of *Brucellae.*
- Early collection of specimens is recommended, preferably before antimicrobial treatment, to ensure successful culture of the organism.
- Serology is the most common method of diagnosis and requires acute- and convalescent-phase blood samples.
- Several serologic tests are available for detection of both IgM and IgG antibodies (~75–80% sensitivity).
- Serum agglutination test is the standard diagnostic assay for brucellosis.

Treatment

- The optimum antimicrobial therapy for brucellosis includes a 6-week course of a combination of antimicrobial agents.
- Antimicrobials most commonly used are doxycycline, rifampin, and streptomycin.

- Precautionary measures are recommended with the choice of drugs for children <8 years of age and pregnant women.
- Relapses may occur with late initiation or premature discontinuation of therapy.

Preventive Measures for Travelers

- No vaccine is available for humans.
- Antimicrobial prophylaxis is not recommended.
- Persons traveling to countries where brucellosis is endemic or enzootic should avoid ingesting unpasteurized dairy products.
- Persons should avoid eating undercooked meat.
- Persons should avoid contact with animals giving birth.
- Persons should use protective clothing and equipment when slaughtering and butchering potentially infected animals.

References

1. Heymann DL, editor. Control of communicable diseases manual: an official report of the American Public Health Association. 18th ed. Washington D.C.: American Public Health Association; 2004.

2. Pappas G, Papadimitriou P, Akritidis N, et al. The new global map of human brucellosis. Lancet Infect Dis. 2006;6(2):91–9.

3. Ariza J, Bosilkovski M, Cascio A, et al.; International Society of Chemotherapy; Institute of Continuing Medical Education of Ioannina. Perspectives for the treatment of brucellosis in the 21st century: the Ioannina recommendations. PLoS Med. 2007;4(12):e317.

4. WHO. Brucellosis [Internet]. Geneva: WHO. [cited 2008 Nov 30]. Available from: http://www.who.int/zoonoses/diseases/brucellosis/en/.

5. American Society for Microbiology. Sentinel laboratory guidelines for suspected agents of bioterrorism: *Brucella* species [Internet]. Snyder JW, editor. Washington D.C.: American Society for Microbiology; 2004. [cited 2008 Nov 30]. Available from: http://www.asm.org/asm/files/leftmarginheaderlist/downloadfilename/000000000523/brucella101504.pdf.

6. Live I, Wolfe B. Response of individuals to injection with ether-killed Brucella abortus. Am J Public Health Nations Health. 1960;50(7):966–75.

7. CDC. Update: Potential Exposures to Attenuated Vaccine Strain *Brucella abortus* RB51 During a Laboratory Proficiency Test—United States and Canada, 2007. MMWR Morb Mortal Wkly Rep. 2008;57(2):36–9.

CAMPYLOBACTER ENTERITIS

Melissa Viray, Michael Lynch

Infectious Agent

Infection is caused by gram-negative, spiral-shaped microaerophilic bacteria of the family *Campylobacteraceae*. Most infections are caused by *Campylobacter jejuni*; other species, including *C. coli*, also cause infection. *C. jejuni* and *C. coli* are carried normally in the intestinal tracts of many domestic and wild animals.

Mode of Transmission

The major modes of transmission include—

- Consuming contaminated foods, especially undercooked chicken and foods contaminated by raw chicken
- Consuming contaminated water or raw (unpasteurized) milk
- Contact with animals, particularly farm animals such as cattle and poultry, as well as cats and dogs.

Occurrence

- *Campylobacter* is a leading cause of bacterial diarrheal disease worldwide; within the United States, it is estimated to affect 2.4 million persons every year.
- Campylobacteriosis is a common cause of travelers' diarrhea (TD). The percentage of bacteria-caused TD due to *Campylobacter* ranges from 1% to 2% in Mexico to 28% in Thailand.

Risk for Travelers

- The infectious dose is thought to be small, typically fewer than 500 organisms.
- The geographic distribution of cases is worldwide; risk for infection is higher in the developing world, especially in areas with poor restaurant hygiene and inadequate sanitation.

Clinical Presentation

- Incubation period is typically 2–4 days.
- Campylobacteriosis is characterized by diarrhea (frequently bloody), abdominal pain, fever, and occasionally, nausea and vomiting. More severe presentations can occur, including bloodstream infection and disease mimicking acute appendicitis or ulcerative colitis.

Diagnosis

- Diagnosis is based on isolation of the organism from stools by using selective media and reduced oxygen tension. Most laboratories also combine this with incubation at 42° C (107.6° F).
- Visualization of motile and curved, spiral or S-shaped rods by stool phase-contrast or darkfield microscopy can provide rapid presumptive evidence for *Campylobacter* enteritis.

Treatment

- Treatment is generally supportive, including oral rehydration solutions (ORS). The disease is generally self-limited and may last up to a week.
- Antibiotic therapy may decrease the duration of symptoms if administered early in the course of disease. Because it is generally not possible to distinguish campylobacteriosis from other etiologies of TD, the use of empiric antibiotics in travelers should follow the guidelines for TD.
- Rates of antibiotic resistance have been on the rise in the past 20 years, in particular for fluoroquinolones; travel abroad has been associated with infection with resistant *Campylobacter*. Clinicians should have a high degree of suspicion for resistant infection in returning travelers. Documented fluoroquinolone resistance has been highest among travelers to Thailand. When fluoroquinolone resistance is proven or suspected, azithromycin is usually the next choice of treatment.
- *Campylobacter* infection can be a trigger for Guillain–Barré syndrome.
- Additional information can be found on the Division of Foodborne, Bacterial and Mycotic Diseases' website: www.cdc.gov/ncidod/dbmd/diseaseinfo/campylobacter_g.htm.

Preventive Measures for Travelers

- No vaccine is available.

- Antibiotic prophylaxis, as used for TD, is likely to be effective, although antibiotic prophylaxis is not routinely recommended
- Preventive measures are aimed at avoiding ingestion of foods at high risk for contamination, as well as safe water practices while traveling.

References

1. Coker AO, Isokpehi RD, Thomas BN, et al. Human campylobacteriosis in developing countries. Emerg Infect Dis. 2002;8(3):237–44.
2. Moore JE, Barton MD, Blair IS, et al. The epidemiology of antibiotic resistance in *Campylobacter*. Microbes Infect. 2006;8(7):1955–66.
3. Tribble DR, Sanders JW, Pang LW, et al. Traveler's diarrhea in Thailand: randomized, double-blind trial comparing single-dose and 3-day azithromycin-based regimens with a 3-day levofloxacin regimen. Clin Infect Dis. 2007;44(3):338–46.
4. Moore JE, Corcoran D, Dooley JS, et al. *Campylobacter*. Vet Res. 2005;36(3):351–82.
5. Altekruse SF, Stern NJ, Fields PI, et al. *Campylobacter jejuni*—an emerging foodborne pathogen. Emerg Infect Dis. 1999;5(1):28–35.
6. Friedman CR, Hoekstra RM, Samuel M, et al. Risk factors for sporadic *Campylobacter* infection in the United States: a case–control study in FoodNet sites. Clin Infect Dis. 2004;38(Suppl 3):S285–96
7. Gupta A, Nelson JM, Barrett TJ, et al. Antimicrobial resistance among *Campylobacter* strains, United States, 1997–2001. Emerg Infect Dis. 2004;10(6):1102–9.
8. Humphrey T, O'Brien S, Madsen M. Campylobacters as zoonotic pathogens: a food production perspective. Int J Food Microbiol. 2007;117(3):237–57.

CHIKUNGUNYA

J. Erin Staples, Marc Fischer, Ann M. Powers

Infectious Agent

Infection is caused by the chikungunya virus (CHIKV), a single-stranded RNA virus that belongs to the family *Togaviridae*, genus *Alphavirus*.

Mode of Transmission

- Transmission is vector-borne, occurring via the bite of an infected mosquito of the *Aedes* spp., predominantly *Ae. aegypti* and less frequently *Ae. albopictus*.
- Nonhuman and human primates are the main reservoirs of the virus, with anthroponotic (human-to-vector-to-human) transmission occurring.
- Blood-borne transmission is possible, with one documented case to date.
- The risk of an individual transmitting the disease to a biting mosquito or through blood is greatest when the patient is viremic during the first 2–6 days of illness.
- Maternal–fetal transmission has been documented during pregnancy. The highest risk occurs when a woman is viremic at the time of delivery, with a vertical transmission rate of 49%.
- CHIKV does not appear to be transmitted through breast milk.

Occurrence

- CHIKV has been identified in many countries in Africa and Asia and is responsible for numerous epidemics in these areas.
- Since a re-emergence of the disease in 2004, millions of cases have occurred throughout countries in and around the Indian Ocean.
- Transmission has also been documented in a limited area of Italy, after an infected traveler transmitted the virus to local *Ae. albopictus* mosquitoes, leading to autochthonous transmission.

- Given the large CHIKV epidemics, high level of viremia in humans, and the worldwide distribution of *Ae. aegypti* and *Ae. albopictus*, there is a risk of importation of chikungunya virus into new areas by infected travelers.
- For information on current outbreaks, consult CDC's Travelers' Health website (www.cdc.gov/travel).

Risk for Travelers

- Risk for travelers to become infected with CHIKV is greatest with travel to areas with ongoing epidemics of the disease.
- Most epidemics occur during the tropical rainy season and abate during the dry season. However, the recent outbreaks in Africa occurred after years of drought where open water-holding containers served as vector-breeding sites.
- Risk of CHIKV infection exists throughout the day, as the primary vector, *Ae. aegypti* breeds in household containers and aggressively bites in the daytime.
- In 2006 and 2007, 52 cases of laboratory-confirmed chikungunya fever were reported in U.S. travelers returning from areas with ongoing disease activity.

Clinical Presentation

- Approximately 3%–25% of persons infected with CHIKV will remain asymptomatic.
- The incubation period is typically 3–7 days (range 2–12 days).
- Disease is most often characterized by sudden onset of high fever (typically greater than 102° F) and severe joint pain. Other symptoms include rash, headache, fatigue, nausea, vomiting, and myalgias.
  - Fevers typically last from several days up to a week. The fever can be biphasic.
  - Joint symptoms are severe and often debilitating. They are usually symmetric and occur most commonly in hands and feet, but they can affect more proximal joints.
  - Rash usually occurs after onset of fever. It is typically maculopapular, involving the trunk and extremities, but can also include palms, soles, and face.
- Rare but serious complications of the disease can occur, including myocarditis, ocular disease (uveitis, retinitis), hepatitis, and neuroinvasive disease, such as meningoencephalitis, Guillain–Barré syndrome, paresis, or palsies.
- Fatalities related to chikungunya virus are rare. Older age and comorbidities are likely risk factors for poor outcomes.
- Following the acute illness, some patients have prolonged fatigue lasting several weeks. Additionally, some patients have reported incapacitating joint pain or tenosynovitis, which may last for weeks or months. Some studies have reported joint stiffness and/or pain more than a year after the initial infection.
- Pregnant women have symptoms and outcomes similar to those of other individuals, and most CHIKV infections that occur during pregnancy will not result in the virus being transmitted to the fetus. However, when intrapartum transmission does occur, it can result in complications for the baby, including neurologic disease, hemorrhagic symptoms, and myocardial disease. There are also rare reports of first-trimester spontaneous abortions following maternal CHIKV infection.

Diagnosis

- Preliminary diagnosis is based on the patient's clinical features, places and dates of travel, and activities.
- Laboratory diagnosis is generally accomplished by testing serum to detect virus-specific IgM and neutralizing antibodies.
- During the first week after onset of symptoms, CHIKV can often be diagnosed by using viral culture or nucleic acid amplification on serum.

- Health-care providers should contact their state or local health department or CDC (970-221-6400) for assistance with diagnostic testing.

Treatment

- There is no specific antiviral treatment currently available for chikungunya fever.
- Treatment is symptomatic and can include rest, fluids, and use of analgesics and antipyretics.
- Infected persons should be protected from further mosquito exposure (staying indoors in areas with screens and/or under a mosquito net) during the first few days of the illness, so they do not contribute to the transmission cycle.

Preventive Measures for Travelers

- There is no vaccine or preventive drug currently available.
- Caution should also be used when advising individuals with significant comorbidities and pregnant women about travel to areas with ongoing outbreaks of the disease, as they or their infants may suffer from more severe disease.
- The best way to prevent chikungunya virus infection is to avoid mosquito bites by—
  - Using insect repellent containing DEET, Picaridin, oil of lemon eucalyptus, or IR3535 on exposed skin. Always follow the directions on the package.
  - Wearing long sleeves, pants, and socks. If possible, treat clothes with permethrin.
  - Staying in screened or air conditioned accommodations to keep mosquitoes out.
  - Getting rid of mosquito sources by emptying standing water from flower pots, buckets and barrels.
- Also see the Protection Against Mosquitoes, Ticks and Other Insects and Arthropods section in Chapter 2.

References

1. Parola P, de Lamballerie X, Jourdan J, et al. Novel chikungunya virus variant in travelers returning from Indian Ocean islands. Emerg Infect Dis. 2006;12(10):1493–9.

2. Gérardin P, Barau G, Michault A, et al. Multidisciplinary prospective study of mother-to-child chikungunya virus infections on the island of La Réunion. PLoS Med. 2008;5(3):e60.

3. Jupp PG, McIntosh BM. Chikungunya virus disease. In: Monath TP, editor. The Arboviruses: epidemiology and ecology. Volume 3. Boca Raton, FL: CRC; 1988. p. 137–57.

4. Powers A, Logue CH. Changing patterns of chikungunya virus: re-emergence of a zoonotic arbovirus. J Gen Virol. 2007;88(Pt 9):2363–77.

5. CDC. Chikungunya distribution and global map [Internet]. Atlanta: Centers for Disease Control and Prevention; 2008. [updated 2008 Mar 11; cited 2008 Nov 30]. Available from: http://www.cdc.gov/ncidod/dvbid/Chikungunya/CH_GlobalMap.html.

6. World Health Organization. Outbreak and spread of chikungunya. Weekly Epidemiol Rec. 2007;82(47):409–15.

7. Rezza G, Nicoletti L, Angelini R, et al. Infection with chikungunya virus in Italy: an outbreak in a temperate region. Lancet. 2007;370(9602):1840–6.

8. Chretien JP, Anyamba A, Bedno SA, et al. Drought-associated chikungunya emergence along coastal East Africa. Am J Trop Med Hyg. 2007;76(3):405–7.

9. CDC. Chikungunya fever diagnosed among international travelers—United States, 2005–2006. MMWR Morb Mortal Wkly Rep. 2006;55(38):1040–2.

10. CDC. Update: Chikungunya fever diagnosed among international travelers—United States, 2006. MMWR Morb Mortal Wkly Rep. 2007;56(12):276–7.

11. Queyriaux B, Simon F, Grandadam M, et al. Clinical burden of chikungunya virus infection. Lancet Infect Dis. 2008;8(1):2–3.

12. Retuya TJA Jr, Ting DL, Dacula BD, et al. Chikungunya fever outbreak in an agricultural village in Indang, Cavite, Philippines. Philippine J Microbiol Infect Dis. 1998;27(3):93–6.

13. Lalitha P, Rathinam S, Banushree K, et al. Ocular involvement associated with an epidemic outbreak of chikungunya virus infection. Am J Ophthalmol. 2007;144(4):552–6.

14. Renault P, Solet JL, Sissoko D, et al. A major epidemic of chikungunya virus infection on Reunion Island, France, 2005–2006. Am J Trop Med Hyg. 2007;77(4):727–31.
15. Brighton SW, Prozesky OW, De La Harpe AL. Chikungunya virus infection: a retrospective study of 107 cases. S Afr Med J. 1983;63(9):313–5.
16. Ramful D, Carbonnier M, Pasquet M, et al. Mother-to-child transmission of chikungunya virus infection. Pediatr Infect Dis J. 2007;26(9):811–5.
17. Touret Y, Randrianaivo H, Michault A, et al. Early maternal–fetal transmission of the chikungunya virus. Presse Med. 2006;35(11 Pt 1):1656–8.
18. Lanciotti RS, Kosoy O, Laven JJ, et al. Chikungunya virus in US travelers returning from India, 2006. Emerg Infect Dis. 2007;13(5):764–7.
19. Panning M, Grywana K, van Esbroeck M, et al. Chikungunya fever in travelers returning to Europe from the Indian Ocean region, 2006. Emerg Infect Dis. 2008;14(3):416–22.

CHOLERA

Eric Mintz

Infectious Agent

Cholera is an acute intestinal infection caused by toxigenic *Vibrio cholerae* O-group 1 or O-group 139.

- Many other serogroups of *Vibrio cholerae*, with or without the cholera toxin gene, can cause a cholera-like illness, as can nontoxigenic strains of the O1 and O139 serogroups.
- Only toxigenic strains of serogroups O1 and O139 have caused widespread epidemics and are reportable to WHO as "cholera."
- *V. cholerae* O1 has two biotypes, Classical and El Tor, and each biotype has two distinct serotypes, Inaba and Ogawa. The symptoms of infection are indistinguishable, although a higher proportion of persons infected with the El Tor biotype remains asymptomatic or has only a mild illness.
- In recent years, infections with the Classical biotype of *V. cholerae* O1 have become quite rare and are limited to parts of Bangladesh and India.

Mode of Transmission

- Toxigenic *V. cholerae* O1 and O139 are free-living organisms found in fresh and brackish water often in association with copepods or other zooplankton, shellfish, and aquatic plants.
- Cholera infections are most commonly acquired from drinking water in which *V. cholerae* is found naturally or into which it has been introduced from the feces of a symptomatic or asymptomatically infected person.
- Other common vehicles include contaminated fish and shellfish, produce, or leftover cooked grains that have not been properly reheated.
- Transmission from person to person, even to health-care workers during epidemics, is rarely documented.

Occurrence

- Since 1961, the seventh pandemic of cholera, caused by *V. cholerae* serogroup O1, biotype El Tor, has spread from Indonesia through most of Asia into Eastern Europe and Africa, and from North Africa to the Iberian Peninsula.
- In 1991, an extensive epidemic began in Peru and spread to neighboring countries in the Western Hemisphere.

- Although few cases of cholera now occur in the Americas, *V. cholerae* O1 remains endemic in much of Africa and South and Southeast Asia.
- *V. cholerae* O139 spread rapidly through Asia in the early 1990s but has since remained localized to a few areas in Bangladesh and India.
- In 2007, 53 countries reported 177,963 cholera cases and 4,031 cholera deaths (case–fatality rate 2.3%) to the WHO. Resource-poor areas continue to report the vast majority of cases; 99% of cases were reported from Africa, continuing a trend.

Risk for Travelers

- Travelers who follow usual tourist itineraries and who observe food safety recommendations while in countries reporting cholera have virtually no risk. The risk is increased for those who drink untreated water or eat poorly cooked or raw seafood in disease-endemic areas.
- From 1996 through 2006, only 40 confirmed cases of cholera in the United States were acquired abroad.
- Two reports of cholera have been associated with food served on board international flights, most recently in 1992, in the midst of the Latin American epidemic, on a flight from Argentina to Los Angeles. CDC consequently advised the International Air Transport Association that oral rehydration solutions should be carried on international flights and that certain food items prepared in cities with cholera epidemics should not be served. Airline flights have not been implicated in any subsequent cases of cholera.

Clinical Presentation

- Cholera infection is most often asymptomatic or results in a mild gastroenteritis.
- Severe cholera is characterized by acute, profuse watery diarrhea, described as "rice-water stools," and often vomiting, leading to volume depletion. Signs and symptoms include tachycardia, loss of skin turgor, dry mucous membranes, hypotension, and thirst. Additional symptoms, including muscle cramps, are secondary to the resulting electrolyte imbalances.
- If untreated, volume depletion can rapidly lead to hypovolemic shock and death.

Diagnosis

- Cholera is confirmed through culture of a stool specimen or rectal swab.
- Cary Blair media is ideal for transport, and the selective thiosulfate–citrate–bile salts agar (TCBS) is ideal for isolation and identification. Reagents for serogrouping *V. cholerae* isolates are available in all state health department laboratories. Commercially available rapid test kits do not yield an isolate for antimicrobial susceptibility testing and subtyping, and should not be used for routine diagnosis.
- All isolates should be sent to CDC via state health department laboratories for cholera toxin-testing and subtyping.
- Cholera is a nationally reportable disease.

Treatment

- Rehydration is the cornerstone of therapy. Oral rehydration salts and, when necessary, intravenous fluids and electrolytes, if administered in a timely manner and in adequate volumes, will reduce case–fatality rates to well under 1%.
- Antibiotics reduce fluid requirements and duration of illness. Antimicrobial therapy is indicated for severe cases, which can be treated with tetracycline, doxycycline, furazolidone, erythromycin, or ciprofloxacin. When possible, antimicrobial susceptibility testing should inform treatment choices.

Preventive Measures for Travelers

- Safe food and water precautions are critical in preventing cholera.
- Chemoprophylaxis is not indicated.

Vaccine

- There is currently no cholera vaccine available in the United States.
- Two oral vaccines are available outside the United States: Dukoral from SBL Vaccin AB and a variant only available in Vietnam, which appears to provide somewhat better immunity and have fewer adverse effects than the previously licensed injectable vaccine. However, CDC does not recommend either of these two vaccines for most travelers because of the low risk of cholera to U.S. travelers and the brief and incomplete immunity that the vaccines confer. Further information on Dukoral can be obtained from SBL Vaccin AB by visiting the website www.sblvaccines.se/en/, or by contacting SBL Vaccin AB via telephone at +46-8-735 10 00, fax at +46-8-82 73 04, or e-mail at info@sblvaccines.se.
- Currently, no country or territory requires vaccination against cholera as a condition for entry.

References

1. Sack DA, Sack RB, Nair B, et al. Cholera. Lancet. 2004;363(9404):223–33
2. World Health Organization. Cholera, 2006. Wkly Epidemiol Rec. 2007;82:273–84.
3. Griffith DC, Kelly-Hope LA, Miller MA. Review of reported cholera outbreaks worldwide, 1995–2005. Am J Trop Med Hyg. 2006;75(5):973–7.
4. Gaffga NH, Tauxe RV, Mintz ED. Cholera: a new homeland in Africa? Am J Trop Med Hyg. 2007;77(4):705–13.
5. Steinberg EB, Greene KD, Bopp CA, et al. Cholera in the United States, 1995–2000: trends at the end of the millennium. J Infect Dis. 2001;184:799–802.
6. CDC. Two cases of toxigenic *Vibrio cholerae* O1 infection after Hurricanes Katrina and Rita—Louisiana, October 2005. MMWR Morb Mortal Wkly Rep. 2006;55(2):31–2.
7. CDC. Summary of Notifiable Diseases—United States, 2006. MMWR Morb Mortal Wkly Rep. 2008;55(53):9 and 45.
8. Sutton RGA. An outbreak of cholera in Australia due to food served in flight on an international aircraft. J. Hyg. 1974;72(3):441–51.
9. CDC. Cholera associated with an international airline flight, 1992. MMWR Morb Mortal Wkly Rep. 1992;41(8):134–5.
10. Kozicki M, Steffen R, Schar M. "Boil it, cook it, peel it, or forget it": does this rule prevent travellers' diarrhoea? Int J Epidemiol. 1985;14:169–72.

COCCIDIOIDOMYCOSIS

Tom Chiller, Benjamin Park

Infectious Agent

Coccidioidomycosis, or "Valley fever," is a disease caused by the fungus *Coccidioides* spp.

Mode of Transmission

The disease is acquired by inhalation of fungal conidia from dust found in ambient air or generated by soil-disrupting human activities or natural disasters. Coccidioidomycosis is not transmitted from person to person.

Occurrence

- *Coccidioides* spp. are primarily endemic in arid regions.

- In the United States, the areas with the highest incidence are primarily in the Sonoran desert in Arizona (Phoenix and Tucson metropolitan areas) and the San Joaquin "Central" Valley in California. Other endemic areas include parts of New Mexico, western Texas, Nevada, and Utah.
- Outside the United States, coccidioidomycosis is endemic in parts of Argentina, Brazil, Colombia, Guatemala, Honduras, Mexico, Nicaragua, Paraguay, and Venezuela.
- Up to 29% of community-acquired pneumonias in endemic areas may be due to *Coccidioides* spp.

Risk for Travelers

- In disease-endemic areas, persons of all ages may be at increased risk for disease if they participate in or are present during activities that disturb the ground and result in exposure to dust, including construction, landscaping, mining, agriculture, archaeologic excavation, military maneuvers, and recreational pursuits, such as dirt biking.
- However, cases may also occur after travel to an endemic area in the absence of these exposures.
- Natural events such as earthquakes or windstorms that result in generation of dust clouds increase the risk of exposure.

Clinical Presentation

- The incubation period ranges from 7 to 21 days.
- Most infections (60%) are asymptomatic.
- Symptomatic persons will generally have disease ranging from a self-limited influenza-like illness characterized by fever, headache, rash, muscle aches, dry cough, weight loss, and malaise, to primary pulmonary coccidioidomycosis, characterized by pneumonia with changes on chest radiography.
- In rare instances, severe lung disease (e.g., cavitary pneumonia) or dissemination to the central nervous system (e.g., meninges), joints, bones, and skin may develop.
- Persons at increased risk for severe pulmonary disease are the elderly and those with diabetes, recent smoking history, and low socioeconomic status.
- Persons at increased risk for disseminated disease include African Americans and Filipinos, those who are immunocompromised (e.g., those with HIV), and women in the third trimester of pregnancy.
- Once infected with *Coccidioides*, a person is immune to reinfection.

Diagnosis

- The diagnosis of coccidioidomycosis is best established by using serologic, histopathologic, and culture methods.
- Serologic tests are useful to confirm diagnoses and provide prognostic information. Because clinical laboratories use different diagnostic test kits, positive results should be confirmed in a reference laboratory.
- Spherules can be visualized in infected body fluid specimens (e.g., pleural fluid, bronchoalveolar lavage) and biopsy specimens of skin lesions or organs. The presence of a mature spherule with endospores is pathognomonic of infection.

Treatment

- The benefit of treating persons with uncomplicated, acute primary coccidioidomycosis has not been well studied. Although some experts feel that persons without risk for severe or disseminated disease do not require treatment because the illness is self-limited, others propose treatment to reduce the intensity or duration of symptoms.

- Persons at high risk for dissemination should receive antifungal therapy when diagnosed with acute coccidioidomycosis.
- Persons with severe acute pulmonary disease, chronic pulmonary infection, or disseminated disease should receive antifungal therapy. Depending on the clinical situation, azole antifungal agents (e.g., fluconazole and itraconazole) or amphotericin B may be used for treatment.
- All patients with clinical signs and symptoms consistent with coccidioidomycosis should be tested for primary infection and followed closely to monitor the course of disease and document improvement.
- An infectious disease specialist should help manage these patients.

Preventive Measures for Travelers

- No vaccine is available.
- Although complete prevention of infection is not possible, travelers, especially those at increased risk for severe and disseminated disease, can decrease their risk by limiting their exposure to outdoor dust in disease-endemic areas.
- Dust-control measures that include wetting soil before disturbing the earth may be effective.
- Other protective measures aimed at reducing exposure to dust, such as wearing well-fitted dust masks capable of filtering particles as small as 0.4 μm and using vehicles with enclosed, air-conditioned cabs, can provide added protection for those with high occupational exposure to dust.

References

1. Chiller TM, Galgiani JN, Stevens DA. Coccidioidomycosis. Infect Dis Clin North Am. 2003;17(1):41–57.
2. Galgiani JN, Ampel NM, Blair JE, et al. Coccidioidomycosis. Clin Infect Dis. 2005;41(9):1217–23.
3. Crum NF, Lederman ER, Stafford CM, et al. Coccidioidomycosis: a descriptive survey of a reemerging disease. Clinical characteristics and current controversies. Medicine (Baltimore). 2004;83(3):149–75.
4. Schneider E, Hajjeh RA, Spiegel RA, et al. A coccidioidomycosis outbreak following the Northridge, California, earthquake. JAMA. 1997;277(11):904–8.
5. Park BJ, Sigel K, Vaz V, et al. An epidemic of coccidioidomycosis in Arizona associated with climate changes, 1998–2001. J Infect Dis. 2005;191(11):1981–7.
6. Galgiani JN. Coccidioidomycosis: a regional disease of national importance. Rethinking approaches for control. Ann Intern Med. 1999:130(4 Pt 1):293–300.
7. Panackal AA, Hajjeh RA, Cetron MS, et al. Fungal infections among returning travelers. Clin Infect Dis. 2002;35(9):1088–95.
8. Valdivia L, Nix D, Wright M, et al. Coccidioidomycosis as a common cause of community-acquired pneumonia. Emerg Infect Dis. 2006;12(6):958–62.
9. Cairns L, Blythe D, Kao A, et al. Outbreak of coccidioidomycosis in Washington state

residents returning from Mexico. Clin Infect Dis. 2000;30(1):61–4.
10. Petersen LR, Marshall SL, Barton-Dickson C, et al. Coccidioidomycosis among workers at an archeological site, northeastern Utah. Emerg Infect Dis. 2004;10(4):637–42.
11. Rosenstein NE, Emery KW, Werner SB, et al. Risk factors for severe pulmonary and disseminated coccidioidomycosis: Kern County, California, 1995–1996. Clin Infect Dis. 2001;32(5):708–15.
12. Woods CW, McRill C, Plikaytis BD, et al. Coccidioidomycosis in human immunodeficiency virus-infected persons in Arizona, 1994–1997: incidence, risk factors, and prevention. J Infect Dis. 2000;181(4):1428–34.
13. Smith CD, Beard RR, Rosenberger HG, et al. Effect of season and dust control on coccidioidomycosis. JAMA. 1946;132:833–8.
14. Fisher FS, Bultman MW, Pappagianis D. Operational guidelines for geological fieldwork in areas endemic for coccidioidomycosis (Valley fever). Reston (VA): US Geological Survey Open-File Report. 2000. Report No:00-348.
15. Galgiani JN, Catanzaro A, Cloud GA, et al. Comparison of oral fluconazole and itraconazole for progressive, nonmeningeal coccidioidomycosis: a randomized, double-blind trial. Mycoses Study Group. Ann Intern Med. 2000;133(9):676–86.

CRYPTOSPORIDIOSIS

Sharon Roy, Michele C. Hlavsa, Michael Beach

Infectious Agent

- Protozoan parasite *Cryptosporidium*.
- Many species of *Cryptosporidium* exist that infect humans and a wide range of animals. The most common species infecting humans are *C. hominis* and *C. parvum*.

Mode of Transmission

Transmission occurs by—

- Ingesting fecally contaminated food or water, including water swallowed while swimming.
- Exposure to fecally contaminated environmental surfaces and objects.
- Fecal–oral, person-to-person contact (e.g., diaper changing, caring for an infected person).

Occurrence

- Cryptosporidiosis transmission occurs worldwide; it is a common cause of childhood diarrhea, especially in developing countries.
- Cryptosporidiosis outbreaks have been reported in North America, Europe, Latin America, Australia, and Asia. Outbreaks have been traced to contaminated recreational water, drinking water, and food; contact with animals (especially calves); hospitals; and daycare settings.

Risk for Travelers

For travelers to developing countries, risk of infection is highest for those with the greatest exposure to potentially contaminated food or water.

Clinical Presentation

- Symptoms usually begin 3–14 days after becoming infected with the parasite and are generally self-limiting.
- The most common symptom is watery diarrhea. Other symptoms can include abdominal cramps, vomiting, dehydration, fever, and weight loss. Some people infected with *Cryptosporidium* have no symptoms at all.
- In immunocompetent persons, symptoms usually last 1–2 weeks but may persist for a month, or rarely, up to 4 months. Some persons may experience a recurrence of symptoms after a brief period of recovery before the illness resolves; symptoms that come and go generally resolve within a month.
- In immunosuppressed persons, such as those with AIDS or patients taking immunosuppressive medications, cryptosporidiosis can become chronic and can be fatal.

Diagnosis

- Tests for *Cryptosporidium* are not routinely done in most laboratories; therefore, health-care providers should specifically request testing for this parasite.

- Because detection of *Cryptosporidium* can be difficult, patients may be asked to submit several stool samples over several days.
- Most often, stool specimens are examined microscopically by using different techniques (e.g., acid-fast staining, direct fluorescent antibody [DFA]—the gold standard) and/or enzyme immunoassays for detection of *Cryptosporidium* spp. antigens).
- Molecular methods (e.g., polymerase chain reaction) are increasingly used in reference diagnostic laboratories, since they can be used to identify *Cryptosporidium* spp. at the species level.

Treatment

- Most immunocompetent persons will recover without treatment. Diarrhea should be managed with adequate fluid replacement to prevent dehydration.
- Nitazoxanide (Alinia, Romark Laboratories, Tampa, FL, USA) has been FDA approved for treatment of diarrhea caused by *Cryptosporidium* in immunocompetent persons and is available by prescription for patients 1 year of age and older. However, the effectiveness of nitazoxanide in immunosuppressed individuals is unclear.

Preventive Measures for Travelers

- No vaccine is available.
- To prevent infection, travelers should be advised to follow strict food precautions. Additionally, travelers should practice good hygiene (e.g., frequent handwashing), avoid swallowing water while swimming, and avoid fecal exposure during sexual activity.
- *Cryptosporidium* is poorly inactivated by chlorine or iodine disinfection. Water can be treated effectively by boiling or filtration with an absolute 1-micron filter. Specific information on preventing cryptosporidiosis through filtration can be found in Cryptosporidiosis: A Guide to Water Filters at www.cdc.gov/crypto/factsheets/filters.html.

References

1. Guerrant RL. Cryptosporidiosis: an emerging, highly infectious threat. Emerg Infect Dis. 1997;3(1):51–7.
2. Kosek M, Alcantara C, Lima AA, et al. Cryptosporidiosis: an update. Lancet Infect Dis. 2001;1(4):262–9.
3. Warren CA, Guerrant RL. Clinical disease and pathology. In: Fayer R, Xiao L, editors. *Cryptosporidium* and cryptosporidiosis. 2nd ed. Boca Raton (FL): CRC Press; 2008. p. 235–53.
4. Roy SL, DeLong SM, Stenzel SA, et al. Risk factors for sporadic cryptosporidiosis among immunocompetent persons in the United States from 1999 to 2001. J Clin Microbiol. 2004;42(7):2944–51.
5. Smith H. Diagnostics. In: Fayer R, Xiao L, editors. *Cryptosporidium* and cryptosporidiosis.

2nd ed. Boca Raton (FL): CRC Press; 2008. p. 173–207.
6. Fox LM, Saravolatz LD. Nitazoxanide: a new thiazolide antiparasitic agent. Clin Infect Dis. 2005;40(8):1173–80.
7. Yoder JS, Beach MJ; CDC. Cryptosporidiosis surveillance—United States, 2003–2005. MMWR Surveill Summ. 2007;56(7):1–10.
8. American Public Health Association. Cryptosporidiosis. In: Heymann DL, editor. Control of communicable disease manual. 18th ed. Washington D.C.: American Public Health Association; 2004. p. 138–42.
9. White, CA Jr. Nitazoxanide: a new broad spectrum antiparasitic agent. Expert Rev Anti Infect Ther. 2004;2(1):43–9.

CUTANEOUS LARVA MIGRANS (CLM)

Susan Montgomery

Infectious Agent

Infection is caused by the larval stages of dog and cat hookworms (*Ancylostoma* spp.). Although other worms, such as *Strongyloides* and *Gnathostoma* spp., can migrate through the skin, this section will deal with the *Ancylostoma* spp.

Mode of Transmission

Infection occurs by contact of skin with contaminated soil or beach sand. Eggs shed in the feces of infected hosts hatch in the soil and develop into third-stage larvae, which penetrate the skin and migrate through the epidermis. In humans, larvae are confined to the dermis, because humans are not their definitive host.

Occurrence

- Dog hookworms are found worldwide and are the species most commonly associated with CLM. Cat hookworms are less commonly implicated.
- Infection is more likely to occur in tropical and semitropical countries where skin exposure is common and environmental conditions are conducive to larval development in the soil. For tourists, beach environments are the most likely risk due to walking and sitting in the sand with bare skin.
- CLM can occur during summer months in northern areas when warmth and moisture are adequate for development of infective larvae in soil.

Risk for Travelers

- Persons of all ages are at risk of infection if they travel to endemic areas.
- Most cases are reported in travelers to the Caribbean, Africa, Asia, and South America. Patients without travel history may have acquired the infection in the United States.
- Walking barefoot, sitting, or lying on contaminated beaches or ground can lead to infection.

Clinical Presentation

- CLM is typically characterized by a serpiginous, erythematous track that appears in the skin, associated with intense itchiness, redness and mild swelling. The larvae causing the tracks can migrate a few millimeters to several centimeters per day depending on parasite species. Typical locations are the bottom or top of the foot or the buttocks.
- Itching can occur as the larvae penetrate the skin. Creeping eruption usually appears 1–5 days later, but the incubation period may be up to a month or longer.
- Infection usually heals spontaneously within weeks to months but has been reported to persist for years in rare cases.
- Bacterial secondary infection can occur.

Diagnosis

CLM is diagnosed clinically on the basis of the presence of characteristic skin lesions. Eosinophilia may not be present, and total immunoglobulin E (IgE) is usually normal. Serologic tests are not helpful in CLM except to rule out other causes of larva migrans syndromes such as toxocariasis or strongyloidiasis. Biopsy is not recommended since the track does not usually correlate with larva location.

Treatment

- Albendazole, 400 mg orally per day for 3 days, is considered the treatment of choice.
- Ivermectin (200 µg/kg orally, daily for 1–2 days) has been shown to be effective but is not FDA approved for this indication.
- For localized lesions, topical 15% thiabendazole cream applied 2–3 times a day for 5 days has been shown to cure most infections within 5–7 days.
- Additional information can be found on the Division of Parasitic Diseases' website: www.cdc.gov/ncidod/dpd/parasites/hookworm/default.htm.

Preventive Measures for Travelers

- Preventive measures include reducing contact with contaminated soil by wearing shoes and protective clothing and using barriers when seated on the ground.
- Infective larvae take about 7 days to develop from eggs passed in dog feces. Regular veterinary attention and antihelminthic treatment controls hookworm infections in dogs and cats, but the risk in many countries is from stray dogs.

References

1. Heukelbach J, Feldmeier H. Epidemiological and clinical characteristics of hookworm-related cutaneous larva migrans. Lancet Infect Dis. 2008;8(5):302–9.
2. Caumes E. Treatment of cutaneous larva migrans. Clin Infect Dis. 2000;30(5):811–4.
3. Gillespie SH. Cutaneous larva migrans. Curr Infect Dis Rep. 2004;6(1):50–3.
4. Hochedez P, Caumes E. Hookworm-related cutaneous larva migrans. J Travel Med. 2007;14(5):326–33.
5. Ansart S, Perez L, Jaureguiberry S, et al. Spectrum of dermatoses in 165 travelers returning from the tropics with skin diseases. Am J Trop Med Hyg. 2007;76(1):184–6.

CYCLOSPORIASIS

David R. Shlim, Barbara L. Herwaldt

Infectious Agent

Cyclosporiasis is caused by *Cyclospora cayetanensis*, which is a protozoan (unicellular), coccidian parasite; oocysts (rather than cysts) are shed in the feces of infected persons.

Mode of Transmission

- Infection results from ingestion of mature (infective) *Cyclospora* oocysts, such as in contaminated food or water.
- Direct person-to-person transmission is unlikely because the oocysts shed in feces must mature in the environment (outside the host) to become infective to someone else. Limited data indicate that the maturation process requires from days to weeks in favorable conditions.

Occurrence

- Cyclosporiasis appears to be most common in tropical and subtropical regions of the world.

- Outbreaks in the United States and Canada have been linked to various types of imported, fresh produce.

Risk for Travelers

- Persons of all ages are at risk for infection.
- Travelers to developing countries can be at increased risk.
- In some regions where cyclosporiasis has been studied, the risk for infection is seasonal. However, no consistent pattern has been discerned with respect to time of year or environmental conditions.

Clinical Presentation

- *Cyclospora* infects the small intestine. Asymptomatic infection has been documented, particularly in settings where cyclosporiasis is endemic.
- Among symptomatic persons, the incubation period averages 1 week (range 2 days to ≥2 weeks).
- Onset of symptoms is often abrupt but can be gradual; some persons have a flu-like prodrome.
- The most common symptom is watery diarrhea, which can be profuse.
- Other common symptoms include anorexia, weight loss, abdominal cramps, bloating, nausea, and body aches. Vomiting and low-grade fever may be noted.
- If untreated, the illness can last for several weeks or months, with a remitting–relapsing course and prolonged fatigue and malaise.

Diagnosis

- Infection is diagnosed by detecting *Cyclospora* oocysts (8–10 μm in diameter) in stool specimens.
- Stool examinations for ova and parasites usually do not include methods for detecting *Cyclospora* unless clinicians specifically request testing for this parasite.
- *Cyclospora* oocysts commonly are shed at low levels, even by persons with profuse diarrhea. This constraint underscores the utility of repeated stool examinations, sensitive recovery methods (particularly concentration procedures), and detection methods that highlight the organism: *Cyclospora* oocysts autofluoresce when viewed by UV fluorescence microscopy and can be stained with modified acid-fast or modified ("hot") safranin techniques.
- For more information about these and other laboratory methods, visit CDC's Division of Parasitic Diseases' DPDx website: www.dpd.cdc.gov/dpdx/HTML/Cyclosporiasis.htm. Diagnostic assistance is available through DPDx (www.dpd.cdc.gov/dpdx/).

Treatment

- The treatment of choice is trimethoprim–sulfamethoxazole (TMP-SMX). The typical regimen for immunocompetent adults is TMP, 160 mg, plus SMX, 800 mg (one double-strength tablet) orally, twice a day for 7–10 days.
- No highly effective alternatives have been identified for persons allergic to (or intolerant of) TMP-SMX. Clinicians may consult CDC about possible approaches for such persons (CDC Public Inquiries, 770-488-7775; parasites@cdc.gov).
- Additional information about clinical issues can be found on the Division of Parasitic Diseases' website at www.cdc.gov/ncidod/dpd/parasites/cyclospora/default.htm.

Preventive Measures for Travelers

- No vaccine is available.

- Travelers to developing countries should be advised to follow the precautions described in the Water Disinfection for Travelers in Chapter 2.
- Disinfection with chlorine or iodine is unlikely to be effective against *Cyclospora* oocysts.

References

1. Herwaldt BL. *Cyclospora cayetanensis*: a review, focusing on the outbreaks of cyclosporiasis in the 1990s. Clin Infect Dis. 2000;31(4):1040–57.

2. Shlim DR. *Cyclospora cayetanensis*. Clin Lab Med. 2002;22(4):927–36.

CYSTICERCOSIS

Caryn Bern, Susan Montgomery

Infectious Agent

Larval stage of the cestode parasite *Taenia solium*.

Mode of Transmission

- By ingestion of eggs excreted by a human carrier of the pork tapeworm, *T. solium*. (Consumption of undercooked pork with cysticerci results in tapeworm infection, not human cysticercosis.)
- Fecally contaminated food can transmit the disease, but epidemiologic studies suggest that close (e.g., household) contact with a tapeworm carrier is the most common risk factor.
- Tapeworm carriers can be infected by ingestion of eggs they themselves have excreted; patients with cysticercosis and their household contacts should have stool specimens examined for eggs.

Occurrence

Common in all countries (Latin America, Asia, and Africa) with poor sanitary conditions, where pigs are raised with access to human feces.

Risk for Travelers

Cysticercosis is very uncommon in returning travelers; three case reports have been published.

Clinical Presentation

- The latent period (before symptoms) is a median of 5 years (range 1–30 years).
- Cysticercosis symptoms depend on the number, location, and stage of cysts. The most common location is brain parenchyma, with late-onset seizures. Other presentations include increased intracranial pressure, encephalitis, symptoms of space-occupying lesion, and hydrocephalus.

Diagnosis

- Based on neuroimaging studies (i.e., CT, MRI) and confirmatory serologic testing.

- The most reliable serologic test is the enzyme-linked immunotransfer blot, but even this test may be negative in up to 30% of patients with a single parenchymal lesion. The test is more sensitive in serum than in cerebrospinal fluid.

Treatment

- Neurocysticercosis is uncommon in the United States, and the inexperienced physician is advised to consult an infectious disease or tropical medicine specialist for diagnosis and treatment.
- Physicians can consult with CDC to obtain information about diagnosis and treatment.
- Albendazole, 15 mg/kg/day for 1 week, is recommended for uncomplicated forms of neurocysticercosis. Longer courses may be indicated for some forms.
- Simultaneous use of dexamethasone (or other steroids) may be indicated.
- For some lesions, surgical intervention may be the treatment of choice.
- Seizures should be managed with conventional anticonvulsant therapy.
- Antiparasitic treatment should **not** be initiated in patients with heavy infections, cysticercotic encephalitis, or increased intracranial pressure, because dying cysts can cause increased inflammation and edema and worsen symptoms. In these cases, neurologic (steroids, mannitol) or neurosurgical management, or both is the priority.

Preventive Measures for Travelers

- No vaccine is available.
- No drugs for preventing infection are available.
- Preventive measures are aimed at avoiding consumption of fecally contaminated food.

References

1. Garcia HH, Del Brutto OH; Cysticercosis Working Group in Peru. Neurocysticercosis: updated concepts about an old disease. Lancet Neurol. 2005;4(10):653–61.

2. Garcia HH, Del Brutto OH, Nash TE, et al. New concepts in the diagnosis and management of neurocysticercosis (Taenia solium). Am J Trop Med Hyg. 2005;72(1):3–9.

DENGUE FEVER (DF) AND DENGUE HEMORRHAGIC FEVER (DHF)

Kay M. Tomashek

Infectious Agent

- Four immunologically related, single positive-stranded RNA viruses known as dengue viruses (DENV-1 through DENV-4) of the genus *Flavivirus*, family *Flaviviridae*, are responsible for causing dengue fever (DF) and dengue hemorrhagic fever (DHF).
- Infection with one DENV produces lifelong immunity against reinfection with that one virus and short-term (≤9 months), partial cross-protection against the other three dengue viruses. An individual may be infected up to four times during his or her lifetime.

Mode of Transmission

- Transmission occurs from the bite of an infected *Aedes aegypti* (rarely *Aedes albopictus*) mosquito. Mosquitoes first become infected with DENV by feeding on the blood of a dengue-infected person. After the virus replicates for 8–12 days in the mosquito, the mosquito can transmit DENV to many other people.

- Direct person-to-person transmission has not been documented. A few case reports have been published of transmission of DENV through exposure to: dengue-infected blood, organs, or other tissues from blood transfusions; solid organ or bone marrow transplants; needlestick injuries; and mucous membrane contact with dengue-infected blood.

Occurrence

- Dengue infections have been reported in over 100 countries and are widespread in most tropical countries of the South Pacific, Asia, the Caribbean, the Americas, and Africa (Maps 5-1 and 5-2). The geographic spread of dengue infections is similar to that of malaria, but unlike malaria, dengue infections are often found in the urban areas of tropical nations, including Thailand, Singapore, Taiwan, Indonesia, Philippines, India, and Brazil. Because the main risk of exposure for the traveler is in populated urban and residential areas, travelers are advised to consult CDC (www.cdc.gov/ncidod/dvbid/dengue) and WHO (www.who.int/topics/dengue/en/) websites for outbreak information.
- Recently, locally acquired dengue infections have been reported in Texas, Hawaii, and the Middle East.

Risk for Travelers

- Cases of DF and DHF are confirmed every year among travelers returning to the United States. Infection rates (based on antidengue serology) among febrile travelers returning from dengue-endemic areas in the tropics range from 2.9% to 8.0%.
- Dengue was the leading cause of systemic febrile illness among travelers returning from the Caribbean, South America, South Central Asia, and Southeast Asia in a recent study of 17,353 ill travelers seen at GeoSentinel surveillance network clinics. In some case studies, dengue is the second most common cause of hospitalization (malaria is the most common) among travelers returning from the tropics.
- The bite of one infected mosquito can result in infection. The risk of being bitten is highest during the early morning, several hours after daybreak, and in the late afternoon several hours before sunset, because the female mosquito typically feeds (bites) during these hours. However, mosquitoes may feed at any time during the day.
- Published data are limited on the health outcomes associated with dengue infection among pregnant women and the effects of maternal dengue infection on a developing fetus. However, if a pregnant woman has dengue at the time of delivery, the infant can be born with dengue infection or acquire dengue during labor and delivery and then develop the clinical manifestations of DF or DHF. Transplacental transfer of maternal antidengue antibodies (from a previous maternal infection) may place infants at greater risk for DHF with their first dengue infection.

Clinical Presentation

- The incubation period is typically 4–7 days (range 3–14 days). Dengue should be considered in the differential diagnosis of febrile patients with a history of travel to the tropics in the 2 weeks prior to symptom onset.
- Most travelers infected with DENV are asymptomatic, as are most people infected with DENV who live in areas where the virus is widespread.
- The clinical manifestation of symptomatic illness ranges from mild, undifferentiated febrile illness to classic DF or DHF. Classic DF presents with a sudden onset of high fever, frontal headache (often accompanied by retro-orbital pain), nausea, backache, muscle aches, and profound weakness. A characteristic rash can be

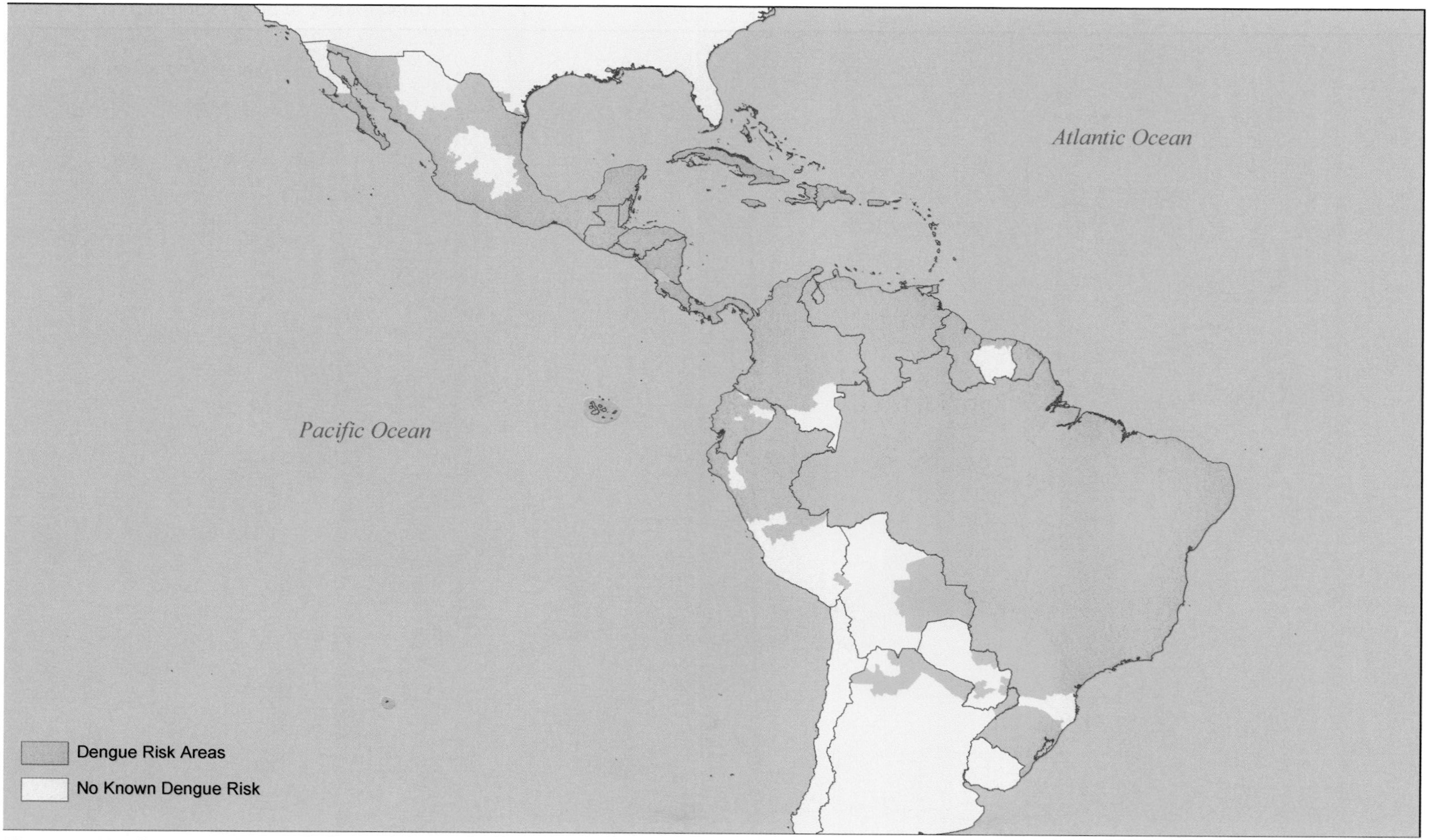

Map 5-1. Distribution of dengue, Western Hemisphere.

Dengue Risk Areas

No Known Dengue Risk

Atlantic Ocean

Pacific Ocean

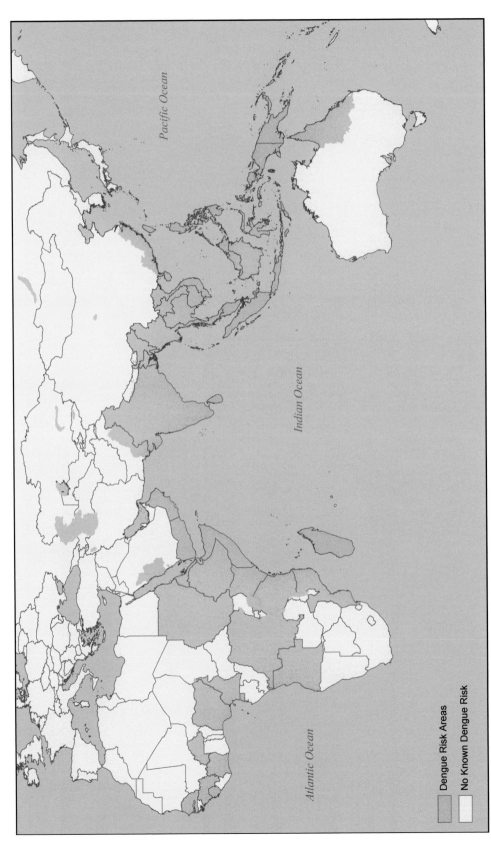

Map 5-2. Distribution of dengue, Eastern Hemisphere.

detected on the second to third day of illness. It is usually a macular, faint red rash that resembles sunburn and occurs mainly on the trunk and upper arms. The rash may not be noticeable until pressure is applied with the hand or a stethoscope, and the skin blanches and only slowly refills over several seconds. The fever persists for 3–6 days. Approximately 1% of patients with DF develop DHF as the fever subsides (usually 3–7 days following the onset of fever).

- The hallmark of DHF is evidence of vascular leakage. DHF is defined by the presence of all of the following symptoms:
  - fever or recent history of fever lasting 2–7 days,
  - any hemorrhagic manifestation,
  - thrombocytopenia (i.e., platelet count <100,000/mm³), and
  - evidence of increased vascular permeability (i.e., hemoconcentration, pleural or abdominal effusion, hypoalbuminemia, or hypoproteinemia).
- Thrombocytopenia is common in classic DF and does not by itself indicate DHF.
- Dengue Shock Syndrome (DSS) is defined as hypotension, narrow pulse pressure (≤20 mm Hg), or frank shock in any case patient whose illness meets the criteria for DHF.

Diagnosis

- A suspected case of dengue infection can be laboratory confirmed by one of the following means:
  - identification of DENV from serum or autopsy tissue samples by reverse transcriptase-polymerase chain reaction (RT-PCR),
  - seroconversion from negative to positive or a four-fold or greater change in anti-dengue antibody titer in paired serum samples taken in the acute- (<6 days after illness onset) and convalescent-phase (6–30 days after onset) of the illness, or
  - dengue viral antigen identification in autopsy tissue samples by immunofluorescence or immunohistochemical analysis.
- In combination with a compatible travel history and symptom profile, anti-dengue IgM positivity in a single serum sample suggests a probable, recent dengue infection. However, antidengue IgG positivity in a single serum sample may only indicate infection at an indeterminate time in the past. Caution should be exercised when using anti-dengue IgM or IgG antibody positivity from a single sample for diagnosis because there is cross-reactivity between anti-dengue IgM and IgG antibodies with antibodies from other flaviviruses such as the West Nile, yellow fever, and Japanese encephalitis viruses. Previous infection or vaccination with another flavivirus may also result in false-positive anti-dengue antibody results.
- If testing at CDC is requested, acute- and convalescent-phase serum samples should be sent through state or territorial health department laboratories to CDC's Dengue Branch at 1324 Calle Cañada, San Juan, Puerto Rico 00920-3860. Serum samples should be accompanied by clinical and epidemiologic information, including the date of disease onset and sample collection and the patient's detailed recent travel history. For additional information, the Dengue Branch can be contacted by telephone 787-706-2399; fax 787-706-2496; or CDC website at www.cdc.gov/ncidod/dvbid/misc/contactus.htm.

Treatment

- No specific therapeutic agents exist for dengue infections.
- Encourage bed rest and maintenance of fluids to prevent dehydration.
- Control fever with acetaminophen. Headache, back pain and muscle aching may be so severe as to require narcotics. Aspirin (acetylsalicylic acid), aspirin-containing drugs, and other nonsteroidal anti-inflammatory drugs (e.g., ibuprofen)

should be avoided because of their anticoagulant properties. Aspirin and other salicylates should be especially avoided in children due to the association with Reye syndrome.

- Ask patients to watch for warning signs of DHF or DSS as fever declines 3–7 days after onset of symptoms. Instruct patients to go to the hospital if they have any of the following warning signs: abrupt change from fever to hypothermia, severe abdominal pain, persistent vomiting, bleeding, difficulties breathing, or altered mental status (e.g., irritability, confusion, lethargy).
- Prompt and judicious administration of intravenous fluids in patients with DHF or DSS can improve outcomes. In patients with DHF or DSS, hospitalization with close monitoring of vital signs, fluid balance, and hematologic parameters (i.e., hematocrit, platelet count) is indicated, as well as additional supportive measures.

Preventive Measures for Travelers

- Neither vaccine nor drugs for preventing infection are available.
- Travelers should be advised to take measures to avoid being bitten by *Aedes* mosquitoes. These preventive measures include the following:
  - Select accommodations with well-screened windows or air-conditioning when possible. *Aedes* mosquitoes typically live indoors and are often found in dark, cool places such as in closets, under beds, behind curtains, and in bathrooms. A traveler should be advised to use insecticides to get rid of mosquitoes in these areas.
  - Wear clothing that adequately covers the arms and legs, especially during the early morning and late afternoon.
  - Apply insect repellent to both skin and clothing (e.g., permethrin). The most effective repellents contain DEET (*N,N*-diethylmetatoluamide) (see the Protection Against Mosquitoes, Ticks, and Other Insects and Arthropods section in Chapter 2).
  - For long-term travelers, empty and clean or cover any standing water that can be mosquito-breeding sites in your accommodation (e.g., water storage barrels).

References

1. Wilder-Smith A, Schwartz E. Dengue in travelers. N Engl J Med. 2005;353(9):924–32.
2. World Health Organization. Dengue haemorrhagic fever: diagnosis, treatment, prevention and control. 3rd ed. Geneva: World Health Organization; 2008.
3. Gubler DJ. The global emergence/resurgence of arboviral diseases as public health problems. Arch Med Res. 2002;33(4):330–42.
4. Potasman I, Srugo I, Schwartz E. Dengue seroconversion among Israeli travelers to tropical countries. Emerg Infect Dis. 1999;5(6):824–7.
5. Freedman DO, Weld LH, Kozarsky PE, et al. Spectrum of disease and relation to place of exposure among ill returned travelers. N Engl J Med. 2006;354(2):119–30.
6. O'Brien D, Tobin S, Brown GV, et al. Fever in returned travelers: review of hospital admissions for a 3-year period. Clin Infect Dis. 2001;33(5):603–9.
7. Schwartz E, Mendelson E, Sidi Y. Dengue fever among travelers. Am J Med. 1996;101(5):516–20.
8. Sabin AB. Viral and ricketsial infections of

man. 3rd ed. Philadelphia: JB Lippincott Company, 1959. p. 361–73.
9. Mohammed H, Linnen JM, Muñoz-Jordán JL, et al. Dengue virus in blood donations, Puerto Rico, 2005. Transfusion. 2008;48(7):1348–54.
10. Ramos MM, Mohammed H, Zielinski-Gutierrez E, et al. Epidemic dengue and dengue hemorrhagic fever at the Texas–Mexico border: results of a household-based seroepidemiologic survey, December 2005. Am J Trop Med Hyg. 2008;78(3):364–9.
11. Effler PV, Pang L, Kitsutani P, et al. Dengue fever, Hawaii, 2001–2002. Emerg Infect Dis. 2005;11(5):742–9.
12. Fakeeh M, Zaki AM. Virologic and serologic surveillance for dengue fever in Jeddah, Saudi Arabia, 1994–1999. Am J Trop Med Hyg. 2001;65(6):764–7.
13. Jelinek T, Dobler G, Hölscher M, et al. Prevalance of infection with dengue virus among international travelers. Arch Intern Med. 1997;157(20):2367–70.
14. Settah SG, Vernazza PL, Morant R, et al. [Imported dengue fever in Switerland—serological evidence for a hitherto

unexpectedly high prevalence.] Article in German. Schweiz Med Wochenschr. 1995;125:1673–8.

15. Wichmann O, Lauschke A, Frank C, et al. Dengue antibody prevalence in German travelers. Emerg Infect Dis. 2005;11(5):762–5.

16. Stienlauf S, Segal G, Sidi Y, et al. Epidemiology of travel-related hospitalization. J Travel Med. 2005;12(3):136–41.

17. Cobelens FG, Groen J, Osterhaus AD, et al. Incidence and risk factors of probable dengue virus infection among Dutch travellers to Asia. Trop Med Int Health. 2002;7(4):331–8.

18. Lindbäck H, Lindbäck J, Tegnell A, et al. Dengue fever in travelers to the tropics, 1998 and 1999. Emerg Infect Dis. 2003;9(4):438–42.

19. García-Rivera EJ, Rigau-Pérez JG. Dengue virus. In: Scott GB, Hutto SC, editors.

Diagnosis of congenital and perinatal infections: a concise guide. Totowa (NJ): Humana Press; 2005. p. 189–99.

20. Kliks SC, Nimmanitya S, Nisalak A, et al. Evidence that maternal dengue antibodies are important in the development of dengue hemorrhagic fever in infants. Am J Trop Med Hyg. 1988;38(2):411–9.

21. Fernández R, Rodríguez T, Borbonet F, et al. Estudio de la relacion dengue-embarazo en un grupo de madres cubanas. Rev Cubana Med Trop. 1994;46(2):76–8.

22. World Health Organization. Dengue hemorrhagic fever: diagnosis, treatment, prevention, and control. 2nd ed. Geneva: World Health Organization; 1997.

ECHINOCOCCOSIS (HYDATID DISEASE)

Peter M. Schantz, Pedro L. Moro

Infectious Agent

- Echinococcosis (hydatid disease) is the infection of humans by the larval stages of taeniid (tapeworm) cestodes of the genus *Echinococcus*.
- Five species have been recognized, but four are of public health concern: *E. granulosus, E. multilocularis, E vogeli,* and *E. oligarthrus.*
- *E. granulosus, E. multilocularis,* and *E vogeli* cause cystic, alveolar, and polycystic echinococcosis, respectively.

Mode of Transmission

- The life cycle of *Echinococcus* species involves carnivores as final hosts and herbivores as intermediate hosts (for a detailed figure of the life cycle, see the CDC website at www.dpd.cdc.gov/dpdx/html/Echinococcosis.htm).
- Humans are an incidental intermediate host, because further development of these cestodes depends on ingestion of their larvae by a carnivore.

Occurrence

- *E. granulosus* is prevalent in broad regions of Eurasia, several South American countries, and Africa.
- *E. multilocularis* is endemic in the central part of Europe, parts of the near East, Russia, and the central Asian Republics, China, northern Japan, and Alaska. Recent findings show major endemic areas for both species, *E. granulosus* and *E. multilocularis,* in China.
- *E. vogeli* is indigenous to the humid tropical forests of central and northern South America.
- Re-emergence seems to have occurred in Bulgaria, where the incidence of cystic echinococcosis in children increased from 0.7 to 5.4/100,000 during the 1970s to the mid-1990s, following the collapse of control efforts.
- In Wales, the prevalence of infected dogs has more than doubled from 1993 (3.4%) to 2002 (8.1%), following policy changes favoring health education over weekly dosing of dogs with praziquantel.

- In North America, most cases are diagnosed in immigrants from endemic countries.
- In endemic areas, hunting dogs are often fed the raw viscera of pacas; dogs infected in this way may then expose humans. A small number of polycystic echinococcosis cases in these geographic areas are caused by *E. oligarthrus*.

Risk for Travelers

- The risk of acquiring hydatid disease during short-term recreational travel is negligible.
- Most cases of hydatid disease seen in nonendemic areas occur in immigrant populations.

Clinical Presentation

Cystic Echinococcosis or Cystic Hydatid Disease

- In humans, hydatid cysts of *E. granulosus* are slowly enlarging masses comparable to benign neoplasms.
- Most human infections remain asymptomatic.
- The clinical manifestations are variable and are determined by the site, size, and condition of the cysts.
- Hydatid cysts in the liver and the lungs together account for 90% of affected localizations.

Alveolar Echinococcosis or Alveolar Hydatid Disease

- The embryo of *E. multilocularis* invariably localizes in the liver of the intermediate host.
- The hepatic parenchyma is gradually invaded and replaced by fibrous tissue in which great numbers of vesicles, many microscopic, are embedded.
- Patients eventually succumb to hepatic failure, invasion of contiguous structures, or, less frequently, metastases to the brain.

Treatment

- Consultation with an infectious disease or tropical medicine specialist for diagnosis and treatment is recommended.
- Surgical removal of hydatid cysts remains the treatment of choice in many countries, and it is the preferred treatment when liver cysts are large (>10 cm in diameter), secondarily infected, or located in the brain, lung or kidney.
- Approximately a third of patients treated with benzimidazole drugs become cured (i.e., complete and permanent disappearance of cysts) and even higher proportions (30%–50%) demonstrate significant regression of cyst size and alleviation of symptoms. However, 20%–40% of cases do not respond favorably.
- Because of its high scolicidal activity, albendazole is recommended as a prophylactic agent 1–3 months before surgical intervention.
- With or without surgery, alveolar hydatid disease has a high mortality rate.
- Long-term treatment with mebendazole or albendazole inhibits growth of larval *E. multilocularis*, reduces metastasis, and enhances both the quality and length of survival; prolonged therapy may eventually be larvicidal in some patients.
- The principles of management for cystic and alveolar echinococcoses also apply to polycystic echinococcosis.

Preventive Measures for Travelers

- No vaccine is available for humans, and no drugs are recommended as chemoprophylactic agents.

- Travelers visiting endemic areas should avoid contact with dogs or wild canids.
- Untreated water from streams, canals, lakes, and rivers may contain echinococcus eggs.
- Heating potentially contaminated food and water at 140° F (>60° C) for at least 30 minutes destroys the eggs.

References

1. Moro P, Schantz PM. Hydatid disease (echinococcosis). In: Wallace R, editor. Public health and preventive medicine. 15th ed. New York: McGraw-Hill Companies, Inc.; 2008. p. 448–60.
2. Moro PL, Schantz PM. Echinococcosis: historical landmarks and progress in research and control. Ann Trop Med Parasitol. 2006;100(8):703–14.
3. Romig T, Dinkel A, Mackenstedt U. The present situation of echinococcosis in Europe. Parasitol Int. 2006;55(Suppl):S187–91.
4. Schantz PM. Progress in diagnosis, treatment and elimination of echinococcosis and cysticercosis. Parasitol Int. 2006;55(Suppl):S7–S13.
5. Filippou D, Tselepis D, Filippou G, et al. Advances in liver echinococcosis: diagnosis and treatment. Clin Gastroenterol Hepatol. 2007;5(2):152–9.
6. Eckert J, Gemmell MA, Meslin F-X, Pawlowski ZS, editors. WHO/OIE manual on echinococcosis in humans and animals: a public health problem of global concern. Paris: World Organisation for Animal Health and World Health Organization; 2001.

FILARIASIS, LYMPHATIC

LeAnne M. Fox

Infectious Agent

Lymphatic filariasis is caused by the filarial nematodes *Wuchereria bancrofti* and *Brugia malayi*.

Mode of Transmission

Vector-borne transmission occurs through the bite of infected *Aedes*, *Culex*, *Anopheles*, and *Mansonia* mosquito species.

Occurrence

- Lymphatic filariasis affects an estimated 120 million persons in tropical areas of the world.
- Lymphatic filariasis is found in sub-Saharan Africa, Egypt, southern Asia, the western Pacific islands, the northeastern coast of Brazil, Guyana, Haiti, and the Dominican Republic.
- Since most infections are asymptomatic, many go unrecognized.

Risk for Travelers

- Short-term travelers to endemic areas are at low risk for this infection.
- Travelers who visit endemic areas for extended periods of time (generally longer than 3 months) and who are intensively exposed to infected mosquitoes are at greater risk of infection.
- Most infections seen in the United States are in immigrants from endemic countries.
- A recent report from the GeoSentinel Surveillance Network showed only 0.62% (N=271 of 43,722) of medical conditions reported during 1995–2004 were caused by any filarial infection, and only 101 (25% of the total) were caused by *W. bancrofti*. Lymphatic filariasis caused by *W. bancrofti* was acquired worldwide, with 32% from South America, 12% from sub-Saharan Africa, 22% from South Central Asia, and

14% from the Caribbean. As expected, the majority of cases (62%) were seen in immigrants or refugees. In the few nonresident visitors with a known trip duration who acquired *W. bancrofti*, the stay was >180 days.

Clinical Presentation

- Most infections are asymptomatic, but living adult worms cause progressive lymphatic vessel dilation and dysfunction. Lymphatic dysfunction may lead to lymphedema of the leg, scrotum, penis, arm, or breast, which can increase in severity as a result of recurrent secondary bacterial infections.
- Tropical pulmonary eosinophilia is a potentially serious progressive lung disease that presents with nocturnal cough, wheezing, and fever, resulting from immune hyperresponsiveness to microfilariae in the pulmonary capillaries.

Diagnosis

- The standard for diagnosis is microscopic detection of microfilariae on a thick blood film. In most endemic areas, the highest concentration of microfilariae in the peripheral blood occurs at night; therefore, blood specimens should be collected between 10 pm and 2 am.
- Determination of serum antifilarial immunoglobulin (IgG) is also a diagnostically useful test. This assay is available through the Parasitic Diseases Laboratory at the National Institutes of Health (NIH) or through CDC's Division of Parasitic Diseases.

Treatment

- The drug of choice for treatment of travelers with *W. bancrofti* or *B. malayi* infection is diethylcarbamazine (DEC). DEC, which is available to physicians licensed in the United States for this purpose, can be obtained from the CDC Parasitic Disease Drug Service at 404-639-3670 under an Investigational New Drug protocol (see www.cdc.gov/ncidod/srp/drugs/drug-service.html). DEC kills circulating microfilariae and is partially effective against the adult worms. DEC is also used to treat tropical pulmonary eosinophilia.
- Although ivermectin kills microfilariae, it does not kill the adult worms.
- Many patients with lymphedema are no longer infected with the filarial parasite and do not benefit from antifilarial drug treatment.
- For chronic manifestations of lymphatic filariasis, such as lymphedema and hydrocele; specific lymphedema treatment, including hygiene, skin care, physiotherapy, and, in some cases, antibiotics; and surgical repair, respectively, are recommended.
- To ensure correct diagnosis and treatment, travelers should be advised to consult an infectious disease or tropical medicine specialist.

Preventive Measures for Travelers

- No vaccine is available.
- No drugs for preventing infection are available.
- Protective measures include avoidance of mosquito bites through the use of personal protection measures against biting insects (see the Protection Against Mosquitoes, Ticks and Other Insects and Arthropods section in Chapter 2).

References

1. Nutman TB, editor. Lymphatic Filariasis. London: Imperial College Press; 2000.

2. Abramowicz M, editor. The Medical Letter Report on Drugs for Parasitic Infections. New

Rochelle, NY: The Medical Letter; 2007.

3. Michael E, Bundy DA, Grenfell BT. Re-assessing the global prevalence and distribution of lymphatic filariasis. Parasitology. 1996;112(Pt 4):409–28.

4. Dreyer G, Addiss D, Roberts J, et al. Progression of lymphatic vessel dilatation in the presence of living adult *Wuchereria bancrofti*. Trans R Soc Trop Med Hyg. 2002;96(2):157–61.

5. Dreyer G, Medeiros Z, Netto MJ, et al. Acute attacks in the extremities of persons living in an area endemic for bancroftian filariasis: differentiation of two syndromes. Trans R Soc Trop Med Hyg. 1999;93(4):413–7.

6. Shenoy RK, Suma TK, Rajan K, et al. Prevention of acute adenolymphangitis in brugian filariasis: comparison of the efficacy of ivermectin and diethylcarbamazine, each combined with local treatment of the affected limb. Ann Trop Med Parasitol. 1998;92(5):587–94.

7. Ottesen EA. Efficacy of diethylcarbamazine in eradicating infection with lymphatic-dwelling filariae in humans. Rev Infect Dis. 1985;7(3):341–56.

8. Dreyer G, Addiss D, Noroes J, et al. Ultrasonographic assessment of the adulticidal efficacy of repeat high-dose ivermectin in bancroftian filariasis. Trop Med Int Health. 1996;1(4):427–32.

9. Dreyer G, Addiss D, Dreyer P, Noroes J. Basic lymphoedema management: Treatment and prevention of problems associated with lymphatic filariasis. Hollis (NH): Hollis Publishing Co.; 2002.

10. Eberhard ML, Lammie PJ. Laboratory diagnosis of filariasis. Clin Lab Med. 1991;11(4):977–1010.

11. Lipner EM, Law MA, Barnett E, et al; GeoSentinel Surveillance Network. Filariasis in travelers presenting to the GeoSentinel Surveillance Network. PLoS Negl Trop Dis. 2007;1(3):e88.

GIARDIA

Sharon Roy, Michele C. Hlavsa, Michael Beach

Infectious Agent

Protozoan parasite *Giardia intestinalis* (formerly known as *Giardia lamblia* or *Giardia duodenalis*).

Mode of Transmission

Transmission occurs by—

- Ingesting fecally contaminated food or water, including water swallowed while swimming.
- Exposure to fecally contaminated environmental surfaces and objects.
- Fecal–oral person-to-person contact (e.g., diaper changing, caring for an infected person, certain sexual practices).

Occurrence

- Giardiasis transmission occurs worldwide.
- Outbreaks have been linked to: contaminated drinking water, recreational water, and food; contact with animals; and daycare settings.

Risk for Travelers

Risk of infection increases with duration of travel and is highest for those who live in or visit rural areas, trek in backcountry areas, or frequently eat, drink, or swim in areas that have poor sanitation and inadequate treatment facilities for drinking water.

Clinical Presentation

- Symptoms usually begin 1–2 weeks after becoming infected with the parasite and are generally self-limiting within 2–4 weeks. However, some patients develop a syndrome of chronic diarrhea that may result in malabsorption. Rarely, reactive arthritis has also occurred, following infection with *Giardia*.

- Giardiasis can cause a variety of intestinal symptoms or signs, which include diarrhea (often with foul-smelling, greasy stools), abdominal cramps, bloating, flatulence, fatigue, anorexia, and nausea. These symptoms may lead to weight loss and dehydration. Fever and vomiting are uncommon. Some people infected with *Giardia* have no symptoms at all.

Diagnosis

- Because detection of *Giardia* can be difficult, patients may be asked to submit several stool samples over several days.
- Most often, stool specimens are examined microscopically by using different techniques (e.g., wet mount with iodine, trichrome, or immunofluorescent antibody staining, and/or enzyme immunoassays for detection of *Giardia* sp. antigens).

Treatment

- Diarrhea should be managed with adequate fluid replacement to prevent dehydration.
- Several antimicrobial drugs (i.e., tinidazole, metronidazole, nitazoxanide, paromomycin, furazolidone, quinacrine) are available by prescription for treatment of giardiasis. Treatment recommendations are available for each of these drugs in textbooks on internal medicine and infectious diseases.

Preventive Measures for Travelers

- No vaccine is available, and there is no recommended chemoprophylaxis.
- To prevent infection, travelers should be advised to follow food and water precautions described elsewhere in this book. Additionally, travelers should practice good hygiene (i.e., frequent handwashing), avoid swallowing water while swimming, and avoid fecal exposure during sexual activity.

References

1. Hill DR, Nash TE. Intestinal flagellate and ciliate infections. In: Tropical infectious diseases. 2nd ed. RL Guerrant, DH Walker, PF Weller, editors. Philadelphia; Churchill Livingstone; 2006. p. 984–1002.
2. Okhuysen PC. Traveler's diarrhea due to intestinal protozoa. Clin Infect Dis. 2001;33(1):110–4.
3. Farthing MJ. Giardiasis. Gastroenterol Clin North Am. 1996;25(3):493–515.
4. Hardie RM, Wall PG, Gott P, et al. Infectious diarrhea in tourist staying in a resort hotel. Emerg Infect Dis. 1999;5(1):168–71.
5. Hill Gaston JS, Lillicrap MS. Arthritis associated with enteric infection. Best Pract Res Clin Rheumatol. 2003;17(2):219–39.
6. Yoder JS, Beach MJ; CDC. Giardiasis surveillance—United States, 2003–2005. MMWR Surveill Summ. 2007;56(7):11–8.
7. Stuart JM, Orr HJ, Warburton FG, et al. Risk factors for sporadic giardiasis: a case-control study in southwestern England. Emerg Infect Dis. 2003;9(2):229–33.

HELICOBACTER PYLORI

Ezra J. Barzilay, Ryan P. Fagan

Infectious Agent

Helicobacter pylori is a small, curved, microaerophilic gram-negative rod.

Mode of Transmission

Exact transmission is unknown, but it is thought to be fecal–oral or possibly oral–oral.

Occurrence

- *H. pylori* infection is one of the most common bacterial infections in the world. Estimated prevalence is 70% in developing countries and 30%–40% in the United States and other industrialized countries.
- Infection usually occurs during childhood and may persist lifelong unless treated.
- Humans are the only known reservoir.

Risk for Travelers

- No increased risk of *H. pylori* seroconversion has been documented among residents of industrialized countries who traveled to developing countries for up to 16 months.
- Among missionaries and long-term travelers to developing countries, the annual incidence of seroconversion is 1.9%, which is relatively higher than the annual incidence of seroconversion (0.3%–1.0%) in industrialized countries.

Clinical Presentation

- Most persons infected with *H. pylori* never develop symptoms.
- *H. pylori* is the major cause of peptic ulcer disease, which most commonly presents as gnawing or burning epigastric pain. Less commonly, symptoms include nausea, vomiting, loss of appetite, or bleeding.
- *H. pylori* infection is a known risk factor for gastritis and duodenal ulcers in children and adults. Rarely and primarily in older adults, *H. pylori* also is associated with a gastric lymphoma of the mucosal-associated lymphoid tissue.

Diagnosis

- Testing is recommended for patients with active gastric or duodenal ulcers, gastric mucosa-associated lymphoid tissue lymphomas, or those who have undergone resection of early-stage gastric cancer.
- Esophago-gastroduodenal endoscopic biopsy is performed to obtain tissue samples for histologic identification of organisms, culture, urease test, antibiotic susceptibility testing, and polymerase chain reaction.
- Active infection can also be diagnosed with a ^{13}C- or ^{14}C-labeled urea breath test or with a fecal antigen detection assay.
- *H. pylori*-specific immunoglobulin G (serum or salivary antibody) is a useful marker for epidemiologic studies of past or current infection, but its sensitivity is suboptimal. A positive antibody screen should be confirmed by a second test (e.g., fecal antigen, urea breath test, or endoscopy).

Treatment

- In the United States, the recommended primary therapies include 14 days of clarithromycin-based triple therapy (proton pump inhibitor [PPI] + clarithromycin + amoxicillin or metronidazole) or 10–14 days of bismuth quadruple therapy (PPI or H2-receptor antagonist + bismuth + metronidazole + tetracycline).
- Detailed information about these and other recommended treatment regimens is available at www.gi.org/physicians/guidelines/ManagementofHpylori.pdf.

Preventive Measures for Travelers

- Because the mode of transmission is not known, there are currently no specific recommendations for the prevention of *H. pylori* infection. Travelers should always eat food that has been properly prepared, cooked, and stored; drink water from a safe and clean source; and perform thorough hand washing.
- No vaccine is currently available.
- No drugs for preventing infection are recommended.

References

1. CDC. *Helicobacter pylori* fact sheet for health care providers [Internet]. Atlanta: Centers for Disease Control and Prevention; 1998. [cited 2008 Nov 30]. Available from: www.cdc.gov/ulcer/files/hpfacts.pdf.

2. Chey WD, Wong BC; Practice Parameters Committee of the American College of Gastroenterology. American College of Gastroenterology guideline on the management of *Helicobacter pylori* infection. Am J Gastroenterol. 2007;102(8):1808–25.

3. Potasman I, Yitzhak A. *Helicobacter pylori* serostatus in backpackers following travel to tropical countries. Am J Trop Med Hyg. 1998;58(3):305–8.

4. Lindkvist P, Wadström T, Giesecke J. *Helicobacter pylori* infection and foreign travel. J Infect Dis. 1995;172(4):1135–6.

5. Becker SI, Smalligan RD, Frame JD, et al. Risk of *Helicobacter pylori* infection among long-term residents in developing countries. Am J Trop Med Hyg. 1999;60(2):267–70.

6. Peterson WL, Fendrick AM, Cave DR, et al. *Helicobacter pylori*-related disease: guidelines for testing and treatment. Arch Intern Med. 2000;160(9):1285–91.

7. Gold BD, Colletti RB, Abbott M, et al. *Helicobacter pylori* infection in children: recommendations for diagnosis and treatment. J Pediatr Gastroenterol Nutr. 2000;31(5):490–7

HELMINTHS, INTESTINAL

Michael Deming

Infectious Agent

Ascaris lumbricoides (roundworm), *Ancylostoma duodenale* (hookworm), *Necator americanus* (hookworm), and *Trichuris trichiura* (whipworm) cause infection in humans.

Mode of Transmission

- Adult female worms in the intestine of infected persons produce eggs that are excreted in the stool of infected persons. Defecation on the ground and use of stool to fertilize crops allow eggs to reach soil—the necessary environment for the next phase of their development. Infection with *Ascaris* and *Trichuris* occurs when eggs in soil have become infective and are ingested.
- Hookworm eggs are not infective; they release larvae in soil that have the ability to penetrate skin. Hookworm infection primarily occurs when skin comes in contact with contaminated soil (e.g., by walking barefoot) but can also occur through the ingestion of larvae.
- *Ascaris* larvae, after they have hatched from eggs in the small intestine, and hookworm larvae, after they have penetrated the skin, begin a migratory phase that takes them through the lungs before they become adult worms in the intestine.

Occurrence

- Widespread, with greatest prevalence in tropical, developing countries.

- In 2002, an estimated 1.5 billion, 1.3 billion and 1.1 billion persons were infected with *Ascaris*, hookworm, and *Trichuris,* respectively.

Risk for Travelers

- The risk of infection is low if travelers ensure that their food is washed, peeled, or cooked and they wear shoes when walking on soil that is potentially contaminated.
- Since adult worms do not multiply in the body, travelers who are diagnosed with intestinal worms generally have very few worms. Sporadic exposure to infection is less likely to produce symptomatic disease.
- Because eggs must pass through a developmental phase in soil before becoming infective or releasing infective larvae, soil-transmitted helminth infections are not transmitted person to person.

Clinical Presentation

- Most infections are asymptomatic, especially when worm burdens are light.
- Pulmonary symptoms occur in a small percentage of patients when *Ascaris* or hookworm larvae pass through the lungs. These symptoms include cough, fever, and chest discomfort.
- The most serious complication of *Ascaris* infection is intestinal obstruction, usually of the small intestine. *Ascaris* and hookworm infection can also cause abdominal discomfort.
- Moderate to heavy *Ascaris* infections can impair the nutritional status of children.
- The most serious effects of hookworm infection are anemia and protein deficiency due to blood loss.
- *Trichuris* infection can also cause blood loss as well as dysentery and rectal prolapse.
- Travelers are almost never at risk for the more severe manifestations of intestinal helminths.

Diagnosis

Diagnosis is made by identifying the eggs of soil-transmitted helminths in the microscopic examination of a stool specimen. Adult *Ascaris* worms may occasionally be coughed up or found in stool or vomit.

Treatment

Soil-transmitted helminth infections are usually treated with albendazole or mebendazole, drugs that are effective and well tolerated.

Preventive Measures for Travelers

- No vaccine is available.
- Drugs are not used to prevent infection.
- Travelers should be reminded to wash hands before eating.
- Travelers should avoid walking barefoot on soil that may be contaminated with sewage, where human feces may have been used as fertilizer, or where people may have defecated.

References

1. Bethony J, Brooker S, Albonico M, et al. Soil-transmitted helminth infections: ascariasis, trichuriasis, and hookworm. Lancet. 2006;367(9521):1521–32.

2. Brooker S, Clements AC, Bundy DA. Global epidemiology, ecology and control of soil-transmitted helminth infections. Adv Parasitol 2006;62:221–61.

3. Cooper E. Trichuriasis. In: Guerrant RL, Walker DH, Weller PF, editors. Tropical infectious diseases: principles, pathogens & practice. 2nd ed. Philadelphia: Elsevier; 2006. p. 1252–56.

4. Gilles HM. Soil-transmitted helminths (geohelminths). In: Cook GC, Zumla A, editors. Manson's tropical diseases. 21st edition. London: Saunders; 2003. p 1527–36.

5. Hotez PJ. Hookworm infections. In: Guerrant RL, Walker DH, Weller PF, editors. Tropical infectious diseases: principles, pathogens & practice. 2nd ed. Philadelphia: Elsevier; 2006. p. 1265–73.

6. Seltzer E, Barry M, Crompton DWT. Ascariasis. In: Guerrant RL, Walker DH,

Weller PF, eds. Tropical infectious diseases: principles, pathogens & practice, 2nd ed. Philadelphia: Elsevier; 2006. p. 1257–64.

7. Brooker S, Bethony J, Hotez PJ. Human hookworm infection in the 21st century. Adv Parasitol. 2004;58:197–288.

8. Crompton DW. Ascaris and ascariasis. Adv Parasitol. 2001;48:285–375.

9. Maguire JH. Intestinal nematodes (roundworms). In: Mandell GL, Bennett JE, Dolin R, editors. Principles and practice of infectious diseases. 6th ed. Philadelphia: Elsevier; 2005. p. 3260–6.

10. WHO Expert Committee. Prevention and control of schistosomiasis and soil transmitted helminthiasis. World Health Organ Tech Rep Ser. 2002;912:1–57.

HEPATITIS C

Scott Holmberg

Infectious Agent

Hepatitis C is caused by the hepatitis C virus (HCV), a spherical, enveloped, positive-strand RNA virus, approximately 50 nm in diameter.

Mode of Transmission

- Transmission of HCV is bloodborne and occurs mainly through sharing drug-injection equipment or from transfusion of unscreened blood or untreated clotting factors.
- Overseas, unsterile medicinal and other injection practices account for many infections.
- HCV is infrequently transmitted through sexual contact.

Occurrence

- Approximately 3% (170 million) of the world's population has been infected with HCV. For most countries, the prevalence of HCV infection is less than 3%. The prevalence is higher (up to 15%) in some countries in Africa and Asia, and highest (over 15%) in Egypt (Map 5-3).
- The most frequent mode of transmission in the United States is through sharing drug-injecting equipment among injecting drug users.
- For international travelers, the principal activities that can result in blood exposure include—
  o Receiving blood transfusions that have not been screened for HCV
  o Having medical or dental procedures
  o Engaging in activities (e.g., acupuncture, tattooing, or injecting drug use) in which equipment has not been adequately sterilized or disinfected or in which contaminated equipment is reused

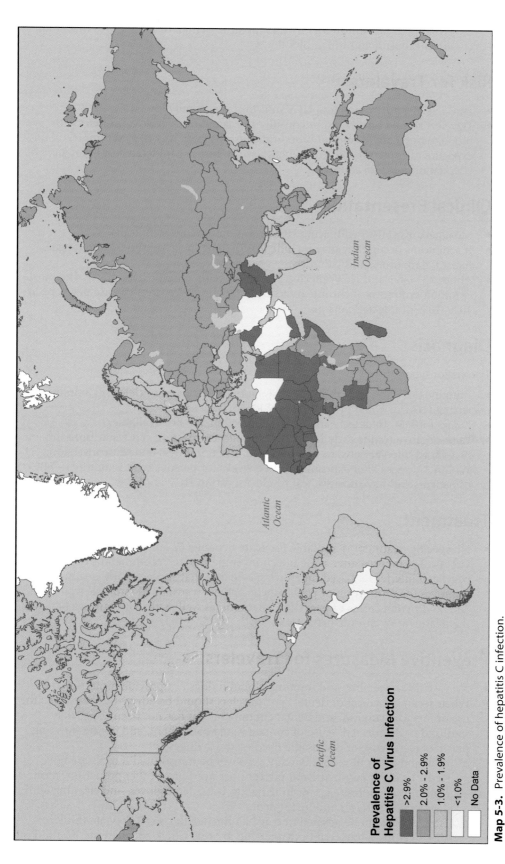

Map 5-3. Prevalence of hepatitis C infection.

(Modified from Perz JF, Farrington LA, Pecoraro C, et al. Estimated global prevalence of hepatitis C virus infection. 42nd Annual Meeting of the Infectious Diseases Society of America; Boston, MA, USA; Sept 30–Oct 3, 2004. Data source: World Health Organization.)

**Prevalence of
Hepatitis C Virus Infection**

- >2.9%
- 2.0% - 2.9%
- 1.0% - 1.9%
- <1.0%
- No Data

   o Working in health-care fields (e.g., medical, dental, or laboratory) that entail direct exposure to human blood.

Risk for Travelers

- Travelers' risk for contracting HCV infection is generally low.
- Travelers should be advised to consider the extent of their direct contact with blood, particularly receipt of blood transfusions from unscreened donors, or exposure to contaminated equipment used in health care-related or cosmetic (e.g., tattooing) procedures.

Clinical Presentation

- Most persons (80%) with acute HCV infection have no symptoms.
- If symptoms occur, they may include loss of appetite, abdominal pain, fatigue, nausea, dark urine, and jaundice.
- About 75%–85% of HCV-infected persons develop chronic hepatitis C. The most common symptom of chronic infection is fatigue; severe liver disease develops in 10%–20% of infected persons.

Diagnosis

Two major types of tests are available:

- Immunoglobulin (IgG) antibody assays for anti-HCV and nucleic acid amplification testing (NAT or NAAT) to detect HCV RNA.
- Assays for IgM, to detect early or acute infection, are not available.
- False-negative results early in the course of acute infection can result from the prolonged interval between exposure and onset of illness and seroconversion. Within 15 weeks after exposure—5 to 6 weeks for persons with symptoms—80% of patients will have positive test results for serum HCV antibody.

Treatment

- No specific treatment is available for acute hepatitis C. For patients who remain viremic 2–4 months after acute infection, some experts recommend treatment with pegylated interferon, based on growing evidence that suggests early treatment improves the proportion of patients who achieve a sustained virologic response.
- Several different forms of pegylated interferon as well as ribavirin are available for the treatment of chronic hepatitis C.

Preventive Measures for Travelers

- No vaccine is available, and immune globulin does not provide protection.
- When seeking medical or dental care, travelers should be advised to be alert to the use of medical, surgical, and dental equipment that has not been adequately sterilized or disinfected, reuse of contaminated equipment, and unsafe injecting practices (e.g., reuse of disposable needles and syringes).
  - o HCV and other bloodborne pathogens can be transmitted if tools are not sterile or if the tattoo artist or piercer does not follow other proper infection-control procedures (e.g., washing hands, using latex gloves, and cleaning and disinfecting surfaces and instruments).
  - o Travelers should be advised to consider the health risks if they are thinking about getting a tattoo or body piercing in areas where adequate sterilization or disinfection procedures might not be available or practiced.

References

1. Prati D. Transmission of hepatitis C by blood transfusions and other medical procedures: a global review. J Hepatol. 2006;45(4):607–16.
2. Perz JF, Farrington LA, Pecoraro C, et al. Estimated global prevalence of hepatitis C virus infection. 42nd Annual Meeting of the Infectious Diseases Society of America; Boston, MA, USA; Sept 30–Oct 3, 2004.
3. Simonsen L, Kane A, Lloyd J, et al. Unsafe injections in the developing world and transmission of bloodborne pathogens: a review. Bull World Health Organ. 1999;77(10):789–800.
4. The Global Burden of Hepatitis C Working Group. Global burden of disease (GBD) for hepatitis C. J Clin Pharmacol. 2004;44(1):20–9.
5. Armstrong GL, Wasley A, Simard EP, et al. The prevalence of hepatitis C virus infection in the United States, 1999 through 2002. Ann Intern Med. 2006;144(10):705–14.
6. Shepard CW, Finelli L, Alter MJ. Global epidemiology of hepatitis C virus infection. Lancet Infect Dis. 2005;5(9):558–67.
7. Strader DB, Wright T, Thomas DL, et al.; American Association for Study of Liver Diseases. Diagnosis, management, and treatment of hepatitis C. Hepatology. 2004;39(4):1147–71.

HEPATITIS E

Chong-Gee Teo

Infectious Agent

Infection is caused by hepatitis E virus (HEV), a single-stranded RNA molecule. It is classified in its own family, *Hepeviridae*.

Mode of Transmission

HEV is transmitted primarily by the fecal–oral route. Epidemics of hepatitis E are principally due to drinking fecally contaminated water. Sporadic disease in Japan is zoonotic and food-borne and is associated with eating meat and viscera of deer, boars, and pigs. Sporadic disease also is observed in other temperate countries, including the United States, but its cause is unknown in most cases. Disease from blood transfusion has been reported, although rare. Perinatal HEV transmission from women infected during pregnancy is common.

Occurrence

- Waterborne outbreaks (often large, involving hundreds to thousands of people) have occurred in South and Central Asia, tropical East Asia, Africa, and Central America (Map 5-4). Clinical attack rates are highest in young adults 15–49 years of age.
- In outbreak-prone areas, interepidemic disease is sporadically encountered.
- In these areas, pregnant women—whether infected sporadically or during an epidemic—are at significant risk of progressing to liver failure and death.
- Sporadic disease also occurs in the Middle East, temperate East Asia (including China), North and South America, and Europe (except Scandinavian countries). Symptomatic disease is observed most frequently in adults >60 years old, especially men.
- Chronic infection has been reported in organ transplant recipients undergoing immunosuppressive therapy.

Risk for Travelers

- Persons of all ages are at risk of HEV infection when they travel to areas where epidemics have occurred, but symptomatic disease is most frequent in young adults.

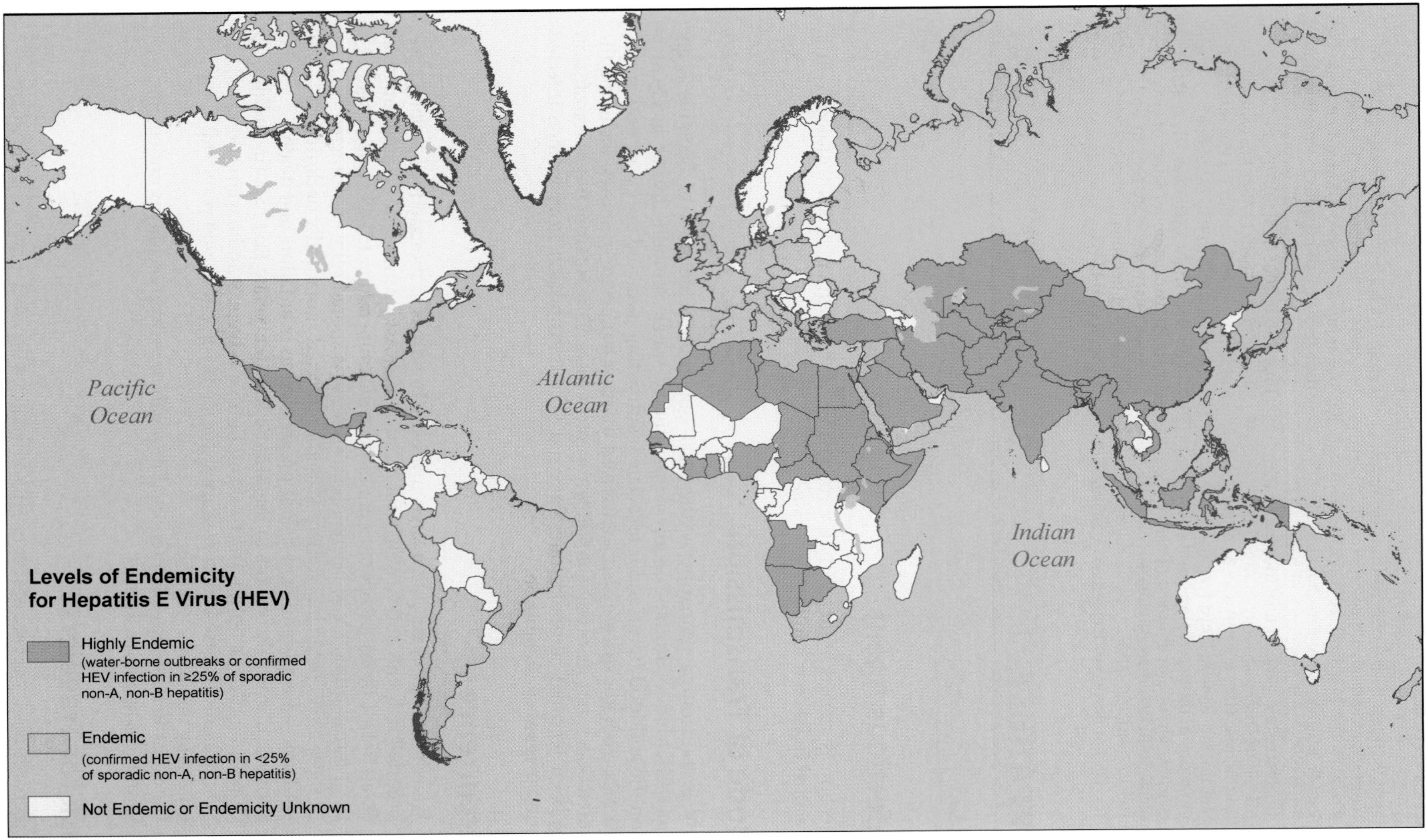
Pacific
Ocean
Atlantic
Ocean
Indian
Ocean
Levels of Endemicity
for Hepatitis E Virus (HEV)
Highly Endemic
(water-borne outbreaks or confirmed
HEV infection in ≥25% of sporadic
non-A, non-B hepatitis)
Endemic
(confirmed HEV infection in <25%
of sporadic non-A, non-B hepatitis)
Not Endemic or Endemicity Unknown

Map 5-4. Distribution of hepatitis E infection, 2008.

- In hyperendemic areas, infection and disease are due to eating and drinking in settings where sanitary conditions are poor.
- When traveling in Japan, eating raw or inadequately cooked venison, boar meat, or pig liver is a significant risk factor for hepatitis E.
- It is unknown if the risk of acquiring hepatitis E in the United States is higher than when traveling to regions outside the United States where sanitation is adequate and sporadic hepatitis E also occurs.

Clinical Presentation

- Incubation period is 2–9 weeks (mean 6 weeks).
- Signs and symptoms of disease during primary infection include jaundice, fever, loss of appetite, abdominal pain, and lethargy.
- Acute hepatitis E is frequently self-limited.
- Pregnant women (particularly those infected during the second or third trimester) may present with or progress to liver failure, and their infants are at risk of spontaneous abortion and premature delivery.
- People with pre-existing chronic liver disease may undergo further hepatic decompensation during HEV infection.

Diagnosis

- The diagnosis of acute hepatitis E is established by the positive detection of both immunoglobulin IgM and IgG anti-HEV antibodies in serum.
- Detection of HEV RNA in serum or stools further confirms the serological diagnosis but is seldom required.
- Longer-term, serial detection of HEV RNA in serum or stools, regardless of the HEV antibody serostatus, suggests chronic HEV infection.
- No FDA-approved diagnostic test is available.

Treatment

Treatment is supportive.

Preventive Measures for Travelers

- No vaccine is available.
- No drugs for preventing infection are available.
- Travelers should avoid drinking unboiled or unchlorinated water and beverages that contain unboiled water or ice.
- Travelers should eat only food that is thoroughly cooked, including seafood, meat, and meat products.

References

1. Appleton H, Banks M, Dentinger CM, Teo CG. Foodborne Viral Hepatitis. In: Foodborne Diseases. Shimjee S, editor. Totowa (NJ): Humana; 2007. p. 175–214.
2. Panda SK, Thakral D, Rehman S. Hepatitis E virus. Rev Med Virol. 2007;17(3):151–80.
3. Teo CG. Hepatitis E indigenous to economically developed countries: to what extent a zoonosis? Curr Opin Infect Dis. 2006;19(5):460–6.
4. Boccia D, Guthmann JP, Klovstad H, et al. High mortality associated with an outbreak of

hepatitis E among displaced persons in Darfur, Sudan. Clin Infect Dis. 2006;42(12):1679–84.
5. Patra S, Kumar A, Trivedi SS, et al. Maternal and fetal outcomes in pregnant women with acute hepatitis E virus infection. Ann Intern Med. 2007;147(1):28–33.
6. Lewis HC, Boisson S, Ijaz S, et al. Hepatitis E in England and Wales. Emerg Infect Dis. 2008;14(1):165–7.
7. Renou C, Moreau X, Pariente A, et al.; ANGH, France. A national survey of acute hepatitis E

in France. Aliment Pharmacol Ther. 2008;27(11):1086–93.

8. Kamar N, Selves J, Mansuy JM, et al. Hepatitis E virus and chronic hepatitis in organ-transplant recipients. N Engl J Med. 2008;358(8):811–7.

9. Feagins AR, Opriessnig T, Guenette DK, Halbur PG, Meng XJ. Detection and characterization of infectious hepatitis E virus from commercial pig livers sold in local grocery stores in the USA. J Gen Virol. 2007; 88:912–7.

10. Albinana-Gimenez N, Clemente-Casares P, Bofill-Mas S, et al. Distribution of human polyomaviruses, adenoviruses, and hepatitis E

virus in the environment and in a drinking-water treatment plant. Environ Sci Technol. 2006;40(23):7416–22.

11. Jeyamani R, Kurian G. Hepatitis E virus and acute-on-chronic liver failure. Indian J Gastroenterol. 2004;23(2):45–6.

12. Emerson SU, Arankalle VA, Purcell RH. Thermal stability of hepatitis E virus. J Infect Dis. 2005;192(5):930–3.

13. Feagins AR, Opriessnig T, Guenette DK, et al. Inactivation of infectious hepatitis E virus present in commercial pig livers sold in local grocery stores in the United States. Int J Food Microbiol. 2008;123(1–2):32–7.

HISTOPLASMOSIS

Tom Chiller

Infectious Agent

Histoplasma capsulatum is a dimorphic fungus growing as a mold in soil and as a yeast in animal and human hosts as an intracellular pathogen.

Mode of Transmission

Histoplasma is acquired via inhalation of spores (conidia) from soil contaminated with bat guano or bird droppings.

Occurrence

- In the United States, *H. capsulatum* is found along the Ohio and Mississippi River valleys, mostly in the central and southeastern states.
- Its occurrence has been described on every continent except Antarctica.
- Indigenous human cases have been reported throughout North, Central, and South America; the Caribbean; parts of the Middle East (Iran and Turkey); parts of Asia (Pakistan, India, China, Thailand, Indonesia, Vietnam, Malaysia, Philippines, Burma, and Japan); parts of Europe (northern Italy, Bulgaria, Spain, Hungary, Austria, France, Portugal, Romania, the countries of the former Soviet Union, Great Britain, Ireland, and Norway); parts of Africa; and Australia.
- Histoplasmosis is not transmitted directly from person to person.

Risk for Travelers

- Overall, histoplasmosis is rare among returning travelers.
- GeoSentinel surveillance data on illness in returning travelers showed that fewer than 0.5% of travelers presenting ill to clinics were diagnosed with histoplasmosis.
- Persons of all ages who visit endemic areas and are exposed to accumulations of bat guano or bird droppings are at increased risk for infection.
- Not all sources of exposure are obvious when visiting endemic areas; however, high-risk activities such as spelunking, mining, construction, excavating, demolishing, roofing, chimney cleaning, farming, gardening, and installing heating and air-conditioning systems are known to be associated with histoplasmosis.

- While in caves or mines, spending time close to the ground or kicking up dirt infested with bat guano containing *H. capsulatum* can increase the risk of infection.
- Other risk-prone activities may become better understood as ecotourism and adventure tourism become more common in endemic areas of Central and South America.

Clinical Presentation

- Incubation period is typically 3–17 days.
- Ninety percent of infections are asymptomatic or result in a mild influenza-like illness.
- Some infections may cause acute pulmonary histoplasmosis, manifested by high fever, headache, nonproductive cough, chills, weakness, pleuritic chest pain, and fatigue.
- Most persons spontaneously recover 2–3 weeks after onset of symptoms, although fatigue may persist longer.
- Dissemination, especially to the gastrointestinal tract and central nervous system, can occur in persons with severe immunocompromising conditions (e.g., HIV infection). Reinfection can occur with sufficient exposure, and in these individuals, the incubation period can be shorter.

Diagnosis

- Culture of *Histoplasma capsulatum* from bone marrow, blood, sputum, and tissue specimens is the definitive method of diagnosis.
- Demonstration of the typical intracellular yeast forms by microscopic examination strongly supports the diagnosis of histoplasmosis when clinical, epidemiologic, and other laboratory studies are compatible.
- An antigen detection test used on urine and serum is a rapid, commercially available diagnostic test. Antigen detection is most sensitive for severe, acute pulmonary infections and for progressive disseminated infections. It often is transiently positive early in the course of acute, self-limited pulmonary infections. A negative test does not exclude infection.
- Serologic testing for antibodies is also available; these tests should be interpreted by an expert.

Treatment

- Antifungal treatment is not usually indicated for healthy, immunocompetant persons with acute, localized pulmonary infection, because this form of the disease is self-limited, often resolving within 3 weeks.
- Persons with persistent symptoms beyond 1 month can be treated with itraconazole or Amphotericin B.
- All persons with severe disease, including diffuse pulmonary and disseminated histoplasmosis, should be treated with either itraconazole or Amphotericin B.
- Persons with immunocompromised conditions and other chronic diseases may require prolonged treatment.
- Consultation with an infectious disease specialist is advised.

Preventive Measures for Travelers

- No vaccine is available.
- Persons at increased risk for severe disease should be advised to avoid high-risk areas, such as bat-inhabited caves.
- If exposure cannot be avoided, persons should be advised to decrease dust generation in infested areas by watering the areas before engaging in dust-generating activities and to wear masks and special protective equipment.

- After engaging in high-risk activities, hosing off footwear and placing clothing in airtight plastic bags to be laundered could also decrease the potential for exposure. Further details about protective equipment can be obtained from www.cdc.gov/niosh/docs/2005-109/.
- Transportation of soil, guano, and other potential fomites should be avoided.

References

1. Buxton JA, Dawar M, Wheat LJ, et al. Outbreak of histoplasmosis in a school party that visited a cave in Belize: role of antigen testing in diagnosis. J Travel Med. 2002;9(1):48–50.

2. Cano MVC, Hajjeh RA. The epidemiology of histoplasmosis: a review. Semin Respir Infect. 2001;16(2):109–18.

3. CDC. Cave-associated histoplasmosis—Costa Rica. MMWR Morb Mortal Wkly Rep. 1988;37(20):312–3.

4. Freedman DO, Weld LH, Kozarsky PE, et al; GeoSentinel Surveillance Network. Spectrum of disease and relation to place of exposure among ill returned travelers. N Engl J Med. 2006;354(2):119–30.

5. Morgan J, Cano MV, Feikin DR, et al.; Acapulco Histoplasmosis Working Group. A large outbreak of histoplasmosis among American travelers associated with a hotel in Acapulco, Mexico, spring 2001. Am J Trop Med Hyg. 2003;69(6):663–9.

6. Nasta P, Donisi A, Cattane A, et al. Acute histoplasmosis in spelunkers returning from Mato Grosso, Peru. J Travel Med. 1997;4(4):176–8.

7. Panackal AA, Hajjeh RA, Cetron MS, et al. Fungal infections among returning travelers. Clin Infect Dis. 2002;35(9):1088–95.

8. Valdez H, Salata RA. Bat-associated histoplasmosis in returning travelers: case presentation and description of a cluster. J Travel Med. 1999;6(4):258–60.

9. Weinberg M, Weeks J, Lance-Parker S, et al. Severe histoplasmosis in travelers to Nicaragua. Emerg Infect Dis. 2003;9(10):1322–5.

10. Wheat LJ. Laboratory diagnosis of histoplasmosis: update 2000. Semin Respir Infect. 2001;16(2):131–40.

11. Wheat LJ. Histoplasmosis: a review for clinicians from non-endemic areas. Mycoses. 2006;49(4):274–82.

12. Wheat J, Freifeld AG, Kleiman MB, et al. Clinical practice guidelines for the management of patients with histoplasmosis: 2007 update by the Infectious Diseases Society of America. Clin Infect Dis. 2007;45(7):807–25.

HIV INFECTION AND ACQUIRED IMMUNODEFICIENCY SYNDROME (AIDS)

John T. Brooks

Infectious Agent

AIDS is a serious disease that represents the late clinical stage of infection with human immunodeficiency virus (HIV). HIV progressively damages the immune system. Without an effective immune system, life-threatening infections and other noninfectious conditions related to failing immunity (such as certain cancers) eventually develop.

Mode of Transmission

HIV can be transmitted through—

- Sexual intercourse
- Needle- or syringe-sharing
- Medical use of blood or blood components
- Organ or tissue transplantation
- Artificial insemination
- Pregnancy (perinatally from an infected woman to her infant).

HIV is not transmitted through casual contact; air, food, or water routes; contact with inanimate objects; or by mosquitoes or other arthropod vectors. The use of any public conveyance (e.g., airplanes, automobiles, boats, buses, or trains) by persons with AIDS or HIV infection does not pose a risk of HIV infection for the crew members or other travelers.

Occurrence

- AIDS and HIV infection occur worldwide.
- As of the end of 2007, over 33 million persons were living with HIV/AIDS. Although sub-Saharan Africa remains the most affected part of the world, notable increases in HIV infection have occurred from 2001 to 2007 in Eastern Europe and throughout Asia (Map 5-5).
- Many countries lack comprehensive surveillance systems, and despite improvements, the true number of cases is likely greater than officially reported, particularly in developing countries.

Risk for Travelers

- The risk of HIV infection for international travelers is generally low.
- Because HIV infection and AIDS are distributed globally, the risk for international travelers is determined less by geographic destination and more by behaviors that put them at risk for becoming infected, such as sexual and drug-using behaviors.
- Factors to consider in assessing risk include the extent of sexual contact with potentially infected persons and the extent of direct contact with blood or other potentially infectious secretions.
- In developing countries, the blood supply might not be adequately screened, thereby increasing the risk of HIV transmission by transfusion.

Diagnosis

- Any person who suspects that she or he may have been exposed to HIV infection should be tested.
- Most HIV tests are antibody tests that measure the antibodies the body makes against HIV. It can take some time for the immune system to produce enough antibodies for the antibody test to detect, and this time period (commonly referred to as the "window period") can vary from person to person.
- Most people will develop detectable antibodies within 2–8 weeks (the average is 25 days). Ninety-seven percent of persons will develop antibodies in the first 3 months following infection. In very rare cases, it can take up to 6 months to develop antibodies to HIV.
- If the initial negative HIV test was conducted within the first 3 months after possible exposure, repeat testing should be considered >3 months after the exposure occurred to account for the possibility of a false-negative result.
- Another type of test is an RNA test, which detects the HIV virus directly. The time from HIV infection to RNA detection is 9–11 days. These tests, which are more costly and used less often than antibody tests, are used in some parts of the United States.
- For information on HIV testing, travelers should talk to their health-care provider or identify the location of an HIV testing site near them by visiting the National HIV Testing Resources website at www.hivtest.org or call CDC-INFO, toll-free at 800-CDC-INFO (800-232-4636) or 888-232-6348 (TTY), in English or Spanish. Both these resources are confidential.
- Diagnosis of HIV infection and AIDS may also be made when a patient presents with an AIDS-compatible diagnosis, such as pneumocystis pneumonia, and is subsequently found to be HIV seropositive.

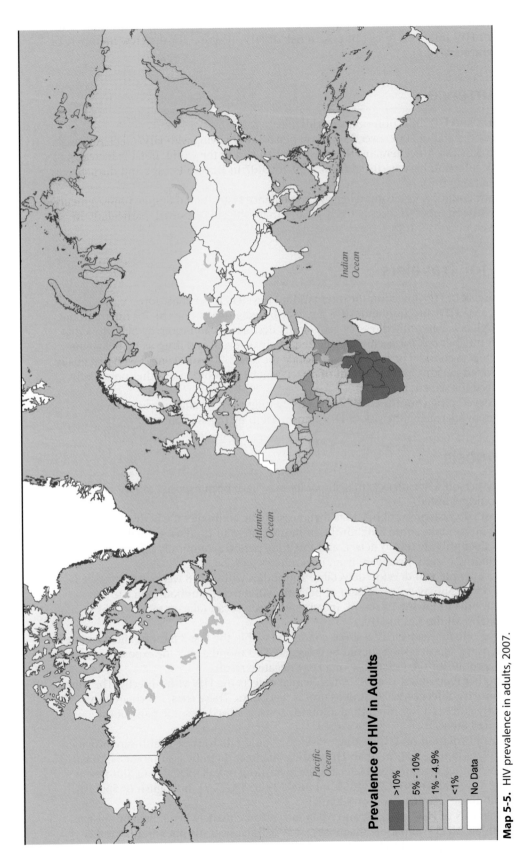

Map 5-5. HIV prevalence in adults, 2007.

(From 2008 Report on the global AIDS epidemic. Data used by kind permission of Joint United Nations Programme on HIV/AIDS (UNAIDS) www.unaids.org.)

Prevalence of HIV in Adults

- >10%
- 5% - 10%
- 1% - 4.9%
- <1%
- No Data

Treatment

- Prompt medical care may delay the onset of AIDS and prevent some life-threatening conditions.
- Travelers who become HIV infected should seek the care of a licensed health-care provider, preferably a provider with experience treating people living with HIV infection, as soon as possible after learning they are infected.
- Detailed information on specific treatments is available from the Department of Health and Human Services' AIDSinfo, see www.aidsinfo.nih.gov/. Information on enrolling in clinical trials is also available at AIDSinfo. Travelers may contact AIDSinfo by phone, toll-free 800-448-0440 (English or Spanish) or 888-480-3739 (TTY).

Preventive Measures for Travelers

- No vaccine is available to prevent infection with HIV.
- Travelers should be advised that they are at risk if they—
  - Have sexual contact (heterosexual or homosexual) with an infected person.
  - Use or allow the use of contaminated, unsterilized syringes or needles for any injections or other procedures that pierce the skin, including acupuncture; use of illicit drugs; steroid or vitamin injections; medical or dental procedures; ear or body piercing; or tattooing.
  - Receive infected blood, blood components, or clotting factor concentrates. HIV infection by this route is rare in countries or cities where donated blood and plasma are screened for antibodies to HIV.
- To reduce their risk of acquiring HIV, travelers should be advised to—
  - Avoid sexual encounters with persons who are infected with HIV or whose HIV infection status is unknown, or who are at high risk for HIV infection, such as intravenous drug users, commercial sex workers (both male and female), and other persons with multiple sexual partners.
  - Use condoms consistently and correctly if sexually active, especially if engaging in vaginal, anal, or oral–genital sexual contact with a person who is HIV-infected or whose HIV status is unknown.
  - Avoid using intravenous drugs.
  - Avoid sharing needles or other devices that can puncture skin for any purpose.
  - Avoid, if at all possible, blood transfusions or use of blood-clotting factor concentrates.

Additional Notes

Condoms

- Persons who are sensitive to latex should use condoms made of polyurethane or other synthetic materials and should carry their own supply of condoms.
- When a male condom cannot be used properly, a female condom should be considered.
- When no condom is available, travelers should abstain from vaginal, anal, and oral–genital sexual contact with persons who are HIV infected or whose HIV status is unknown. Barrier methods other than condoms have not been shown to be effective in the prevention of HIV transmission.
- Spermicides alone have also not been shown to be effective. The widely used spermicide nonoxynol-9 can increase the risk of HIV transmission and should not be used.

Needles

- Needles used to draw blood or administer injections should be sterile, single use, disposable, and prepackaged in a sealed container.

- If at all possible, travelers should avoid receiving medications from multidose vials, which may have become contaminated by used needles.
- Travelers with insulin-dependent diabetes, hemophilia, or other conditions that necessitate routine or frequent injections should be advised to carry a supply of medication, syringes, needles, and disinfectant swabs (e.g., alcohol wipes) sufficient to last their entire stay abroad. Before traveling, such persons should consider requesting documentation of the medical necessity for traveling with these items (e.g., a doctor's letter) in case their need is questioned by inspection personnel at ports of entry.

Transfusions

- In many developed countries, the risk of transfusion-associated HIV infection has been virtually eliminated through required testing of all donated blood for HIV.
- Developing countries may have no formal program or inadequate technology for testing blood or biological products for contamination with HIV.
- If transfusion is necessary, the blood should be tested, if at all possible, for HIV antibody by trained laboratory technicians using a reliable test.

Postexposure Prophylaxis

- Persons who in the course of their travel (e.g., nurse volunteer drawing blood or medical missionary performing surgeries) may have contact with HIV-infected or potentially infected biological materials should ensure that they will have access to all personal protective equipment necessary (e.g., latex gloves, goggles, face shield, gowns) and that this equipment meets established international quality standards.
- Such travelers may also wish to consider familiarizing themselves with the principles of postexposure prophylaxis and, in the event of a high-risk exposure, establishing a plan for seeking medical consultation and bringing a supply of antiretroviral medication of sufficient quantity to provide postexposure prophylaxis until medical care can be obtained (see the Occupational Exposure to HIV section in Chapter 2).
- The efficacy of postexposure prophylaxis with antiretrovirals for nonoccupational exposures to HIV (e.g., sexual, injecting drug use) has not been established. CDC recommends it be considered as an unproven clinical intervention, after careful consideration of potential risks and benefits and with full awareness of gaps in current knowledge.

HIV Testing Requirements for U.S. Travelers Entering Foreign Countries

- International travelers should be advised that some countries screen incoming travelers for HIV infection and may deny entry to persons with AIDS or evidence of HIV infection. These countries usually screen only persons planning extended visits, such as for work or study.
- Persons intending to visit a country for an extended stay should be informed of that country's policies and requirements. This information is usually available from the consular officials of the individual nations. Information about entry and exit requirements compiled by the U.S. Department of State can be found at http://travel.state.gov/travel/tips/tips_1232.html#requirement.

References

1. UNAIDS; WHO. AIDS epidemic update: 2007 [Internet]. Geneva: UNAIDS; 2007. [cited 2008 Nov 30]. Available from: http://data.unaids.org/pub/EPISlides/2007/2007_epiupdate_en.pdf.

2. Memish ZA, Osoba AO. Sexually transmitted diseases and travel. Int J Antimicrob Agents. 2003;21(2):131–4.

3. Wright ER. Travel, tourism, and HIV risk

among older adults. J Acquir Immune Defic Syndr. 2003;33(Suppl 2):S233–7.

4. CDC. HIV Prevention bulletin: medical advice for persons who inject illicit drugs [Internet]. Atlanta: Centers for Disease Control and Prevention. [updated 2007 Dec 26; cited 2006 May 31]. Available from: http://www.cdc.gov/idu/pubs/hiv_prev.htm.

5. Panlilio AL, Cardo DM, Grohskopf LA, et al.; U.S. Public Health Service. Updated U.S. Public Health Service guidelines for the management of occupational exposures to HIV and recommendations for postexposure

prophylaxis. MMWR Recomm Rep. 2005;54(RR-9):1–17.

6. CDC. Management of possible sexual, injecting-drug-use, or other nonoccupational exposure to HIV, including considerations related to antiretroviral therapy. Public Health Service statement. MMWR Recomm Rep. 1998;47(RR-17):1–14.

7. UNAIDS; WHO. 2008 Report on the global AIDS epidemic [Internet]. Geneva: UNAIDS; 2008. [cited 2008 Nov 30]. Available from: www.unaids.org/en/KnowledgeCentre/HIVData/GlobalReport/2008/.

LEGIONELLOSIS (LEGIONNAIRES' DISEASE AND PONTIAC FEVER)

Lauri A. Hicks, Nicole T. Alexander

Infectious Agent

Legionellosis is caused by gram-negative bacteria of the genus *Legionella*.

Mode of Transmission

Transmission occurs by inhalation of a water aerosol containing the bacteria. The bacterium grows in warm freshwater environments.

Occurrence

- Legionellae are ubiquitous worldwide. Most cases of legionellosis are caused by *L. pneumophila*.
- Disease occurs following exposure to aquatic settings that promote bacterial growth—the aquatic environment is somewhat stagnant, the water is warm (77° F–108° F, 25° C–42° C), and the water must be aerosolized so that the bacteria can be inhaled into the lungs. These three conditions are met almost exclusively in developed or industrialized settings.
- Disease does not occur in association with natural settings such as waterfalls, lakes, or streams.
- Outbreaks of legionellosis have been described in numerous countries throughout the world.
  - In Australia and the United States, rare cases of legionellosis caused by *L. longbeacheae* have been associated with exposure to potting soil.
  - The largest outbreak (449 cases) ever reported was traced to a cooling tower on the roof of a city hospital in Murcia, Spain, in 2001.
  - Outbreaks have been reported on cruise ships.
  - CDC conducts enhanced surveillance for travel-associated legionellosis cases in an effort to identify clusters and recommend measures to prevent ongoing transmission.
- Person-to-person transmission does not occur with either Legionnaires' disease or Pontiac fever.

Risk for Travelers

- U.S. legionellosis patients frequently report overnight stays at hotels and travel outside their state of residence.
- Travelers who are exposed to aerosolized, warm water are at risk for infection.
- Despite the presence of *Legionella* bacteria in many aquatic environments, the risk of developing legionellosis for most individuals is low.
- Elderly and immunocompromised travelers, such as those being treated for cancer, are at higher risk.
- Exposures can occur during recreation in or near a whirlpool spa (e.g., on a cruise ship), while showering in a hotel, or touring in cities with buildings that have cooling towers.

Clinical Presentation

- Legionnaires' disease typically presents with pneumonia, which usually requires hospitalization and can be fatal in 10%–15% of cases.
- Symptom onset occurs 2–14 days after exposure.
- In outbreak settings, fewer than 5% of persons exposed to the source of the outbreak develop Legionnaires' disease.
- Pontiac fever differs from Legionnaires' disease in that Pontiac fever presents as an influenza-like illness, with fever, headache, and myalgias, but no signs of pneumonia. Pontiac fever can affect healthy individuals as well as those with underlying illnesses, and symptoms occur within 72 hours of exposure. Full recovery is the rule. Up to 95% of people exposed in outbreak settings can develop symptoms of Pontiac fever.

Diagnosis

- Isolation of *Legionella* from respiratory secretions, lung tissue, pleural fluid, or a normally sterile site is an important method for diagnosis of Legionnaires' disease. Clinical isolates are often necessary to interpret the findings of an environmental investigation. Culture cannot be used to confirm Pontiac fever.
- The most common diagnostic method is the *Legionella* urinary antigen assay. However, the assay can only detect *L. pneumophila* serogroup 1, the most common cause of legionellosis.
- Paired serology showing a four-fold rise in antibody titer between acute- and convalescent-phase specimens confirms the diagnosis. A single antibody titer of any level is not diagnostic of legionellosis.
- Additional information can be found at CDC's Legionellosis Resource Site (www.cdc.gov/legionella/index.htm).

Treatment

- For travelers with Legionnaires' disease, specific antibiotic treatment is necessary and should be administered promptly while diagnostic tests are being processed.
- Appropriate antibiotics include fluoroquinolones and macrolides.
- Treatment may be necessary for up to 3 weeks. In severe cases, patients may have prolonged stays in intensive care units.
- Consultation with an infectious diseases specialist is advised.
- Pontiac fever is a self-limited illness that requires supportive care only; antibiotics have no benefit.

Preventive Measures for Travelers

- There is no vaccine for legionellosis, and antibiotic prophylaxis is not effective.

- Travelers at increased risk for infection, such as the elderly or those with immunocompromising conditions (e.g., cancer, diabetes), may choose to avoid high-risk areas, such as whirlpool spas.
- If exposure cannot be avoided, travelers should be advised to seek medical attention promptly if they develop symptoms of Legionnaires' disease or Pontiac fever.

References

1. Fields BS, Benson RF, Besser RE. Legionella and Legionnaires' disease: 25 years of investigation. Clin Microbiol Rev. 2002;15:506–26.
2. CDC. Legionnaires' disease associated with potting soil—California, Oregon, and Washington, May–June 2000. MMWR Morb Mortal Wkly Rep. 2000;49:777–8.
3. Steele TW, Lanser J, Sangster N. Isolation of *Legionella longbeachae* serogroup 1 from potting mixes. Appl Environ Microbiol. 1990;56:49–53.
4. CDC. Surveillance for travel-associated Legionnaires' disease—United States, 2005–2006. MMWR Morb Mortal Wkly Rep. 2007;56:1261–3.
5. Jernigan DB, Hofmann J, Cetron MS, et al. Outbreak of Legionnaires' disease among cruise ship passengers exposed to a contaminated whirlpool spa. Lancet. 1996;347:494–9.
6. CDC. Cruise-ship-associated Legionnaires disease, November 2003–May 2004. MMWR Morb Mortal Wkly Rep. 2005;54:1153–5.
7. Burnsed, LJ, Hicks LA, Smithee LM, et al.; the Legionellosis Outbreak Investigation Team. A large, travel-associated outbreak of legionellosis among hotel guests: utility of the urine antigen assay in confirming Pontiac fever. Clin Infec Dis. 2007;44:222–8.
8. Garcia-Fulgueiras A, Navarro C, Fenoll D, et al. Legionnaires' disease outbreak in Murcia, Spain. Emerg Infect Dis. 2003;9:915–21.
9. Mandell LA, Wunderink RG, Anzueto A, et al. Infectious Diseases Society of America/ American Thoracic Society consensus guidelines on the management of community-acquired pneumonia in adults. Clin Infect Dis. 2007;44(Suppl 2):S27–72.

LEISHMANIASIS, CUTANEOUS (CL)

Barbara L. Herwaldt, Alan J. Magill

Leishmaniasis is a parasitic disease found in parts of the tropics, subtropics, and southern Europe. Leishmaniasis has several different forms. This section focuses on cutaneous leishmaniasis (CL), the most common form, both in general and in travelers.

Infectious Agent

Obligate intracellular protozoan parasites of the genus *Leishmania*; approximately 20 species cause CL.

Mode of Transmission

Vector-borne, through the bite of infected female phlebotomine sand flies. CL also can occur after accidental occupational (laboratory) exposures to *Leishmania* parasites.

Occurrence

- In the Old World (Eastern Hemisphere), CL is found in parts of the Middle East, Asia (particularly Southwest and Central Asia), Africa (particularly the tropical region and North Africa), and southern Europe.
- In the New World (Western Hemisphere), CL is found in parts of Mexico, Central America, and South America. Occasional cases have been reported in Texas and Oklahoma. CL is not found in Chile, Uruguay, or Canada.

- Overall, CL is found in focal areas of ~90 countries. Most (>90%) of the world's cases of CL occur in eight countries: Afghanistan, Algeria, Iran, Iraq, Saudi Arabia, and Syria (in the Old World); and Brazil and Peru (in the New World).

Risk for Travelers

- The geographic distribution of cases of CL evaluated in countries such as the United States reflects travel and immigration patterns. CDC is consulted about cases acquired in many different areas of the world; however, >75% of the cases in U.S. civilians are acquired in Latin America, including popular tourist destinations such as Costa Rica. Cases in U.S. service personnel reflect military activities (e.g., in Iraq).
- CL usually is more common in rural than urban areas. However, it is found in some periurban and urban areas (e.g., in Baghdad, Iraq, and Kabul, Afghanistan). The ecologic settings range from rainforests to arid regions.
- The risk is highest from dusk to dawn because sand flies typically feed (bite) at night and during twilight hours. Although sand flies are less active during the hottest time of the day, they may bite if they are disturbed (e.g., if hikers brush up against tree trunks or other sites where sand flies are resting). Vector activity can easily be overlooked: sand flies do not make any noise ("buzz"), they are small (about one-third the size of mosquitoes), and their bites might not be noticed.
- Examples of types of travelers who might have an increased risk for CL include ecotourists, adventure travelers, bird watchers, Peace Corps volunteers, missionaries, soldiers, construction workers, and persons who do research outdoors at night or twilight. However, even very short-term travelers in endemic areas have developed CL.

Clinical Presentation

- CL is characterized by the presence of one or more skin lesions (open or closed sores), which typically develop within several weeks or months of the exposure. In some persons, the sores first appear months or years later, in the context of trauma (e.g., skin wounds or surgery).
- The sores can change in size and appearance over time. They typically progress from small papules, to nodular plaques, to open sores, with a raised border and central crater (ulcer), which can be covered with scales or crust. The lesions usually are painless but can be painful, particularly if open sores become infected with bacteria.
- Satellite lesions, regional lymphadenopathy (swollen glands), and nodular lymphangitis can be noted.
- The sores usually heal eventually, even without treatment. However, they can last for months or years and typically result in scarring.
- Another potential concern applies to some of the *Leishmania* species in South and Central America—occasionally, these parasites spread from the skin to the mucosal surfaces of the nose or mouth and cause sores there. This form of leishmaniasis, mucosal leishmaniasis (ML), might not be noticed until years after the original skin sores appear to have healed. Although ML is uncommon, it has occurred in travelers and expatriates whose cases of CL were not treated or were inadequately treated. The initial clinical manifestations typically involve the nose (e.g., chronic stuffiness, bleeding, and inflamed mucosa/sores) and less often the mouth; in advanced cases, ulcerative destruction of the nose, mouth, and pharynx can be noted (e.g., perforation of the nasal septum).

Diagnosis

- Clinicians should consider the possibility of CL in persons with chronic (nonhealing) skin lesions who have been in areas where leishmaniasis is found.

- Laboratory confirmation of the diagnosis is achieved by detecting *Leishmania* parasites (or DNA) in infected tissue, through light-microscopic examination of stained specimens, culture techniques, or molecular methods.
- CDC can assist in all aspects of the diagnostic evaluation. Identification of the *Leishmania* species can be important, particularly if more than one species is found where the patient traveled and if the species can have different clinical and prognostic implications (e.g., *L. mexicana* versus *L. [V.] braziliensis*).
- Serologic testing generally is not useful for CL but can provide supportive evidence for the diagnosis of ML.

Treatment

- Decisions about whether and how to treat CL should be individualized. (All cases of ML should be treated.) Clinicians may consult with CDC staff about the relative merits of various approaches.
- The pentavalent antimonial compound sodium stibogluconate (Pentostam) is available to U.S.-licensed physicians through the CDC Drug Service (404-639-3670), for intravenous (or intramuscular) administration under an Investigational New Drug protocol (see www.cdc.gov/ncidod/srp/drugs/drug-service.html).

Preventive Measures for Travelers

- No vaccines or drugs to prevent infection are available.
- Preventive measures are aimed at reducing contact with sand flies by using personal protective measures (see the Protection Against Mosquitoes, Ticks, and Other Insects and Arthropods section in Chapter 2).
- Travelers should be advised to:
  - Avoid outdoor activities, especially from dusk to dawn, when sand flies generally are the most active.
  - Wear protective clothing, and apply repellent with DEET (*N,N*-diethylmeta-toluamide) to exposed skin and under the edges of clothing, such as sleeves and pant legs, according to the manufacturer's instructions.
  - Sleep in air-conditioned or well-screened areas. Spraying the quarters with insecticide might provide some protection. Fans or ventilators might inhibit the movement of sand flies, which are weak fliers.

Sand flies are so small (~2–3 mm; <1/8th of an inch) that they can pass through the holes in ordinary bed nets; "mosquito nets" typically have 12–15 holes per linear inch (120–200 holes per square inch). Although closely woven nets (>30 holes per linear inch; >10,000 holes per square inch) are available, they may be uncomfortable in hot climates. The effectiveness of bed nets can be enhanced by treatment with a pyrethroid-containing insecticide (permethrin or deltamethrin). The same treatment can be applied to window screens, curtains, bed sheets, and clothing.

Contact Information for CDC

For consultative services, contact CDC Public Inquiries (770-488-7775; parasites@cdc.gov). Additional information can be found on the Division of Parasitic Diseases' website at www.cdc.gov/ncidod/dpd/parasites/leishmania/default.htm.

References

1. Murray HW, Berman JD, Davies CR, et al. Advances in leishmaniasis. Lancet. 2005;366:1561–77.

2. Herwaldt BL. Leishmaniasis. Lancet. 1999;354:1191–9.

3. Magill AJ. Cutaneous leishmaniasis in the returning traveler. Infect Dis Clin North Am. 2005;19:241–66.
4. Herwaldt BL, Stokes SL, Juranek DD. American cutaneous leishmaniasis in U.S. travelers. Ann Intern Med. 1993;118:779–84.
5. Ahluwalia S, Lawn SD, Kanagalingam J, et al. Mucocutaneous leishmaniasis: an imported

infection among travellers to central and South America. BMJ. 2004;329:842–4.
6. Blum J, Desjeux P, Schwartz E, et al. Treatment of cutaneous leishmaniasis among travellers. J Antimicrob Chemother. 2004;53:158–66.
7. Schwartz E, Hatz C, Blum J. New World cutaneous leishmaniasis in travellers. Lancet Infect Dis. 2006;6:342–9.

LEISHMANIASIS, VISCERAL (VL)

Barbara L. Herwaldt, Alan J. Magill

Leishmaniasis is a parasitic disease found in parts of the tropics, subtropics, and southern Europe. Leishmaniasis has several different forms. This section focuses on visceral leishmaniasis (VL), which affects some of the internal organs of the body (e.g., spleen, liver, bone marrow).

Infectious Agent

Obligate intracellular protozoan parasites of the genus *Leishmania*, particularly, *Leishmania donovani* and *L. infantum/L. chagasi*.

Mode of Transmission

Predominantly vector-borne, through the bite of infected female phlebotomine sand flies. Congenital and parenteral transmission (through blood transfusions and needle sharing) have been reported.

Occurrence

- VL usually is more common in rural than urban areas; but it is found in some periurban areas (e.g., in northeastern Brazil).
- In the Old World (Eastern Hemisphere), VL is found in parts of Asia (particularly the Indian subcontinent and Southwest/Central Asia), the Middle East, Africa (particularly East Africa), and southern Europe.
- In the New World (Western Hemisphere), most cases occur in Brazil; some cases occur in scattered foci elsewhere in South and Central America.
- Overall, VL is found in focal areas of approximately 65 countries. Most (>90%) of the world's cases of VL occur in the Indian subcontinent (India, Bangladesh, and Nepal), Sudan, and Brazil; none of the affected areas in these five countries are common tourist destinations.

Risk for Travelers

- The geographic distribution of cases of VL evaluated in countries such as the United States reflects travel and immigration patterns.
- VL is uncommon in U.S. travelers and expatriates. Occasional cases have been diagnosed in short-term travelers (tourists) in southern Europe and also in longer-term travelers (e.g., expatriates, deployed soldiers) in the Mediterranean region and other areas where VL is found.

Clinical Presentation

- Among symptomatic persons, the incubation period typically ranges from weeks to months. The onset of illness can be abrupt or gradual.
- Stereotypical manifestations of VL include fever, weight loss, hepatosplenomegaly (especially splenomegaly), and pancytopenia (anemia, leukopenia, and thrombocytopenia).
- If untreated, severe (advanced) cases of VL typically are fatal.
- Latent visceral infection can become clinically manifest years to decades after exposure in persons who become immunocompromised due to other medical reasons.

Diagnosis

- Clinicians should consider the possibility of VL in persons with a relevant travel history (even in the distant past) and a persistent, unexplained febrile illness, especially if accompanied by other suggestive manifestations (e.g., splenomegaly, pancytopenia).
- Laboratory confirmation of the diagnosis is achieved by detecting *Leishmania* parasites or DNA in infected tissue (e.g., bone marrow, liver, lymph node, blood), through light-microscopic examination of stained specimens, culture techniques, or molecular methods. Serologic testing can provide supportive evidence for the diagnosis.
- CDC can assist in all aspects of the diagnostic evaluation, including species identification.

Treatment

- Travelers should be advised to consult an infectious disease or tropical medicine specialist. Therapy of VL should be individualized with expert consultation. The relative merits of various approaches can be discussed with CDC staff.
- Liposomal amphotericin B (AmBisome) is approved by the U.S. Food and Drug Administration for treatment of VL.
- The pentavalent antimonial compound sodium stibogluconate (Pentostam) is available to U.S.-licensed physicians through the CDC Drug Service (404-639-3670) under an Investigational New Drug protocol (see www.cdc.gov/ncidod/srp/drugs/drug-service.html).

Preventive Measures for Travelers

- No vaccines or drugs to prevent infection are available.
- Preventive measures for travelers are aimed at reducing contact with sand flies by using Personal Protective Measures (see the Protection Against Mosquitoes, Ticks, and Other Insects and Arthropods section in Chapter 2 and Preventive Measures for Travelers in the previous section on Cutaneous Leishmaniasis).
  - ○ In particular, travelers should be advised to avoid outdoor activities, especially from dusk to dawn, when sand flies generally are the most active, and to sleep in air-conditioned or well-screened quarters.
  - ○ Preventive measures also include wearing protective clothing, applying insect repellent to exposed skin, using bed nets treated with a pyrethroid-containing insecticide, and spraying dwellings with residual-action insecticides.

Contact Information for CDC

For consultative services, contact CDC Public Inquiries (770-488-7775; parasites@cdc.gov). Additional information can be found on the Division of Parasitic Diseases' website at www.cdc.gov/ncidod/dpd/parasites/leishmania/default.htm.

References

1. Murray HW, Berman JD, Davies CR, et al. Advances in leishmaniasis. Lancet. 2005;366:1561–77.
2. Herwaldt BL. Leishmaniasis. Lancet. 1999;354:1191–9.
3. Malik AN, John L, Bruceson AD, et al. Changing pattern of visceral leishmaniasis, United Kingdom, 1985–2004. Emerg Infect Dis. 2006;12:1257–9.
4. Weisser M, Khanlari B, Terracciano L, et al. Visceral leishmaniasis: a threat to immunocompromised patients in non-endemic areas? Clin Microbiol Infect. 2007;13:751–3.
5. Myles O, Wortmann GW, Cummings JF, et al. Visceral leishmaniasis: clinical observations in 4 US Army soldiers deployed to Afghanistan or Iraq, 2002–2004. Arch Intern Med. 2007;167:1899–901.

LEPTOSPIROSIS

Robyn Stoddard, Sean V. Shadomy

Infectious Agent

Leptospirosis is caused by obligate aerobic spirochete bacteria in the genus *Leptospira*, with optimal growth occurring at 28° C–30° C.

Mode of Transmission

Infection occurs through abrasions or cuts in the skin or through the conjunctiva and mucous membranes. Humans may be infected by direct contact with urine or reproductive fluids from infected animals or with water or soil contaminated with those fluids. Prolonged immersion in contaminated water increases the risk for infection. Infection rarely occurs through animal bites or human-to-human contact.

Occurrence

- Leptospirosis has worldwide distribution, with a higher incidence in tropical climates.
- Domestic, peridomestic, and wild animals serve as maintenance hosts of the bacteria and excrete the bacteria in their urine, amniotic fluid, or placental tissue, which can contaminate the soil and water.
- Most *Leptospira* species proliferate in fresh water, damp soil, or mud.
- The occurrence of flooding after hurricanes or heavy rainfall facilitates the spread of the organism, contributing to outbreaks. This is especially true in regions with high endemic rates of infection.
- Leptospirosis is associated with animal husbandry.
- Rodent-borne leptospirosis may be a risk to persons exposed to rat urine in infested urban areas.

Risk for Travelers

- Travelers participating in recreational water activities, such as whitewater rafting, adventure racing, kayaking, or triathlon events may be at increased risk for leptospirosis, particularly following periods of heavy rainfall or flooding.
- Outbreaks of leptospirosis have occurred in the United States after flooding in both Hawaii and Puerto Rico. Leptospirosis has also been reported in international travelers to regions experiencing epidemics following heavy rainfall or flooding (CDC, unreported data).

Clinical Presentation

- The incubation period is 2 days to 3 weeks.
- The symptoms of leptospirosis are broad and often biphasic. The acute or bacteremic phase lasts a week, followed by the immune phase that is characterized by both antibody production and the presence of leptospires in the urine.
- The acute, generalized illness mimics other acute febrile illnesses such as dengue fever, malaria, or typhus. Common symptoms include headache, fever, chills, myalgia, nausea, diarrhea, abdominal pain, uveitis, adenopathy, conjunctival suffusion without purulent discharge, and occasionally a skin rash. The headache is often severe and includes retro-orbital pain and photophobia. Aseptic meningitis occurs in up to 25% of cases.
- The icteric or severe form of the disease (Weil's disease) occurs in 5%–10% of patients with leptospirosis. Symptoms include jaundice, renal failure, hemorrhage, cardiac arrhythmias, pneumonitis, and hemodynamic collapse. The mortality rate in patients with severe leptospirosis ranges from 5% to 15%.

Diagnosis

- Diagnosis of leptospirosis is usually based on serology. Antibodies may be detected in the blood within 5–7 days of symptom onset. Culture or demonstration of the organism under darkfield microscopy are both relatively insensitive. No PCR assay has been validated with clinical specimens.
- Confirmation of leptospirosis requires seroconversion between acute- and convalescent-phase serum specimens, as demonstrated by the microscopic agglutination test (MAT); culture of the organism from clinical specimens; or demonstration of *Leptospira* in a clinical specimen by immunofluorescence.
- MAT, the recognized standard reference test for serologic diagnosis of leptospirosis, is performed only in reference laboratories. Although MAT is not specific for diagnosis of acute cases, a single elevated MAT titer in a patient with a compatible febrile illness and suspected exposure suggests acute leptospirosis. Seroconversion with a four-fold or greater rise in titer between acute- and convalescent-phase serum specimens obtained ≥2 weeks apart confirms the diagnosis.
- Several rapid, reliable serologic assays are commercially available for diagnostic screening for an acute infection. A recent evaluation of four of these assays concluded that both a microplate IgM ELISA and an IgM dot-ELISA dipstick test exhibited high sensitivity and specificity on acute samples.

Treatment

- Missed or delayed diagnosis of leptospirosis is common due to its nonspecific clinical presentation and a low index of suspicion among health-care providers seeing returned travelers.
- Antimicrobial therapy should be initiated early in the course of the disease if leptospirosis is suspected.
- Intravenous penicillin is the drug of choice for patients with severe leptospirosis. As with other spirochete infections, a Jarisch–Herxheimer reaction (an acute febrile reaction that can range from rash to anaphylaxis) can develop after initiation of penicillin therapy. Various methods have been described to prevent or control Jarisch–Herxheimer reactions, and management should follow the appropriate standards for patient care.
- Oral doxycycline is effective in decreasing the severity and duration of leptospirosis and the occurrence of leptospiruria in acute or mild disease. Doxycycline should not be used in pregnant women or children younger than 8 years of age because of the risk for dental staining.

- Parenteral third-generation cephalosporins (e.g., ceftriaxone or cefotaxime), doxycycline, or azithromycin may also be used for the treatment of severe leptospirosis.
- Due to the risk for potential complications, including cardiac arrhythmia, renal failure, pulmonary involvement and respiratory distress, or myocarditis, patients with leptospirosis may require hospitalization, supportive therapy, and close monitoring.

Preventive Measures for Travelers

- No vaccine is available in the United States.
- Travelers who might be at an increased risk for infection due to recreational water activities or exposure to contaminated surface waters and soil should be advised to consider preventive measures such as wearing protective clothing, especially footwear, and covering cuts and abrasions with occlusive dressings. They should avoid contact with, submersion in, or swallowing potentially contaminated water.

Antibiotic Chemoprophylaxis

- Travelers at risk because of destination or activities during travel may benefit from chemoprophylaxis. Until further data become available, CDC recommends that adult travelers who might be at increased risk for leptospirosis be advised to consider chemoprophylaxis with doxycycline (200 mg orally, weekly), begun 1–2 days before and continuing through the period of exposure. Indications for prophylactic doxycycline use for children have not been established.
- Travelers at increased risk for leptospirosis and in need of malaria chemoprophylaxis should consider using doxycycline for both indications.

References

1. Levett PN. Leptospirosis. Clin Microbiol Rev. 2001;14(2):296–326.
2. Vinetz JM, Glass GE, Flexner CE, et al. Sporadic urban leptospirosis. Ann Intern Med. 1996;125(10):794–8.
3. Haake DA, Dundoo M, Cader R, et al. Leptospirosis, water sports, and chemophrophylaxis. Clin Infect Dis. 2002;34(9):e40–3.
4. Morgan J, Bornstein SL, Karpati AM, et al.; Leptospirosis Working Group. Outbreak of leptospirosis among triathlon participants and community residents in Springfield, Illinois, 1998. Clin Infect Dis. 2002;34(12):1593–9.
5. Gaynor K, Katz AR, Park SY, et al. Leptospirosis on Oahu: an outbreak associated with flooding of a university campus. Am J Trop Med Hyg. 2007;76(5):882–5.
6. Sanders EJ, Rigau-Pérez JG, Smits HL, et al. Increase of leptospirosis in dengue-negative patients after a hurricane in Puerto Rico in 1996. Am J Trop Med Hyg. 1999;61(3):399–404.
7. Bajani MD, Ashford DA, Bragg SL, et al. Evaluation of four commercially available rapid serologic tests for diagnosis of leptospirosis. J Clin Microbiol. 2003;41(2):803–9.
8. Griffith ME, Hospenthal DR, Murray CK. Antimicrobial therapy of leptospirosis. Curr Opin Infect Dis. 2006;19(6):533–7.
9. Pappas G, Cascio A. Optimal treatment of leptospirosis: queries and projections. Int J Antimicrob Agents. 2006;28(6):491–6.
10. Phimda K, Hoontrakul S, Suttinont C, et al. Doxycycline versus azithromycin for treatment of leptospirosis and scrub typhus. Antimicrob Agents Chemother. 2007;51(9):3259–63.
11. Guidugli F, Castro AA, Atallah AN. Antibiotics for preventing leptospirosis. Cochrane Database Syst Rev. 2000;(4):CD001305. Review.

LYME DISEASE

Paul S. Mead

Infectious Agent

Lyme disease is caused by spirochetes belonging to the *Borrelia burgdorferi* sensu lato complex, including:

- *B. afzelii*
- *B. burgdorferi* sensu stricto
- *B. garinii*

Mode of Transmission

Infection occurs by vector-borne transmission via bite of infected ticks of the *Ixodes ricinus* complex.

Occurrence

- Temperate forested regions throughout Europe and northern Asia; more common in eastern and central Europe than western Europe.
- Northeastern, north central, and Pacific coastal regions of North America; about 20,000 cases are reported yearly in the United States. Lyme disease is the most common vector-borne disease in the United States and Europe.
- Transmission has not been documented in the tropics.

Risk for Travelers

- Lyme disease is rarely reported in returning travelers.
- All ages are at risk for infection with travel to endemic areas.
- Infection is associated with exposure to tick habitats (e.g., wooded, brushy, or grassy areas).
- Vector ticks are very small; infected persons are often unaware that they have been bitten.

Clinical Presentation

- Infection can result in dermatologic, rheumatologic, neurologic, or cardiac abnormalities.
- Incubation period is 3–32 days.
- In 70%–80% of cases, patients develop a characteristic rash, erythema migrans (EM), within 30 days of exposure to *B. burgdorferi*. EM is a red expanding rash, with or without central clearing, that is often accompanied by symptoms of fatigue, fever, headache, mild stiff neck, arthralgia, or myalgia.
- Within days or weeks, infection can spread to other parts of the body, causing more serious neurologic conditions (meningitis, radiculopathy, and facial palsy) or cardiac abnormalities (carditis with atrioventricular heart block).
- Untreated, infection can progress over a period of months to cause mono- or oligoarticular arthritis, peripheral neuropathy, or encephalopathy. Long-term sequelae can be typically observed over a number of months; range from 1 week to a few years.

Diagnosis

- Lyme disease is diagnosed on the basis of physician-observed clinical manifestations and a history of likely exposure to infected ticks.
- Culture may be done (e.g., from EM lesion) early in disease; PCR is more reliable from areas such as joint fluid.
- Serologic testing is often negative in the first few weeks of illness and is therefore not recommended to confirm the diagnosis in patients with recent onset (2–3 weeks) of a characteristic EM rash.
- Serologic testing may be helpful in patients with musculoskeletal, neurologic, or cardiac symptoms.

- Patients suspected of acquiring Lyme disease overseas should be tested by using a C6-based assay, as other serologic tests may not detect infection with European species of *Borrelia*.

Treatment

- Guidelines for treatment of Lyme disease have been published by the Infectious Diseases Society of America and are available at www.journals.uchicago.edu/doi/full/10.1086/508667.
- Depending on the stage of disease, most patients can be treated with either oral doxycycline or intravenous ceftriaxone.
- Physicians unfamiliar with Lyme disease may wish to consult an infectious disease specialist for further guidance.
- Additional information about Lyme disease can be found at www.cdc.gov/ncidod/dvbid/lyme/index.htm.

Preventive Measures for Travelers

- No vaccine is currently available.
- Measures to prevent Lyme disease and other tick-borne infections include avoidance of tick habitat, use of insect repellent (see the Protection Against Mosquitoes, Ticks, and Other Insects and Arthropods section in Chapter 2) on exposed skin and clothing, and carefully checking every day for attached ticks.
- Remove ticks by grasping them firmly with tweezers as close to the skin as possible and lifting gently.
- Ideally, tick removal should be done within 24 hours of attachment; 24–72 hours of attachment is necessary before transmission of the spirochete occurs.
- Prophylactic antibiotics are not recommended for travelers.
- Postexposure prophylaxis is generally not recommended unless the traveler sustained a tick bite(s) in a highly endemic area.

References

1. Wormser GP, Dattwyler RJ, Shapiro ED, et al. The clinical assessment, treatment, and prevention of Lyme disease, human granulocytic anaplasmosis, and babesiosis: clinical practice guidelines by the Infectious Diseases Society of America. Clin Infect Dis. 2006;43:1089–134.
2. Weber K. Aspects of Lyme borreliosis in Europe. Eur J Clin Microbiol Infect Dis. 2001;20:6–13.
3. Steere AC. Lyme disease. N Engl J Med. 2001;345:115–25.
4. Stanek G, Strle F. Lyme borreliosis. Lancet. 2003;362:1639–47.
5. Gern L, Humair PF. Ecology of *Borrelia burgdorferi* sensu lato in Europe. In: Gray JS,

Kahl O, Lane RS, Stanek G, editors. Lyme borreliosis: biology, epidemiology and control. New York: CABI Publishing; 2002. p. 149–74.
6. Korenberg EI, Gorelova NB, Kovalevskii YV. Ecology of *Borrelia burgdorferi* sensu lato in Russia. In: Gray JS, Kahl O, Lane RS, Stanek G, editors. Lyme borreliosis: biology, epidemiology and control. New York: CABI Publishing; 2002. p. 175–200.
7. Miyamoto K, Masuzawa T. Ecology of *Borrelia burgdorferi* sensu lato in Japan and East Asia. In: Gray JS, Kahl O, Lane RS, Stanek G, editors. Lyme borreliosis: biology, epidemiology and control. New York: CABI Publishing; 2002. p. 201–22.

MELIOIDOSIS

Theresa L. Smith, Jay E. Gee, Mary D. Ari

Infectious Agent

Burkholderia pseudomallei is a saprophytic, gram-negative bacillus widely distributed in tropical soil and water.

Mode of Transmission

Usually human infection with *B. pseudomallei* occurs by inhalation or subcutaneous inoculation, but rarely by ingestion or by person-to-person transmission via contact with the blood and body fluids of an infected person.

Occurrence

- Melioidosis is an infectious disease endemic in Southeast Asia and northern Australia (Map 5-6).
- In northern Australia, melioidosis accounts for 20% of all community-acquired septicemias.
- Melioidosis has been reported in Puerto Rico, suspected in El Salvador, and may be underdiagnosed in India, the Caribbean, and Central and South America.
- In northern Brazil, melioidosis has recently been recognized and is associated with periods of heavy rainfall.

Risk For Travelers

- All ages are at risk of infection with travel to areas endemic for melioidosis.
- The highest risk for melioidosis exists for military personnel, adventure travelers, eco-tourists, construction and resource extraction workers, and other persons whose contact with contaminated soil or water may expose them to the bacteria. *B. pseudomallei* has been isolated from ill troops of all nationalities who had served in areas with endemic disease, with a latency of as long as 62 years.
- As much as 85% of cases occur during the rainy season, when exposure to the organism is believed to be greatest. Melioidosis has been diagnosed among travelers who contracted the disease while staying in endemic areas during the rainy season. Following the 2004 Southeast Asian tsunami, an increase in the number of melioidosis cases was observed among repatriated tourists.

Clinical Presentation

- Melioidosis is emerging as a significant cause of community-acquired sepsis in the tropics, with a variety of presentations, including abscesses and organ system failure. The incubation period ranges from 1–21 days; however, with a high inoculum, symptoms can develop in a few hours.
- Melioidosis occurs as a localized infection, acute pulmonary infection, acute systemic infection, chronic suppurative infection, or subclinical infection.
- Most cases present as an acute febrile illness with severe pneumonia and sepsis. Patients are overwhelmed by the infection and die from septic shock within 48 hours of developing symptoms.
- Meningoencephalitis with flaccid paraparesis or peripheral motor weakness occurs in 4% of cases in northern Australia. Cerebral abscess is occasionally reported.
- Melioidosis should be considered in the differential diagnosis of unusual subacute to chronic suppurative cutaneous lesions in a febrile patient returning from an area endemic for the disease. Local infections may progress to systemic disease if left untreated.
- The possibility of melioidosis must be kept in mind in any unexplained suppurative disease, especially cavitating pulmonary disease, in patients living in or returned from areas endemic for melioidosis, even many years after exposure.
- The morbidity and mortality rates of melioidosis are greater in persons with underlying diseases such as diabetes mellitus, renal dysfunction, chronic pulmonary disease, or compromised immune system. However, HIV infection does not appear to be a major risk factor for developing melioidosis.

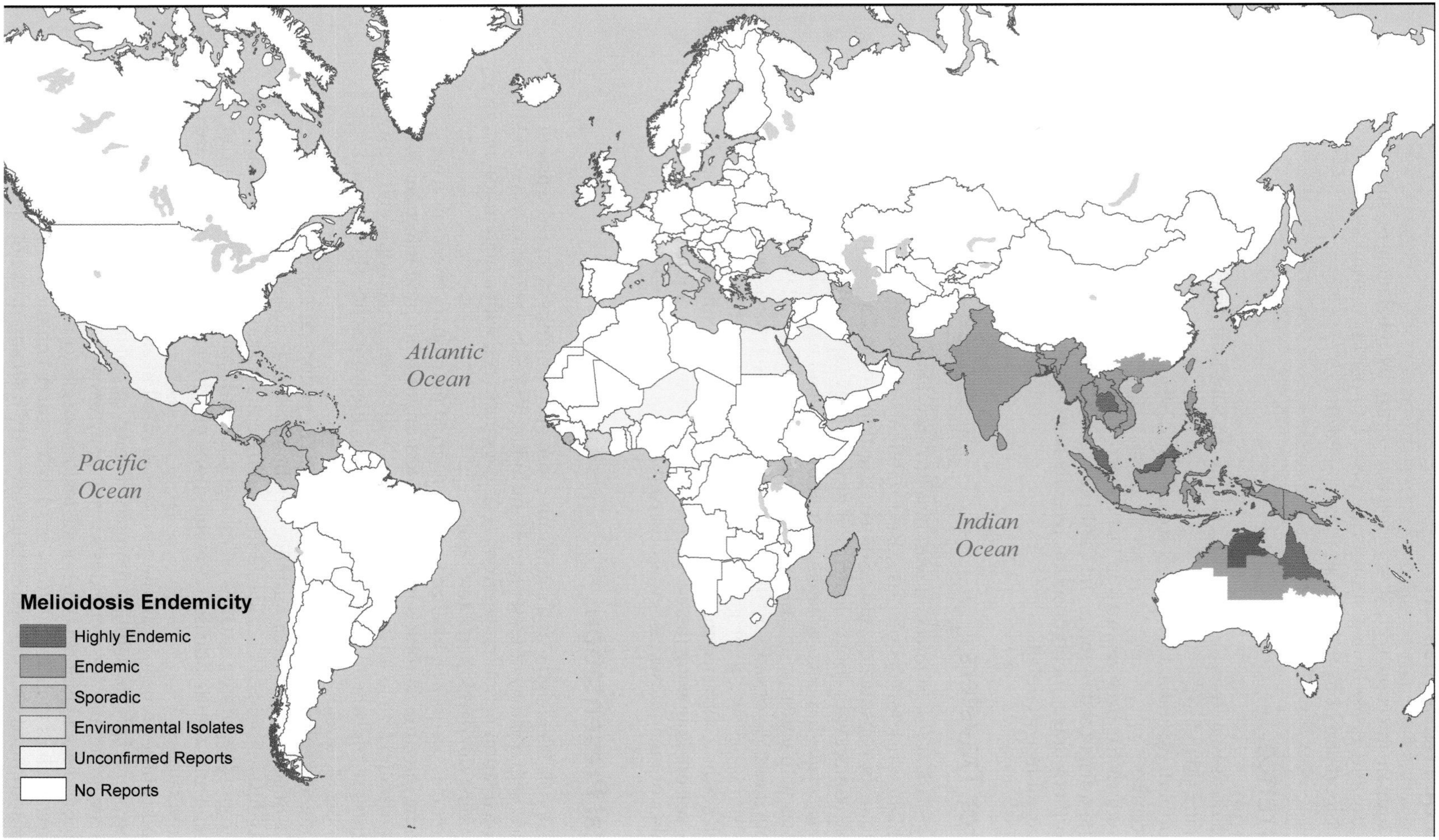

Map 5-6. Endemicity of melioidosis infection.

(Modified from Cheng AC, Currie BJ. Melioidosis: epidemiology, pathophysiology, and management. Clin Microbiol Rev. 2005;18:383–416. With permission from American Society for Microbiology Journals Department).

Melioidosis Endemicity

- Highly Endemic
- Endemic
- Sporadic
- Environmental Isolates
- Unconfirmed Reports
- No Reports

Pacific Ocean

Atlantic Ocean

Indian Ocean

Diagnosis

- Culture of the organism may be done from blood, sputum, pus, urine, synovial fluid, peritoneal fluid and pericardial fluid.
- The most widely used serologic test for melioidosis is the indirect hemagglutination assay (IHA).

Treatment

- Melioidosis requires long courses of antimicrobial therapy. Initial treatment consists of supportive measures and 10 days of intensive-phase therapy with intravenous ceftazidime, imipenem, or meropenem.
- Following intensive-phase therapy, ambulatory eradication-phase therapy consists of 20–24 weeks of oral trimethoprim–sulfamethoxazole, with or without doxycycline.

Preventive Measures for Travelers

- There is no vaccine available for protection against melioidosis.
- In areas of endemic disease, skin lacerations, abrasions or burns that have been contaminated with soil or surface water should be immediately and thoroughly cleaned.
- Persons with chronic diseases, including diabetes, and those with traumatic wounds should avoid exposure to soil or water in areas endemic for melioidosis.

References

1. White NJ. Melioidosis. Lancet. 2003;361:1715–22.
2. Cheng AC, Currie BJ. Melioidosis: epidemiology, pathophysiology, and management. Clin Microbiol Rev. 2005;18:383–416.
3. Inglis TJ, Sagripanti JL. Environmental factors that affect the survival and persistence of *Burkholderia pseudomallei*. Appl Environ Microbiol. 2006;72:6865–75.
4. Inglis TJ, Rolim DB, Sousa Ade Q. Meliodosis in the Americas. Am J Trop Med Hyg. 2006;75:947–54.
5. Ngauy V, Lemeshev Y, Sadkowski L, et al. Cutaneous melioidosis in a man who was taken as a prisoner of war by the Japanese during World War II. J Clin Microbiol. 2005;43:970–2.
6. Ko WC, Cheung BM, Tang HJ, et al. Melioidosis outbreak after typhoon, southern Taiwan. Emerg Infect Dis. 2007;13:896–8.
7. Currie BJ, Fisher DA, Howard DM, et al. Endemic melioidosis in tropical northern Australia: a 10-year prospective study and review of the literature. Clin Infect Dis. 2000;31:981–6.
8. Dance DA. Ecology of *Burkholderia pseudomallei* and the interactions between environmental *Burkholderia* spp. and human–animal hosts. Acta Trop. 2000;74:159–68.
9. Peacock SJ. Melioidosis. Curr Opin Infect Dis. 2006;19(5):421–8.
10. Currie BJ. Advances and remaining uncertainties in the epidemiology of *Burkholderia pseudomallei* and melioidosis. Trans R Soc Trop Med Hyg. 2008;102:225–7.

NOROVIRUS

Aron J. Hall, Marc-Alain Widdowson

Infectious Agent

Norovirus infection is caused by nonenveloped, single-stranded RNA viruses of the genus *Norovirus*, also referred to as "Norwalk-like viruses," Norwalk viruses, human caliciviruses, and small round-structured viruses.

Mode of Transmission

Transmission occurs primarily through the fecal–oral route, either directly from person to person via contaminated hands or indirectly via contaminated food or water. Norovirus is also indirectly spread through aerosols of vomitus and contaminated environments.

Occurrence

- Norovirus infections are found worldwide and can occur year round.
- In the United States, norovirus infections are estimated to cause 23 million illnesses a year and may cause up to 50% of all foodborne outbreaks.
- Seroprevalence studies in the Amazon, southern Africa, Mexico, Chile, and Canada have shown that norovirus infections are common throughout the world, and most children will have experienced at least one infection by the age of 5 years.
- Case–control studies of norovirus as a cause of travelers' diarrhea (TD) have not been done. Norovirus has been looked for in the stools of visitors to Guatemala and Mexico, with positive findings ranging from 17% to 65% of stools. However, concomitant infection with known pathogens was common, and the rate of norovirus in asymptomatic controls tested in the same manner was not determined. The viral etiology of TD in studies in Asia was found to be 5%–8%, but the increasing prevalence of norovirus recognition around the world may change these statistics.

Risk for Travelers

- Travelers of all ages are potentially at risk for norovirus infection, and previous infection does not reliably result in subsequent immunity.
- Risk for infection is present anywhere food is prepared in an unsanitary manner and may become contaminated or where drinking water is inadequately treated.
- Of particular risk are "ready-to-eat" cold foods, such as sandwiches and salads. Raw shellfish, especially oysters, are also a frequent source of infection, because virus from contaminated water concentrates in the gut of these filter feeders.
- Large outbreaks of gastroenteritis are associated with settings where persons are living in close quarters, such as hotels, cruise ships, and camps, and can easily infect each other over several days.
- Inapparent viral contamination of inanimate objects may persist during outbreaks and act as a source of infection. On cruise ships, for instance, such environmental contamination has caused recurrent outbreaks of illness on successive cruises with newly boarded passengers.
- Transmission of norovirus on an airplane may be limited if vomiting is confined to restrooms and sick persons are kept separate from others.

Clinical Presentation

- Infected persons usually have acute-onset, violent vomiting and nonbloody diarrhea after an incubation period of 24–48 hours. Other symptoms include abdominal cramps, nausea, and occasionally a low-grade fever.
- Illness is generally self-limited, and full recovery can be expected in 1–4 days. In some cases, dehydration, especially in those who are very young or elderly, may require medical attention.

Diagnosis

- Generally diagnosed by clinical presentation. Laboratory testing is currently not FDA approved in the United States for clinical management, but is used during outbreak investigations by public health agencies. Norovirus diagnostic testing is usually not available in developing countries.
- The most common diagnostic test used at state public health laboratories and CDC is reverse transcriptase polymerase chain reaction (RT-PCR), which provides rapid and reliable detection of the virus in stool specimens.
- Several commercial enzyme immunoassays (EIAs) are available for detection of the virus in stool specimens. The specificity and sensitivity of these assays are relatively poor or unknown. These tests have been used occasionally by cruise lines during outbreaks on ships.

Treatment

- The mainstay of management is supportive care, such as rest and oral rehydration.
- No antiviral medication is available for treating norovirus infection.

Preventive Measures for Travelers

- No vaccines are available.
- Noroviruses are very common and highly contagious, but the risk for infection can be minimized by frequent and proper handwashing and avoidance of possibly contaminated food and water.
- In addition to handwashing, measures to prevent transmission of noroviruses between persons traveling together include careful clean up of fecal material or vomit and disinfection of contaminated surfaces and toilet areas with products approved for norovirus disinfection by the Environmental Protection Agency, or a high concentration of domestic bleach (at least a 1:50 solution of bleach and water). Soiled articles of clothing should be washed promptly and thoroughly and machine-dried at high heat.
- Confinement of ill persons to help prevent the spread of noroviruses has occasionally been implemented on cruise ships.

References

1. Widdowson MA, Vinjé J. Food-borne viruses—state of the art. In: Koopmans MP, Cliver DO, Bosch A, editors. Food-borne viruses: progress and challenges. Washington, DC: ASM Press; 2008. p. 29–64.
2. Widdowson MA, Cramer EH, Hadley L, et al. Outbreaks of acute gastroenteritis on cruise ships and on land: identification of a predominant circulating strain of norovirus—United States, 2002. J Infect Dis. 2004;190:27–36.
3. Bresee JS, Widdowson MA, Monroe SS, et al. Foodborne viral gastroenteritis: challenges and opportunities. Clin Infect Dis. 2002;35:748–53.
4. Ko G, Garcia C, Jiang ZD, et al. Noroviruses as a cause of traveler's diarrhea among students from the United States visiting Mexico. J Clin Microbiol. 2005;43:6126–9.
5. Mead PS, Slutsker L, Dietz V, et al. Food-related illness and death in the United States. Emerg Infect Dis. 1999;5:607–25.
6. Chapin AR, Carpenter CM, Dudley WC, et al. Prevalence of norovirus among visitors from the United States to Mexico and Guatemala who experience traveler's diarrhea. J Clin Microbiol. 2005;43:1112–7.
7. CDC. Norovirus activity—United States, 2006–2007. MMWR Morb Mortal Wkly Rep. 2007;56:842–6.
8. Widdowson MA, Glass R, Monroe S, et al. Probable transmission of norovirus on an airplane. JAMA. 2005;293:1859–60.
9. CDC. "Norwalk-like viruses." Public health consequences and outbreak management. MMWR Recomm Rep. 2001;50:(RR-9):1–17.

ONCHOCERCIASIS (RIVER BLINDNESS)

LeAnne M. Fox

Infectious Agent

Onchocerciasis, also known as river blindness, is caused by the filarial nematode, *Onchocerca volvulus*.

Mode of Transmission

Infection occurs through vector-borne transmission by the bite of female blackflies of the genus *Simulium*, that bite during the day and are found near rapidly flowing rivers and streams.

Occurrence

- Onchocerciasis is endemic in more than 25 nations located in a broad band across the central part of Africa. Small endemic foci are also present in the Arabian Peninsula (Yemen) and in the Americas (Brazil, Colombia, Ecuador, Guatemala, southern Mexico, and Venezuela).
- An estimated 17 million people are infected worldwide.

Risk for Travelers

- Short-term travelers to endemic areas are at low risk for this infection.
- Travelers who visit endemic areas for extended periods of time (generally greater than 3 months) and live or work near blackfly habitats are at greater risk for infection.
- Most infections seen in the United States occur in expatriate groups, such as missionaries, field scientists, and Peace Corps volunteers.

Clinical Presentation

- Infection with *O. volvulus* can result in a highly pruritic, papular dermatitis; subcutaneous nodules; lymphadenitis; and ocular lesions, which can progress to visual loss and blindness.
- Symptoms in travelers are primarily dermatologic and may occur months to years after departure from endemic areas.
- Immigrants from endemic areas may present with skin and/or ocular disease.

Diagnosis

- Diagnosis is made by finding either the microfilariae in superficial skin shavings or punch biopsy, adult worms in histologic sections of excised nodules, or characteristic eye lesions.
- Serologic testing is most useful for detecting infection in specific groups, such as expatriates with a brief exposure history, when microfilariae are not identifiable. Determination of serum antifilarial immunoglobulin (IgG) is available through the Parasitic Diseases Laboratory at the National Institutes of Health (NIH) or through the Division of Parasitic Diseases, CDC.

Treatment

- Ivermectin (150–200 µg/kg orally, once or twice per year) is the drug of choice for onchocerciasis. Repeated annual or semiannual doses may be required, because the drug kills the microfilariae but not the adult worms, which can live for many years.
- Antibiotic trials, with doxycycline (100 mg orally per day), directed against *Wolbachia*, an endosymbiont of *O. volvulus*, have demonstrated a decrease in onchocercal microfiladermia with 6 weeks of therapy.
- Diethylcarbamazine (DEC) is contraindicated in onchocerciasis, as it has been associated with severe and fatal post-treatment reactions.
- Any subcutaneous nodules should be excised if their anatomic location allows it to be done safely.
- To ensure correct diagnosis and treatment, travelers should be advised to consult with an infectious diseases or tropical medicine specialist.

Preventive Measures for Travelers

- No vaccine is available.
- No drugs for preventing infection are available.
- Protective measures include avoidance of blackfly habitats and the use of personal protection measures against biting insects (see the Protection Against Mosquitoes, Ticks, and Other Insects and Arthropods section in Chapter 2).

References

1. Burnham G. Onchocerciasis. Lancet. 1998;351:1341–6.
2. Drugs for parasitic infections. Med Lett Drugs Ther. 2007;5(Suppl):e1–15.
3. World Health Organization. Onchocerciasis and its control. Report of a WHO Expert Committee on Onchocerciasis Control. World Health Organ Tech Rep Ser. 1995;852:1–104.
4. Murdoch ME, Asuzu MC, Hagan M, et al. Onchocerciasis: the clinical and epidemiological burden of skin disease in Africa. Ann Trop Med Parasitol. 2002;96:283–96.
5. Albiez EJ, Büttner DW, Duke BO. Diagnosis and extirpation of nodules in human onchocerciasis. Trop Med Parasitol. 1988;39(Suppl 4):331–46.
6. Abiose A. Onchocercal eye disease and the impact of Mectizan treatment. Ann Trop Med Parasitol. 1998;92(Suppl 1):S11–22.
7. Brieger WR, Awedoba AK, Eneanya CI, et al. The effects of ivermectin on onchocercal skin disease and severe itching: results of a multicentre trial. Trop Med Int Health. 1998;3:951–61.
8. Tielsch JM, Beeche A. Impact of ivermectin on illness and disability associated with onchocerciasis. Trop Med Int Health. 2004;9(4):A45–56.
9. Hoerauf H, Mand S, Adjei O, et al. Depletion of *Wolbachia* endobacteria in *Onchocerca volvulus* by doxycycline and microfilaridermia after ivermectin treatment. Lancet. 2001;357:1415–6.

PINWORM (ENTEROBIASIS, OXYURIASIS, THREADWORM)

John C. Watson

Infectious Agent

The intestinal nematode (roundworm), *Enterobius vermicularis* causes pinworm infection.

Mode of Transmission

- Fecal–oral ingestion of the egg, direct person-to-person, or indirect via contaminated hands, dust, food, or objects (e.g., bedding, clothing, toys, bathwater, toilet seats) serve as modes of transmission.

- Incubation period from egg ingestion to migration of adult worm to anus is 1–2 months, but may be longer.
- Eggs can remain infective indoors for 2–3 weeks.
- Humans are the only known natural host; animal pinworms do not infect humans.

Occurrence

- Pinworm infection is found worldwide, in all races and social classes, and is the most frequent worm infection in the United States.
- Infections cluster in households; are common in school-age and preschool-age children and their household members, caregivers, and playmates; and are common in child care and institutional care settings.
- Crowded living conditions facilitate transmission.

Risk for Travelers

- Persons of all ages are at risk.
- Primary settings of risk include—
  - Poor hygiene (e.g., failure to follow proper handwashing practices, poor toileting hygiene)
  - Unsanitary or inadequate toilet facilities
  - Crowded living conditions or living in same household as infected person(s)
  - Close day-to-day contact (i.e., living and working) with the local population, particularly institutionalized persons or preschool- and school-age children (e.g., Peace Corps volunteers, mission or volunteer workers, expatriates)
- Dustborne infection (inhalation with ingestion) can occur in heavily contaminated settings.

Clinical Presentation

- Although infections can be asymptomatic, common symptoms include nocturnal perianal and perineal pruritus and restless sleep.
- Urethritis, vaginitis, salpingitis, hepatitis, or peritonitis may occur from aberrant migration of adult worm from perineum to ectopic site.
- Secondary bacterial infection of skin may occur from scratching.

Diagnosis

- Diagnosis is made by identifying the worm or its eggs by:
  - Direct visualization of female adult worm(s) near anus or on sheets or underclothing or pajamas at night, about 2–3 hours after patient falls asleep
  - Microscopic identification of worm eggs by using the "cellophane tape test" on three consecutive mornings (i.e., firmly pressing adhesive side of clear transparent, not translucent, cellophane tape to the skin around the anus when patient first awakens, before washing or bathing; tape is then directly affixed to microscope slide and examined under low power for eggs)
- Eosinophilia is unusual (due to absence of tissue invasion); serologic testing is not useful or widely available.
- Eggs and worms are rarely found in routine stool samples.

Treatment

- Administer an antihelminthic as a single oral dose; repeat in 2 weeks. Drugs of choice are mebendazole, albendazole, or pyrantel pamoate (available without prescription).

- Treat all household contacts and caretakers at same time as patient.
- Daily morning bathing removes a large proportion of eggs; change underclothing and bedding frequently and launder in hot water.
- Reinfection occurs easily; instruction about prevention is mandatory to eliminate continued infection and spread.

Preventive Measures for Travelers

- Strict observance of good hand hygiene is essential (i.e., proper handwashing, maintaining clean short fingernails, avoiding or preventing nail biting, avoiding or preventing scratching the perianal and perineal region).
- Daily morning bathing, as well as careful handling and frequent changing and laundering of underclothing and bedding with hot water can help reduce infection and prevent reinfection and environmental contamination with eggs.

References

1. American Academy of Pediatrics. Pinworm infection *(Enterobius vermicularis)*. In: Pickering LK, Baker CJ, Long SS, McMillan JA, editors. Red book: 2006 Report of the Committee on Infectious Diseases. 27th ed. Elk Grove Village (IL): American Academy of Pediatrics; 2006. p. 520–2.
2. American Public Health Association. Enterobiasis. In: Heyman DL, editor. Control of communicable diseases manual. 18th ed. Washington, DC: American Public Health Association; 2004. p. 194–6.
3. Kucik CJ, Martin GL, Sortor BV. Common intestinal parasites. Am Fam Physician. 2004;69:1161–8.
4. Meinking TL, Burkhart CN, Burkhart CG. Changing paradigms in parasitic infections: common dermatological helminthic infections and cutaneous myiasis. Clin Dermatol. 2003;21:407–16.
5. St Georgiev V. Chemotherapy of enterobiasis (oxyuriasis). Expert Opin Pharmacother. 2001;2(2):267–75.

PLAGUE (BUBONIC, PNEUMONIC, SEPTICEMIC)

Paul S. Mead, Ingrid B. Weber

Infectious Agent

Plague is caused by gram-negative bacterium, *Yersinia pestis*.

Mode of Transmission

- Zoonotic disease is usually transmitted to humans by the bites of infected rodent fleas.
- Less common exposures include handling infected animal tissues (hunters, wildlife personnel); inhalation of infectious droplets from cats with plague; and, rarely, contact with a pneumonic plague patient.

Occurrence

- 1,000 to 2,000 cases occur globally each year.
- Rural areas in central and southern Africa, central Asia and the Indian subcontinent, the northeastern part of South America, and parts of the southwestern United States.
- Although rare, urban outbreaks of plague have been reported in Majunga, Madagascar.

Risk for Travelers

- All ages are at risk for infection; however, risk to travelers is largely restricted to rural endemic areas.
- Only one case associated with international travel has been reported in the United States in the past two decades.

Clinical Presentation

- Incubation period is typically 1–6 days.
- History is suggestive of exposure to rodents, rodent fleas, wild rabbits, sick or dead carnivores, or patients with pneumonic plague.
- Symptoms and signs of the three clinical presentations of plague illness include:
  - Bubonic (>80%)—rapid onset of fever; painful, swollen and tender lymph node, usually inguinal, axillary, or cervical
  - Pneumonic—high fever; overwhelming pneumonia; cough; bloody sputum; chills
  - Septicemic—prostration, hemorrhagic and/or thrombotic phenomena progressing to acral gangrene

Diagnosis

- Specimens: bubo aspirates; blood cultures; sputum culture if pneumonic
- Microscopic identification, culture confirmation; confirmatory and rapid assays available through public health laboratories
- Serologic tests: fourfold change in antibody titer to F1 antigen between acute- and convalescent-phase sera

Treatment

- Physicians should report all suspected plague cases to state or local health departments and/or consult with CDC to obtain information and access diagnostic services.
- Parenteral antibiotic therapy with streptomycin is the recommended first-line therapy; alternatively, gentamicin; or where treatment is limited to oral therapy, doxycycline.
- Additional information can be found on the Division of Vector-Borne Infectious Diseases website at www.cdc.gov/ncidod/dvbid/plague/index.htm.

Preventive Measures for Travelers

- No vaccine is currently available in the United States.
- Preventive measures are aimed at reducing contact with fleas and potentially infected rodents and other wildlife.
- Health-care workers should follow droplet precautions while working with suspected plague patients, especially if patient is coughing.
- Prophylactic antibiotic treatment is given only in the event of exposure to bites of wild rodent fleas during an outbreak, exposure to tissues of a plague-infected animal, or close exposure to another person or animal with suspected plague pneumonia.

References

1. Inglesby TV, Dennis DT, Henderson DA, et al. Plague as a biological weapon: medical and public health management. Working Group on Civilian Biodefense. JAMA. 2000;283:2281–90.

2. Dennis DT, Campbell GL. Plague and other *Yersinia* infections. In: Fauci AS, Braunwald E, Kasper DL, Hauser SL, Longo DL, Jameson JL, Loscalzo J, editors. Harrison's principles of internal medicine. 17th ed. New York:

McGraw-Hill Medical Publishing Division; 2008. p. 980–6.

3. Gage KL. Plague. In: Collier L, editor. Microbiology and microbial infections. 9th ed. New York: Arnold; 1998.

4. Perry RD, Fetherston JD. *Yersinia pestis*— etiologic agent of plague. Clin Microbiol Rev. 1997;10(1):35–66.

5. CDC. Human plague—India, 1994. MMWR Morb Mortal Wkly Rep. 1994;43(38):689–91.

6. Boisier P, Rasolomaharo M, Ranaivoson G, et al. Urban epidemic of bubonic plague in Majunga, Madagascar: epidemiological aspects. Trop Med Int Health. 1997;2(5):422–7.

7. Boulanger LL, Ettestad P, Fogarty JD, et al. Gentamicin and tetracyclines for the treatment of human plague: review of 75 cases in New Mexico, 1985–1999. Clin Infect Dis. 2004;38(5):663–9.

8. CDC. Prevention of plague: recommendations of the Advisory Committee on Immunization Practices (ACIP). MMWR Recomm Rep. 1996;45(RR-14):1–15.

9. Kool JL. Risk of person-to-person transmission of pneumonic plague. Clin Infect Dis. 2005;40(8):1166–72.

Q FEVER

Alicia Anderson, Jennifer McQuiston

Infectious Agent

Q fever is caused by the organism *Coxiella burnetii*, which is an obligate intracellular bacterial parasite of the genus *Coxiella*.

Mode of Transmission

Q fever is a zoonotic disease that is often associated with exposure to cattle, sheep, and goats. Infection typically occurs by inhalation of the organism in small droplets or inhalation of dust contaminated with *C. burnetii*. Although direct animal contact appears to carry the highest risk for infection, windborne spread through contaminated dust has been reported. Infections via ingestion of contaminated dairy products, tick bites, and human-to-human transmission via sexual contact or during parturition have been less commonly reported.

Occurrence

- Q fever is found worldwide. Human cases of Q fever have been reported from across the United States and are most commonly reported in those who are occupationally exposed to livestock.
- On average, approximately 50–60 cases of Q fever are reported in the United States each year, and the average annual reported incidence is 0.28 cases per million persons. The incidence in the United Kingdom also appears to be low (2 cases per million), whereas the reported incidence in France (500 cases per million) and Australia (38 cases per million) is much higher. Q fever is believed to be underdiagnosed and underreported throughout the world, so the number of reported cases likely does not reflect the true incidence of disease.

Risk for Travelers

- Travelers who visit rural areas or farms with cattle, sheep, goats, or other livestock may be exposed to Q fever. Transmission is also possible through infected ticks or consumption of unpasteurized milk.
- Occupational exposure to infected animals (e.g., farmers, veterinarians, butchers, meat packers, seasonal or migrant farm workers), particularly during parturition, poses a high risk for disease transmission.

- Recent cases of Q fever in military personnel returning from deployments to Iraq and Afghanistan should alert physicians to consider this diagnosis among persons presenting with compatible symptoms.

Clinical Presentation

- Approximately half of infected persons will be asymptomatic.
- Symptomatic illness typically occurs within 2–3 weeks after exposure. Variable incubation periods may be dose-dependent, with shorter incubation periods after exposure to high organism numbers.
- The most common presentation is a mild and self-limiting influenza-like illness. Other potential manifestations include pneumonia, hepatitis, myocarditis, encephalitis, osteomyelitis, and miscarriage in pregnant women.
- Chronic Q fever is uncommon (<5% of acutely infected patients). The majority of chronic cases (60%–70%) present as culture-negative endocarditis, particularly in a patient who is immunosuppressed or has a previous valvulopathy.

Diagnosis

Whenever possible, specimens for lab testing of acutely ill patients should be obtained before starting antimicrobial therapy.

- Diagnosis relies mainly on serology. The indirect immunofluorescence assay is the most dependable and widely used method. Testing of paired (acute- and convalescent-phase) serum specimens, taken 2–3 weeks apart, is preferred, because changes in antibody titers provide the best evidence of recent infection. In some cases, a single high serum antibody titer may be considered evidence of probable infection.
- *C. burnetii* may be detected in infected tissues by using immunohistochemical staining and DNA detection methods or by direct isolation of the agent via culture. PCR assays may be used on blood samples.

Treatment

- Doxycycline is the treatment of choice for acute Q fever. Chronic Q fever endocarditis is much more difficult to treat effectively and often requires the use of multiple drugs.
- Additional information can be found on the CDC website at http://emergency.cdc.gov/agent/qfever/clinicians/.

Preventive Measures for Travelers

- A human vaccine for Q fever has been developed and used successfully in Australia. No vaccine is commercially available in the United States.
- No drugs for preventing infection are available.
- Preventive measures are aimed at restricting access to areas where potentially infected animals are kept and at properly disposing birth products from livestock. Persons at highest risk for developing chronic Q fever (i.e., those with pre-existing valvulopathy or immunosuppression) should be educated on the risks and sources of infection.
- Travelers should also avoid consumption of unpasteurized dairy products and take precautions to prevent tick attachment.

References

1. Maurin M, Raoult D. Q fever. Clin Microbiol Rev. 1999;12(4): 518–53.

2. McQuiston JH, Childs JE, Thompson HA. Q fever. J Am Vet Med Assoc. 2002;221(6):796–9.

3. McQuiston JH, Holman RC, McCall CL, et al. National surveillance and the epidemiology of human Q fever in the United States, 1978–2004. Am J Trop Med Hyg. 2006;75:36–40.
4. Anderson AD, Smoak B, Shuping E, et al. Q fever and the US military. Emerg Infect Dis. 2005;11(8):1320–2.
5. Leung-Shea C, Danaher PJ. Q fever in members of the United States armed forced returning from Iraq. Clin Infect Dis. 2006;43(8):77–82.
6. Gleeson TD, Decker CF, Johnson MD, et al. Q fever in U.S. military returning from Iraq. Am J Med. 2007;120(9):e11–2.
7. Karakousis PC, Trucksis M, Dumler JS. Chronic Q fever in the United States. J Clin Microbiol. 2006;44(6):2283–7.

RICKETTSIAL (SPOTTED AND TYPHUS FEVERS) AND RELATED INFECTIONS (ANAPLASMOSIS AND EHRLICHIOSIS)

Jennifer Adjemian, Marina E. Eremeeva, Gregory A. Dasch

Infectious Agent

- Rickettsial infections are caused by a variety of obligate intracellular, gram-negative bacteria from the genera *Rickettsia, Orientia, Ehrlichia, Neorickettsia,* and *Anaplasma* (Table 5-1).
- *Rickettsia* are further classified into the typhus group and spotted fever group (SFG), and *Orientia* comprises the classic scrub typhus group.

Mode of Transmission

- Most rickettsial pathogens are transmitted by ectoparasites such as fleas, lice, mites, and ticks during bloodfeeding or from scarification of infectious feces from these vectors that may be deposited on the skin.
- Many rickettsiae of concern to travelers, including *Ehrlichia* sp., *Anaplasma* sp., and most SFG rickettsiae, are transmitted by ticks.
- Mites transmit the SFG rickettsia *R. akari,* which causes rickettsialpox.
- Chiggers, the immature stage of *Leptotrombidium* mites, transmit *Orientia tsutsugamushi,* the etiologic agent of scrub typhus.
- Fleas serve as vectors for *R. typhi* and *R. felis,* which cause endemic or murine typhus and cat flea rickettsiosis, respectively.
- Human body lice and the ectoparasites of flying squirrels can transmit *R. prowazekii,* the causative agent of epidemic or louse-borne typhus.
- *Neorickettsia sennetsu* causes sennetsu fever and is likely transmitted by the ingestion of infected trematodes in raw fish.
- Transmission of rickettsiae following blood transfusion is rare but has been reported during the asymptomatic incubation period of those diseases.

Occurrence

- SFG and typhus group rickettsiae have been reported worldwide. SFG rickettsial infections among travelers include African tick-bite fever (ATBF) from Africa and the Caribbean islands; Mediterranean (or Boutonneuse) spotted fever from southern Europe and Africa; Indian tick typhus from India; Astrakhan fever from southeastern Europe and Central Africa; Israeli tick typhus from Mediterranean basin; Thai tick typhus from Asia and Australia; Queensland tick typhus and Australian spotted fever from eastern Australia; tick-borne lymphadenopathy from European countries; North Asian tick typhus from China and Russia; and Rocky Mountain spotted fever (RMSF) and *R. parkeri* from North, Central, and South America.

- Rickettsialpox, transmitted by house-mouse mites, circulates in urban centers in Ukraine, South Africa, Korea, Balkan states, and the United States. The agent may spill over and occasionally be found within some wild rodent populations.
- Scrub typhus is endemic in northern Japan, Southeast Asia, the western Pacific islands, eastern Australia, China, maritime and several parts of south-central Russia, India and Sri Lanka. More than one million cases occur annually. Unusual travel-associated cases of scrub typhus have been diagnosed in individuals returning from Ghana to Japan and from Dubai to Australia.
- Flea-borne rickettsioses caused by *R. typhi* and *R. felis* are widely distributed, especially throughout the tropics and subtropics and in port cities and coastal regions with rodents. Murine typhus has been reported among travelers returning from Asia, Africa, and southern Europe and has also been reported from Hawaii, California, and Texas in the United States.
- Epidemic typhus occurs in communities and populations where body lice are prevalent. Outbreaks have often been tied to periods of war, poverty, and natural disasters, especially during the colder months when infested clothing is not laundered. Active foci of endemic typhus are known in the Andes regions of South America and in Burundi and Ethiopia. Sylvatic epidemic typhus is also endemic among flying squirrels in the eastern United States. Tick-associated reservoirs of *R. prowazekii* have been described in Ethiopia, Mexico, and Brazil.
- Ehrlichiosis is most commonly reported in the southeastern and south-central United States where the lonestar tick, *Amblyomma americanum*, and white-tailed deer are commonplace. It is also found in Brazil and Panama. In Europe and Asia, transmission of monocytic ehrlichiosis may be due to *E. chaffeensis* or related organisms such as *E. muris* that are associated with ticks of the *Ixodes persulcatus* complex, found on small rodents and passerine birds.
- Anaplasmosis occurs worldwide, corresponding with the ranges of *Ixodes persulcatus* group ticks. Known endemic regions include the United States, Europe, China, Siberia, Russia, and Korea.
- Sennetsu fever occurs in Japan, Malaysia, and possibly other parts of Asia.
- Refer to Table 5-1 for additional details about rickettsiae known to cause disease in humans.

Risk for Travelers

- All ages are at risk for rickettsial infections with travel to endemic areas, especially when participating in outdoor activities during spring and summer months when ticks and fleas are most active, but infection can occur throughout the year.
- Game hunting, traveling to southern Africa, and traveling during November through April represent specific risk factors for ATBF in travelers. One study estimated that the risk of a traveler contracting a rickettsiosis in southern Africa is four to five times higher than that of acquiring malaria.
- Contact with tick-infested dogs in areas endemic for certain SFG rickettsiae increases risk of acquiring disease.
- Outbreaks of rickettsialpox most often occur following contact with infected rodents and their mites, especially during natural die-offs or extermination of infected rodents that cause the mites to seek out new hosts, such as humans.
- Most travel-acquired cases of scrub typhus occur during visits to rural areas in endemic countries for activities such as camping, hiking, or rafting.
- Humans exposed to flea-infested cats, dogs, and peridomestic animals while traveling in endemic regions are at greatest risk for flea-borne rickettsioses.
- Travelers at greatest risk for epidemic typhus include those who may work with and/or visit areas with large homeless populations, impoverished areas or refugee camps, and regions that have recently experienced war or natural disasters, especially during the colder months. Sylvatic epidemic typhus cases occur only from direct contact with flying squirrels or their nesting materials.
- Sennetsu fever can be contracted from consuming raw infected fish.

Table 5-1. Classification, primary vector, and reservoir occurrence of rickettsiae known to cause disease in humans and clinical symptoms of the rickettsial diseases

Antigenic Group	Disease	Species	Vector	Animal Reservoir(s)	Geographic Distribution	Clinical Symptoms
Anaplasma	Human granulocytic anaplasmosis	*Anaplasma phagocytophilum*	Tick	Deer, elk, small mammals, and rodents	Worldwide	Fever, headache, malaise, myalgia, vomiting
Ehrlichia	Human monocytic ehrlichiosis	*Ehrlichia chaffeensis*	Tick	Deer, wild and domestic dogs domestic ruminants, and rodents	Worldwide	Fever, headache, malaise, myalgia
	Ehrlichiosis	*Ehrlichia ewingii*	Tick	Deer, wild and domestic dogs, and rodents	North America	Fever, headache, malaise, myalgia, nausea, vomiting
Neorickettsia	Sennetsu fever	*Neorickettsia sennetsu*	Trematode	Fish	Japan, Malaysia, possibly other parts of Asia	Fever, headache, myalgia
Scrub typhus	Scrub typhus	*Orientia tsutsugamushi*	Larval mite (chigger)	Rodents	Asia-Pacific region from Maritime Russia and China to Indonesia and North Australia to Afghanistan	Fever, headache, myalgia, possibly a maculopapular rash
Spotted fever	Rickettsiosis	*Rickettsia aeschlimannii*	Tick	Unknown	South Africa, Morocco, Mediterranean littoral	Fever, eschar, maculopapular rash
	African tick-bite fever	*Rickettsia africae*	Tick	Rodents	Sub-Saharan Africa, West Indies	Fever, eschar(s)
	Rickettsialpox	*Rickettsia akari*	Mite	House mice, wild rodents	Former Soviet Union, South Africa, Korea, Turkey, Balkan countries, North and South America	Fever, eschar, adenopathy, disseminated vesicular rash
	Queensland tick typhus	*Rickettsia australis*	Tick	Rodents	Australia, Tasmania	Fever, eschar, regional adenopathy, rash on extremities

(Continued)

Table 5-1. Classification, primary vector, and reservoir occurrence of rickettsiae known to cause disease in humans and clinical symptoms of the rickettsial diseases *(Continued)*

Antigenic Group	Disease	Species	Vector	Animal Reservoir(s)	Geographic Distribution	Clinical Symptoms
Spotted fever *(Continued)*	Mediterranean spotted fever or Boutonneuse fever	*Rickettsia conorii*[1]	Tick	Dogs, rodents	Southern Europe, southern and western Asia, Africa, India	Fever, eschar, regional adenopathy, maculopapular rash on extremities
	Cat flea rickettsiosis	*Rickettsia felis*	Cat and dog flea	Domestic cats, rodents, opossums	Europe, North and South America, Africa, Asia	Headache, chills, fever, prostration, confusion, photophobia, vomiting, rash (generally originating on trunk)
	Far Eastern spotted fever	*Rickettsia heilongjiangensis*	Tick	Rodents	Far East of Russia, Northern China, Eastern Asia	Fever, eschar, maculopapular rash, lymph-adenopathy, enlarged lymph nodes
	Aneruptive fever	*Rickettsia helvetica*	Tick	Rodents	Central and northern Europe, Asia	Fever, headache, myalgia
	Flinders Island spotted fever, Thai tick typhus	*Rickettsia honei*	Tick	Unknown	Australia, Thailand	Mild spotted fever; eschar and adenopathy are rare
	Japanese spotted fever	*Rickettsia japonica*	Tick	Rodents	Japan	Fever, eschar(s), regional adenopathy, rash on extremities
	Australian spotted fever	*Rickettsia marmionii*	Tick	Rodents, reptiles	Australia	Fever, eschar, maculopapular or vesicular rash, adenopathy
	Mediterranean spotted fever-like disease	*Rickettsia massiliae*	Tick	Unknown	France, Greece, Spain, Portugal, Switzerland, Sicily, Central Africa, and Mali	Fever, maculopapular rash, necrotic eschar
	Maculatum infection	*Rickettsia parkeri*	Tick	Rodents	North and South America	Fever, eschar, maculopapular or vesicular rash

(Continued)

Table 5-1. Classification, primary vector, and reservoir occurrence of rickettsiae known to cause disease in humans and clinical symptoms of the rickettsial diseases *(Continued)*

Antigenic Group	Disease	Species	Vector	Animal Reservoir(s)	Geographic Distribution	Clinical Symptoms
Spotted fever *(Continued)*	Rocky Mountain spotted fever, febre maculosa, Sao Paulo exanthematic typhus, Minas Gerais exanthematic typhus, Brazillian spotted fever	*Rickettsia rickettsii*	Tick	Rodents	North, Central, and South America	Fever, headache, abdominal pain, maculopapular rash progressing into papular or petechial rash (generally originating on extremities)
	North Asian tick typhus, Siberian tick typhus	*Rickettisa sibirica*	Tick	Rodents	Russia, China, Mongolia	Fever, eschar(s), regional adenopathy, maculopapular rash
	Lymphangitis-associated rickettsiosis	*Rickettsia siberica mongolotimonae*	Tick	Rodents	Southern France, Portugal, China, sub-Saharan Africa	Fever, multiple eschars, regional adenopathy and lymphangitis, maculopapular rash
	Tick-borne lymphadeno-pathy (TIBOLA), *Dermacentor*-borne necrosis and lymph-adenopathy (DEBONEL)	*Rickettsia slovaca*	Tick	Lagomorphs, rodents	Southern and eastern Europe, Asia	Necrosis erythema, cervical lymph-adenopathy and enlarged lymph nodes, rare maculopapular rash
Typhus fever	Epidemic typhus, Sylvatic typhus	*Rickettsia prowazekii*	Human body louse, flying squirrel ectopara-sites, *Amblyomma* ticks	Humans, flying squirrels	Central Africa, Asia, Central, North, and South America	Headache, chills, fever, prostration, confusion, rash, photophobia
	Murine typhus	*Rickettsia typhi*	Flea	Rodents	Tropical and subtropical areas worldwide	Same as above, but milder

1 Includes four different subspecies that can be distinguished serologically and by PCR assay, and respectively are the etiologic agents of Boutonneuse fever and Mediterranean tick fever in Southern Europe and Africa (*R. conorii* subsp. *conorii*), Indian tick typhus in South Asia (*R. conorii* subsp. *indica*), Israeli tick typhus in Southern Europe and Middle East (*R. conorii* subsp. *israelensis*), and Astrakhan spotted fever in the North Caspian region of Russia (*R. conorii* subsp. *caspiae*).

Clinical Presentation

- Although the clinical presentation varies by pathogen, some common symptoms that typically develop within 1–2 weeks of exposure include fever, headache, malaise, and sometimes nausea and vomiting.
- Most tick-transmitted rickettsioses are accompanied by a macupapular, vesicular or petechial rash, and/or an eschar at the site of the tick bite.
- While many rickettsial diseases cause mild or moderate illness, epidemic typhus and RMSF can be quite severe and may be fatal in 20%–60% of untreated cases.
- Most symptoms associated with rickettsial infections are very nonspecific and require further tests to make an accurate diagnosis.

Diagnosis

- If clinical symptoms and the epidemiologic history are compatible with rickettsial infections, the following diagnostic tests should be utilized:
  - PCR test
  - Specific immunohistologic detection of rickettsiae
  - Isolation of a rickettsial agent by culture during the acute stage of illness and before antibiotic treatment.
- The diagnosis can be confirmed at a later time by obtaining acute- and convalescent-phase serum from the patient.
- In patients suspicious for rickettsial disease, an acute-phase serum should be drawn and held in case serology becomes necessary at a later time. Most serum specimens collected during the acute stage of rickettsial diseases do not contain antirickettsial antibodies, although immune responses to scrub typhus rickettsiae can be very rapid.

Treatment

- Diagnosing a rickettsial infection can be difficult, but rapid treatment with appropriate antibiotic therapy is critical for rapid recovery.
- Treatment must be based on clinical suspicion and not be delayed pending results of laboratory tests.
- Antibiotics of the tetracycline class (doxycycline in particular) have a high degree of efficacy and low toxicity in treating rickettsial infections, even in children. Depending on the specific pathogen, chloramphenicol, azithromycin, fluoroquinolones, and rifampin may also be considered, but these are not universally effective for all rickettsial agents, nor have they been evaluated by controlled clinical trials.
- The standard treatment regimen consists of 200 mg of doxycycline daily for 3–14 days or 2.2 mg/kg body weight per dose administered twice daily (orally or intravenously) for children weighing <100 lbs. (45.4 kg). However, the specific type and duration of antibiotic administered may vary, depending on the disease and kinetics of defervescence.
- Physicians can consult with CDC to obtain further information and access diagnostic services.

Preventive Measures for Travelers

- No vaccines or drugs are available for preventing infection.
- The best prevention is to minimize exposure to fleas, ticks, and animal reservoirs when traveling in endemic areas.
- The proper use of insect repellents, avoiding vector-infested areas, and wearing protective clothing are important ways to reduce risk.

- These precautions are especially important for persons with underlying conditions that may compromise their immune systems, as these individuals may be more susceptible to severe disease.

References

1. Raoult D, Parola P, editors. Rickettsial diseases. New York: Informa Healthcare USA, Inc.; 2007.
2. Walker DH. Rickettsial diseases in travelers. Travel Med Infect Dis. 2003;1:35–40.
3. Jensenius M, Fournier PE, Raoult D. Tick-borne rickettsioses in international travellers. Int J Infect Dis. 2004;8:139–46.
4. Parola P, Paddock CD, Raoult D. Tick-borne rickettsioses around the world: emerging diseases challenging old concepts. Clin Microbiol Rev. 2005;18(4):719–56.
5. Nachega JB, Bottieau E, Zech F, et al. Travel-acquired scrub typhus: emphasis on the differential diagnosis, treatment, and prevention strategies. J Travel Med. 2007;14(5):352–5.
6. Dumler JS, Madigan JE, Pusterla N, et al. Ehrlichiosis in humans: epidemiology, clinical presentation, diagnosis, and treatment. Clin Infect Dis. 2007;45(Suppl 1):S45–51.
7. Jensenius M, Fournier PE, Vene S, et al. African tick bite fever in travelers to rural sub-Equatorial Africa. Clin Infect Dis. 2003;36:1411–7.
8. Jensenius M, Fournier PE, Raoult D. Rickettsioses and the international traveler. Clin Infect Dis. 2004;39:1493–9.
9. Paddock CD, Eremeeva ME. Rickettsialpox. In: Raoult D, Parola P, editors. Rickettsial diseases. New York: Informa Healthcare USA, Inc.; 2007. p. 63–86.
10. Dumler JS, Barbet AF, Bekker CP, et al. Reorganization of genera in the families *Rickettsiaceae* and *Anaplasmataceae* in the order *Rickettsiales*: unification of some species of *Ehrlichia* with *Anaplasma*, *Cowdria* with *Ehrlichia* and *Ehrlichia* with *Neorickettsia*, descriptions of six new species combinations and designation of *Ehrlichia equi* and 'HGE agent' as subjective synonyms of *Ehrlichia phagocytophila*. Int J Syst Evol Microbiol. 2001;51(Pt 6):2145–65.

SCABIES (SARCOPTIC ITCH, SARCOPTIC ACARIASIS)

John C. Watson

Infectious Agent

Scabies is caused by the microscopic human itch mite (*Sarcoptes scabiei* var. *hominis*).

Mode of Transmission

Transmission occurs—

- Directly via prolonged skin-to-skin contact with a person with conventional scabies or via brief skin-to-skin contact with a person with crusted (Norwegian) scabies.
- Indirectly via contact with objects (e.g., bedding, clothing, furniture) contaminated by a person with crusted (Norwegian) scabies; rarely via contact with fomites used by a person with conventional scabies.
- Human scabies is not spread by pets or other animals.

Occurrence

- Scabies occurs worldwide; it is epidemic in much of the developing world and common in the tropics.
- Infection occurs in all races and social classes.
- Outbreaks are reported most commonly in nursing-care facilities, prisons, and schools.

Risk for Travelers

- All ages are at risk.

- Household members and sexual partners of infested persons are at high risk.
- Exposure to crusted (Norwegian) scabies is more likely in institutions (e.g., nursing homes, extended-care facilities) caring for the elderly, the immunocompromised (e.g., HIV/AIDS), or the mentally or physically disabled (e.g., cognitive deficiency, neurologic injury).
- Exposure to crowded living conditions and/or where close body and skin contact are common (e.g., refugee/displaced person settings, schools/child-care facilities).
- Close day-to-day contact (living/working) with local populations in high prevalence areas/situations (e.g., Peace Corps volunteers, mission/volunteer work, adventure travel, expatriates).

Clinical Presentation

- Symptom onset occurs from 2 weeks to 2 months after exposure for first infestation; symptom onset occurs 1–4 days after exposure for subsequent infestations. A patient is contagious from the time of exposure, even while asymptomatic, until successfully treated and all mites and eggs are killed.
- Head, neck, palms/soles are usually not affected in older children and adults in temperate climates.
- *Conventional scabies:*
  - Intense pruritus (itching), particularly at night, and papular (pimple-like) or papulovesicular, pruritic (itchy) erythematous rash; common sites are wrists, elbows, axillae, groin/genitals, breasts/nipples, beltline, buttocks, between fingers/shoulder blades; itching can be generalized; papules are often excoriated; secondary bacterial infection can occur.
  - Tiny, raised, greyish or skin colored, serpiginous lines on skin surface represent mite burrows; most commonly seen on wrist, penis, between fingers; often few and difficult to find.
- *Crusted (Norwegian) scabies:*
  - Pruritus is often mild or absent; exfoliating hyperkeratotic scales/crusts (contain large numbers of mites).

Diagnosis

Diagnosis can be made through—

- Pruritus and characteristic rash in patient and household members/associates
- Identification of characteristic burrow(s)
- Microscopic identification of mites, mite eggs, or scybala (mite feces) in skin scrapings of fresh lesions (intact papules/burrows); placing a drop of mineral oil on the skin can facilitate scraping and subsequent microscopic examination; excoriated lesions rarely contain mites.

Treatment

- Permethrin (5%) cream is considered by many to be drug of choice; not FDA-approved for use in children <2 months of age.
- Ivermectin, an oral antiparasitic agent, is reported safe and effective for treatment of scabies, including crusted (Norwegian) scabies; two or more doses may be necessary to eliminate infestation; it should be considered for patients in whom treatment has failed or who cannot tolerate other approved medications; not FDA-approved for treatment of scabies.
- Crotamiton (10%) lotion or cream: associated with frequent treatment failure; not FDA-approved for use in children.

- Lindane (1%) lotion: not recommended as first-line therapy because of neurotoxicity; use restricted to patients in whom treatment has failed or who cannot tolerate other medications that pose less risk; it should not be used to treat premature infants, persons with a seizure disorder, women who are pregnant or breastfeeding, persons who have very irritated skin or sores where lindane will be applied, infants, children, the elderly, and persons who weigh less than 110 pounds (less than 50 kg).
- Other medications used in some geographic locations: topical precipitated sulfur in petrolatum; benzyl benzoate solution/emulsion.
- All household members and intimate contacts should be treated at the same time.
- To prevent reinfestation, exposed clothing and bed linen should be washed in hot water (at least 122° F or 50° C), or dry clean, at same time as treatment.
- Additional information can be found on the Division of Parasitic Diseases website at www.cdc.gov/scabies.

Preventive Measures for Travelers

- No vaccine is available.
- Preventive measures are aimed at reducing prolonged direct skin-to-skin contact with infested persons and with items such as clothing and bed linen used by an infested person.
- Environmental fumigation generally is not necessary and is not recommended.

References

1. American Academy of Pediatrics. Scabies. In: Pickering LK, Baker CJ, Long SS, McMillan JA, editors. Red book: 2006 Report of the Committee on Infectious Diseases. 27th ed. Elk Grove Village (IL): American Academy of Pediatrics; 2006. p. 584–7.

2. Strother MS, Colven R. Ectoparasites, cutaneous parasites, and cnidarian envenomation. In: Jong EC, McMullen WR, editors. The travel and tropical medicine manual. 3rd ed. Philadelphia: Saunders; 2003. p. 459–70.

3. Ansart S, Perez L, Jaureguiberry S, et al. Spectrum of dermatoses in 165 travelers returning from the tropics with skin diseases. Am J Trop Med Hyg. 2007;76:184–6.

4. Chosidow O. Clinical practices. Scabies. N Engl J Med. 2006;354:1718–27.

5. Hengge UR, Currie BJ, Jäger G, et al. Scabies: a ubiquitous neglected skin disease. Lancet Infect Dis. 2006;6:769–79.

6. Heukelbach J, Feldmeier H. Scabies. Lancet. 2006;367:1767–74.

7. Meinking TL. Infestations. Curr Probl Dermatol. 1999;11(3):73–118.

8. Strong M, Johnstone PW. Interventions for treating scabies. Cochrane Database Syst Rev. 2007 Jul 18;(3):CD000320.

9. Wilson ME, Chen LH. Dermatologic infectious diseases in international travelers. Curr Infect Dis Rep. 2004;6:54–62.

SCHISTOSOMIASIS

Susan Montgomery

Infectious Agent

Schistosomiasis is caused by helminth parasites of the genus *Schistosoma*.

Mode of Transmission

Waterborne transmission occurs via penetration of larval cercariae in contaminated bodies of fresh water.

Occurrence

- An estimated 85% of the world's cases of schistosomiasis are in Africa, where prevalence rates can exceed 50% in local populations.
- *S. mansoni* and *S. haematobium* are distributed throughout Africa; only *S. haematobium* is found in areas of the Middle East, while *S. japonicum* is found in Indonesia and parts of China and Southeast Asia (Map 5-7).
- Two other species can infect humans: *S. mekongi*, found in Cambodia and Laos, and *S. intercalatum*, found in parts of Central and West Africa. These two species are rarely reported causes of infection.

Risk for Travelers

- All ages are at risk for infection with travel to endemic areas and freshwater exposure.
- Swimming, bathing and wading into contaminated freshwater can result in infection. Human schistosomiasis cannot be acquired by contact with saltwater (oceans or seas).
- The distribution of schistosomiasis is very focal and determined by the presence of competent snail vectors, inadequate sanitation, and infected humans. The geographic distribution of cases of schistosomiasis acquired by travelers reflects travel and immigration patterns. Most travel-associated cases of schistosomiasis are acquired in sub-Saharan Africa.
- The specific snail vectors can be difficult to identify, and snail infection with human schistosome species must be determined in the laboratory.
- The types of travelers and expatriates potentially at increased risk for infection include adventure travelers, Peace Corps volunteers, missionaries, soldiers, and ecotourists.
- Outbreaks of schistosomiasis have occurred among adventure travelers on river trips in Africa.

Clinical Presentation

- Incubation period is typically 14–84 days for acute schistosomiasis (Katayama syndrome), but chronic infection can remain asymptomatic for years.
- Penetration of cercariae can be associated with a rash that develops within hours or up to a week after contaminated water exposures.
- Acute schistosomiasis is characterized by fever, headache, myalgia, and respiratory symptoms. Eosinophilia is present, as well as often painful hepato- and/or spenomegaly.
- The clinical manifestations of chronic schistosomiasis are the result of host immune responses to schistosome eggs. Eggs secreted by adult worm pairs enter the circulation and lodge in organs and cause granulomatous reactions. Eosinophilia may be present.
- *S. mansoni* and *S. japonicum* eggs most commonly lodge in the blood vessels of the liver or intestine and can cause diarrhea, constipation, and blood in the stool. Chronic inflammation can lead to bowel wall ulceration, hyperplasia, and polyposis and, with heavy infections, to periportal liver fibrosis.
- *S. haematobium* eggs typically lodge in the urinary tract and can cause dysuria and hematuria. Calcifications in the bladder may appear late in the disease. *S. haematobium* infection has been associated with increased risk of bladder cancer.
- Rarely, central nervous system schistosomiasis may develop; this form is thought to result from aberrant migration of adult worms or eggs depositing in the spinal cord or brain. Signs and symptoms are related to the site of the granulomas in the central nervous system and can present as transverse myelitis.

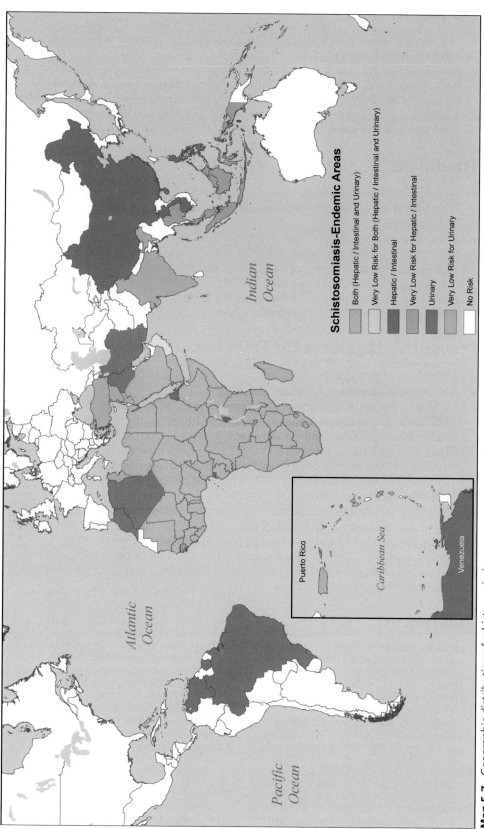

Schistosomiasis-Endemic Areas

- Both (Hepatic / Intestinal and Urinary)
- Very Low Risk for Both (Hepatic / Intestinal and Urinary)
- Hepatic / Intestinal
- Very Low Risk for Hepatic / Intestinal
- Urinary
- Very Low Risk for Urinary
- No Risk

Indian Ocean

Atlantic Ocean

Pacific Ocean

Caribbean Sea

Puerto Rico

Venezuela

Map 5-7. Geographic distribution of schistosomiasis.

Diagnosis

- Microscopic identification of parasite eggs in stool (*S. mansoni* or *S. japonicum*) or urine (*S. haematobium*).
- Serologic tests are useful to diagnose light infections where egg shedding may not be consistent and in travelers and others who have not had schistosomiasis previously. Antibody tests do not distinguish between past and current infection. Available test sensitivity and specificity vary, depending on the antigen preparation used and how the test is performed.

Treatment

- Schistosomiasis is uncommon in the United States, and the inexperienced physician is advised to consult an infectious disease or tropical medicine specialist for diagnosis and treatment.
- Physicians can consult with CDC to obtain information and access diagnostic services.
- Praziquantel is used for the treatment of schistosomiasis. Praziquantel is most effective against adult forms of the parasite and requires an immune response to the adult worm to be fully effective.
- Additional information can be found on the Division of Parasitic Diseases' website at www.cdc.gov/ncidod/dpd/parasites/schistosomiasis/default.htm.

Preventive Measures for Travelers

- No vaccine is available.
- No drugs for preventing infection are available.
- Preventive measures are primarily avoiding wading, swimming, or other contact with freshwater in disease-endemic countries. Untreated piped water coming directly from freshwater sources may contain cercariae, but filtering with fine-mesh filters, heating bathing water to 50° C (122° F) for 5 minutes, or allowing water to stand for at least 24 hours before exposure can eliminate risk of infection.
- Swimming in adequately chlorinated swimming pools is virtually always safe, even in disease-endemic countries.
- Vigorous towel-drying after accidental exposure to water has been suggested as a way to remove cercariae before they can penetrate, but this may only prevent some infections and should not be recommended as a preventive measure.
- Topical applications of the insect repellent DEET can block penetrating cercariae, but the effect depends on the repellent formulation and may be short lived and cannot reliably prevent infection.

References

1. Ross AG, Bartley PB, Sleigh AC, et al. Schistosomiasis. N Engl J Med. 2002;346(16):1212–20.
2. Ross A, Vickers D, Olds G, et al. Katayama syndrome. Lancet. 2007;7:218–24.
3. Bierman W, Wetsteyn JC, van Gool T. Presentation and diagnosis of imported schistosomiasis: relevance of eosinophilia, microscopy for ova, and serology. J Travel Med. 2005;12:9–13.
4. Fenwick A, Keiser J, Utzinger J. Epidemiology, burden and control of schistosomiasis with particular consideration to past and current treatment trends. Drugs Fut. 2006;31(5):413–25.
5. WHO Expert Committee. Prevention and control of schistosomiasis and soil-transmitted helminthiasis. World Health Organ Tech Rep Ser. 2002;912:1–57.
6. Jordan P, Webb G, Sturrock RF, editors. Human schistosomiasis. Wallingford (CT): CAB International; 1993.
7. Corachan M. Schistosomiasis and international travel. Clin Infect Dis. 2002;35:446–50.
8. King C, Sturrock R, Kariuki H, et al. Transmission control for schistosomiasis—why it matters now. Trends Parasitol. 2006; 22(12): 575–82.
9. Meltzer E, Artom G, Marva E, et al. Schistosomiasis among travelers: new aspects of an old disease. Emerg Infect Dis. 2006;12:1696–700.

SEXUALLY TRANSMITTED DISEASES (STDs)

Kimberly Workowski

Infectious Agent

Sexually transmitted diseases (STDs) are the infections and resulting clinical syndromes caused by more than 25 infectious organisms.

Mode of Transmission

Sexual activity is the predominant mode of transmission, through genital, anal, or oral mucosal contact.

Occurrence

- STDs are among the most common infections. Annually an estimated 340 million infections occur worldwide, and 18.9 million infections in the United States.
- Travelers who have sexual interactions with core groups of efficient transmitters (commercial sex workers) in endemic areas may have high rates of acquisition of some STDs, such as gonorrhea.
- Some STDs are more prevalent in developing countries (chancroid, lymphogranuloma venereum, granuloma inguinale) and may be more likely to be imported into developed countries by travelers returning from such locales.

Risk for Travelers

- International travelers are at risk of contracting STDs, including HIV, if they have sexual contact with partners in locales with high STD prevalence.
- Increased sexual promiscuity and casual sexual relationships tend to occur during travel abroad to foreign countries and are frequently detected in long-term overseas travelers.
- Commercial sexual service in various destinations (Southeast Asia) attracts many foreign travelers; knowledge of the clinical presentation, frequency of infection, and antimicrobial resistance patterns (quinolone-resistant *Neisseria gonorrhoeae*) is important in the management of STDs that occur in travelers to specific destinations.
- Assessment of sexual risk for men who have sex with men (MSM) is important because of the recent increased rates of infectious syphilis, quinolone-resistant gonorrhea, and lymphogranuloma venereum in various geographic locations.

Clinical Presentation

- As many infections may be asymptomatic (chlamydia, gonorrhea), screening for such infections at anatomic sites of contact and serologic testing for syphilis should be encouraged among travelers who have had sexual exposure.
- Any traveler who might have been exposed to an STD and who develops vaginal, urethral, or rectal discharge, an unexplained rash or genital lesion, or genital or pelvic pain should be advised to cease sexual activity and promptly seek medical evaluation.

Diagnosis

- Genital ulcer evaluation should include a serologic test for syphilis, a culture or antigen test for genital herpes, and a culture for chancroid (if exposure occurred in areas where chancroid is prevalent, such as Africa, Asia, and Latin America). Lymphadenopathy can accompany genital ulceration with these infections, as well as with lymphogranuloma venereum (LGV) and donovanosis. LGV should be suspected in a traveler with tender unilateral inguinal or femoral lymphadenopathy or protocolitis. Genital and lymph node specimens should be tested for *Chlamydia trachomatis* by culture, direct immunofluorescence, or nucleic acid testing. Donovanosis is endemic in some areas, including India, Papua New Guinea, central Australia, and southern Africa, and is diagnosed with a crush preparation from the lesion.

- Chlamydia and gonorrhea testing at the anatomic site of exposure with nucleic acid amplification testing or culture is available for the detection of *C. trachomatis* and *N. gonorrhoeae*. The use of culture and antibiotic susceptibility testing is especially important when gonorrhea is suspected, due to geographic differences in antimicrobial susceptibility.
- Various diagnostic methods are available to identify the etiology of an abnormal vaginal discharge, including microscopic evaluation and pH of vaginal secretions, DNA probe-based testing, and culture.
- All persons who seek evaluation and treatment for STDs should be screened for HIV infection.

Treatment

- Etiologic treatment directed toward the specific pathogen is the historical norm for most STDs in industrialized countries.
- Syndromic management, of interest in developing countries, requires broad clinical manifestations with risk assessment, followed by treatment of the main causes of the syndrome without identification of a specific pathogen.
- Evaluation and management of STDs should be based on standard guidelines (CDC, World Health Organization) with consideration of the high frequency of antimicrobial resistance in different geographic areas.
- Early detection and treatment are important. STDs can often result in serious and long-term complications, including pelvic inflammatory disease, infertility, stillbirths and neonatal infections, genital cancers, and an increased risk for HIV acquisition and transmission.

Preventive Measures for Travelers

- The prevention and control of STDs are based on education and counseling. Specific messages to avoid acquiring or transmitting STDs should be part of the health advice given to travelers.
- Abstinence or mutual monogamy is the most reliable way to avoid acquisition and transmission of STDs.
- For persons whose sexual behaviors place them at risk for other STDs, correct and consistent use of the male latex condom can reduce the risk of HIV infection and some STDs, including chlamydia, gonorrhea, and trichomoniasis, and might protect women from developing pelvic inflammatory disease. Condoms might afford protection against transmission of herpes simplex virus-2, although data are more limited.
- Only water-based lubricants (e.g., K-Y Jelly or glycerine) should be used with latex condoms, because oil-based lubricants (e.g., petroleum jelly, shortening, mineral oil, or massage oils) can weaken latex condoms.
- Vaginal spermacides containing nonoxynol-9 are not recommended for STD/HIV prevention.
- Prompt evaluation of sexual partners is necessary to prevent reinfection and disrupt transmission of many STDs.

- Pre-exposure vaccination against hepatitis A and B is recommended, as these infections can be sexually transmissible. Hepatitis A vaccine is recommended for all unvaccinated sexually active MSM or those using injection drugs. Hepatitis B vaccine is recommended for all unvaccinated persons with a history of STD, multiple sexual partners, a sexual partner with injection drug use, or for MSM.
- A quadravalent vaccine against human papillomavirus (HPV) is available for females 9–26 years of age.

References

1. Abdullah AS, Ebrahim SH, Fielding R, et al. Sexually transmitted infections in travelers: implications for prevention and control. Clin Infect Dis. 2004;39:533–8.
2. CDC. Sexually transmitted diseases treatment guidelines, 2006. MMWR Recomm Rep. 2006;55:(RR-11):1–94.
3. Ward BJ, Plourde P. Travel and sexually transmitted infections. J Travel Med. 2006;13(5):300–17.
4. Workowski KA, Berman SM, Douglas JM Jr. Emerging antimicrobial resistance in *Neisseria gonorrhoeae*: urgent need to strengthen prevention strategies. Ann Intern Med. 2008;148:606–13.
5. Weinstock H, Berman S, Cates W. Sexually transmitted diseases among American youth: incidence and prevalence estimates, 2000. Perspect Sex Reprod Health. 2004;36:6–10.
6. Memish ZA, Osoba AO. Sexually transmitted diseases and travel. Int J Antimicrob Agents. 2003;21:131–4.
7. Matteelli A, Carosi G. Sexually transmitted
diseases in travelers. Clin Infect Dis. 2001;32:1063–7.
8. Ward H, Martin I, Macdonald N, et al. Lymphogranuloma venereum in the United Kingdom. Clin Infect Dis. 2007;44:26–32.
9. Peterman TA, Heffelfinger JD, Swint EB, et al. The changing epidemiology of syphilis. Sex Transm Dis. 2005;32(10 Suppl):S4–10.
10. Wald A, Langenberg AG, Krantz E, et al. The relationship between condom use and herpes simplex virus acquisition. Ann Intern Med. 2005;143:707–13.
11. Holmes KK, Levine R, Weaver M. Effectiveness of condoms in preventing sexually transmitted infections. Bull World Health Organ. 2004;82:454–61.
12. Schmid G, Steen R, N'Dowa F. Control of bacterial sexually transmitted diseases in the developing world is possible. Clin Infect Dis. 2005;41:1313–5.
13. Tietz A, Davies SC, Moran JS. Guide to sexually transmitted disease resources on the Internet. Clin Infect Dis. 2004;38:1304–10.

Perspectives: **Sexual Tourism**

Alan J. Magill

SEXUAL TOURISM AND THE EXPLOITATION OF WOMEN AND CHILDREN

The term "sexual tourism" has been defined as travel specifically planned and arranged to facilitate the procurement of sex by travelers, who can be referred to in this context as "sex tourists." Sexual tourism may involve travel specifically arranged to gain access to full-time commercial sex workers or underage individuals in destination countries. Sex tourism is a very lucrative industry that spans the globe. In 1998, the International Labour Organization reported that 2%–14% of the gross domestic product of Indonesia, Malaysia, the Philippines, and Thailand derived from sex tourism. Asian countries, including Thailand, India, and the Philippines, have long been prime destinations for child-sex tourists, but in recent years, Mexico and Central America have been increasingly popular destinations as well.

THE TRAVEL MEDICINE PROVIDER AND SEX TOURISM

The pre-travel visit should ideally include counseling for prevention of STDs for all travelers and in particular for those who can be considered at higher likelihood of having casual sex while abroad.

What should a provider do if one has a suspicion the purpose of travel is to engage in child sex tourism? These individuals can be informed that this behavior is illegal, and in certain cases— and depending on confidentiality policies—one may also consider contacting the appropriate authorities (see below). Travel medicine providers need to be aware of this global phenomenon and promote actions individual travelers and travel providers can take to minimize its effects.

RESPONSE TO CHILD SEX TOURISM

Travel medicine practitioners may want to provide certain groups of travelers with the following information about what they can do if they suspect or are confronted with child sex tourism:

- Report to the authorities abroad and/or to the U.S. Department of Homeland Security's Immigration and Customs Enforcement if you suspect children are being commercially sexually exploited in tourist destinations. If you have information regarding a person who has sexually exploited a child or suspect someone of child sex tourism, e-mail the U.S. Immigration and Customs Enforcement (ICE), Operation Predator: operation.predator@DHS.gov or call the ICE hotline: 866-347-2423.

- Federal law prohibits adult U.S. residents/citizens from engaging in sexual acts with persons under age 18 outside the United States (18 USC 2423). Be aware that any U.S. citizen or permanent legal resident arrested in a foreign country for sexually abusing minors may be subject to return to the United States, and if convicted, can face up to 30 years in prison.

- Be aware of the efforts of nongovernmental organizations (NGOs) and other governments working to protect children from commercial sexual exploitation.

- If immediate assistance is needed, contact the regional security officer at the local American embassy or consulate, or foreign law enforcement officials.

REFERENCES

1. U.S. Department of Justice, Child Exploitation and Obscenity Section. Child sex tourism [Internet]. Washington D.C.: U.S. Department of Justice. [updated 2007 Nov 6; cited 2008 Nov 30]. Available from: http://www.usdoj.gov/criminal/ceos/sextour.html.

2. U.S. Department of State. Office to Monitor and Combat Trafficking in Persons [Internet]. Washington D.C.: U.S. Department of State. [cited 2008 Nov 20]. Available from: http://www.state.gov/g/tip/.

3. International Labour Organization, International Programme on the Elimination of Child Labour. Commercial Sexual Exploitation of Children [Internet]. Geneva: International Labour Organization. [cited 2008 Nov 20]. Available from: http://www.ilo.org/ipec/areas/CSEC/lang--en/index.htm.

4. Pan-American Health Organization, Women, Health and Development Program. Trafficking of Women and Children for Sexual Exploitation in the Americas [Internet]. 2001. [cited 2008 Nov 30]. Available from: http://www.paho.org/English/AD/GE/TraffickingPaper.pdf.

5. Sexual tourism: implications for travelers and the destination culture. Marrazzo JM. Infect Dis Clin North Am. 2005 Mar;19(1):103–20.

SHIGELLOSIS

Eric Mintz, Katharine Schilling

Infectious Agent

Shigellosis is an acute infection of the intestine caused by the bacteria *Shigella*.

- There are four species of *Shigella*: *Shigella dysenteriae*, *S. flexneri*, *S. boydii*, and *S. sonnei* (also referred to as Group A, B, C, and D, respectively). Several distinct serotypes are recognized within the first three species.
- Disease severity varies according to species and serotype.
- *Shigella dysenteriae* serotype 1 (Sd1) is the agent of epidemic dysentery, while *S. sonnei* is a common cause of mild diarrheal illness.

Mode of Transmission

Transmission occurs via the fecal–oral route, either indirectly through contaminated food, water, or fomites, or via direct person-to-person contact. As few as 10 to 100 organisms are sufficient to cause infection. Only humans and higher primates carry *Shigella*. Outbreaks have been traced to contaminated produce and other foods, contaminated drinking water, swimming in contaminated water, and men who have sex with men. In the United States, outbreaks of *S. sonnei* among young children in day care settings are common.

Occurrence

- Worldwide, *Shigella* is estimated to cause 80–165 million cases and 600,000 deaths annually.
- *Shigella* is endemic in temperate and tropical climates.
- *Shigella sonnei* are found most frequently in industrialized countries; *S. flexneri* more commonly affects the developing world.

Risk for Travelers

- *Shigella* sp. are an uncommon cause of travelers' diarrhea (TD) among travelers to Mexico but are common among travelers to Asia.
- The exact number of cases contracted internationally is unknown, but a recent FoodNet study suggests that approximately 26% of U.S. residents with sporadic shigellosis reported international travel in the week before symptom onset.
- Travelers at increased risk include those staying in areas with nonexistent or inadequate sanitation, drinking water, and hygiene facilities and in areas of overcrowding.

Clinical Presentation

- Disease onset occurs 12–96 hours after exposure.
- The symptoms of shigellosis range from mild to severe and typically last 4–7 days.
- The disease is characterized by watery, bloody or mucoid diarrhea, fever, stomach cramps, and nausea.
- On rare occasions, patients experience toxemia, vomiting, tenesmus, or postinfectious arthritis.

Diagnosis

- Shigellosis is confirmed through culture of a stool specimen or rectal swab.
- To effectively isolate *Shigella*, samples must be processed rapidly, because it cannot survive outside the body for long periods of time. *Shigella* isolates may then be speciated and serotyped and their antimicrobial susceptibilities determined.

Treatment

- In healthy adults, shigellosis will typically resolve within 4–7 days, even without treatment.
- In severe cases, fluid and electrolyte replenishment are essential in preventing dehydration, and appropriate antimicrobial treatment given early in the course will shorten the duration of symptoms and of carriage. Where possible, treatment should be guided by antimicrobial susceptibility testing.
- Cases of dysentery (bloody diarrhea) should be promptly treated with an appropriate antimicrobial, such as a fluoroquinolone.

Preventive Measures for Travelers

- Currently no vaccines are available for *Shigella*.
- The best defense against shigellosis is proper hygiene and strict adherence to standard food and water safety recommendations.

References

1. Kotloff KL, Winickoff JP, Ivanoff B, et al. Global burden of *Shigella* infections: implications for vaccine development and implementation of control strategies. Bull World Health Organ. 1999;77:651–66.

2. Ram PK, Crump JA, Gupta SK, et al. Part II. Analysis of data gaps pertaining to *Shigella* infections in low and medium human development index countries, 1984–2005. Epidemiol Infect. 2008;136:577–603.

3. American Public Health Association. Shigellosis. In: Heymann DL, editor. Control of communicable diseases manual. 18th ed. Washington, DC.: American Public Health Association; 2004. p. 487–91.

4. American Academy of Pediatrics. *Shigella* infections. In: Pickering L, Baker CJ, Long SS, McMillan JA, editors. Red book: 2006 report of the Committee on Infectious Diseases. 27th ed. Elk Grove Village (IL): American Academy of Pediatrics; 2006. p. 589–90.

5. Gaynor K, Park SY, Kanenaka R, et al. International foodborne outbreak of *Shigella sonnei* infection in airline passengers. Epidemiol Infect. 2008;4:1–7.

6. CDC. *Shigella* surveillance: annual summary, 2004. Atlanta: U.S. Department of Health and Human Services; 2005.

7. Dutta S, Dutta S, Dutta P, et al., *Shigella dysenteriae* serotype 1, Kolkata, India. Emerg Infect Dis. 2003;9:1471–4.

SMALLPOX AND OTHER ORTHOPOXVIRUS-ASSOCIATED INFECTIONS

Noelle A. Benzekri, Mary G. Reynolds

Infectious Agent

Smallpox is caused by variola virus, a member of the Poxvirus family, genus orthopoxvirus. Other members of this genus known to cause infection in humans are vaccinia virus, cowpox virus, and monkeypox virus.

As a result of the Smallpox Eradication Program (1967–1980), smallpox was declared eradicated by the WHO in 1980.

Mode of Transmission

- Infection with vaccinia virus is a rare adverse event that can occur among social contacts of persons recently vaccinated for smallpox.
- Other orthopoxvirus infections result largely from zoonotic exposures.
- Monkeypox virus infection can occur following contact with infected animals or from persons who are currently ill with monkeypox.
  - Multiple species of African rodents and primates are known to carry the virus, although the precise reservoir host for monkeypox virus remains unknown.
  - Human-to-human transmission occurs by way of large respiratory droplets and contact with lesions or infected materials.

Occurrence

- The last reported case of endemic smallpox occurred in Somalia in 1977, and the last reported case of laboratory-acquired smallpox occurred in the United Kingdom in 1978.

- Infections with wild vaccinia-like viruses have been reported among dairy workers in Brazil.
- Human infections with cowpox virus have been reported in Europe.
- Monkeypox virus is endemic in tropical forested regions of Africa, notably the Congo Basin.

Risk for Travelers

- Smallpox is not considered a risk for international travelers.
- International travelers may be at risk of infection with other orthopoxviruses.
  - Both infections with wild, vaccinia-like viruses and human infections with cowpox virus are rare, although those who are immunocompromised may have a higher risk.

Clinical Presentation

- Infections with wild vaccinia-like viruses and human infections with cowpox virus are most often self-limited, characterized by localized lesions.
- Monkeypox virus causes illness clinically identical to smallpox.
  - Results in fever, marked lymphadenopathy, and widespread vesiculopustular rash involving the palms and soles.
  - Monkeypox case–fatality rate is approximately 10%.

Diagnosis

Orthopoxvirus infection is confirmed by PCR or virus isolation.

Treatment

- Treatment is mainly supportive, to include prevention of secondary infections.
- To prevent human-to-human transmission, patients should be isolated and cared for by someone who has received the smallpox vaccine.

Preventive Measures for Travelers

- Smallpox vaccine is not recommended for international travelers.
  - Live vaccinia virus is the main component of the smallpox vaccine.
  - Because of the elimination of smallpox, routine smallpox vaccination ceased worldwide in 1980.
  - Smallpox vaccination is recommended only for laboratory workers who handle variola virus (the agent of smallpox) or viruses closely related to variola virus, and health-care and public health officials who would be designated first-responders in the event of an intentional release of variola virus. In addition, members of the U.S. military may be required to receive the vaccine.
- Travelers are advised to avoid contact with rodents and sick or dead animals.
- No vaccines for other orthopoxviruses are available for travelers.
- No drugs for preventing infection are available.

For more information about monkeypox and other orthopoxviruses, contact the CDC Poxvirus Inquiry Line: 404-639-4129.

References

1. Rotz LD, Dotson DA, Damon IK. Vaccinia (smallpox) vaccine: recommendations of the Advisory Committee on Immunization Practices (ACIP), 2001. MMWR Recomm Rep. 2001;50(RR-10):1–25.

2. Nagasse-Sugahara TK, Kisielius JJ, Ueda-Ito

M., et al. Human vaccinia-like virus outbreaks in São Paulo and Goiás States, Brazil: virus detection, isolation and identification. Rev Inst Med Trop São Paulo. 2004;46(6):315–22.

3. Vorou RM, Papavassiliou VG, Pierroutsakos IN. Cowpox virus infection: an emerging health threat. Curr Opin Infect Dis. 2008;21(2):153–6.

4. CDC. Human monkeypox—Kasai Oriental, Democratic Republic of Congo, February 1996—October 1997. MMWR Morb Mortal Wkly Rep. 1997;46:1168–71.

5. Learned LA, Reynolds MG, Wassa DW, et al. Extended interhuman transmission of

monkeypox in a hospital community in the Republic of Congo, 2003. Am J Trop Med Hyg. 2005;73:428–34.

6. Reynolds mg, Davidson WB, Curns AT, et al. Spectrum of infection and risk factors for human monkeypox, United States, 2003. Emerg Infect Dis. 2007;13:1332–9.

7. Damon IK, Roth CE, Chowdhary V. Discovery of monkeypox in Sudan. N Engl J Med. 2006;355(9):962–3.

8. Levine RS, Peterson AT, Yorita KL, et al. Ecological niche and geographic distribution of human monkeypox in Africa. PLoS ONE. 2007;2(1):e176.

STRONGYLOIDIASIS

LeAnne M. Fox

Infectious Agent

Strongyloidiasis is caused by an intestinal nematode, *Strongyloides stercoralis*.

Mode of Transmission

- Filariform larvae found in infected soil in the tropics and subtropics penetrate human skin.
- Person-to-person transmission is rare, but has been documented.

Occurrence

- *Strongyloides* is endemic in the tropics and subtropics and in limited foci in the southeastern United States, Europe, Australia, and Japan.
- Estimates of global prevalence vary between 3 million and 100 million.

Risk for Travelers

- Travelers who visit endemic areas and have contact with contaminated soil through bare skin are at risk for infection.
- Most infections seen in the United States occur in immigrants, refugees, and military veterans who have lived in endemic areas for long periods of time.
- Risk for short-term travelers appears to be very low, but can occur.

Clinical Presentation

- Most infections are asymptomatic.
- With acute infections, a localized, pruritic, erythematous papular rash can develop at the site of skin penetration followed by pulmonary symptoms (a Loëffler-like pneumonitis), diarrhea, abdominal pain, and eosinophilia. Migrating larvae in the skin can cause *larva currens*, a serpiginous urticarial rash.
- Immunocompromised individuals, especially those receiving systemic corticosteroids or patients with HTLV-1 infection, are at risk for hyperinfection or disseminated disease, characterized by abdominal pain, diffuse pulmonary infiltrates, and septicemia or meningitis from enteric gram-negative bacilli. Untreated disseminated strongyloidiasis has high mortality.
- Unexplained eosinophilia may be a presenting sign of strongyloidiasis.

Diagnosis

- Diagnosis is made by finding rhabditiform larvae on microscopic examination of the stool, either directly or by culture on agar plates. Repeated stool examinations or examination of duodenal contents may be necessary, given the low sensitivity of a single stool examination.
- Serologic testing using an immunoassay is useful and is available through the Division of Parasitic Diseases, CDC.
- Hyperinfection and disseminated strongyloidiasis are readily diagnosed by examining stool, sputum, cerebrospinal fluid, and other body fluids and tissues, which typically contain high numbers of larvae.

Treatment

- Ivermectin (200 µg/kg orally for 2 days) is the treatment of choice for both chronic infection and disseminated disease with hyperinfection.
- Albendazole is an alternative agent, although associated with slightly lower cure rates.
- Prolonged or repeated treatment may be necessary in patients with hyperinfection and disseminated strongyloidiasis, and relapse can occur.

Preventive Measures for Travelers

- No vaccine is available.
- No drugs for preventing infection are available.
- Protective measures include proper sewage disposal and wearing shoes to reduce the risk of infection through bare skin.

References

1. Siddiqui AA, Berk SL. Diagnosis of *Strongyloides stercoralis* infection. Clin Infect Dis. 2001;33:1040–7.
2. Drugs for parasitic infections. Med Lett Drugs Ther. 2007;5(Suppl):e1–15.
3. Grove DI. Human strongyloidiasis. Adv Parasitol. 1996;38:251-309.
4. Keiser PB, Nutman TB. *Strongyloides stercoralis* in the immunocompromised population. Clin Microbiol Rev. 2004;17:208–17.
5. Cappello M, Hotez PJ. Disseminated strongyloidiasis. Semin Neurol. 1993;13:169–74.
6. Adedayo O, Grell G, Bellot P. Hyperinfective strongloidiasis in the medical ward: review of 27 cases in 5 years. South Med J. 2002;95:711–6.
7. Zaha O, Hirata T, Kinjo F, Saito A. Strongyloidiasis—progress in diagnosis and treatment. Intern Med. 2000;39:695–700.
8. Gyorkos TW, Genta RM, Viens P, et al. Seroepidemiology of *Strongyloides* infection in the Southeast Asian refugee population in Canada. Am J Epidemiol. 1990;132:257–264.
9. Genta RM, Weesner R, Douce RW, et al. Strongyloidiasis in US veterans of the Vietnam and other wars. JAMA. 1987;258:49–52.
10. Arthur RP, Shelley WB. Larva currens; a distinctive variant of cutaneous larva migrans due to *Strongyloides stercoralis*. AMA Arch Derm. 1958;78:186–190.

TAENIASIS

Jeffrey L. Jones

Infectious Agent

- Intestinal infection with adult stage of tapeworms *Taenia solium* (pork tapeworm) and *T. saginata* (beef tapeworm).
- Cysticercosis is a tissue infection with the larval stage of the pork tapeworm (see the Cysticercosis section earlier in this chapter).

Mode of Transmission

Taenia solium

- Humans acquire the organism when they eat raw or undercooked pork contaminated with *T. solium*; the adult worm then develops in the intestine.
- Eggs passed by humans in the stool are infectious to pigs; the larval stage lives in the flesh of pigs (pig cysticercosis). Eggs passed by humans in the feces are also infectious to humans and can be transferred by the fecal–oral route.
- When humans ingest *T. solium* eggs, the larvae penetrate the intestinal wall and spread to the tissues via the blood and lymphatics (human cysticercosis). Eggs are infectious when shed.

Taenia saginata

- Eggs passed in the stool of an infected person are infectious only to cattle; the larval stage lives in the flesh of cattle (cysticercosis bovis) and infects humans when they eat raw or undercooked beef contaminated with the organism.
- *T. asiatica* is a third species, more similar to *T. saginata*.

Occurrence

- Worldwide; more common where pigs and cattle have access to human feces.
- Highest prevalence rates occur in Latin America, Africa, and south and southeastern Asia.
- The disease has been reported, but at lower rates, from Eastern Europe, Spain, and Portugal.
- Immigrants from these areas may have taeniasis or cysticercosis.
- Transmission of *T. solium* is rare in the United States, Canada, Western Europe and many areas of Asia and the Pacific.

Risk for Travelers

A higher risk for infection exists in developing countries where inadequate sanitation leads to pork and beef contamination with larvae, as well as food and water contamination with *Taenia* eggs.

Clinical Presentation

- Taeniasis (intestinal tape worm) may be asymptomatic or associated with abdominal discomfort, weight loss, anorexia, insomnia, weakness, perianal pruritis, and nervousness. Tapeworms can live in the intestine 30 years or longer. Eosinophilia is often present, but the duration and magnitude is not well described.
- Incubation period (time for eggs to appear in stool): *T. solium* 8–10 weeks; *T. saginata* 10–14 weeks.

Diagnosis

- Adult tapeworm infection is identified by eggs, proglottids (segments), or tapeworm antigens in the feces or on anal swabs.
- Differentiation of *T. solium* from *T. saginata* is based on morphology of the scolex and gravid proglottids.

Treatment

- Praziquantel for intestinal infections with *T. solium* or *T. saginata*.
- Niclosimide is an alternative but not as widely available.

Preventive Measures for Travelers

- Cook meat to safe temperatures (at least 150° F [65° C] throughout).
- Peel or wash fruits and vegetables thoroughly in clean water before eating.
- Wash hands after soil contact.
- Freezing (23° F, −5°C) meat for 4 or more days will kill cysticerci.
- Identify and treat persons who become infected with tapeworms.
- Avoid ingestion of untreated water.

References

1. CDC. Taeniasis [Internet]. In: CDC. DPDx: laboratory identification of parasites of public health concern. [cited 2008 Nov 28]. Available from: http://www.dpd.cdc.gov/dpdx/HTML/Taeniasis.htm
2. CDC. Cysticercosis [Internet]. In: CDC. DPDx: laboratory identification of parasites of public health concern. [cited 2008 Nov 28]. Available from: http://www.dpd.cdc.gov/dpdx/HTML/Cysticercosis.htm
3. Drugs for parasitic infections. Med Lett Drugs Ther. 2007;5(Suppl):e1–15.
4. Wittner M, Tanowitz HB. *Taenia* and other tapeworms. In: Guerrant RL, Walker DH, Weller PF, editors. Tropical infectious diseases: principles, pathogens, and practice. 2nd ed. Philadelphia: Churchill Livingstone; 2006. p. 1327–30

TICK-BORNE ENCEPHALITIS (TBE)

Marc Fischer, Anne Griggs, J. Erin Staples

Infectious Agent

Tick-borne encephalitis virus (TBEV) is a single-stranded RNA virus that belongs to the genus *Flavivirus* and is closely related to Powassan virus. TBEV has three subtypes: European, Siberian, and Far Eastern.

Mode of Transmission

- Transmitted to humans through the bite of an infected tick of the *Ixodes* species, primarily *I. ricinus* (European subtype) or *I. persulcatus* (Siberian and Far Eastern subtypes). The virus is maintained in discrete areas of deciduous forest where both the tick vectors and animal hosts (mainly rodents) are found.
- Can also be acquired by ingesting unpasteurized dairy products from infected goats, sheep, or cows. TBEV transmission has also been reported through a laboratory exposure and the slaughtering of a viremic goat.
- Direct person-to-person spread of TBEV does not occur except rarely through blood transfusion or breastfeeding.

Occurrence

- TBE is endemic in temperate regions of Europe and Asia (from eastern France to northern Japan and from northern Russia to Albania) and up to about 1,400 m in altitude.
- The highest incidences are reported in Austria, Czech Republic, Estonia, Germany, Hungary, Latvia, Lithuania, Poland, Russia, Slovenia, Sweden, and Switzerland.
- European countries with no reported cases are Belgium, Ireland, Luxembourg, the Netherlands, Portugal, Spain, and the United Kingdom.
- Most cases occur during April–November, with peaks in early and late summer when ticks are active.

- The incidence and severity of disease are highest in persons >50 years of age.
- Over the last 30 years, the geographic range of TBEV and the number of reported TBE cases have increased significantly. These trends are likely due to a complex combination of changes in the ecology and climate, increased human activity in affected areas, and increased recognition.

Risk for Travelers

- The overall risk of acquiring TBE for an unvaccinated visitor to an endemic area during the TBEV transmission season has been estimated at 1 case per 10,000 person-months of exposure.
- Most TBEV infections result from tick bites acquired in forested areas through activities such as camping, hiking, fishing, bicycling; collecting mushrooms, berries, or flowers; and outdoor occupations such as forestry or military training. The risk is negligible for persons who remain in urban or unforested areas and who do not consume unpasteurized dairy products.
- Vector tick density and infection rates in TBEV-endemic foci are highly variable. For example, TBEV infection rates in *I. ricinus* in central Europe vary from less than 0.1% to approximately 5%, depending on geographic location and time of year, while rates of up to 40% have been reported in *I. persulcatus* in Siberia.
- The number of TBE cases reported from a country depends on the ecology and geographic distribution of TBEV, the intensity of diagnosis and surveillance, and the vaccine coverage in the population. Therefore, the number of human TBE cases reported from an area may not be a reliable predictor of a traveler's risk for infection.

Clinical Presentation

- Approximately two-thirds of infections are asymptomatic.
- The median incubation period for TBE is 8 days (range 4–28 days). The incubation period for milk-borne exposure is usually shorter (3–4 days).
- Acute neuroinvasive disease is the most commonly recognized clinical manifestation of TBEV infection. However, TBE disease often presents with milder forms of the disease or a biphasic course.
  - First phase: nonspecific febrile illness with headache, myalgia, and fatigue. Usually lasts for several days and may be followed by an afebrile and relatively asymptomatic period. Up to two-thirds of patients may recover without any further illness.
  - Second phase: central nervous system involvement resulting in aseptic meningitis, encephalitis, or myelitis. Cranial nerve involvement, bulbar syndrome, and acute flaccid paralysis of the upper extremities have also been described.
- Among patients who develop central nervous system involvement, approximately 10% require intensive care and 5% need mechanical ventilation.
- Clinical course and long-term outcome varies by subtype of TBEV.
  - The European subtype is associated with milder disease, a case–fatality ratio of <2%, and neurologic sequelae in up to 30% of patients.
  - The Far Eastern subtype is often associated with a more severe disease course, including a case–fatality ratio of 20%–40% and higher rates of severe neurologic sequelae.
  - The Siberian subtype is more frequently associated with chronic or progressive disease and has a case–fatality ratio of 2%–3%.

Diagnosis

- TBE should be suspected in travelers who develop a nonspecific febrile illness that progresses to neuroinvasive disease within 4 weeks of arriving from an endemic area. Approximately 30% of TBE patients do not recall a tick bite.

- Serology is typically used for laboratory diagnosis. IgM-capture ELISA performed on serum or cerebrospinal fluid is virtually always positive during the neuroinvasive phase of the illness.
- Vaccination history, date of onset of symptoms, and information regarding other flaviviruses known to circulate in the geographic area that may cross-react in serologic assays need to be considered when interpreting results.
- During the first phase of the illness, TBEV or TBEV RNA can sometimes be detected in serum samples by virus isolation or nucleic acid amplification tests (NAAT). However, by the time neurologic symptoms are recognized, the virus or viral RNA is usually undetectable. Therefore, virus isolation and NAAT should not be used for ruling out a diagnosis of TBE.
- Health-care providers should contact their state or local health department or CDC's Division of Vector Borne Infectious Diseases (970-221-6400) for assistance with diagnostic testing.

Treatment

There is no specific antiviral treatment for TBE; therapy consists of supportive care and management of complications.

Preventive Measures for Travelers

Personal Protection Measures

- Avoid consumption of unpasteurized dairy products.
- Use all measures to avoid tick bites (see the Protection Against Mosquitoes, Ticks, and Other Insects and Arthropods section in Chapter 2).

TBE Vaccine

- No TBE vaccines are licensed or available in the United States.
- Two safe, effective inactivated TBE vaccines are available in Europe, in adult and pediatric formulations: FSME-IMMUN (Baxter, Austria) and Encepur (Novartis, Germany). The adult formulation of FSME-IMMUN is also licensed in Canada. Two other TBE vaccines are produced in Russia, but little information has been published about their safety and efficacy.
- Immunogenicity studies suggest that the European vaccines, produced using the TBEV European subtype, should also provide cross-protection against the Far Eastern subtype.

Table 5-2. Tick-borne encephalitis (TBE) vaccination schedules[1,2]

Vaccination	Age	Vaccination schedules		
		Conventional	Accelerated	
			FSME-IMMUN[3]	Encepur[4]
Primary series (3 doses)	≥1 year	0, 1–3 months, 9–12 months	0, 14 days, 5–12 months	0, 7, 21 days
1st booster	≥1 year	3 years	3 years	12–18 months
Subsequent boosters	<50 years	5 years	5 years	5 years
	≥50 years	3 years	3 years	3 years

1 Modified from Rendi-Wagner P. Advances in vaccination against tick-borne encephalitis. Expert Rev Vaccines. 2008;7:589-96.
2 No TBE vaccines are licensed or available in the United States.
3 Different formulation and dose for children 1–15 years of age.
4 Different formulation and dose for children 1–11 years of age.

- For both FSME-IMMUN and Encepur, the recommended primary vaccination series consists of three doses (the second given 1–3 months after the first, and the third given 9–12 months after the second (Table 5-2). Although no formal efficacy trials of these vaccines have been conducted, indirect evidence suggests that their efficacy is above 95%.

- Regardless of age, the first booster dose should be given 3 years following the primary series. Recommended intervals for subsequent booster doses vary by age and should be given every 5 years for persons <50 years of age and every 3 years for those ≥50 years of age.

- Because the primary vaccination series requires at least 9 months for completion, most travelers to TBE-endemic areas will find tick-bite prevention to be more practical than vaccination. However, an accelerated vaccination schedule has been evaluated for both European vaccines and shown to result in seroconversion rates similar to those observed with the standard vaccination schedule. For Encepur, the accelerated schedule is a three-dose primary series on days 0, 7, 21, with the first booster at 12–18 months. For FSME-IMMUN, the accelerated schedule is a three-dose primary series on days 0 and 14 and at 5–12 months; the first booster dose is administered at 3 years, according to the conventional schedule.

- Travelers anticipating high-risk exposures, such as working or camping in forested areas or farmland, adventure travel, or living in TBE-endemic countries for an extended period of time, may wish to be vaccinated in Canada or Europe.

References

1. Lindquist L, Vapalahti O. Tick-borne encephalitis. Lancet. 2008;371:1861–71.

2. Süss J. Epidemiology and ecology of TBE relevant to the production of effective vaccines. Vaccine. 2003;21(Suppl 1):S19–35.

3. Barrett PN, Dorner F, Ehrlich H, Plotkin SA. Tick-borne encephalitis virus vaccine. In: Plotkin SA, Orenstein WA, editors. Vaccines. 4th ed. Philadelphia: WB Saunders Company; 2004. p. 1039–55.

4. Süss J. Tick-borne encephalitis in Europe and beyond—the epidemiological situation as of 2007. Euro Surveill. 2008;13(26). pii: 18916.

5. International Scientific Working Group on Tick-Borne Encephalitis (ISW TBE). Tick-borne encephalitis in the golden agers: A conference report of the International Scientific Working Group on Tick-Borne Encephalitis (ISW TBE). Vaccine. 2006;24:1236–7.

6. Rendi-Wagner P. Risk and prevention of tick-borne encephalitis in travelers. J Travel Med. 2004;11:307–12.

7. Dumpis U, Crook D, Oksi J. Tick-borne encephalitis. Clin Infect Dis. 1999;28:882–90.

8. Haglund M, Günther G. Tick-borne encephalitis—pathogenesis, clinical course and long-term follow-up. Vaccine. 2003;21(Suppl 1):S11–8.

9. Kaiser R. The clinical and epidemiological profile of tick-borne encephalitis in southern Germany 1994–98: a prospective study of 656 patients. Brain. 1999;122(Pt 11):2067–78.

10. Holzmann H. Diagnosis of tick-borne encephalitis. Vaccine. 2003;21(Suppl 1):S36–40.

11. Committee to Advise on Tropical Medicine and Travel (CATMAT). Statement on tick-borne encephalitis. An Advisory Committee Statement (ACS). Can Commun Dis Rep. 2006;32(ACS-3):1–18.

12. Zent O, Bröker M. Tick-borne encephalitis vaccines: past and present. Expert Rev Vaccines. 2005;4:747–55.

13. Rendi-Wagner P. Advances in vaccination against tick-borne encephalitis. Expert Rev Vaccines. 2008;7:589–96.

14. Leonova GN, Ternovoi VA, Pavlenko EV, et al. Evaluation of vaccine Encepur® Adult for induction of human neutralizing antibodies against recent Far Eastern subtype strains of tick-borne encephalitis virus. Vaccine. 2007;25:895–901.

15. Kunz C. TBE vaccination and the Austrian experience. Vaccine. 2003;21(Suppl 1):S50–5.

16. Loew-Baselli A, Poellabauer EM, Fritsch S, et al. Immunogenicity and safety of FSME-IMMUN® 0.5ml using a rapid immunization schedule. Int J Med Microbiol. 2006;S1:213–14.

17. Schöndorf I, Beran J, Cizkova D, et al. Tick-borne encephalitis (TBE) vaccination: applying the most suitable vaccination schedule. Vaccine. 2007;25:1470–5.

18. Schoendorf I, Ternak G. Oroszlàn G, et al. Tick-borne encephalitis (TBE) vaccination in children: advantage of the rapid immunization schedule (i.e., days 0, 7, 21). Hum Vacc. 2007;3:42–7.

TOXOPLASMOSIS

Jeffrey L. Jones

Infectious Agent

Toxoplasma gondii is an intracellular coccidian protozoan parasite of cats.

Mode of Transmission

Toxoplasmosis is transmitted by—

- Oocysts in cat feces, or soil or water contaminated with cat feces
- Undercooked meat
- Congenitally when a woman becomes newly infected during pregnancy
- Blood transfusion and organ transplantation

Occurrence

Human infection with *T. gondii* occurs worldwide. The prevalence in adults ranges from <10% to >90%; higher prevalence rates tend to occur at lower elevations and in latitudes closer to the equator.

Risk for Travelers

The risk for infection is higher in many developing and tropical countries, especially when there is ingestion of undercooked meat, extensive soil exposure, or drinking of untreated water.

Clinical Presentation

- The incubation period ranges from 5 to 23 days.
- Acute infection in children and adults with normal immunity is often asymptomatic. When illness occurs, it is usually mild with "flu-like" symptoms (e.g., tender lymph nodes, muscle aches, etc.) that last for several weeks.
- An infectious mononucleosis-like syndrome has been described in febrile returning travelers, characterized by prolonged fever, lymphadenopathy, elevated liver enzymes, and lymphocytosis. Protracted fever and asthenia are common.
- Among acutely infected persons, 0.5% to 2% of develop ocular disease, usually retinochoroiditis; symptoms include blurred vision, pain, photophobia, tearing, and loss of vision.
- In severely immunosuppressed persons, including those with HIV infection, severe and even fatal toxoplasmic encephalitis, pneumonitis, and other systemic illnesses can occur, most often from reactivation of a previous infection. Immunosuppressed persons with HIV infection are routinely prescribed prophylactic medication active against *T. gondii*.
- In 70% to 90% of cases, infants with congenital toxoplasmosis are asymptomatic or have mild symptoms not recognized at birth. However, learning disabilities, mental retardation, or visual impairment often occur later in life. Congenital infection can result in maculopapular rash, generalized lymphadenopathy, hepatomegaly, splenomegaly, jaundice, and thrombocytopenia. In addition, hydrocephalus, microcephaly, seizures, retinochoroiditis, and deafness can occur. Cerebral calcifications may be seen on radiography or ultrasonography of the head.

Diagnosis

- For acutely infected children and adults: serologic testing (*Toxoplasma* specific IgM and IgG).
- Ocular disease: characteristic retinal lesions, serum testing for *T. gondii* antibodies; ocular fluid can be tested for *T. gondii* antibodies.
- Immunosuppressed persons: serologic testing (usually but not always *Toxoplasma* IgG antibody positive), typical clinical course, and identification of one or more mass lesions by CT, MRI, or other radiographic testing. Biopsy may be needed to make a definitive diagnosis.
- Congenital infection: testing should be done at a *Toxoplasma* reference laboratory.
- To determine infection status and help to estimate the timing of infection in the mother: serologic testing (for example, IgM, IgG, avidity, and at some laboratories, differential agglutination [AC/HS test], IgA, and IgE). Some commercial IgM tests have high false-positive rates.
- Fetal infection: detecting parasite DNA in amniotic fluid or fetal blood or by isolating the organism by mouse or tissue inoculation. Congenital infection in infants is determined by serologic testing (IgM, IgA, IgG western blot pattern comparison with mother), and PCR of white blood cells, cerebrospinal fluid, or amniotic fluid at a reference laboratory. Isolation of *Toxoplasma* by mouse inoculation can be attempted from the placenta, umbilical cord, or blood from the infant. Persistently positive IgG titers beyond 12 months of age confirm congenital infection.

Treatment

Acute Infection

- Adult: Pyrimethamine, 25–100 mg/d orally for 3–4 weeks, plus sulfadiazine, 1–1.5 g orally four times a day for 3–4 weeks, plus leucovorin, 10–25 mg orally with each dose of pyrimethamine. Pyrimethamine should be taken with food to minimize adverse gastrointestinal effects. Sulfadiazine should be taken on an empty stomach with adequate water.
- Pediatric: Pyrimethamine, 2 mg/kg/day, orally for 3 days, then 1 mg/kg/day (to a maximum of 25 mg/day) for 4 weeks, plus sulfadiazine, 100–200 mg/kg/d orally for 3–4 weeks, plus leucovorin, 10–25 mg orally with each dose of pyrimethamine.

Patients with Specific Concerns

- Ocular disease should be treated in consultation with an ophthalmologist. Corticosteroids may be added to regimens of pyrimethamine, sulfadiazine, and folinic acid (or other combinations of drugs active against *T. gondii*) when retinochoroiditis threatens vision.
- Immunosuppressed persons with active toxoplasmosis should be treated in consultation with a physician experienced in treating immunosuppressed persons.
- Toxoplasmosis during pregnancy and congenital infection in the infant should be treated in consultation with fetal medicine and pediatric specialists.

Preventive Measures for Travelers

Travelers should be advised to—

- Cook meat to safe temperatures (at least 160° F [71° C] throughout).
- Peel or wash fruits and vegetables thoroughly before eating.
- Wash cutting boards, dishes, counters, utensils, and hands with hot soapy water after contact with raw meat or with unwashed fruits or vegetables.

- Freeze meat for several days before cooking to greatly reduce chance of infection.
- Wear gloves when gardening and during any contact with soil or sand, because it might be contaminated with cat feces that contain *T. gondii*. Wash hands thoroughly after gardening or contact with soil or sand.
- Avoid drinking untreated water. *T. gondii* is not killed by chlorine levels used for water treatment, so in developing countries water must be treated and filtered or boiled; alternatively, use safe bottled water.
- Change the litter box daily. *T. gondii* does not become infectious until 1–5 days after it is shed in a cat's feces.
- Pregnant or immunocompromised persons should—
  - Avoid changing cat litter if possible. If no one else can perform the task, wear disposable gloves and wash hands thoroughly with soap and water afterwards.
  - Keep cats indoors.
  - Do not adopt or handle stray cats, especially kittens. Do not get a new cat while you are pregnant.
- Feed cats only canned or dried commercial food or well-cooked table food, not raw or undercooked meats.
- Keep outdoor sandboxes covered.

References

1. CDC. Toxoplasmosis [Internet]. In: CDC. DPDx: laboratory identification of parasites of public health concern. [cited 2008 Nov 28]. Available from: http://www.cdc.gov/toxoplasmosis/.
2. Montoya JG, Liesenfeld O. Toxoplasmosis. Lancet. 2004;363:1965–76.
3. Benson CA, Kaplan JE, Masur H, et al. Treating Opportunistic Infections Among HIV-Infected Adults and Adolescents: Recommendations from CDC, the National Institutes of Health, and the HIV Medicine Association/Infectious Diseases Society of America [Internet]. Rockville (MD): AIDS*Info*; 2004. [cited 2008 Nov 28]. Available from: http://www.aidsinfo.nih.gov/Guidelines/GuidelineDetail.aspx?GuidelineID=14.
4. Bottieau E, Clerinx J, Van den Enden E, et al. Infectious mononucleosis-like syndromes in febrile travelers returning from the tropics. J Travel Med. 2006;13(4):191–7.

TRYPANOSOMIASIS, HUMAN AFRICAN (HAT, AFRICAN SLEEPING SICKNESS)

Anne Moore

Infectious Agent

Two subspecies of the protozoan parasite *Trypanosoma brucei* (*T. b. rhodesiense* and *T. b. gambiense*) cause infection.

Mode of Transmission

Infection occurs through vector-borne transmission by the bite of an infected tsetse fly (*Glossina* spp.). Transmission via bloodborne or congenital routes can occur but is rarely reported.

Occurrence

- HAT is transmitted only in rural sub-Saharan Africa. The two human-infective subspecies of *T. brucei* do not overlap in geographic distribution.
- *T. b. rhodesiense* is found in eastern and southeastern Africa. Over 95% of the cases of *T. b. rhodesiense* infection occur in Tanzania, Uganda, Malawi, and Zambia.

- *T. b. gambiense* is found predominately in central Africa and in limited areas of West Africa. Over 95% of the cases of *T. b. gambiense* infection are reported from the Democratic Republic of Congo, Angola, Sudan, Central African Republic, Republic of Congo, Chad, and northern Uganda.

Risk for Travelers

- Infection of international travelers occurs but is rare. On average, a single case per year is reported among U.S. travelers.
- Most infections in U.S. travelers are caused by *T. b. rhodesiense* and are acquired in East Africa game parks.
- Tsetse flies inhabit rural areas, living in the woodlands and thickets of the savannah and the dense vegetation along streams. Less than 1% of flies are infected in a typical endemic area.
- Tsetse flies bite during daylight hours. Most bites that occur on the African savannah are quite painful, and travelers often recall the bite.
- Travelers to urban areas are not at risk.

Clinical Presentation

- Presentation is variable and depends on the infecting subspecies. Infection with *T. b. rhodesiense* is more acute clinically and progresses more rapidly than *T. b. gambiense*.
- Symptoms and signs of *T. b. rhodesiense* infection generally appear within 1–3 weeks of the infective bite. These may include high fever, a chancre at the site of the infective bite, skin rash, headache, myalgia, thrombocytopenia, and less commonly, splenomegaly, renal failure, or cardiac dysfunction. Central nervous system involvement can occur within the first month of infection.
- Symptoms of *T. b. gambiense* infection are nonspecific, and patients may remain paucisymptomatic for many months after infection. Symptoms and signs may include fever, headache, malaise, myalgia, facial edema, pruritus, lymphadenopathy, and weight loss. Central nervous system involvement occurs after months of infection and is characterized by somnolence, severe headache, and a wide range of neurologic manifestations, including mood disorders, behavior change, focal deficits, and endocrine disorders.
- Untreated HAT infection is eventually fatal.

Diagnosis

- Microscopic identification of parasites in specimens of blood, chancre fluid or tissue, lymph node aspirate, or cerebrospinal fluid. Buffy coat preparations concentrate the parasite. Parasitemias are higher in *T. b. rhodesiense* than in *T. b. gambiense* infection.
- Serologic tests are not helpful for diagnosis of *T. b. rhodesiense*. CDC can provide information for arranging for serologic testing for *T. b. gambiense*, which is not available in the United States.
- Diagnostic assistance is available through CDC DPDx (www.dpd.cdc.gov/dpdx).

Treatment

- Travelers who sustain tsetse fly bites and become ill with high fever or other manifestations of African trypanosomiasis are advised to seek early medical attention. The infection can usually be cured by a course of antitrypanosomal therapy.
- HAT is rare in the United States, and the inexperienced physician is advised to consult with an infectious disease or tropical medicine specialist for diagnosis and treatment.

- Physicians can consult with CDC for assistance with diagnosis and clinical management (DPD Public Inquiries, 770-488-7775, ncidpbdpi@cdc.gov).
- Treatment drugs (suramin, melarsoprol, eflornithine) are provided by CDC under investigational protocols.

Preventive Measures for Travelers

- No vaccine or drug for prophylaxis is available.
- Preventive measures are aimed at reducing contact with tsetse flies. Areas of heavy infestation tend to be sporadically distributed and are usually well known to local residents. Avoidance of these areas is the best means of protection.
- Tsetse flies are attracted to moving vehicles and bright, dark colors. Permethrin-impregnated clothing and use of DEET repellent may reduce the number of fly bites. The flies can bite through lightweight clothing. Travelers are advised to wear clothing of wrist and ankle length made of medium-weight fabric in neutral colors that blend with the background environment.

References

1. Braakman HM, van de Molengraft FJ, Hubert WW, Boerman DH. Lethal African trypanosomiasis in a traveler: MRI and neuropathology. Neurology. 2006;66:1094–6.
2. Moore DA, Edwards M, Escombe R, et al. African trypanosomiasis in travelers returning to the United Kingdom. Emerg Infect Dis. 2002;8:74–6.
3. Moore AC, Ryan ET, Waldron MA. Case records of the Massachusetts General Hospital. Weekly clinicopathological exercises. Case 20-2002. A 37-year-old man with fever, hepatosplenomegaly, and a cutaneous foot lesion after a trip to Africa. N Engl J Med. 2002;346:2069–76.
4. Sholdt LL, Schreck CE, Mwangelwa MI, et al.Evaluations of permethrin-impregnated clothing and three topical repellent formulations of DEET against tsetse flies in Zambia. Med Vet Entomol. 1989;3(2):153–8.

TRYPANOSOMIASIS, AMERICAN (CHAGAS DISEASE)

Alicia I. Hidron, Carlos Franco-Paredes

Infectious Agent

American Trypanosomiasis is caused by the protozoan parasite, *Trypanosoma cruzi*.

Mode of Transmission

Infection occurs—

- Through vector-borne transmission in endemic counties via the feces of the triatomine insect (reduviid bug), which may be inadvertently inoculated into the skin, the mucosa of eye, nose, or mouth when the insect's bite is scratched and rubbed
- Through transfusion or organ transplantation
- From mother to infant
- By ingestion of contaminated food or drink
- Through occupational exposure in research workers

Occurrence

Approximately 7.6 million people are infected with Chagas disease, according to the most recent estimates. The disease is endemic in Mexico, Central and South America.

Rare cases of Chagas disease attributed to local vector-borne transmission have been reported in the United States.

Risk for Travelers

- No cases have been documented of Chagas disease acquired during travel; the risk of acquiring Chagas disease while traveling is assumed to be extremely low.
- Travelers could be at risk for Chagas disease if staying in poor-quality housing (for example, mud walls with cracks) in endemic areas.
- Chagas disease could be acquired through blood transfusion in areas with poor screening or through the ingestion of contaminated food or drink.

Clinical Presentation

The acute phase of Chagas disease lasts up to 90 days, followed by asymptomatic chronic infection, usually undetectable by parasitologic methods. Most infected individuals never develop symptoms but remain infected throughout their lives. Those who develop acute illness will do so at least one week following exposure. A chagoma may develop, which is an area of edema and erythema at the site of infection; the classic picture is Romaña's sign, which presents as edema of the lid and ocular tissues when the entry site was the conjunctiva. Approximately 20%–30% of infected patients will develop manifestations of chronic Chagas disease, usually involving the heart. Clinical signs include conduction system abnormalities, ventricular arrhythmias, and in late stage disease, congestive cardiomyopathy. Chronic gastrointestinal problems may ensue when Chagas causes megaesophagus or megacolon. Reactivation disease can occur in immunocompromised patients.

Diagnosis

Diagnosis requires consideration of both test results and patient exposure history. During the acute phase, parasites may be detectable in fresh preparations of buffy coat or stained peripheral blood specimens. After the acute phase, diagnosis relies on the use of at least two different serologic tests (most commonly, enzyme-linked immunosorbent assays and the immunofluorescent antibody test). Infected individuals should be evaluated for symptoms and signs of cardiac and gastrointestinal disease.

Treatment

- Consultation with an infectious disease or tropical medicine specialist for the diagnosis and treatment of Chagas disease should be advised.
- Antitrypanosomal drug treatment is always recommended for acute, early congenital, and reactivated *T. cruzi* infection and for chronic *T. cruzi* infection in children up to 18 years old. In adults, treatment is usually recommended, based on recent data suggesting that a course of antitrypanosomal treatment delays progression of cardiomyopathy and decreases mortality.
- In the United States, the only source of the antitrypanosomal drugs, benznidazole and nifurtimox, is through CDC. The drugs are not licensed in the United States and are provided only under investigational new drug protocols. Health-care providers should contact the Division of Parasitic Diseases Public Inquiries line (770-448-7775), the CDC Drug Service (404-639-3670), or, outside business hours, the CDC Emergency Operations Center (770-488-7100). CDC also provides guidance on diagnostic testing and clinical evaluation.

Preventive Measures for Travelers

- No vaccine is available.

- Preventive measures include insecticide spraying of sleeping quarters or infested houses.
- Travelers who cannot avoid camping, sleeping outdoors, or sleeping in poorly constructed houses in endemic areas should use insecticide-impregnated bed nets and tuck in the edges to provide a physical barrier to the vectors.
- Compliance with food and water precautions in endemic areas is also recommended to prevent the extremely rare occurrence of foodborne Chagas disease.
- Blood transfusion and organ transplantation should be avoided in endemic countries (see the Medical Tourism section in Chapter 2).

References

1. Magill AJ, Reed SG. American trypanosomiasis. In: Strickland GT, editor. Hunter's tropical edicine and emerging infectious diseases. 8th ed. Philadelphia: WB Saunders Company; 2000. p. 653–64.
2. Schmunis GA. Epidemiology of Chagas disease in non-endemic countries: the role of international migration. Mem Inst Oswaldo Cruz. 2007;102 Suppl 1:75–85.
3. CDC. Chagas disease after organ transplantation—United States, 2001. MMWR Morb Mortal Wkly Rep. 2002;51:210–2.
4. ProMED-mail. Trypanosomiasis, foodborne— Brazil (Santa Catarina) [Internet]. ProMED-mail. 2005; 24 Mar:20050324.0847. [cited 2008 May 27]. Available from: http://www.promedmail.org/pls/otn/f?p= 2400:1202:4024327548670824::NO::F2400_ P1202_CHECK_DISPLAY,F2400_P1202_ PUB_MAIL_ID:X,28451.
5. Dorn PL, Perniciaro L, Yabsley MJ, et al. Autochthonous transmission of *Trypanosoma cruzi*, Louisiana. Emerg Infect Dis. 2007;13(4):605–7.
6. Schmunis GA, Cruz JR. Safety of the blood supply in Latin America. Clin Microbiol Rev. 2005;18(1):12–29.
7. Dias JC. The indeterminate form of human chronic Chagas' disease: a clinical epidemiological review. Rev Soc Bras Med Trop. 1989;22(3):147–56.
8. Rassi A Jr., Rassi A, Little WC. Chagas' heart disease. Clin Cardiol. 2000;23(12):883–9.
9. Bern C, Montgomery SP, Herwaldt BL, et al. Evaluation and treatment of Chagas disease in the United States: a systematic review. JAMA. 2007;298(18):2171–81.
10. Marin-Neto JA, Cunha-Neto E, Maciel BC, Simões MV. Pathogenesis of chronic Chagas heart disease. Circulation. 2007;115:1109–23.

TUBERCULOSIS (TB)

Philip LoBue

Infectious Agent

Mycobacterium tuberculosis is a rod-shaped, nonmotile, acid-fast bacterium.

Mode of Transmission

- Tuberculosis (TB) transmission occurs when a contagious patient coughs, spreading the bacilli through the airborne route to a person sharing the same air space.
- Bovine TB (caused by the closely related *Mycobacterium bovis)* can be transmitted by ingestion of contaminated, unpasteurized dairy products from infected cattle.

Occurrence

- Globally there are nearly 9 million new TB cases and nearly 2 million TB-related deaths each year.
- TB occurs throughout the world, but the incidence varies greatly (see Map 5-8). In the United States, the annual incidence is less than 5 per 100,000 persons, but in some countries in sub-Saharan Africa and Asia the annual incidence is several hundred per 100,000.
- Drug-resistant TB is of increasing concern. Multidrug-resistant or MDR TB is TB resistant to at least two of the most effective drugs, isoniazid and rifampin (also

called first-line drugs). Extensively resistant or XDR TB is resistant to at least these two drugs and any fluoroquinolone and at least one of three injectable drugs (i.e., amikacin, kanamycin, or capreomycin). Although MDR TB occurs globally, it is less common than drug-susceptible TB. There are nearly 500,000 new cases of MDR TB each year, with some countries having proportions of MDR TB as high as 20% (see Map 5-9). MDR and XDR TB are of particular concern among HIV-infected or other immunocompromised persons.

Risk for Travelers

- To become infected, a person usually has to spend a relatively long time in a closed environment where the air was contaminated by a person with untreated TB who was coughing and who had numerous *M. tuberculosis* organisms (or tubercle bacilli) in secretions from the lungs.
- Documented sites of MDR and XDR TB include crowded hospitals, prisons, homeless shelters, and other settings where susceptible persons come in contact with infected persons with TB disease.
- Travelers who anticipate possible prolonged exposure to TB (e.g., those who could be expected to come in contact routinely with hospital, prison, or homeless shelter populations) or those who may have an extended stay over a period of years in an endemic country should be advised to have a two-step tuberculin skin test (TST) or an interferon-gamma release assay (IGRA), such as the QuantiFERON TB test (Gold or Gold In-Tube versions), before leaving the United States (see *Perspectives:* PPD Testing of Travelers in Chapter 2).
- Because persons with HIV infection or other immunocompromising conditions are more likely to have an impaired response to the test, travelers should be advised to inform their physicians about such conditions.
- Except for travelers with impaired immunity, travelers who have already been infected are unlikely to be reinfected.
- The risk of TB transmission on an airplane does not appear to be greater than in any other enclosed space. To prevent the possibility of exposure to TB on airplanes, CDC and WHO recommend that persons known to have infectious TB not travel by commercial airplanes or other commercial conveyances. WHO has issued guidelines for notifying passengers who might have been exposed to TB aboard airplanes. Passengers concerned about possible exposure to TB should be advised to see their primary health-care provider for evaluation.
- Risk for bovine TB (*M. bovis*) in travelers exists for those who consume unpasteurized dairy products in countries where *M. bovis* in cattle is common (Mexico is one of the more common places of infection for U.S. travelers).

Clinical Presentation

- Infection is manifested by development of a positive TST or IGRA, which usually occurs 8–10 weeks after exposure.
- Overall, only 5%–10% persons progress from infection to disease during their lifetime. In the remainder, the infection remains in a latent state (latent tuberculosis infection or LTBI). The risk of progression is much greater in immunosuppressed persons (e.g., 8%–10% per year in HIV-infected persons).
- LTBI is an asymptomatic condition, and persons with LTBI do not transmit TB.
- Progression to disease can occur weeks to decades after initial infection.
- TB disease can affect any organ, but most commonly occurs in the lungs, known as pulmonary TB (70%–80%).
- The most common types of extrapulmonary disease include lymphadenitis, pleuritis, bone and joint disease, meningitis, and genitourinary disease.
- Common TB symptoms include prolonged cough, fever, anorexia, weight loss, night sweats, and hemoptysis.

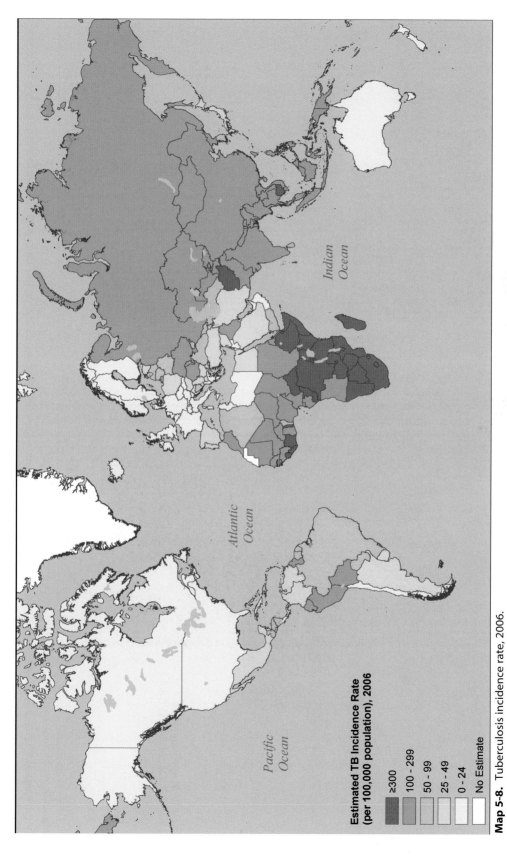

Map 5-8. Tuberculosis incidence rate, 2006.

(From WHO. Global tuberculosis control—surveillance, planning, financing: WHO Report 2008. Geneva: World Health Organization; 2008.)

**Estimated TB Incidence Rate
(per 100,000 population), 2006**

≥300

100 - 299

50 - 99

25 - 49

0 - 24

No Estimate

*Pacific
Ocean*

*Atlantic
Ocean*

*Indian
Ocean*

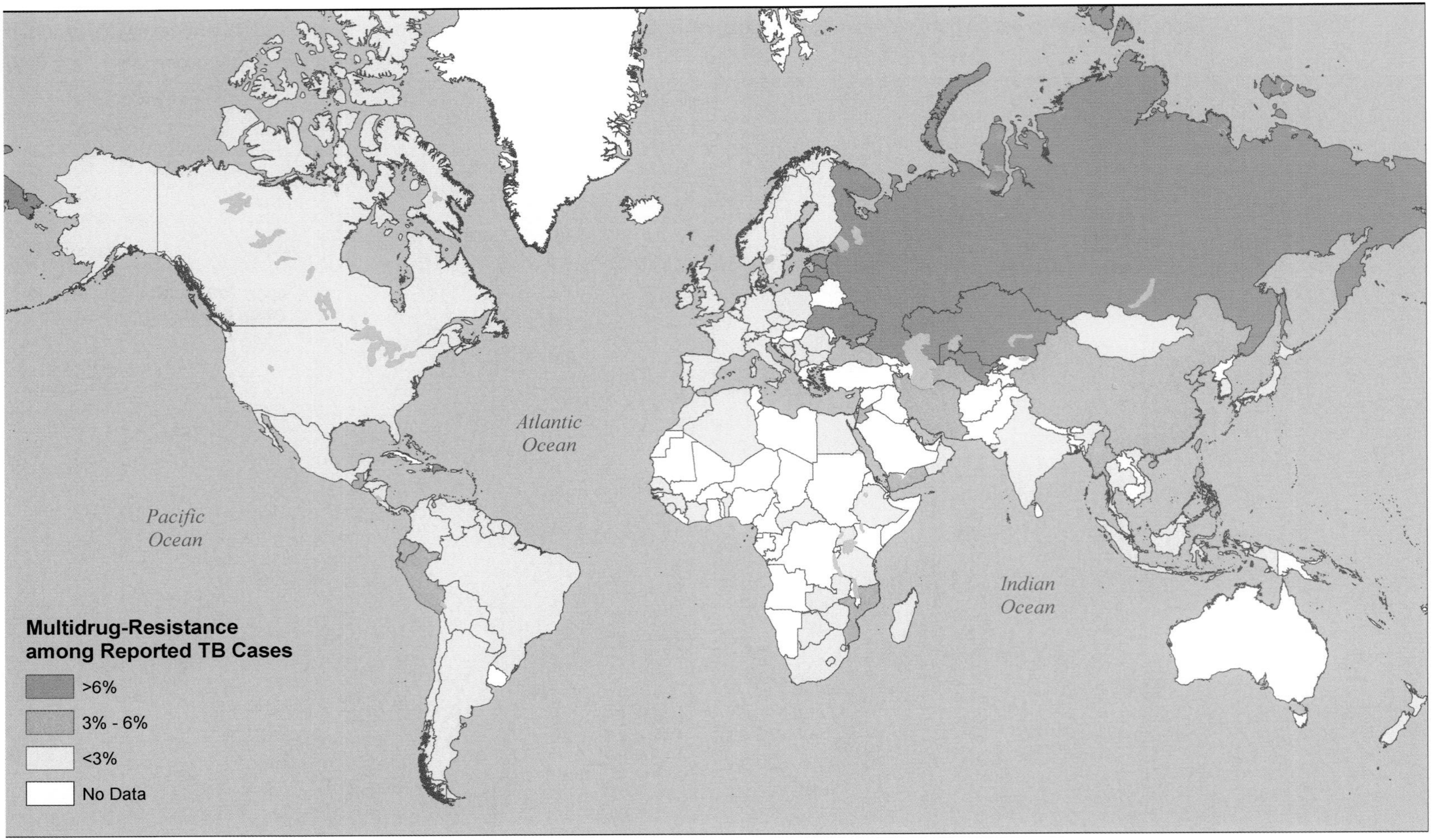

Map 5-9. Multidrug-resistance among reported tuberculosis cases, 2006.

(From WHO/IUATLD Global Project on Anti-Tuberculosis Drug Resistance Surveillance. Anti-tuberculosis drug resistance in the world: fourth global report. Geneva: World Health Organization; 2008.)

Multidrug-Resistance among Reported TB Cases

>6%

3% - 6%

<3%

No Data

Diagnosis

- Diagnosis of TB disease is confirmed by culturing *M. tuberculosis* from sputum or other respiratory specimens for pulmonary TB and from other affected body tissues or fluids for extrapulmonary TB. On average, it takes about 2 weeks to culture and identify *M. tuberculosis*, even with rapid culture techniques.
- A preliminary diagnosis of TB can be made when acid-fast bacilli (AFB) are seen on sputum smear or in other body tissues or fluids. However, microscopy cannot distinguish between *M. tuberculosis* and nontuberculous mycobacteria. This is particularly problematic in low TB incidence countries such as the United States.
- Nucleic acid amplification tests are more rapid than culture and very specific for *M. tuberculosis*. They are also more sensitive than the AFB smear, but less sensitive than culture.
- A diagnosis of TB disease can be made by using clinical criteria in the absence of microbiologic confirmation.
- LTBI is diagnosed by a positive TST or IGRA.

Treatment

- Persons with LTBI can be treated to prevent progression to TB disease. American Thoracic Society (ATS)/CDC guidelines for treatment of LTBI recommend 9 months of isoniazid as the preferred treatment and suggest that 4 months of rifampin is a reasonable alternative.
- Travelers who suspect that they have been exposed to TB should be advised to inform their physicians of the possible exposure and receive medical evaluation. CDC and ATS have published guidelines for targeted testing and treatment of LTBI. Recent data from the WHO suggest that drug resistance is relatively common in some parts of the world. Travelers who have TST or IGRA conversion associated with international travel should consult experts in infectious diseases or pulmonary medicine.
- TB disease is treated with a multiple drug regimen for 6–9 months (usually isoniazid, rifampin, ethambutol and pyrazinamide for 2 months, followed by isoniazid and rifampin for 4 months) if the TB is not MDR TB. MDR TB treatment is more difficult, requiring 4–6 drugs for 18–24 months; it should be managed by an expert in MDR TB. ATS/CDC/Infectious Diseases Society of America have published guidelines on TB treatment.

Preventive Measures for Travelers

- Travelers should be advised to avoid exposure to known TB patients in crowded environments (e.g., hospitals, prisons, or homeless shelters).
- Travelers who will be working in hospitals or health-care settings where TB patients are likely to be encountered should be advised to consult infection control or occupational health experts about procedures for obtaining personal respiratory protective devices (e.g., N-95 respirators), along with respirator selection and training.
- Based on WHO recommendations, the Bacille Calmette–Guérin (BCG) vaccine is used once at birth in most developing countries to reduce the severe consequences of TB in infants and children. However, BCG vaccine has variable efficacy in preventing the adult forms of TB and interferes with testing for LTBI with the TST. Therefore, BCG is not routinely recommended for use in the United States.
- Travelers should avoid eating or drinking any unpasteurized dairy products.

References

1. WHO. Global tuberculosis control— surveillance, planning, financing: WHO Report 2007. Geneva: World Health Organization; 2007.

2. American Thoracic Society; CDC. Targeted tuberculin testing and treatment of latent tuberculosis infection. Am J Respir Crit Care Med. 2000;161(4 Pt 2):S221–47.

3. American Thoracic Society, CDC, Infectious Diseases Society of America. Treatment of tuberculosis. MMWR Recomm Rep. 2003;52(RR-11):1–77.

4. WHO/IUATLD Global Project on Anti-Tuberculosis Drug Resistance Surveillance. Anti-tuberculosis drug resistance in the world: fourth global report. Geneva: World Health Organization; 2008.

5. CDC. Guidelines for using the QuantiFERON-TB Gold test for detecting *Mycobacterium tuberculosis* infection, United States. MMWR Recomm Rep. 2005;54(RR-15):49–55.

6. Jensen PA, Lambert LA, Iademarco MF, et al. Guidelines for preventing the transmission of *Mycobacterium tuberculosis* in health-care settings, 2005. MMWR Recomm Rep. 2005;54(RR-17):1–141.

7. WHO; International Civil Aviation;

Organization, the International Air Transport Association. Tuberculosis and air travel: guidelines for prevention and control. 2nd ed. Wook KJ, editor. Geneva: World Health Organization; 2006.

8. Villarino ME, Huebner RE, Lanner AH, Geiter LJ. The role of BCG vaccine in the prevention and control of tuberculosis in the United States: a joint statement by the Advisory Council for the Elimination of Tuberculosis and the Advisory Committee on Immunization Practices. MMWR Recomm Rep. 1996;45(RR-4):1–18.

9. National Tuberculosis Controllers Association, CDC. Guidelines for the investigation of contacts of persons with infectious tuberculosis. Recommendations from the National Tuberculosis Controllers Association and CDC. MMWR Recomm Rep. 2005;54(RR-15):1–47.

10. American Thoracic Society; CDC. Diagnostic standards and classification of tuberculosis in adults and children. Am J Respir Crit Care Med. 2000;161:1376–95.

VIRAL HEMORRHAGIC FEVERS

Eileen C. Farnon, Pierre E. Rollin

Infectious Agent

Viral hemorrhagic fevers (VHFs) are caused by several families of enveloped RNA viruses: filoviruses (Ebola and Marburg viruses), arenaviruses (including Lassa fever and Guanarito, Machupo, Junin, and Sabia viruses), bunyaviruses (Rift Valley fever [RVF], Crimean–Congo hemorrhagic fever [CCHF], and hantaviruses), and flaviviruses (dengue, yellow fever, Omsk hemorrhagic fever, and Kyasanur Forest disease [KFD] viruses) (see the Yellow Fever section in Chapter 2 and the Dengue Fever section in Chapter 5).

Mode of Transmission

- VHFs are spread person-to-person through direct contact with symptomatic patients, body fluids, cadavers, or inadequate infection control (filoviruses, arenaviruses, CCHF virus).
- Zoonotic spread includes—
  - Livestock via slaughter, or consumption of raw milk or meat from infected animals (CCHF, RVF viruses)
  - Bushmeat, likely via slaughter or consumption of infected animals (Ebola, Marburg viruses)
  - Rodent-borne (arenaviruses, Hantaan, Omsk, and KFD viruses) via inhalation of or contact with materials contaminated with rodent excreta
  - Other reservoir species, such as bats (Ebola, Marburg viruses)
- Vector-borne transmission also occurs via mosquitoes (RVF virus) or ticks (CCHF, Omsk, and KFD viruses).

Occurrence

The viruses that cause VHF are distributed over much of the globe. Each virus is associated with one or more nonhuman host or vector species, restricting the virus and the disease it causes to the areas inhabited by these species. These viruses are initially transmitted to humans when the habitats of infected reservoir hosts or vectors and humans overlap. Humans are incidental hosts for these enzootic diseases; however, person-to-person transmission of some viruses can result in large human outbreaks. Specific viruses are addressed below.

Ebola and Marburg: Filoviral Diseases

- Ebola and Marburg viruses cause hemorrhagic fever in humans and nonhuman primates.
- Five species of Ebola virus have been identified: Côte d'Ivoire, Sudan, Zaire, Bundibugyo, and Reston. Ebola-Reston has not been shown to cause human disease.
- Occurrence: tropical regions in Africa. Countries with confirmed human cases of Ebola hemorrhagic fever: Republic of Congo, Côte d'Ivoire, Democratic Republic of Congo, Gabon, Sudan, and Uganda; Marburg hemorrhagic fever: Uganda, Kenya, Democratic Republic of Congo, Angola, and possibly Zimbabwe.
- Reservoir host species: Growing evidence indicates that fruit bats are the natural reservoir for filoviruses. Outbreaks occur when an index case-patient becomes infected after exposure to the reservoir species or an infected nonhuman primate and transmits the virus to other people in the community.

Lassa Fever and Other Arenaviral Diseases

- Arenaviruses are transmitted from rodents to humans, except Tacaribe virus, which is found in bats. Most infections are mild, but some result in hemorrhagic fever with high fatality rates.
- Occurrence: Old and New World viruses, causing the following diseases:
  - Old World viruses: Lassa virus (Lassa fever) and lymphocytic choriomeningitis (LCM) virus (meningitis, encephalitis, and congenital fetal infection in normal hosts, hemorrhagic fever in organ transplant recipients). Lassa fever occurs in rural West Africa, with hyperendemic areas in Sierra Leone, Guinea, Liberia, and Nigeria.
  - New World viruses: Junin (Argentine hemorrhagic fever), Machupo (Bolivian hemorrhagic fever), Guanarito (Venezuelan hemorrhagic fever), Sabia (Brazilian hemorrhagic fever), and recently discovered viruses (Chapare, Flexal).
- Reservoir host species: New World rats and mice (family Muridae, subfamily Sigmodontinae); Old World rats and mice (family Muridae, subfamily Murinae). These rodent types are found worldwide, including Europe, Asia, Africa, and the Americas.
- Transmission: inhalation of aerosols from rodent urine, ingestion of rodent-contaminated food, or direct contact of broken skin with rodent excreta. Risk of Lassa infection is associated with peridomestic rodent exposure. Inappropriate food storage increases the risk for exposure. Nosocomial transmission of Lassa and Machupo viruses has occurred through droplet and contact. One anecdotal report of possible airborne transmission exists.

Rift Valley Fever and Other Bunyaviral Diseases

- RVF causes fever, hemorrhage, encephalitis, and retinitis in humans, but primarily affects livestock. RVF is endemic to sub-Saharan Africa. Sporadic outbreaks have occurred in humans in Egypt, Madagascar, and Mauritania. Large epidemics occurred in Kenya, Somalia, and Tanzania in 1997–1998 and 2006–2007 and in Saudi Arabia and Yemen in 2000. RVF virus is transmitted by mosquito, percutaneous inoculation, and slaughter or consumption of infected animals.
- CCHF is endemic where ticks of the genus *Hyalomma* are found in Africa and Eurasia, including South Africa, the Balkans, the Middle East, Russia, and western China, and is highly endemic in Afghanistan, Iran, Pakistan, and Turkey. CCHF virus is transmitted to humans by infected ticks or direct handling and preparation

of fresh carcasses of infected animals, usually domestic livestock. Nosocomial transmission often occurs.

- Hantaviruses cause hantavirus pulmonary syndrome (HPS) and hemorrhagic fever with renal syndrome (HFRS). The viruses that cause HPS are present in the New World; those that cause HFRS occur worldwide. Both HPS and HFRS are transmitted to humans through contact with urine, feces, or saliva of infected rodents.

Risk for Travelers

- The risk of acquiring VHF is generally very low for international travelers.
- Viruses with rodent reservoirs are transmitted when humans have contact with excreta from infected rodents. Several cases of Lassa fever have been confirmed in international travelers living in traditional dwellings in the countryside. Travelers staying in rodent-infested dwellings are at risk for HPS and HFRS.
- Viruses associated with arthropod vectors are transmitted through mosquito or tick bites or by crushing infected ticks. Some vectors also infect animals, including livestock, and humans can be infected through care, slaughter, or consumption of infected animals.
- Travelers at increased risk for exposure include those engaging in animal research, health-care workers, and others providing care for patients in the community, particularly where outbreaks of VHF are occurring.
- Three cases of Marburg hemorrhagic fever have occurred in travelers to caves harboring bats, including Kitum cave in Kenya and Python cave in Maramagambo Forest, Uganda. Miners have also acquired Marburg infection from working in underground mines harboring bats in the Democratic Republic of Congo and Uganda.

Clinical Presentation

- Signs and symptoms vary by disease, but in general, patients with VHF present with abrupt onset of fever, myalgias, and prostration, followed by coagulopathy with a petechial rash or ecchymoses, and sometimes overt bleeding. Vascular endothelial damage leads to shock and pulmonary edema, and liver injury is common.
- Signs seen with specific viruses include renal failure (HFRS), ecchymoses (CCHF), hearing loss, anasarca and shock in newborns (Lassa fever), and spontaneous abortion (Lassa and LCM viruses).
- Because the incubation period may be as long as 21 days, patients may not develop illness until returning from travel, and a thorough travel and exposure history is critical.

Diagnosis

- U.S.-based clinicians should notify CDC's Special Pathogens Branch immediately of any suspected cases of viral hemorrhagic fever occurring in patients residing in or requiring evacuation to the United States: 404-639-1115 or 404-639-2888 after hours. CDC also provides consultation for international clinicians and health ministries.
- Whole blood or serum may be tested for virologic (RT-PCR, antigen detection, virus isolation) and immunologic (IgM, IgG) evidence of infection. Tissue may be tested by immunohistochemistry, RT-PCR, and virus isolation. Postmortem skin biopsies fixed in formalin and blood collected within a few hours after death by cardiac puncture can be used for diagnosis. Samples should be sent for testing to a reference laboratory with Biosafety level 3 and 4 capability.

Treatment

- Supportive care. Ribavirin is effective for treating Lassa fever, New World arenaviruses, and likely for CCHF, but is not approved by FDA for these indications. Convalescent-phase plasma is effective in treating Argentine hemorrhagic fever.

- Intravenous ribavirin can be obtained for compassionate use through FDA, from Valeant Pharmaceuticals (Aliso Viejo, California), via 1) single-patient emergency Investigational New Drug (IND) or 2) protocol (for multiple uses). Requests should be provider-initiated through FDA, with simultaneous notification to Valeant: 800-548-5100, extension 5 (domestic telephone) or 949-461-6456 (international telephone). The IND process is explained on FDA's website: www.fda.gov/cder/regulatory/applications/ind_page_1.htm#emergency.

Preventive Measures for Travelers

- Prevention should focus on avoiding contact with host or vector species. Travelers should not visit locations where an outbreak is occurring. Contact with rodents should be avoided. Travelers should avoid contact with livestock in RVF and CCHF-endemic areas, and they should use insecticide-treated bed nets and insect repellent to prevent vector-borne disease.
- Standard precautions and contact and droplet precautions for suspected VHF case-patients are recommended to avoid health care-associated transmission.
- Direct contact should be avoided with corpses of patients suspected of having died of Ebola, Marburg, or Old World arenavirus infection.
- Contact with or consumption of primates, bats, and other bushmeat should be avoided.
- Investigational vaccines exist for Argentine hemorrhagic fever and RVF; however, neither is FDA-approved nor commonly available in the United States.

References

1. Geisbert TW, Jahrling PB. Exotic emerging viral diseases: progress and challenges. Nature Med. 2004;10(Suppl 12):S110–21.

2. Marty AM, Jahrling PB, Geisbert TW. Viral hemorrhagic fevers. Clin Lab Med. 2006;26:345–86, viii.

3. Bausch DG, Ksiazek TG. Viral hemorrhagic fevers including hantavirus pulmonary syndrome in the Americas. Clin Lab Med. 2002;22:981–1020.

4. Peters CJ, Zaki SR. Overview of viral hemorrhagic fevers. In: Guerrant RL, Walker DH, Weller PF, editors. Tropical infectious diseases: principles, pathogens and practice. 2nd ed. Philadelphia: Churchill Livingstone; 2006. p. 726–33.

5. Watts DM, Flick R, Peters CJ, et al. Bunyaviral fevers: Rift valley fever and Crimean–Congo hemorrhagic fever. In: Guerrant RL, Walker DH, Weller PF, editors. Tropical infectious diseases: principles, pathogens and practice. Philadelphia: Churchill Livingstone; 2006. p. 756–61.

6. Wahl-Jensen V, Feldmann H, Sanchez A, et al. Filovirus infections. In: Guerrant RL, Walker DH, Weller P, editors. Tropical infectious diseases: principles, pathogens and practice. 2nd ed. Philadelphia: Churchill Livingstone; 2006. p. 784–96.

7. Bausch DG, Borchert M, Grein T, et al. Risk factors for Marburg hemorrhagic fever, Democratic Republic of the Congo. Emerg Infect Dis. 2003;9:1531–7.

8. Günther S, Lenz O. Lassa virus. Crit Rev Clin Lab Sci. 2004;41:339–90.

9. De Manzione N, Salas RA, Paredes H, et al. Venezuelan hemorrhagic fever: clinical and epidemiological studies of 165 cases. Clin Infect Dis. 1998;26:308–13.

10. Madani TA, Al-Mazrou YY, Al-Jeffri MH, et al. Rift Valley fever epidemic in Saudi Arabia: epidemiological, clinical, and laboratory characteristics. Clin Infect Dis. 2003;37:1084–92.

11. Vapalahti O, Mustonen J, Lundkvist A, et al. Hantavirus infections in Europe. Lancet Infect Dis. 2003;3:653–61.

12. Rouquet P, Froment JM, Bermejo M, et al. Wild animal mortality monitoring and human Ebola outbreaks, Gabon and Republic of Congo, 2001–2003. Emerg Infect Dis. 2005;11:283–90.

13. Peters CJ, Jahrling PB, Khan AS. Patients infected with high-hazard viruses: scientific basis for infection control. Arch Virol Suppl. 1996;11:141–68.

14. Feldmann H, Jones SM, Schnittler HJ, Geisbert T. Therapy and prophylaxis of Ebola virus infections. Curr Opin Investig Drugs. 2005;6:823–30.

15. Ozkurt Z, Kiki I, Erol S, et al. Crimean–Congo hemorrhagic fever in Eastern Turkey: clinical features, risk factors and efficacy of ribavirin therapy. J Infect. 2006;52:207–15.

YERSINIA

Amy L. Boore, L. Hannah Gould

Infectious Agent

- Yersinia is caused by facultative anaerobic gram-negative coccobacillus of the genus *Yersinia*.
- Most human infections are associated with *Y. entercolitica* serogroups O:3, O:5,27, O:8, and O:9; infection with *Y. pseudotuberculosis* can also occur, but is uncommon.

Mode of Transmission

Yersinia is transmitted by consumption of contaminated food products (most commonly raw or undercooked pork products), unpasteurized or inadequately pasteurized milk, untreated water, or by direct or indirect contact with animals.

Occurrence

- Favors cooler months in temperate climates.
- Highest incidence reported in Northern Europe (particularly Scandinavia), Japan, and Canada.

Risk for Travelers

- In developed countries, infections are primarily seen among infants and young children, although all ages are at risk.
- Persons with high iron levels, such as those with chronic hemolysis, sickle-cell disease, or beta-thalassemia or who are using deferoxamine, are at higher risk of infection and severe disease.
- The incidence among travelers to developing countries has been reported as very low in the few studies that specifically looked for *Yersinia*.

Clinical Presentation

- Incubation period is typically 4–6 days but may range from 1 to 14 days. Illness typically resolves spontaneously.
- Young children usually have fever, abdominal pain, and diarrhea, which may be bloody. The duration of diarrhea varies, but it can persist for several weeks. Relapsing disease and, rarely, necrotizing enterocolitis have been described.
- Older children and adults commonly present with pseudoappendicitis, including fever, right-sided abdominal pain, and leukocytosis.
- Bacteremia is rare and occurs most commonly in young children and infants with predisposing conditions such as excessive iron storage and immunosuppressive states.
- Focal manifestations may rarely occur, including pharyngitis, meningitis, osteomyelitis, pyomyositis, conjunctivitis, pneumonia, empyema, endocarditis, acute peritonitis, abscesses of the liver and spleen, and primary cutaneous infection.
- Postinfectious sequelae are sometimes reported, predominantly in adults. Reactive arthritis affecting the wrists, knees, and ankles can occur, with onset usually 1 month after the initial diarrhea episode and symptoms typically resolving after 1–6 months. Erythema nodosum can also occur, manifesting as painful raised red or purple lesions along the trunk and legs. This condition is more commonly reported among women; symptoms usually resolve spontaneously within 1 month.

Diagnosis

- Isolation of organism from stool, blood, or bile.
- Can also be cultured from wounds, throat swabs, mesenteric lymph nodes, cerebrospinal fluid, and peritoneal fluid.
- Most laboratories do not routinely test for *Y. enterocolitica*. If suspected, laboratories should be notified and instructed to culture on CIN agar.
- Postinfectious sequelae, reactive arthritis, and erythema nodosum are diagnosed serologically.
- Tests for *Y. entercolitica* serogroup O:9 may cross-react with tests for *Brucella* and *Escherichia coli* O157:H7.

Treatment

- Fluid and electrolyte replacement for enteritis.
- Symptomatic treatment for abdominal pain.
- Antibiotic treatment may reduce the duration of fecal shedding; however, the benefits of antibiotic therapy in uncomplicated cases are not well established. Antibiotic treatment should be given for severe cases, including patients with septicemia, metastatic focal infections, or underlying immunosuppression. *Y. enterocolitica* is usually susceptible to trimethoprim–sulfamethoxazole, aminoglycosides, cefotaxime, fluoroquinolones, tetracycline, doxycycline (for children ≥8 years old), and chloramphenicol. *Y. enterocolitica* isolates typically are resistant to first-generation and most second-generation cephalosporins and most penicillins. Antimicrobial therapy has no effect on postinfectious sequelae.

Preventive Measures for Travelers

- No vaccine is available.
- No drugs for preventing infection are recommended.
- Travelers should avoid raw or undercooked pork products, unpasteurized milk products, and untreated water.

References

1. Dennis DT, Campbell GL. Plague and other *Yersinia* infections. In: Fauci AS, Braunwald E, Kasper DL, Hauser SL, Longo DL, Jameson JL, Loscalzo J, editors. Harrison's principles of internal medicine. 17th ed. New York: McGraw-Hill Medical; 2008. p. 980–6.
2. Bottone EJ. *Yersinia enterocolitica*: overview and epidemiologic correlates. Microb Infect. 1999;1(4):323–33.
3. Bottone EJ. *Yersinia enterocolitica*: the charisma continues. Clin Microbiol Rev. 1997;10(2):257–76.
4. Perdikogianni C, Galanakis E, Michalakis M, et al. *Yersinia enterocolitica* infection mimicking surgical conditions. Pediatr Surg Int. 2006;22(7):589–92.
5. Vantrappen G, Geboes K, Ponette E. *Yersinia* enteritis. Med Clin North Am.1982;66(3):639–53.
6. American Academy of Pediatrics. *Yersinia enterocolitica* and *Yersinia pseudotuberculosis* infections (enteritis and other illnesses). In: Pickering LK, Baker CJ, Long SS, McMillan JA, editors. Red book: 2006 Report of the Committee on Infectious Diseases. 27th ed. Elk Grove Village (IL): American Academy of Pediatrics; 2006. p. 732–4.
7. Adamkiewicz TV, Berkovitch M, Krishnan C, et al. Infection due to *Yersinia enterocolitica* in a series of patients with beta-thalassemia: incidence and predisposing factors. Clin Infect Dis. 1998;27(6):1367–8.
8. Kapperud G. *Yersinia enterocolitica* in food hygiene. Int J Food Microbiol. 1991;12:53–65.
9. Lee LA, Taylor J, Carter GP, et al. *Yersinia enterocolitica* O:3: an emerging cause of pediatric gastroenteritis in the United States. The *Yersinia enterocolitica* Collaborative Study Group. J Infect Dis. 1991;163(3):660–3.
10. Ostroff SM, Kapperud G, Hutwagner LC, et al. Sources of sporadic *Yersinia enterocolitica* infections in Norway: a prospective case–control study. Epidemiol Infect. 1994;112(1):133–41.
11. Schiemann DA. *Yersinia enterocolitica* in milk and dairy products. J Dairy Sci. 1987;70:383–91.
12. Tauxe RV, Vandepitte J, Wauters G, et al. *Yersinia enterocolitica* infections and pork: the missing link. Lancet. 1987;1(8542):1129–32.

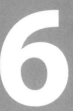

Conveyance and Transportation Issues

AIR TRAVEL

Nancy M. Gallagher, Karen J. Marienau, Petra A. Illig, Phyllis E. Kozarsky

Travelers often have concerns about the health risks of flying in airplanes. Illness that occurs as a direct result of air travel is uncommon, but the main concerns are—

- Exacerbations of chronic medical problems due to changes in air pressure, humidity, and oxygen concentration
- Relative immobility during flights (risk of thromboembolic disease)
- Close proximity to other passengers with certain communicable diseases
- Spraying of airplane cabins with insecticides (disinsection) prior to landing in certain destinations

Exacerbation of Chronic Disease

During flight, the aircraft cabin pressure is usually maintained at the equivalent of 1,500–2,500 m (5,000–8,000 ft) above sea level. Most healthy travelers will not notice any effects. However, for travelers with cardiopulmonary diseases (especially those who normally require supplemental oxygen), cerebrovascular disease, anemia, and sickle cell disease, conditions in an aircraft can increase the risk of exacerbations of their underlying conditions. Aircraft cabin air is typically very dry, usually 10%–20% humidity, which can cause dryness of the mucous membranes of the eyes and airways.

People with chronic illnesses, particularly those whose conditions may be unstable, should be evaluated by a physician to ensure they are fit for travel. For those who require supplemental in-flight oxygen, the following must be taken into consideration:

- Federal regulations prohibit airlines from allowing passengers to bring their own oxygen aboard; passengers requiring in-flight supplemental oxygen should notify the airline at least 72 hours before departure.
- Information regarding the screening of respiratory equipment (e.g., oxygen canisters or Portable Oxygen Concentrators [POCs]) at airports in the United States and regulations regarding oxygen use on aircraft can be found at www.tsa.gov/travelers/airtravel/.
- Airlines may not offer in-flight supplemental oxygen on all aircraft or flights; some airlines permit only POCs.

- Travelers must arrange their own oxygen supply while on the ground, at departure, during layovers, and on arrival. The National Home Oxygen Patients Association provides a brochure, *Airline Travel with Oxygen* (available at www.homeoxygen.org/airtrav.html) to assist patients who require supplemental oxygen during travel.

Barotrauma during Flight

Air in the middle ear and sinuses, as well as intra-abdominal gas, expands during ascent. Air in the middle ear and sinuses can usually equalize during ascent. More problems occur as the low-pressure air within these spaces needs to be equalized by air that flows in the eustachean tube or sinus passages.

The following suggestions may help avoid potential barotrauma:

- People with ear, nose, and sinus infections or severe congestion may wish to temporarily avoid flying to prevent pain and injury. This is particularly true for infants and toddlers, in whom obstruction occurs more readily.
- Oral pseudoephedrine 30 minutes before flight departure or a nonsteroidal anti-inflammatory agent may alleviate symptoms.
- Travelers sensitive to abdominal bloating should avoid carbonated beverages and foods that can increase gas production.
- Patients who have had recent surgery, particularly intra-abdominal, neurologic, intrapulmonary or intraocular procedures, should consult with their physicians before flying.

Ventilation and Air Quality

All commercial jet aircraft built after the late 1980s and a few modified older aircraft recirculate 10%–50% of the air in the cabin mixed with outside air. The recirculated air passes through a series of filters 20–30 times per hour. In most newer model airplanes, the recycled air passes through high-efficiency particulate air (HEPA) filters, which capture 99.9% of particles (bacteria, fungi, and larger viruses) between 0.1 and 0.3 microns. Air flow occurs horizontally across the plane in limited bands, and air is not forced up and down the length of the plane.

In-Flight Transmission of Communicable Diseases

Communicable diseases may be transmitted to other travelers during air travel, therefore—

- Persons who are acutely ill, or still within the infectious period for a specific disease, should be discouraged from traveling.
- Travelers should be reminded to wash their hands frequently and cover their noses and mouths when coughing or sneezing.

If a passenger with a communicable disease is identified as having flown on a particular flight (or flights), passengers who may have been exposed will be contacted by public health authorities for possible screening or prophylaxis.

For certain communicable diseases, public health authorities will obtain contact information from the airline for potentially exposed travelers so they may be contacted and offered appropriate intervention. To assist in this process, travelers can provide airlines with current contact information such as a telephone number and state of residence. Travel agencies will not share passenger contact information with the airline or public health authorities.

Tuberculosis

Although the risk of transmission of *Mycobacterium tuberculosis* on board aircraft is low, international TB experts agree that contact investigations for flights >8 hours are warranted when the ill traveler meets WHO criteria for being infectious during flight. The concern is greatest when a person may have flown with a highly resistant strain of TB. People known to have infectious TB should not travel by commercial air (or any other commercial means) until criteria for no longer being infectious are met. State health department TB controllers are valuable resources for advice (www.phf.org/links.htm#State-Health).

Neisseria meningitidis

Meningococcal disease is potentially rapidly fatal, thus rapid identification of close contacts and provision of prophylactic antimicrobials are critical. Antimicrobial prophylaxis should be considered for—

- household members traveling with a patient,
- travel companions with close contact, and
- passengers seated directly next to the ill traveler on flights of >8 hours.

Measles

Most measles cases diagnosed in the United States are imported from countries where measles is endemic.

- An ill traveler is considered infectious during a flight of any duration if he or she traveled during the 4 days before rash onset through 4 days after rash onset.
- Intervention may prevent or mitigate measles in susceptible contacts if—
  o MMR vaccine is given within 72 hours of flight exposure **or**
  o Immunoglobulin is given within 6 days of flight exposure.
- International travelers should ensure they are immune to measles prior to travel.

Influenza

Transmission of the influenza virus aboard aircraft has been documented, but data are limited. Transmission is thought to be primarily due to large droplets; therefore, passengers seated closest to the source case are believed to be most at risk for exposure (see the Influenza section in Chapter 2 and www.cdc.gov/flu for more information).

The avian influenza virus (H5N1) has infected hundreds of humans since 1997, primarily associated with direct contact with infected birds or bird products. No cases have yet been associated with air travel. See www.cdc.gov/travel for more general information and up-to-date, specific guidelines for travelers and the airline industry.

Severe Acute Respiratory Syndrome (SARS)

SARS can potentially be transmitted anywhere people are gathered, including aircraft cabins. The last known case of person-to-person transmission occurred in 2003. If SARS were to re-emerge, www.cdc.gov/travel will provide up-to-date information for travelers and flight crews.

Disinsection

To reduce the accidental spread of mosquitoes and other vectors via airline cabins and luggage compartments, a number of countries require disinsection of all inbound flights. WHO and the International Civil Aviation Organization (ICAO) specify two approaches for aircraft disinsection—

- Spraying the aircraft cabin with an aerosolized insecticide (usually 2% phenothrin) while passengers are on board
- Treating the aircraft's interior surfaces with a residual insecticide while the aircraft is empty

Some countries use a third method, in which aircraft are sprayed with an aerosolized insecticide while passengers are not on board.

Disinsection is not routinely done on incoming flights to the United States. Although disinsection, when done appropriately, was declared safe by the WHO in 1995, there is still much debate about the safety of the agents and methods used. Guidelines for disinsection have been updated for the revised International Health Regulations (www2a.cdc.gov/phlp/docs/58assembly.pdf). Many countries, including the United States, reserve the right to increase the use of disinsection in case of increased threat of vector or disease spread. An updated list of countries that require disinsection and the types of methods used are available at the U.S. Department of Transportation website: (http://ostpxweb.ost.dot.gov/policy/safetyenergyenv/disinsection.htm).

References

1. Bagshaw M, Nicolls DJ. Aircraft cabin environment. In: Keystone JS, Kozarsky PE, Freedman DO, Nothdurft HO, Connor BA, editors. Travel medicine. 2nd ed. Philadelphia: Mosby. 2008. p. 447–62.
2. Kenyon TA, Valway SE, Ihle WW, et al. Transmission of multidrug-resistant *Mycobacterium tuberculosis* during a long airplane flight. N Engl J Med. 1996;334(15):933–8.
3. World Health Organization. 2008. Tuberculosis and air travel: guidelines for prevention and control, 3rd ed. [cited 2008 Jun 24]. Available from: www.who.int/entity/tb/publications/2008/WHO_HTM_TB_2008.399_eng.pdf.
4. CDC. Exposure to patients with meningococcal disease on aircrafts—United States, 1999–2001. MMWR Morb Mortal Wkly Rep. 2001;50(23);485–9.
5. Moser MR, Bender TR, Margolis HS, et al. An outbreak of influenza aboard a commercial airliner. Am J Epidemiol. 1979;110(1):1–6.
6. Vogt TM, Guerra MA, Flagg EW, et al. Risk of SARS-associated coronavirus transmission aboard commercial aircraft. J Travel Med. 2006;13(5):268–72.
7. CDC. Multistate Measles Outbreak Associated with an International Youth Sporting Event—Pennsylvania, Michigan, and Texas, August–September 2007. MMWR Morb Mortal Wkly Rep. 2008;57(07);169–173.
8. Marsden AG. Influenza outbreak related to air travel. Med J Aust 2003;179(3):172–3.
9. Wilder-Smith A, Paton N, Goh KT. Experience of severe acute respiratory syndrome in Singapore: importation of cases, and defense strategies at the airport. J Travel Med. 2003;10(5):259–62.

CRUISE SHIP TRAVEL

Kiren Mitruka

The continued popularity of cruise travel, along with the expansion of cruise itineraries to areas not easily accessible otherwise, promotes the exposure of travelers to multiple global destinations in a short period of time. Passengers and crew from around the world bring together a diversity of cultures, medical risk factors, and health risk behaviors.

- About 12 million passengers worldwide took a cruise vacation in 2007, a 7% increase over 2006.
- The North American cruise industry makes up the majority of the global cruise market and since 1980 has had an average annual passenger growth rate of 8.1%.
- U.S. ports handle about 75% of all embarkations.
- The Caribbean is the top cruise destination, followed by the Mediterranean, Europe, Alaska, and Mexico.
- A typical cruise is about 7 days long and includes 3,000 passengers and 1,000 crew members.
- Approximately 78% of cruise passengers are U.S. residents. About 50 nationalities are represented among crew members, most of whom are from developing countries.

Challenges of Cruise Ship Travel and Infectious Diseases

- Densely populated, semi-enclosed cruise ship environments may permit repeated and prolonged exposure to communicable diseases, resulting in their transmission between passengers and crew members.

- Differences in sanitation standards and disease prevalence between seaports may also lead to communicable disease exposure and spread.
- The risk of acquiring an infectious disease during cruise travel is difficult to quantify due to the diverse activities of crew and passengers, as well as the wide range of potential disease exposures.
- Senior citizens (an estimated one-third of cruise travelers) and travelers with underlying chronic health problems are at increased risk of illness from infections such as influenza, *Legionella*, and noroviruses.
- Early detection and prevention of infectious diseases are important, not only to protect the health of cruise travelers, but also to avoid global dissemination of diseases in home communities through disembarking passengers and crew members.

Medical Care Aboard Cruise Ships

Medical facilities on cruise ships can vary, depending on the size of the ship, its itinerary, number of crew and passengers, and the mean age and health status of passengers.

The American College of Emergency Physicians (ACEP) *Health Care Guidelines for Cruise Ship Medical Facilities* is a consensus report on appropriate facilities and staffing requirements for basic shipboard medical and emergency services, given the recognized limitations of offshore environments. Shipboard health care recommended in these guidelines includes provision of—

- A medical infirmary with licensed medical staff (physician and registered nurse) on call 24 hours per day
- One intensive care unit (ICU) room
- One bed per 1,000 passengers and crew members
- One isolation room or the capability to isolate patients with communicable diseases
- Emergency and portable medical equipment, such as a bag valve mask, oxygen tank, endotracheal tube, defibrillator, and a cardiac monitor or external cardiac pacer
- Medications to handle medical emergencies
- Basic diagnostic and laboratory supplies for blood chemistry analyses, complete blood counts, urinalyses, chest x-rays, and electrocardiograms (EKGs)
- A medical record and communication system
- Health, hygiene, and safety program for medical personnel

Large cruise lines that operate in the United States or are members of Cruise Lines International Organization (CLIA) meet or exceed ACEP guideline standards. However, medical care on these ships should be equated to that of community urgent-care centers, not full-service hospitals. Small ships or those run by independent ship operators may not follow the ACEP guidelines. Therefore, on such ships, medical provisions might not be available onboard.

Primary Health Concerns on Cruise Ships

General

In a retrospective study of four cruise ship medical logs maintained by a major cruiseline, 7,147 new patient visits occurred among 196,171 cruise passengers on 172 voyages.

- Over half of shipboard infirmary visits are made by passengers over the age of 65.
- The most common diagnosis was respiratory tract infection (29.1%), followed by injuries (18.2%), seasickness (9.1%), and gastrointestinal (GI) illness (8.9%).
- An estimated 95% of illnesses seen in cruise ship medical facilities can be treated onboard. However, passengers with serious problems, such as myocardial infarction

or cerebrovascular accidents, need to be transferred to shoreside hospitals after stabilization.

Communicable Diseases

Communicable diseases occurring onboard cruise ships are similar to those that occur onshore. Detecting illnesses of public health significance is aided by heightened cruise line surveillance efforts in cooperation with public health authorities, and passenger reporting.

- The most frequently documented cruise ship outbreaks involve respiratory infections (influenza and *Legionella*) and gastrointestinal infections (norovirus).
- In the past decade, clusters of illnesses due to vaccine-preventable diseases other than influenza, such as rubella and varicella (chickenpox), have also been reported.

Respiratory Illnesses

Influenza

- Outbreaks of influenza A and B can occur year-round, despite seasonality in the destination regions for cruises.
- Respiratory illness outbreaks usually result from the importation of influenza by embarking passengers and crew; the infection subsequently spreads person to person on the ship.
- Onboard control measures include isolation, infection control, and antiviral treatment of ill individuals as well as those exposed to the illness.
- One of the largest and most protracted influenza outbreaks occurred among land- and sea-based tourists to Alaska and the Yukon during the summer of 1998.

Legionnaires' Disease

- Legionnaires' disease has led to pneumonia outbreaks on multiple occasions, sometimes on consecutive cruises.
- Although contaminated ships' whirlpool spas and potable water supply systems are the most commonly implicated sources of *Legionella* outbreaks, exposure to other sources may also occur during port stops.
- Pinpointing the source of these outbreaks has proved difficult because diagnoses in returned travelers may be delayed and clinical specimens may be unavailable for culture at the time of diagnosis.
- Culture-based diagnostic tests for cruise travel-associated Legionnaires' disease are of public health importance.
- Improvements in ship design and standardization of spa and water supply disinfection have reduced the risk of *Legionella* growth and colonization.

Gastrointestinal (GI) Illnesses

The estimated likelihood of contracting gastroenteritis on an average 7-day cruise is less than 1%. GI illness accounts for fewer than 10% of shipboard passenger infirmary visits. In recent years, outbreaks of gastroenteritis on cruise ships have increased, despite good cruise ship environmental health standards.

Noroviruses

- The increase in gastroenteritis on cruise ships is primarily attributed to noroviruses, also the main cause of acute viral gastroenteritis in the United States.
- Large, consecutive cruise ship outbreaks have resulted from noroviruses, due to their—
  ○ low infective dose,
  ○ easy person-to-person transmissibility, and
  ○ ability to survive routine cleaning procedures.
- Prompt implementation of disease control measures, such as the isolation of ill persons, strict application of food and water sanitation measures, and disinfection of surfaces with suitable disinfectants, are key to controlling norovirus outbreaks.

Other pathogens

Other known causes of GI illness clusters on cruise ships include food or water contaminated with *Salmonella* spp., enterotoxigenic *Escherichia coli*, *Shigella* spp., *Vibrio* spp., *Staphylococcus aureus*, *Clostridium perfringens*, *Cyclospora* sp., and *Trichinella spiralis*.

Vaccine-Preventable Diseases on Cruises

Other than influenza, clusters of rubella and varicella have been investigated on cruises originating in the United States, highlighting the potential global dissemination of vaccine-preventable diseases through cruise travel.

- During a cruise ship outbreak investigation of rubella, 11% of the crew was found to be acutely infected with or susceptible to rubella and 33% of passengers onboard were women of childbearing age—a high-risk group for congenital rubella syndrome if infected during pregnancy.
- One investigation of varicella outbreak aboard a cruise ship found that 13% of the crew, most foreign-born from tropical countries, were either acutely infected or susceptible.
- Vaccine administration to crew members without documented immunity to vaccine-preventable diseases and notification of all passengers at risk for exposure serve as important control measures.

Other Health Concerns

Injuries

- Are among the most common reasons for passengers to seek medical care on cruise ships.
- Account for about 18% of passenger infirmary visits.
- Occurring most frequently on cruise ships include sprains, contusions, and superficial wounds.

Seasickness

- Is also a common reason for cruise passenger infirmary visits.
- May not be reduced by the central location of a cabin.
- See the Motion Sickness section in Chapter 2 for more information.

Exacerbation of Chronic Conditions

- Cruise ship travelers with chronic health conditions may experience complications due to—
  - Climatic variations
  - Environmental exposure to pollutants
  - Changes in diet and physical activity levels
  - An increased level of stress due to being in an unfamiliar environment
- Special cruises are available for travelers with certain medical conditions, including persons on dialysis.

Preventive Measures for Cruise Ship Travelers

Due to multiple port visits and potential exposures, cruise ship travelers may be uncertain about which prevention medications, immunizations, and behaviors are appropriate for them and for their itineraries. Pre-travel advice for cruise ship travelers should include a complete review of the health status of the traveler, duration of travel, countries to be visited, and shore side activities. Box 6-1 summarizes recommendations for cruise travelers

---

Box 6-1. Healthy cruise ship travel tips

Considerations for Health-Care Professionals (During Pre-travel Consultation)

General:
- Cruise ship itinerary, including planned activities at port stops.
- Travelers' underlying medical conditions.

Vaccine-preventable diseases:
- Routine age-specific vaccines.
- Destination- and activity-specific recommendations or required vaccines. Note: Proof of yellow fever vaccine may be required for entry into certain countries.

Medications based on risk and need:
- Antimalarial (consider risks at port stops).
- Antiviral (for travelers at high risk of severe influenza).
- Motion sickness medication.
- Antibiotic for travelers' diarrhea.

Documentation:
- Written summary of medical history-including pertinent diagnostics, such as EKG and chest x-ray, to facilitate overseas medical care should it be required.
- Vaccines and prescriptions given.

Traveler Pre-Travel Preparations

- Assess cruise ship medical facilities, sanitation scores, and presence of acute gastroenteritis outbreaks.
- Cruise ship travelers with chronic diseases, special needs, or those who may require comprehensive medical care during travel should notify the cruise line of special needs before travel (e.g., wheelchair access, oxygen tank, and dialysis needs).
- Ensure adequate medical insurance coverage for receiving health care overseas and medical evacuation (see the Travel Insurance and Evacuation Insurance section in Chapter 2).

Traveler Precautions During Travel

- Wash hands often with soap and water. If soap and water are not available, use an alcohol-based gel containing at least 60% alcohol.
- Practice respiratory hygiene by using a tissue to cover coughs and sneezes.
- Take food and water precautions by eating foods that are thoroughly cooked and of appropriate temperature.
- Prevent mosquito and other insect bites by using DEET or picaridin-containing repellents and clothing that provides complete coverage.
- Use sun protection and drink plenty of water to avoid heat-related illness.
- Other—avoid excessive alcohol, get plenty of rest, avoid contact with ill persons and report illnesses to cruise staff, and practice safe sex.

---

and health-care providers advising cruise travelers in pre-travel preparation and healthy behaviors during travel.

After Travel

Health-care providers can contribute to healthy cruise ship environments by questioning ill returned travelers about recent cruise vacations and promptly reporting any suspected communicable disease to public health authorities.

Contacts for concerns about illnesses on cruise ships:

- GI illnesses concerns should be directed to CDC Vessel Sanitation Program—
  - Phone: 800-CDC-INFO (800-232-4636)
  - E-mail: CDCINFO@cdc.gov
- Other illnesses suggestive of a communicable disease should be reported to the nearest CDC quarantine station with jurisdiction nearest to the cruise ship's port of arrival.

References

1. Minooee, A, Rickman LS. Infectious diseases on cruise ships. Clin Infect Dis. 1999;29(4):737–43.

2. Maloney SA, Cetron M. Investigation and management of infectious diseases on international conveyances (airplanes and cruise ships). In: Dupont HL, Steffen R, editors. Textbook of travel medicine and health. 2nd ed. Hamilton, Ontario: BC Decker; 2001. p.519–30.

3. Cruise Lines International Association (CLIA). Cruise Industry Overview—Marketing Edition 2005. [cited 2998 Aug 6]. Available from: http://www.cruising.org/press/overview/ind_overview.cfm.

4. Cruise Lines International Association (CLIA). About CLIA.[cited 2008 Aug 6]. Available from: http://www.cruising.org/about.cfm.

5. CDC. Rubella among crew members of commercial cruise ships—Florida, 1997. MMWR. Morb Mortal Wkly Rep 1998;46(52):1247–50.

6. Miller JM, Tam TW, Maloney S, et al. Cruise ships: high-risk passengers and the global spread of new influenza viruses. Clin Infect Dis. 2000;31(2):433–8.

7. Rowbotham TJ. Legionellosis associated with ships: 1977 to1997. Comm Dis Public Health. 1998;1(3):146–51.

8. Isakbaeva ET, Widdowson MA, Beard RS, et al. Norovirus transmission on cruise ships. Emerg Infect Dis. 2005;11(1):154–8.

9. ACEP. Healthcare Guidelines for Cruise Ship Medical Facilities. [cited 2008 Aug 6]. Available from: http://www3.acep.org/practres.aspx?id=29980.

10. Wheeler RE. Travel health at sea: cruise ship medicine. In: Zuckerman JN, editor. Principle and practices of travel medicine. New York: John Wiley and Sons; 2001. p. 275–87.

11. Peake DE, Gray CL, Ludwig MR, et al. Descriptive epidemiology of injury and illness among cruise ship passengers. Ann Emerg Med. 1999;33(1):67–72.

12. CDC. Vessel sanitation program. [cited 2008 Aug 6]. Available from: http://www.cdc.gov/nceh/vsp/.

13. Cramer EH, Blanton CJ, Blanton LH, et al. Epidemiology of gastroenteritis on cruise ships, 2001–2004. Am J Prev Med. 2006;30(3):252–7.

14. Uyeki TM, Zane SB, Bodnar UR, et al. Large summertime influenza A outbreaks among tourists in Alaska and the Yukon Territory. Clin Infect Dis. 2003;36(9):1095–102.

15. Public Health Agency of Canada. Statement on cruise ship travel. Canada Communicable Disease Report 15 October 2005: 31-ACS—8 and 9. [cited 2008 Nov 29]. Available from: http://www.phac-aspc.gc.ca/publicat/ccdr-rmtc/05pdf/acs-dcc310809.pdf.

16. CDC. Prevention and control of influenza: recommendations of the Advisory Committee on Immunization Practices (ACIP). MMWR Morb Mortal Wkly Rep. 2005;54(RR08):1–40.

17. CDC. Quarantine station jurisdictions and contact information. [cited 2008 Aug 6]. Available from: http://www.cdc.gov/ncidod/dq/resources/Quarantine_Station_Contact_List.pdf.

DEATH DURING TRAVEL

Clare A. Dykewicz, Xiaohong Mao Davis, Carl Lawson

Traveling abroad is an exciting event for many travelers. Fortunately, Americans die only rarely during international travel. Cardiovascular events, followed by injuries, have been the leading cause of deaths; in contrast, infectious diseases other than pneumonias have caused just 1% of deaths. Not surprisingly, injury-related deaths occur at a higher proportion abroad than in the United States (see the Injuries and Safety section in Chapter 2). In a recent review of injury-related deaths in U.S. travelers abroad, the most common causes of death were motor vehicle accidents, homicides, drowning, and suicides. This section provides some highlights regarding recommendations for preventing death during travel and explains regulations on the importation of human remains into the United States.

Recommendations for Preventing Death During Travel Abroad

Cardiovascular Events

* Persons with known or suspected cardiovascular conditions—such as angina,

congestive heart failure, arrhythmias, or hypertension—should refer to the Traveling with Chronic Medical Illnesses section in Chapter 8.

- Persons with cardiovascular disease (as well as all other travelers) should consider purchasing supplemental insurance such as that covering trip cancellation, health care overseas and medical evacuation. The problem of deep vein thrombosis is receiving greater attention as it relates to travelers; see the Deep Vein Thrombosis and Pulmonary Embolism section in Chapter 2 for a complete review.

Motor Vehicle Injury

- Travelers should be cautioned about the risks of motor-vehicle injuries during travel, including those caused by unfamiliar road environments, poorly maintained roads, and unavailable passenger restraints. This is especially important for travelers visiting less-developed countries.
- Travelers should be advised to use seatbelts and child restraints, take mass transportation such as trains and subways whenever possible, avoid road travel at night, avoid drinking and driving, avoid speeding, and wear helmets when riding bicycles, mopeds, and motorcycles (see the Injuries and Safety section in Chapter 2).

Drowning

- Travelers should be advised that the use of alcohol or illicit drugs may increase the risk of assault or injuries, including drowning. It is advisable for them to swim in areas supervised by a lifeguard if at all possible.
- Personal flotation devices should be used by adults and children, while operating personal watercraft, and during whitewater boating, waterskiing, and sailboarding.

Homicide

The U.S. Department of State offers the following guidance for reduction of crime, including homicide. Travelers should take the following precautions:

- Avoid drawing personal attention when traveling by not wearing expensive clothes or jewelry.
- Carry as little baggage as possible, so movement can be quick and easy.
- Leave valuables at home, or at least keep them well hidden.
- Use travelers' cheques and credit cards rather than carrying large quantities of cash.
- Avoid short cuts, narrow alleys, or poorly lit streets.
- Do not travel alone at night.
- Avoid discussing travel plans with strangers.
- Never attend public demonstrations and civil disturbances.
- Beware of pickpockets who might jostle or try to distract.
- Know how to use a local telephone, and have emergency numbers readily available.
- Give up valuables or car if confronted.
- Keep hotel doors locked at all times and meet visitors in the lobby.
- Do not get in an elevator alone with suspicious-looking persons.
- Do not accept food or drink from strangers.

For detailed information on safety abroad, the State Department's website, Safe Trip Abroad, is extremely helpful (see http://travel.state.gov/travel/tips/safety/safety_1747.html). For additional assistance, U.S. Embassies or Consulates can give assistance or referrals to local services.

Suicide

- Psychological problems are not uncommon in travelers, and often travel can precipitate problems that had been previously masked. See the Mental Health and Travel section in Chapter 2 for more detailed information. Fortunately, suicide can be prevented. People who are experiencing thoughts of suicide should get help as soon as possible.

- The following signs and symptoms may indicate a person is suicidal:
  - Withdrawing from friends, family, and society
  - Anxiety, agitation, inability to sleep, or sleeping much more than usual
  - Dramatic mood changes
  - Rage, uncontrolled anger, and seeking revenge
  - Acting recklessly or engaging in risky activities, seemingly without thinking
  - Increasing alcohol or drug use
  - Feelings of hopelessness
  - Feeling trapped, like there's no way out
  - Feeling that there is no reason to live and having no sense of purpose in life

When U.S. Citizens Die Abroad

Obtaining U.S. Department of State Assistance

- Family members of U.S. citizens who die abroad are advised to contact the nearest U.S. Consulate for assistance.
- In case of emergencies abroad, the Office of Overseas Citizen Services in the Department of State's Bureau of Consular Affairs may be contacted from 8 am to 8 pm Eastern Time, Monday through Friday, by calling 888-407-4747 from the United States or Canada or 202-501-4444 if calling from overseas. For emergency assistance after working hours or on weekends and holidays, call the Department of State Switchboard at 202-647-4000 and ask to speak with the Overseas Citizens Duty Officer.

Importation of Human Remains

General Guidance

Persons wishing to import human remains, including cremated remains, into the United States must obtain clearance from CDC's Division of Global Migration and Quarantine (DGMQ).

- Clearance can be obtained by presenting copies of the foreign death certificate and if needed, a CDC/DGMQ permit to the CDC Quarantine Station with jurisdiction for the U.S. port of entry.
- A CDC/DGMQ permit may be needed to import human remains if the deceased is known or suspected to have died from a quarantinable communicable disease.
- A copy of the foreign death certificate and the CDC/DGMQ permit must accompany the human remains at all times during shipment. The foreign death certificate should state the cause of death and must be translated into English.

The U.S. mortician handling the remains is subject to the regulations of state and local health authorities for interstate and intrastate shipment. The U.S. mortician handling the importation and disposition of the remains will afterwards submit a letter to CDC/DGMQ certifying that the human remains were imported, handled, and disposed of according to the terms of the CDC permit.

Human Remains of a Person Known or Suspected to Have Died from a Quarantinable Communicable Disease

Federal quarantine regulations (42 CFR Part 71) state that the remains of a person who is known or suspected to have died from a quarantinable communicable disease may not be brought into the United States unless the remains are—

- properly embalmed and placed in a hermetically sealed casket,
- cremated, or
- accompanied by a permit issued by the CDC Director.

Quarantinable communicable diseases include cholera; diphtheria, infectious tuberculosis; plague; smallpox, yellow fever; viral hemorrhagic fevers (Lassa, Marburg, Ebola, Congo-

Crimean, or others not yet isolated or named); severe acute respiratory syndrome (SARS); and influenza caused by novel or re-emergent influenza viruses that are causing or have the potential to cause a pandemic.

A CDC permit may be required when the remains are not embalmed or cremated, especially if the person is suspected or known to have died from a communicable disease.

- If a CDC permit is obtained for importation of human remains, CDC may impose additional conditions for importation beyond those listed above.
- Permits for importation of human remains may be obtained through CDC/DGMQ by calling 866-694-4867 or the CDC Director's Emergency Operation's Center at 770-488-7100.

Human Remains of a Person Who Died of a Nonquarantinable Communicable Disease

Federal regulations also give CDC the authority to restrict the importation of the remains of a person who died of a nonquarantinable communicable disease when necessary to prevent the spread of communicable disease.

Human Remains of a Person Who Died of a Noncommunicable Disease

CDC places no restrictions on the importation of the remains of a person who died of a noncommunicable disease, although other federal, state, or local regulations may apply.

Exportation of Human Remains

CDC places no restrictions on the exportation of human remains outside the United States, although other federal, state, and local regulations may apply. Travelers should also be advised that the requirements of the country of destination must be met. Information regarding these requirements may be obtained from the appropriate foreign embassy or consulate.

References

1. Hargarten SW, Baker TD, Guptill K. Overseas fatalities of United States citizen travelers: an analysis of deaths related to international travel. Ann Emerg Med. 1991;20(6):622–6.

2. U.S. Department of State. Statistical Summary: Total Number of Non-Natural Deaths by Region, January 1, 2005-December 31, 2007. [cited 2008 Jun 5]. Available from: http://travel.state.gov/law/family_issues/death/death_3753.html.

3. Possick SE, Barry M. Evaluation and management of the cardiovascular patient embarking on air travel. Ann Intern Med. 2004;141(2):148–54.

4. Leon MN, Lateef M, Fuentes F. Prevention and management of cardiovascular events during travel. J Travel Med. 1996;3(4):227–30.

5. Hill DR, Ericsson CD, Pearson RD, et al. The practice of travel medicine: guidelines by the Infectious Diseases Society of America. Clin Infect Dis. 2006;43(12):1499–539.

6. Guse CE, Cortés LM, Hargarten SW, et al. Fatal injuries of U.S. citizens abroad. J Travel Med. 2007;14(5):279–87.

7. Dinh-Zarr TB, Hargarten SW. Road crash deaths of American travelers: the make roads safe report. An analysis of U.S. State Department Data on Unnatural Causes of Death to U.S. Citizens Abroad (2004–2006).

[cited 2008 Jun 22]. Available from: http://www.makeroadssafe.org/documents/make_roads_safe_us_report_4_25_07.pdf.

8. Cortés LM, Hargarten SW, Hennes HM. Recommendations for water safety and drowning prevention for travelers. J Travel Med. 2006;13(1):21–34.

9. American Association of Suicidology. [homepage on internet]. [cited 2008 Jul 22]. Available from: http://www.suicidology.org/displaycommon.cfm?an=2.

10. U.S. Department of State. Death of a U.S. citizen abroad. [cited 2008 Jun 5]. Available from: http://travel.state.gov/travel/tips/emergencies/emergencies_1205.html#death.

11. CDC. Quarantine Station jurisdictions and contact information. [cited 2008 Jun 27]. Available from: http://www.cdc.gov/ncidod/dq/resources/Quarantine_Station_Contact_List.pdf.

12. U.S. Department of Health and Human Services. Title 42, Part 71. Foreign quarantine. Washington, DC: Government Printing Office; 2003 [cited 2004 Oct 25]. Available from: http://www.access.gpo.gov/nara/cfr/waisidx_03/42cfr71_03.html.

13. Executive Order 13295. Revised list of quarantinable communicable diseases. Federal Register 68(68):17255 (April 4, 2003) and Executive Order 13325. Amendment to

Executive Order 13295 Relating to Certain Influenza Viruses and Quarantinable Communicable Diseases. Federal Register 70(64):17299 (April 4, 2005). [cited 2008 Jun 27]. Available from: http://a257.g.akamaitech.net/7/257/2422/ 14mar20010800/edocket.access.gpo.gov/ 2003/pdf/03-8832.pdf and http:// a257.g.akamaitech.net/7/257/2422/ 01jan20051800/edocket.access.gpo.gov/2005/ pdf/05-6907.pdf.

TAKING ANIMALS ACROSS INTERNATIONAL BORDERS

G. Gale Galland, Robert J. Mullan, Heather Bair-Brake

Travelers should be advised that CDC restricts the importation of animals that may pose an infectious disease threat to humans. These restrictions apply to some pets, such as dogs and cats, as well as turtles, nonhuman primates, African rodents, birds, civets, bats, and other animals and animal products capable of causing human disease (see www.cdc.gov/yellowbook/AnimalImportation and www.cdc.gov/yellowbook/AnimalFaq).

Upon return, animals taken out of the United States are subject to the same regulations as those entering for the first time. The U.S. Department of Agriculture (USDA) and the U.S. Fish and Wildlife Service (FWS) also have jurisdiction over the importation of some animals. States may have additional restrictions on the importation of animals (see www.agr.wa.gov/FoodAnimal/AnimalHealth/StateVets.htm for additional information).

Health Certificates

- CDC regulations do not require general health certificates for animals (including dogs or cats) entering the United States
- Health certificates may be required for entry into some states
- Health certificates may be required by airlines for pet travel
- Travelers should check with officials in their state of destination and with the airline prior to the travel date

Dogs

Dogs are subject to inspection and may be denied entry into the United States if they have evidence of an infectious disease that can be transmitted to humans. If a dog appears to be ill, further examination by a licensed veterinarian at the owner's expense may be required before entry.

Unless a dog is being imported from a country considered "rabies-free" by the World Health Organization (see Table 2-16), it must be accompanied by a valid rabies vaccination certificate that includes the following information:

- The breed, sex, age, color, markings, and other identifying information
- A vaccination date at least 30 days before importation
- A vaccination date reflecting that the dog was at least 3 months of age at the time of vaccination
- The vaccination expiration date (if not shown, the date of vaccination must be within 12 months of date of importation)
- The signature of a licensed veterinarian

A dog not accompanied by a current rabies vaccination certificate may be admitted provided the importer completes a confinement letter agreeing to the following:

- Dogs must be kept confined at a place of the owner's choosing, including their home until proper rabies vaccination is obtained. Confinement is defined as isolation away from other animals and people except for contact necessary for the dog's care. If the dog is allowed out of its enclosure, the owner must muzzle the dog and use a leash.

- The dog must be vaccinated within 4 days of arrival at its destination and remain in confinement for at least 30 days after the date of vaccination.
- The dog may not be sold or transferred from the responsibility of the importer during the time of confinement.
- A copy of the confinement agreement (Form CDC 75.37) can be found on the CDC website at www.cdc.gov/yellowbook/ConfinementAgreement.
- Puppies <3 months of age are not considered old enough for rabies vaccination. Puppies <3 months of age may be admitted provided the importer completes a confinement agreement, vaccinates the animal at 3 months of age, and keeps the animal in confinement for at least 30 days after vaccination.
- Routine rabies vaccination of dogs is recommended in the United States and required by most state and local health authorities.
- Check with state authorities at the final destination to determine the local requirements for rabies vaccination.
- All pet dogs arriving in the state of Hawaii and the territory of Guam, even from the U.S. mainland, are subject to locally imposed quarantine requirements. For more information, consult http://hawaii.gov/hdoa/ai/aqs/info or call 808-483-7151 (Hawaii), or see http://k9.gov.gu/ or call 671-475-1426 (Guam).

Cats

- Cats are subject to inspection at ports of entry and may be denied entry into the United States if they have evidence of an infectious disease that can be transmitted to humans. If a cat appears to be ill, further examination by a licensed veterinarian at the owner's expense may be required at the port of entry.
- Cats are not required to have proof of rabies vaccination for importation into the United States.
- States may require rabies vaccination for cats, so it is a good idea to check with state and local health authorities at the final destination.
- All pet cats arriving in the state of Hawaii and the territory of Guam, even from the U.S. mainland, are subject to locally imposed quarantine requirements. For more information, consult http://hawaii.gov/hdoa/ai/aqs/info or call 808-483-7151 (Hawaii), or see http://k9.gov.gu/ or call 671-475-1426 (Guam).

Other Animals, Animal Products, and Vectors

Nonhuman Primates (Monkeys, Apes, etc.)

- Nonhuman primates can transmit a variety of serious diseases to humans, including Ebola and tuberculosis. Nonhuman primate entry into the United States is restricted, see—
  - www.cdc.gov/yellowbook/AnimalFaq
  - www.cdc.gov/yellowbook/Primates
- Nonhuman primates may only be imported into the United States by a CDC registered importer and only for scientific, educational, or exhibition purposes. Nonhuman primates may not be imported as pets.
- All nonhuman primates are considered endangered or threatened and require additional permits issued by FWS for import. More information is available at www.fws.gov/le/Travelers/TipsforTravelers.htm.
- Nonhuman primates that leave the United States may only return through a registered importer and only if they are imported for science, education, or exhibition.

Turtles

- Turtles can transmit *Salmonella* to humans, and because small turtles are often kept

as pets, restrictions apply to their importation. More information is available at—
- o   www.cdc.gov/yellowbook/AnimalFaq
- o   www.cdc.gov/yellowbook/FederalRegs42CFR71
- An individual may import no more than six viable turtle eggs or six live turtles with a carapace (shell) length of less than 4 inches.
- Seven or more turtles may be imported with permission from CDC and only for scientific, educational, or exhibition purposes.
- CDC has no restrictions on the importation of live turtles with a carapace length ≥4 inches. Check with USDA or U.S. Fish and Wildlife regarding additional requirements to import turtles.

African Rodents and Civets

- To reduce the risk of introducing monkeypox and the SARS-coronavirus, live African rodents and civets, as well as potentially infectious products made from these animals, may not be imported into the United States. More information is available at—
- o   www.cdc.gov/ncidod/monkeypox/embargoqa.htm
- o   http://edocket.access.gpo.gov/2003/03-27557.htm
- Exceptions may be made for scientific, exhibition, or educational purposes with a valid permit issued by CDC.
- African rodent and civet products that have been processed in a way to render them noninfectious do not require CDC permission for importation; however, these items should be accompanied by a statement indicating how they have been treated to render them noninfectious.

Birds from Countries with Highly Pathogenic Avian Influenza (H5N1)

- To reduce the risk of introducing highly pathogenic avian influenza (HPAI) H5N1 into the United States, CDC restricts the importation of birds and unprocessed bird products from countries where HPAI H5N1 has been confirmed in poultry (see www.cdc.gov/flu/avian/outbreaks/embargo.htm).
- Current details on the countries affected by the CDC restrictions may be found at www.cdc.gov/flu/avian/outbreaks/embargo.htm.
- These restrictions are subject to change at any time, depending on the current situation regarding the geographic range of this disease in birds and other animals, and the virus' transmissibility.
- USDA maintains similar restrictions. The CDC and USDA import restrictions allow U.S.-origin pet birds to return following quarantine for 30 days at a USDA facility. CDC and USDA allow import of processed bird products that have been rendered noninfectious. These products must be accompanied by a USDA permit and government certification confirming that the products were treated according to USDA requirements.

Bats

- Bats have been shown to be reservoirs of many viruses that can infect humans, including rabies virus, Nipah virus, SARS-coronavirus, and others. To reduce the risk of introducing these viruses, the importation of all live bats requires a permit from CDC.
- Because they may be endangered species, bats also require additional permits issued by FWS. The applications for a CDC import permit for these animals can be found at www.cdc.gov/yellowbook/bats.

Other Animals, Trophies, Animal Products, and Vectors

- Certain live animals, hosts, or vectors of human disease, including insects, biological materials, tissues, and other unprocessed animal products, may pose an infectious disease risk to humans and be restricted from entry.

○ For example, goatskin souvenirs (such as goatskin drums) from Haiti have been associated with human anthrax cases, and CDC restricts these items from entry into the United States.

○ Potentially infectious nonhuman primate trophies may be imported only with a permit issued by CDC and must be taken to a USDA-licensed taxidermist for processing. More information on import restrictions for nonhuman primate trophies may be found at www.cdc.gov/od/ohs/biosfty/IP_NHP_Guidance013004.pdf.

• In some circumstances, restricted items may be admitted with a permit from CDC for scientific, educational or exhibition purposes (see www.cdc.gov/od/eaipp/).

Measures at Ports of Entry

The goal of these restrictions is to prevent the importation into the United States of communicable diseases transmissible from animals to humans or other animals. Persons who violate these requirements may be subject to criminal and/or civil penalties. For additional information regarding importation of these animals, travelers should be advised to contact CDC, Attention: Division of Global Migration and Quarantine, Mailstop E03, Atlanta, Georgia 30333 (404-639-3441), or visit www.cdc.gov/yellowbook/AnimalFaq.

Travelers planning to import horses, ruminants, swine, poultry, birds, and dogs used for handling livestock should be advised to contact the USDA Animal Plant Health Inspection Service (301-734-8364) or at www.aphis.usda.gov regarding additional requirements.

Travelers planning to import fish, reptiles, spiders, wild birds, rabbits, bears, wild members of the cat family, or other wild or endangered animals should be advised to contact FWS (800-358-1949) or at www.fws.gov/le.

Traveling Abroad with a Pet

Travelers planning to take a companion animal to a foreign country should be advised to meet the entry requirements of the country of destination and transportation guidelines of the airline. To obtain this information, travelers should contact the country's embassy in Washington, D.C., or the nearest consulate (see www.state.gov/s/cpr/rls/fco/).

There are several ways to travel with a companion animal. The animal may be allowed in the cabin if it meets certain size and weight restrictions, may be checked in with luggage, or may be placed into cargo. Travelers intending to bring their pets onboard with them should check with the airline for space and size/weight restrictions. For the health of the animal, pets are allowed to travel in checked luggage or cargo only if weather conditions permit. The airline will be able to help determine the best dates and times for traveling with pets.

References

1. CDC. Compendium of animal rabies prevention and control, 2005: National Association of State Public Health Veterinarians, Inc. (NASPHV). MMWR Recomm Rep. 2005;54(RR-3):1–7.

2. CDC. Human rabies prevention—United States, 1999: recommendations of the Advisory Committee on Immunization Practices (ACIP). MMWR Recomm Rep. 1999;48(RR-1):1–21.

3. Demarcus TA, Tipple MA, Ostrowski SR. US policy for disease control among imported nonhuman primates. J Infect Dis. 1999;179(Suppl 1):S281–2.

4. Stam F, Romkens TE, Hekker TA, Smulders YM. Turtle-associated human salmonellosis. Clin Infect Dis. 2003;37(11):e167–9.

5. CDC. Update: Multistate outbreak of monkeypox—Illinois, Indiana, Kansas, Missouri, Ohio, and Wisconsin, 2003. MMWR Morb Mortal Wkly Rep. 2003;52(27):642–6.

6. Wu D, Tu C, Xin C, et al. Civets are equally susceptible to experimental infection by two different severe acute respiratory syndrome coronavirus isolates. J Virol. 2005;79(4):2620–5.

7. Dobson AP. Virology: What links bats to emerging infectious diseases? Science. 2005;310(5748):628–9.

8. Editorial: Bongo-drum disease. Lancet. 1974;1(7867):1152.

7

International Travel with Infants and Children

TRAVELING SAFELY WITH INFANTS AND CHILDREN

Nicholas Weinberg, Michelle Weinberg, Susan Maloney

Introduction

The number of children who travel or live outside their home countries has increased dramatically. An estimated 1.9 million children travel overseas each year. Although data about the incidence of pediatric illnesses associated with international travel are limited, the risks that children face while traveling are likely similar to the risks that their parents face.

The most common reported health problems among children are—

- Diarrheal illnesses,
- Malaria, and
- Motor vehicle- and water-related accidents.

Clinicians should—

- Review routine childhood and travel-related vaccinations. The pre-travel visit is an opportunity to assure that children are up-to-date on routine vaccinations.
- Obtain a complete assessment of travel-related activities.
- Provide preventive counseling and interventions tailored to specific risks, including special travel preparations and treatment that may be required for children with underlying conditions, chronic diseases, or immunocompromising conditions.
- Give special consideration to the risks of children who are visiting friends and relatives living in developing countries. These conditions may include increased risk of malaria, intestinal parasites, and tuberculosis.
- Consider counseling adults and older children to take a course in basic first aid prior to travel.

Diarrhea and Dehydration

Diarrhea and associated gastrointestinal illness are among the most common travel-related problems affecting children. Young children and infants are at high risk for diarrhea and other food- and waterborne illnesses because of limited pre-existing immunity and behavioral factors such as frequent hand-to-mouth contact. Infants and children with diarrhea can become dehydrated more quickly than adults.

Prevention

The etiology of travelers' diarrhea (TD) in children is similar to that in adults.

- For young infants, breastfeeding is the best way to reduce the risk of food- and waterborne illness.
- Travelers should use only purified water for drinking, preparing ice cubes, brushing teeth, and mixing infant formula and foods.
- Scrupulous attention should be paid to handwashing and cleaning pacifiers, teething rings, and toys that fall to the floor or are handled by others.
- When proper handwashing facilities are not available, an alcohol-based hand sanitizer can be used as a disinfecting agent. Alcohol does not remove organic material; visibly soiled hands should be washed with soap and water.
- Fresh dairy products in developing countries may not be pasteurized and may be diluted with untreated water.
- For short trips, parents may want to bring a supply of safe snacks from home for times when the children are hungry and the available food may not be appealing or safe.

Management of Diarrhea in Infants and Young Children

Adults traveling with children should be counseled about the signs and symptoms of dehydration and the proper use of World Health Organization (WHO) oral rehydration solutions (ORS).

Medical attention may be required for an infant or young child with diarrhea who has—

- signs of moderate to severe dehydration (Table 7-1),
- bloody diarrhea,
- fever higher than 101.5° F (38.5° C), or
- persistent vomiting (unable to maintain oral hydration).

ORS should be provided to the infant by bottle, oral syringe, or spoon while medical attention is being obtained. See more details about the use of ORS below.

Diarrheal stools in infants in diapers may induce a painful, red, eczematous rash on the buttocks. This rash does not respond to ordinary diaper rash preparations but clears up dramatically with the application of 1% hydrocortisone cream.

Table 7-1. Assessment of dehydration levels in infants

Signs	Severity		
	Mild	Moderate	Severe
General condition	Thirsty, restless, agitated	Thirsty, restless, irritable	Withdrawn, somnolent, or comatose; rapid deep breathing
Pulse	Normal	Rapid, weak	Rapid, weak
Anterior fontanelle	Normal	Sunken	Very sunken
Eyes	Normal	Sunken	Very sunken
Tears	Present	Absent	Absent
Mucous membranes	Slightly dry	Dry	Dry
Skin turgor	Normal	Decreased	Decreased with tenting
Urine	Normal	Reduced, concentrated	None for several hours
Weight loss	4%–5%	6%–9%	>10%

Assessment and Treatment of Dehydration

The greatest risk to the infant with diarrhea and vomiting is dehydration. Fever or increased ambient temperature increases fluid losses and speeds dehydration.

- Parents should be advised that dehydration is best prevented and treated by use of ORS, in addition to the infant's usual food (see Table 2-25).
- Rice and other cereal-based ORS, in which complex carbohydrates are substituted for glucose, are also available and may be more acceptable to young children.
- Adults traveling with children should be counseled that sports drinks, which are designed to replace water and electrolytes lost through sweat, do not contain the same proportions of electrolytes as the solution recommended by WHO for rehydration during diarrheal illness. However, if ORS is not readily available, children should be offered whatever palatable liquid they will take until ORS is obtained.

Oral Rehydration Solution (ORS) Use and Availability

ORS packets are available at stores or pharmacies in almost all developing countries. (See information below regarding ORS availability in the United States.)

- ORS is prepared by adding one packet to boiled or treated water. Travelers should be advised to check packet instructions carefully to ensure that the salts are added to the correct volume of water.
- ORS solution should be consumed or discarded within 12 hours if held at room temperature or 24 hours if kept refrigerated.
- A dehydrated child will drink ORS avidly; travelers should be advised to give it to the child as long as the dehydration persists. As dehydration lessens, the salty-tasting ORS solution may be refused, and another liquid can be offered. An infant or child who vomits the ORS will usually keep it down if it is offered by spoon in frequent small sips.
- Children weighing <10 kg who have mild to moderate dehydration should be administered 60–120 mL of ORS for each diarrheal stool or vomiting episode. Children who weigh 10 kg or more should receive 120–240 mL of ORS for each diarrheal stool or vomiting episode.
- Oral syringes that are available in most pharmacies for oral medications can be useful for the administration of ORS and can be included as part of the travelers' health kit for young children.
- Severe dehydration is a medical emergency that usually requires administration of fluids by IV or intraosseous routes.

ORS packets are available in the United States from Jianas Brothers Packaging Company, 2533 Southwest Boulevard, Kansas City, Missouri 64108, USA (816-421-2880). ORS packets may also be available at stores that sell outdoor recreation and camping supplies.

In addition, Cera Products, 9017 Mendenhall Court, Columbia, Maryland 21045, USA (410-309-1000 or 888-Ceralyte; www.ceraproductsinc.com), markets a rice cereal rather than a glucose-based product, Ceralyte, in different flavors.

Dietary Modification

- Breastfed infants should continue nursing on demand.
- Formula-fed infants should continue their usual formula during rehydration. They should receive a volume that is sufficient to satisfy energy and nutrient requirements. Lactose-free or lactose-reduced formulas are usually unnecessary. Diluting formula may slow resolution of diarrhea and is not recommended.
- Older infants and children receiving semisolid or solid foods should continue to receive their usual diet during the illness. Recommended foods include starches, cereals, yogurt, fruits, and vegetables. Foods that are high in simple sugars, such as soft drinks, undiluted apple juice, gelatins, and presweetened cereals, can exacerbate diarrhea by osmotic effects and should be avoided. In addition, foods high in fat may not be tolerated because of their tendency to delay gastric emptying.

- The practice of withholding food for 24 hours or more is not recommended. Early feeding can decrease changes in intestinal permeability caused by infection, reduce illness duration and improve nutritional outcome.
- Highly specific diets (e.g., the BRAT [bananas, rice, applesauce, and toast] diet) have been commonly recommended; however, similar to juice-centered and clear fluid diets, such severely restrictive diets have no scientific basis and should be avoided.
- Parents should be particularly careful to wash hands well after diaper changes for infants with diarrhea to avoid spreading infection to themselves and other family members.

Antibiotics

Few data are available regarding empiric administration of antibiotics for TD in children. The antimicrobial options for empiric treatment in children are limited.

- In practice, some clinicians prescribe azithromycin as a single dose (10 mg/kg) for 1–2 days when an antibiotic is indicated.
- Flavored oral suspension of azithromycin is available. Parents can obtain the unreconstituted powder, with clear instructions from the pharmacist as to how to mix it up if it becomes necessary to use it.
- Fluoroquinolones are frequently used for the empiric treatment of TD in adults. The use of fluoroquinolones is not generally recommended for children and adolescents <18 years of age because of cartilage damage seen in animals tested.
  - The only indication for fluoroquinolone use in children that has been approved by the Federal Drug Administration is for complicated urinary tract infections.
  - The American Academy of Pediatrics suggests some special circumstances for fluoroquinolone use, including the treatment of gastrointestinal infection caused by multidrug-resistant *Shigella* species, *Salmonella* species, *Vibrio cholerae*, or *Campylobacter jejuni*.
  - The routine use for empiric treatment for TD is not recommended.

Malaria

Malaria is one of the most serious, life-threatening diseases affecting pediatric international travelers, especially children who are visiting friends and relatives.

- Children with malaria can rapidly develop a high level of parasitemia.
- They are at increased risk for severe complications of malaria, including shock, seizures, coma, and death.
- Initial symptoms of malaria in children may mimic many other common causes of pediatric febrile illness and therefore may result in delayed diagnosis and treatment.
- Clinicians should counsel adults traveling in malarious areas with children to be aware of the signs and symptoms of malaria and to seek prompt medical attention if they develop.

Detailed information about malaria risk and chemoprophylaxis, as well as precautions for avoiding mosquito bites, is presented in the Protection Against Mosquitoes, Ticks, and Other Insects and Arthropods section in Chapter 2.

Antimalarial Drugs

Pediatric doses for malaria chemoprophylaxis are provided in Table 2-23. Pediatric doses of medications used for self-treatment are included in Table 2-22. All dosing should be calculated based on body weight. Medications used for infants and young children are the same as those recommended for adults, except under the following circumstances:

- Doxycycline should not be given to children <8 years of age due to the risk of teeth staining.
- Atovaquone/proguanil (Malarone) should not be used for prophylaxis in children weighing <5 kg (11 lbs) because of lack of data on safety and efficacy.

Chloroquine, mefloquine, and atovaquone/proguanil have a bitter taste. Before departure, pharmacists can be asked to pulverize tablets and prepare gelatin capsules with calculated pediatric doses.

- Mixing the powder in a small amount of food or drink can facilitate the administration of antimalarial drugs to infants and children.
- Additionally, any compounding pharmacy can alter the flavoring of malaria medication tablets so that they are more willingly ingested by children. Assistance with finding a compounding pharmacy is available on the International Academy of Compounding Pharmacists' website at www.iacprx.org/site/PageServer?pagename=home_page.

Because overdose of antimalarial drugs, particularly chloroquine, can be fatal, medication should be stored in childproof containers and kept out of the reach of infants and children.

Insect and Other Arthropod Precautions

Personal protection against mosquitoes and other biting insects is an important part of prevention of disease, particularly for such diseases as yellow fever, Japanese encephalitis, and dengue, for which no treatment is available.

General Protective Measures

- Children should sleep in rooms with air conditioning, screened windows, or under bed nets, when available.
- Mosquito netting should be used over infant carriers.
- Children can wear clothing that covers more skin, such as long pants and long sleeves, while outdoors.
- Clothing and mosquito nets can be treated with permethrin, a repellent and insecticide that repels and kills ticks, mosquitoes, and other arthropods. Permethrin remains effective through multiple washings. Clothing and bednets should be retreated according to the product label. Permethrin should not be applied to the skin.
- For more information on protecting against insect and other arthropod bites, see the Protection Against Mosquitoes, Ticks, and Other Insects and Arthropods section in Chapter 2.

Repellent Use

CDC recommends the use of repellents, with active ingredients registered with the United States Environmental Protection Agency (EPA), according to the product labels.

- Most repellents can be used on children >2 months of age, with the following considerations:
  - Products containing oil of lemon eucalyptus specify that they should not be used on children under the age of 3 years.
  - Repellent products must state any age restriction. If there is none, EPA has not required a restriction on the use of the product.
  - The American Academy of Pediatrics (AAP) recommends that repellents with DEET should not be used on infants <2 months old.
- Protect infants <2 months of age from biting mosquitoes by using an infant carrier draped with mosquito netting with an elastic edge for a tight fit.
- Apply repellents only to exposed skin.
- Never use repellents over cuts, wounds, or irritated skin.
- Do not allow young children to handle the product.
- When using repellent on a child, an adult should apply it to his or her own hands and then rub them on the child. Avoid the child's eyes and mouth, and apply sparingly around the ears.
- Do not apply repellent to children's hands. (Children tend to put their hands in their mouths.)

- Do not apply repellent under clothing.
- Heavy application and saturation are generally unnecessary for effectiveness. If biting insects do not respond to a thin film of repellent, then apply a bit more.
- After returning indoors, wash treated skin with soap and water or bathe. This is particularly important when repellents are used repeatedly in a day or on consecutive days.
- Keep repellents out of reach of children.

Products that contain repellents and sunscreen are generally **not** recommended because instructions for use are different, and the need to reapply sunscreen is usually more frequent than with repellent alone. Mosquito coils should be used with caution in the presence of children to avoid burns and inadvertent ingestion.

Infection and Infestation from Soil Contact

Children are more likely than adults to have contact with soil or sand and therefore may be exposed to infectious stages of parasites present in soil, including ascariasis, hookworm, cutaneous larva migrans, trichuriasis, and strongyloidiasis.

- Children and infants should wear protective footwear and play on a sheet or towel rather than directly on the ground.
- Clothing should not be dried on the ground. Clothing or diapers dried in the open air should be ironed before use to prevent infestation with fly larvae (i.e., myiasis), in areas where that might be a risk.

Animal Bites and Rabies

Worldwide, rabies is more common in children than adults. In addition to the potential for increased contact with animals, children are also more likely to be bitten on the head or neck, leading to more severe injuries.

- Children and their families should be counseled to avoid all stray or unfamiliar animals and to inform adults of any contact or bites.
- Mammal-associated injuries should be washed thoroughly with water and soap (and povidone iodine if available), and the child should be evaluated promptly to assess the need for rabies postexposure prophylaxis. Bats throughout the world are considered to have the potential of transmitting rabies virus.

Air Travel

Although air travel is safe for healthy newborns, infants, and children, a few issues should be considered in preparation for travel.

- Children with chronic heart or lung problems may be at risk for hypoxia during flight, and a physician should be consulted before travel.
- Making sure that children can be safely restrained during a flight is an important safety consideration. Severe turbulence or a nonfatal crash can create enough momentum that a parent cannot hold onto a child.
  - Children should be placed in a rear-facing Federal Aviation Authority (FAA)-approved child-safety seat until they are at least 1 year old and weigh at least 20 pounds.
  - Children >1 year of age and 20–40 pounds in body weight should use a forward-facing FAA-approved child safety seat, while children weighing more than 40 pounds can be secured in the aircraft seat belt.
- Ear pain can be very troublesome for infants and children during descent. Equalization of pressure in the middle ear can be facilitated by swallowing or chewing.
  - Infants should nurse or suck on a bottle.

- o Older children can try chewing gum.
- o Antihistamines and decongestants have not been shown to be of benefit in this situation.
- There is no evidence that air travel exacerbates the symptoms or complications associated with otitis media.
- Travel to different time zones, "jet lag," and schedule disruptions can disturb sleep patterns in infants and children, as well as adults. After arrival, children should be encouraged to be active outside during daylight hours to promote adjustment.

Accidents

Vehicle-Related

Vehicle-related accidents are the leading cause of death in children who travel.

- While traveling in automobiles and other vehicles, children weighing <40 pounds should be restrained in age-appropriate car seats or booster seats, as described above. These seats often must be carried from home, since availability of well-maintained and approved seats may be limited abroad.
- In general, children are safest traveling in the rear seat; no one should ever travel in the bed of a pick-up truck.
- Families should be counseled that in many developing countries cars may lack front or rear seatbelts.

Drowning and Water-Related Illness and Injuries

Drowning is the second leading cause of death in young travelers. Children may not be familiar with hazards in the ocean or in rivers. Swimming pools may not have protective fencing to keep toddlers from falling into the pool.

- Close supervision of children around water is essential.
- Appropriate water safety devices such as life vests may not be available abroad, and families should consider bringing these from home.
- Protective footwear is important to avoid injury in many marine environments.

Schistosomiasis is a risk to children and adults in endemic areas. While in schistosomiasis-endemic areas (see Map 5-7), children should not swim in fresh, unchlorinated water.

Accommodations

Conditions at hotels and other lodging may not be as safe as those in the United States, and accommodations should be carefully inspected for exposed wiring, pest poisons, paint chips, or inadequate stairway or balcony railings.

Altitude

Children are as susceptible to altitude illness as adults. Young children who cannot talk can show nonspecific symptoms, such as loss of appetite and irritability. They may present with unexplained fussiness and change in sleep and activity patterns. Older children may complain of headache or shortness of breath.

If a child demonstrates unexplained symptoms after an ascent to altitude, it may be necessary to descend to see if they improve. Acetazolamide (Diamox) is not approved for pediatric use for altitude illness, but it is generally safe in children when used for other indications.

Sun Exposure

Sun exposure and particularly sunburn before age 15 are strongly associated with melanoma and other forms of skin cancer. Exposure to UV light is highest near the equator, at high altitudes, during midday (10 am to 4 pm), and where light is reflected off water or snow.

- Sunscreens are generally recommended for use in children >6 months of age. Sunscreens (or sun blocks), either physical (e.g., titanium or zinc oxides) or chemical, at least SPF 15 and providing protection from both UVA and UVB, should be applied as directed, and re-applied as needed after sweating and water exposure.
- Babies <6 months of age require extra protection from the sun because of their thinner and more sensitive skin; severe sunburn for this age group is considered a medical emergency. Babies should be kept in the shade and wear clothing that covers the entire body; a minimal amount of sunscreen can be applied to small exposed areas, including the infant's face and hands.
- There are sun-blocking shirts available that are made for swimming and preclude having to smear sunscreens over the entire trunk.
- Hats and sunglasses also reduce sun injury to skin and eyes.
- If both sunscreen and insect repellent are applied, the efficacy of the sunscreen is diminished by one third, and covering attire should be worn or time in the sun decreased accordingly.

Other General Considerations

Travel Stress

Changes in schedule, activities, and environment can be stressful for children. Including children in planning for the trip and bringing along familiar toys or other objects can decrease these stresses. For children with chronic illnesses, decisions regarding timing and itinerary should be made in consultation with their health-care provider(s).

Insurance

As for any traveler, insurance coverage for illnesses and accidents while abroad should be verified before departure. Consideration should be given to purchasing special travel insurance for airlifting or air ambulance to an area with adequate medical care.

Identification

In case family members become separated, each infant or child should carry identifying information and contact numbers in their own clothing or pockets.

Because of concerns about illegal transport of children across international borders, if only one parent is traveling with the child he or she may need to carry relevant custody papers or a notarized permission letter from the other parent.

Pediatric Travel Health Kit

In addition to the travel health kit items listed in Chapter 2, parents with children may also consider the following items:

- Safe water and snacks
- Child-safe hand wipes
- ORS packets
- Oral syringes for administration of medications and ORS
- Diapers and diaper rash ointment—if the child still wears diapers. Parents should try to ascertain whether reliable supplies of disposable diapers are available at their destination. If not, they will need to carry enough for the duration of their trip.
- Any medications the child takes regularly, bringing enough for the entire trip
- Other medications occasionally used (e.g., acetaminophen) if illness develops (Locally purchased medications and health products may not be available or may be counterfeit.)

CHAPTER
7
International Travel with Infants and Children
Traveling Safely with Infants and Children

References

1. King C, Glass R, Bresee J, et al. Managing acute gastroenteritis among children: oral rehydration, maintenance, and nutritional therapy. MMWR Recomm Rep. 2003;52(RR-16):1–16.
2. American Academy of Pediatrics. Antimicrobial agents and related therapy. In: Pickering LK,

Baker CJ, Long SS, McMillan JA, editors. Red book: 2006 Report of the Committee on Infectious Diseases. 27th ed. Elk Grove Village, IL: American Academy of Pediatrics; 2006. p.735–6.

VACCINE RECOMMENDATIONS FOR INFANTS AND CHILDREN

Sheila M. Mackell

Vaccinating children for travel requires careful evaluation. Whenever possible, children should complete the routine immunizations of childhood on a normal schedule. However, travel at an earlier age may require accelerated schedules.

- Not all travel-related vaccines are effective in infants, and some are specifically contraindicated.

The recommended childhood and adolescent immunization schedules are depicted in Tables 7-2 and 7-3. Table 7-4 depicts the catch-up schedule for children and adolescents who start their vaccination schedule late or who are >1 month behind. This table also describes the recommended minimal intervals between doses for children who need to be vaccinated on an accelerated schedule, which may be necessary prior to international travel. Proof of yellow fever vaccination is required for entry into certain countries.

Modifying the Immunization Schedule for Inadequately Immunized Infants and Younger Children Before International Travel

Several factors influence recommendations for the age at which a vaccine is administered, including age-specific risks of the disease and its complications, the ability of people of a given age to develop an adequate immune response to the vaccine, and potential interference with the immune response by passively transferred maternal antibody.

The routine immunization recommendations and schedules for infants and children in the United States do not provide specific guidelines for those traveling internationally before the age when specific vaccines and toxoids are routinely recommended. Recommended age limitations are based on potential adverse events (yellow fever), lack of efficacy or inadequate immune response (polysaccharide vaccines and influenza), maternal antibody interference (measles, mumps, rubella), or lack of safety data. In deciding when to travel with a young infant or child, parents should be advised that the earliest opportunity to receive routinely recommended immunizations in the United States (except for the dose of hepatitis B vaccine at birth) is at 6 weeks of age.

Routine Infant and Childhood Vaccinations

Hepatitis B Vaccine

Hepatitis B virus (HBV) is a cause of acute and chronic hepatitis, cirrhosis, and hepatocellular carcinoma. There are more than 200 million chronically infected persons worldwide. The risk of chronic infection is highest when infection occurs in infancy or childhood and declines with age.

- Infants and children who have not previously been vaccinated and who are traveling

Table 7-2. Recommended immunization schedule for ages 0–6 years—United States, 2009

Recommended Immunization Schedule for Persons Aged 0 Through 6 Years—United States • 2009

For those who fall behind or start late, see the catch-up schedule

Vaccine ▼ Age ▶	Birth	1 month	2 months	4 months	6 months	12 months	15 months	18 months	19–23 months	2–3 years	4–6 years
Hepatitis B[1]	HepB	HepB		see footnote 1		HepB					
Rotavirus[2]			RV	RV	RV[2]						
Diphtheria, Tetanus, Pertussis[3]			DTaP	DTaP	DTaP		see footnote 3	DTaP			DTaP
Haemophilus influenzae type b[4]			Hib	Hib	Hib[4]	Hib					
Pneumococcal[5]			PCV	PCV	PCV	PCV				PPSV	
Inactivated Poliovirus			IPV	IPV		IPV					IPV
Influenza[6]						Influenza (Yearly)					
Measles, Mumps, Rubella[7]						MMR		see footnote 7			MMR
Varicella[8]						Varicella		see footnote 8			Varicella
Hepatitis A[9]						HepA (2 doses)				HepA Series	
Meningococcal[10]										MCV	

■ Range of recommended ages

■ Certain high-risk groups

This schedule indicates the recommended ages for routine administration of currently licensed vaccines, as of December 1, 2008, for children aged 0 through 6 years. Any dose not administered at the recommended age should be administered at a subsequent visit, when indicated and feasible. Licensed combination vaccines may be used whenever any component of the combination is indicated and other components are not contraindicated and if approved by the Food and Drug Administration for that dose of the series. Providers should consult the relevant Advisory Committee on Immunization Practices statement for detailed recommendations, including high-risk conditions: http://www.cdc.gov/vaccines/pubs/acip-list.htm. Clinically significant adverse events that follow immunization should be reported to the Vaccine Adverse Event Reporting System (VAERS). Guidance about how to obtain and complete a VAERS form is available at http://www.vaers.hhs.gov or by telephone, 800-822-7967.

1. Hepatitis B vaccine (HepB). *(Minimum age: birth)*
At birth:
• Administer monovalent HepB to all newborns before hospital discharge.
• If mother is hepatitis B surface antigen (HBsAg)-positive, administer HepB and 0.5 mL of hepatitis B immune globulin (HBIG) within 12 hours of birth.
• If mother's HBsAg status is unknown, administer HepB within 12 hours of birth. Determine mother's HBsAg status as soon as possible and, if HBsAg-positive, administer HBIG (no later than age 1 week).
After the birth dose:
• The HepB series should be completed with either monovalent HepB or a combination vaccine containing HepB. The second dose should be administered at age 1 or 2 months. The final dose should be administered no earlier than age 24 weeks.
• Infants born to HBsAg-positive mothers should be tested for HBsAg and antibody to HBsAg (anti-HBs) after completion of at least 3 doses of the HepB series, at age 9 through 18 months (generally at the next well-child visit).
4-month dose:
• Administration of 4 doses of HepB to infants is permissible when combination vaccines containing HepB are administered after the birth dose.

2. Rotavirus vaccine (RV). *(Minimum age: 6 weeks)*
• Administer the first dose at age 6 through 14 weeks (maximum age: 14 weeks 6 days). Vaccination should not be initiated for infants aged 15 weeks or older (i.e., 15 weeks 0 days or older).
• Administer the final dose in the series by age 8 months 0 days.
• If Rotarix® is administered at ages 2 and 4 months, a dose at 6 months is not indicated.

3. Diphtheria and tetanus toxoids and acellular pertussis vaccine (DTaP). *(Minimum age: 6 weeks)*
• The fourth dose may be administered as early as age 12 months, provided at least 6 months have elapsed since the third dose.
• Administer the final dose in the series at age 4 through 6 years.

4. Haemophilus influenzae type b conjugate vaccine (Hib). *(Minimum age: 6 weeks)*
• If PRP-OMP (PedvaxHIB® or Comvax® [HepB-Hib]) is administered at ages 2 and 4 months, a dose at age 6 months is not indicated.
• TriHiBit® (DTaP/Hib) should not be used for doses at ages 2, 4, or 6 months but can be used as the final dose in children aged 12 months or older.

5. Pneumococcal vaccine. *(Minimum age: 6 weeks for pneumococcal conjugate vaccine [PCV]; 2 years for pneumococcal polysaccharide vaccine [PPSV])*
• PCV is recommended for all children aged younger than 5 years. Administer 1 dose of PCV to all healthy children aged 24 through 59 months who are not completely vaccinated for their age.

• Administer PPSV to children aged 2 years or older with certain underlying medical conditions (see *MMWR* 2000;49[No. RR-9]), including a cochlear implant.

6. Influenza vaccine. *(Minimum age: 6 months for trivalent inactivated influenza vaccine [TIV]; 2 years for live, attenuated influenza vaccine [LAIV])*
• Administer annually to children aged 6 months through 18 years.
• For healthy nonpregnant persons (i.e., those who do not have underlying medical conditions that predispose them to influenza complications) aged 2 through 49 years, either LAIV or TIV may be used.
• Children receiving TIV should receive 0.25 mL if aged 6 through 35 months or 0.5 mL if aged 3 years or older.
• Administer 2 doses (separated by at least 4 weeks) to children aged younger than 9 years who are receiving influenza vaccine for the first time or who were vaccinated for the first time during the previous influenza season but only received 1 dose.

7. Measles, mumps, and rubella vaccine (MMR). *(Minimum age: 12 months)*
• Administer the second dose at age 4 through 6 years. However, the second dose may be administered before age 4, provided at least 28 days have elapsed since the first dose.

8. Varicella vaccine. *(Minimum age: 12 months)*
• Administer the second dose at age 4 through 6 years. However, the second dose may be administered before age 4, provided at least 3 months have elapsed since the first dose.
• For children aged 12 months through 12 years the minimum interval between doses is 3 months. However, if the second dose was administered at least 28 days after the first dose, it can be accepted as valid.

9. Hepatitis A vaccine (HepA). *(Minimum age: 12 months)*
• Administer to all children aged 1 year (i.e., aged 12 through 23 months). Administer 2 doses at least 6 months apart.
• Children not fully vaccinated by age 2 years can be vaccinated at subsequent visits.
• HepA also is recommended for children older than 1 year who live in areas where vaccination programs target older children or who are at increased risk of infection. See *MMWR* 2006;55(No. RR-7).

10. Meningococcal vaccine. *(Minimum age: 2 years for meningococcal conjugate vaccine [MCV] and for meningococcal polysaccharide vaccine [MPSV])*
• Administer MCV to children aged 2 through 10 years with terminal complement component deficiency, anatomic or functional asplenia, and certain other high-risk groups. See *MMWR* 2005;54(No. RR-7).
• Persons who received MPSV 3 or more years previously and who remain at increased risk for meningococcal disease should be revaccinated with MCV.

The Recommended Immunization Schedules for Persons Aged 0 Through 18 Years are approved by the Advisory Committee on Immunization Practices (www.cdc.gov/vaccines/recs/acip), the American Academy of Pediatrics (http://www.aap.org), and the American Academy of Family Physicians (http://www.aafp.org).

DEPARTMENT OF HEALTH AND HUMAN SERVICES • CENTERS FOR DISEASE CONTROL AND PREVENTION

---

to areas with intermediate and high HBV endemicity are at risk if they are directly exposed to blood (or body fluids containing blood) from the local population.

• Circumstances in which HBV transmission could occur in children include receipt of blood transfusions not screened for HBV surface antigen (HBsAg), exposure to unsterilized medical or dental equipment, or continuous close contact with local residents who have open skin lesions (impetigo, scabies, or scratched insect bites).

Hepatitis B vaccine is recommended for all infants in the United States, with the first dose administered soon after birth and before hospital discharge.

Table 7-3. Recommended immunization schedule for ages 7–18 years—United States, 2009

Recommended Immunization Schedule for Persons Aged 7 Through 18 Years—United States • 2009
For those who fall behind or start late, see the schedule below and the catch-up schedule

Vaccine ▼ Age ►	7–10 years	11–12 years	13–18 years	
Tetanus, Diphtheria, Pertussis[1]	see footnote 1	Tdap	Tdap	Range of recommended ages
Human Papillomavirus[2]	see footnote 2	HPV (3 doses)	HPV Series	
Meningococcal[3]	MCV	MCV	MCV	
Influenza[4]	Influenza (Yearly)			Catch-up immunization
Pneumococcal[5]	PPSV			
Hepatitis A[6]	HepA Series			
Hepatitis B[7]	HepB Series			Certain high-risk groups
Inactivated Poliovirus[8]	IPV Series			
Measles, Mumps, Rubella[9]	MMR Series			
Varicella[10]	Varicella Series			

This schedule indicates the recommended ages for routine administration of currently licensed vaccines, as of December 1, 2008, for children aged 7 through 18 years. Any dose not administered at the recommended age should be administered at a subsequent visit, when indicated and feasible. Licensed combination vaccines may be used whenever any component of the combination is indicated and other components are not contraindicated and if approved by the Food and Drug Administration for that dose of the series. Providers should consult the relevant Advisory Committee on Immunization Practices statement for detailed recommendations, including high-risk conditions: http://www.cdc.gov/vaccines/pubs/acip-list.htm. Clinically significant adverse events that follow immunization should be reported to the Vaccine Adverse Event Reporting System (VAERS). Guidance about how to obtain and complete a VAERS form is available at http://www.vaers.hhs.gov or by telephone, 800-822-7967.

1. Tetanus and diphtheria toxoids and acellular pertussis vaccine (Tdap). *(Minimum age: 10 years for BOOSTRIX® and 11 years for ADACEL®)*
- Administer at age 11 or 12 years for those who have completed the recommended childhood DTP/DTaP vaccination series and have not received a tetanus and diphtheria toxoid (Td) booster dose.
- Persons aged 13 through 18 years who have not received Tdap should receive a dose.
- A 5-year interval from the last Td dose is encouraged when Tdap is used as a booster dose; however, a shorter interval may be used if pertussis immunity is needed.

2. Human papillomavirus vaccine (HPV). *(Minimum age: 9 years)*
- Administer the first dose to females at age 11 or 12 years.
- Administer the second dose 2 months after the first dose and the third dose 6 months after the first dose (at least 24 weeks after the first dose).
- Administer the series to females at age 13 through 18 years if not previously vaccinated.

3. Meningococcal conjugate vaccine (MCV).
- Administer at age 11 or 12 years, or at age 13 through 18 years if not previously vaccinated.
- Administer to previously unvaccinated college freshmen living in a dormitory.
- MCV is recommended for children aged 2 through 10 years with terminal complement component deficiency, anatomic or functional asplenia, and certain other groups at high risk. See *MMWR* 2005;54(No. RR-7).
- Persons who received MPSV 5 or more years previously and remain at increased risk for meningococcal disease should be revaccinated with MCV.

4. Influenza vaccine.
- Administer annually to children aged 6 months through 18 years.
- For healthy nonpregnant persons (i.e., those who do not have underlying medical conditions that predispose them to influenza complications) aged 2 through 49 years, either LAIV or TIV may be used.
- Administer 2 doses (separated by at least 4 weeks) to children aged younger than 9 years who are receiving influenza vaccine for the first time or who were vaccinated for the first time during the previous influenza season but only received 1 dose.

5. Pneumococcal polysaccharide vaccine (PPSV).
- Administer to children with certain underlying medical conditions (see *MMWR* 1997;46[No. RR-8]), including a cochlear implant. A single revaccination should be administered to children with functional or anatomic asplenia or other immunocompromising condition after 5 years.

6. Hepatitis A vaccine (HepA).
- Administer 2 doses at least 6 months apart.
- HepA is recommended for children older than 1 year who live in areas where vaccination programs target older children or who are at increased risk of infection. See *MMWR* 2006;55(No. RR-7).

7. Hepatitis B vaccine (HepB).
- Administer the 3-dose series to those not previously vaccinated.
- A 2-dose series (separated by at least 4 months) of adult formulation Recombivax HB® is licensed for children aged 11 through 15 years.

8. Inactivated poliovirus vaccine (IPV).
- For children who received an all-IPV or all-oral poliovirus (OPV) series, a fourth dose is not necessary if the third dose was administered at age 4 years or older.
- If both OPV and IPV were administered as part of a series, a total of 4 doses should be administered, regardless of the child's current age.

9. Measles, mumps, and rubella vaccine (MMR).
- If not previously vaccinated, administer 2 doses or the second dose for those who have received only 1 dose, with at least 28 days between doses.

10. Varicella vaccine.
- For persons aged 7 through 18 years without evidence of immunity (see *MMWR* 2007;56[No. RR-4]), administer 2 doses if not previously vaccinated or the second dose if they have received only 1 dose.
- For persons aged 7 through 12 years, the minimum interval between doses is 3 months. However, if the second dose was administered at least 28 days after the first dose, it can be accepted as valid.
- For persons aged 13 years and older, the minimum interval between doses is 28 days.

The Recommended Immunization Schedules for Persons Aged 0 Through 18 Years are approved by the Advisory Committee on Immunization Practices (www.cdc.gov/vaccines/recs/acip), the American Academy of Pediatrics (http://www.aap.org), and the American Academy of Family Physicians (http://www.aafp.org).
DEPARTMENT OF HEALTH AND HUMAN SERVICES • CENTERS FOR DISEASE CONTROL AND PREVENTION

- Infants and children who will travel should receive three doses of HBV vaccine before traveling.
  - The interval between doses one and two should be at least 4 weeks.
  - Between doses two and three, the interval should be a minimum of 8 weeks; the interval between doses one and three should be at least 16 weeks. The third dose should not be given before the infant is at least 24 weeks of age.
- Adolescents not previously vaccinated with hepatitis B vaccine should be vaccinated at 11–12 years of age.
  - For adolescents, the usual schedule is two doses separated by at least 4 weeks, followed by a third dose 4–6 months after the second dose.

Table 7-4. Recommended childhood catch-up immunization schedule—United States, 2009. Children and adolescents who start late or who are more than 1 month behind.

Catch-up Immunization Schedule for Persons Aged 4 Months Through 18 Years Who Start Late or Who Are More Than 1 Month Behind—United States • 2009

The table below provides catch-up schedules and minimum intervals between doses for children whose vaccinations have been delayed. A vaccine series does not need to be restarted, regardless of the time that has elapsed between doses. Use the section appropriate for the child's age.

Vaccine	Minimum Age for Dose 1	Minimum Interval Between Doses			
		Dose 1 to Dose 2	Dose 2 to Dose 3	Dose 3 to Dose 4	Dose 4 to Dose 5
CATCH-UP SCHEDULE FOR PERSONS AGED 4 MONTHS THROUGH 6 YEARS					
Hepatitis B[1]	Birth	4 weeks	**8 weeks** (and at least 16 weeks after first dose)		
Rotavirus[2]	6 wks	4 weeks	4 weeks[2]		
Diphtheria, Tetanus, Pertussis[3]	6 wks	4 weeks	4 weeks	6 months	6 months[3]
Haemophilus influenzae type b[4]	6 wks	**4 weeks** if first dose administered at younger than age 12 months **8 weeks** (as final dose) if first dose administered at age 12-14 months **No further doses needed** if first dose administered at age 15 months or older	**4 weeks**[4] if current age is younger than 12 months **8 weeks** (as final dose)[4] if current age is 12 months or older and second dose administered at younger than age 15 months **No further doses needed** if previous dose administered at age 15 months or older	**8 weeks** (as final dose) This dose only necessary for children aged 12 months through 59 months who received 3 doses before age 12 months	
Pneumococcal[5]	6 wks	**4 weeks** if first dose administered at younger than age 12 months **8 weeks** (as final dose for healthy children) if first dose administered at age 12 months or older or current age 24 through 59 months **No further doses needed** for healthy children if first dose administered at age 24 months or older	**4 weeks** if current age is younger than 12 months **8 weeks** (as final dose for healthy children) if current age is 12 months or older **No further doses needed** for healthy children if previous dose administered at age 24 months or older	**8 weeks** (as final dose) This dose only necessary for children aged 12 months through 59 months who received 3 doses before age 12 months or for high-risk children who received 3 doses at any age	
Inactivated Poliovirus[6]	6 wks	4 weeks	4 weeks	4 weeks[6]	
Measles, Mumps, Rubella[7]	12 mos	4 weeks			
Varicella[8]	12 mos	3 months			
Hepatitis A[9]	12 mos	6 months			
CATCH-UP SCHEDULE FOR PERSONS AGED 7 THROUGH 18 YEARS					
Tetanus, Diphtheria/ Tetanus, Diphtheria, Pertussis[10]	7 yrs[10]	4 weeks	**4 weeks** if first dose administered at younger than age 12 months **6 months** if first dose administered at age 12 months or older	**6 months** if first dose administered at younger than age 12 months	
Human Papillomavirus[11]	9 yrs	Routine dosing intervals are recommended[11]			
Hepatitis A[9]	12 mos	6 months			
Hepatitis B[1]	Birth	4 weeks	**8 weeks** (and at least 16 weeks after first dose)		
Inactivated Poliovirus[6]	6 wks	4 weeks	4 weeks	4 weeks[6]	
Measles, Mumps, Rubella[7]	12 mos	4 weeks			
Varicella[8]	12 mos	**3 months** if the person is younger than age 13 years **4 weeks** if the person is aged 13 years or older			

1. Hepatitis B vaccine (HepB).
- Administer the 3-dose series to those not previously vaccinated.
- A 2-dose series (separated by at least 4 months) of adult formulation Recombivax HB® is licensed for children aged 11 through 15 years.

2. Rotavirus vaccine (RV).
- The maximum age for the first dose is 14 weeks 6 days. Vaccination should not be initiated for infants aged 15 weeks or older (i.e., 15 weeks 0 days or older).
- Administer the final dose in the series by age 8 months 0 days.
- If Rotarix® was administered for the first and second doses, a third dose is not indicated.

3. Diphtheria and tetanus toxoids and acellular pertussis vaccine (DTaP).
- The fifth dose is not necessary if the fourth dose was administered at age 4 years or older.

4. *Haemophilus influenzae* type b conjugate vaccine (Hib).
- Hib vaccine is not generally recommended for persons aged 5 years or older. No efficacy data are available on which to base a recommendation concerning use of Hib vaccine for older children and adults. However, studies suggest good immunogenicity in persons who have sickle cell disease, leukemia, or HIV infection, or who have had a splenectomy; administering 1 dose of Hib vaccine to these persons is not contraindicated.
- If the first 2 doses were PRP-OMP (PedvaxHIB® or Comvax®), and administered at age 11 months or younger, the third (and final) dose should be administered at age 12 through 15 months and at least 8 weeks after the second dose.
- If the first dose was administered at age 7 through 11 months, administer 2 doses separated by 4 weeks and a final dose at age 12 through 15 months.

5. Pneumococcal vaccine.
- Administer 1 dose of pneumococcal conjugate vaccine (PCV) to all healthy children aged 24 through 59 months who have not received at least 1 dose of PCV on or after age 12 months.
- For children aged 24 through 59 months with underlying medical conditions, administer 1 dose of PCV if 3 doses were received previously or administer 2 doses of PCV at least 8 weeks apart if fewer than 3 doses were received previously.
- Administer pneumococcal polysaccharide vaccine (PPSV) to children aged 2 years or older with certain underlying medical conditions (see *MMWR* 2000;49[No. RR-9]), including a cochlear implant, at least 8 weeks after the last dose of PCV.

6. Inactivated poliovirus vaccine (IPV).
- For children who received an all-IPV or all-oral poliovirus (OPV) series, a fourth dose is not necessary if the third dose was administered at age 4 years or older.
- If both OPV and IPV were administered as part of a series, a total of 4 doses should be administered, regardless of the child's current age.

7. Measles, mumps, and rubella vaccine (MMR).
- Administer the second dose at age 4 through 6 years. However, the second dose may be administered before age 4, provided at least 28 days have elapsed since the first dose.
- If not previously vaccinated, administer 2 doses with at least 28 days between doses.

8. Varicella vaccine.
- Administer the second dose at age 4 through 6 years. However, the second dose may be administered before age 4, provided at least 3 months have elapsed since the first dose.
- For persons aged 12 months through 12 years, the minimum interval between doses is 3 months. However, if the second dose was administered at least 28 days after the first dose, it can be accepted as valid.
- For persons aged 13 years and older, the minimum interval between doses is 28 days.

9. Hepatitis A vaccine (HepA).
- HepA is recommended for children older than 1 year who live in areas where vaccination programs target older children or who are at increased risk of infection. See *MMWR* 2006;55(No. RR-7).

10. Tetanus and diphtheria toxoids vaccine (Td) and tetanus and diphtheria toxoids and acellular pertussis vaccine (Tdap).
- Doses of DTaP are counted as part of the Td/Tdap series.
- Tdap should be substituted for a single dose of Td in the catch-up series or as a booster for children aged 10 through 18 years; use Td for other doses.

11. Human papillomavirus vaccine (HPV).
- Administer the series to females at age 13 through 18 years if not previously vaccinated.
- Use recommended routine dosing intervals for series catch-up (i.e., the second and third doses should be administered at 2 and 6 months after the first dose). However, the minimum interval between the first and second doses is 4 weeks. The minimum interval between the second and third doses is 12 weeks, and the third dose should be given at least 24 weeks after the first dose.

Information about reporting reactions after immunization is available online at http://www.vaers.hhs.gov or by telephone, 800-822-7967. Suspected cases of vaccine-preventable diseases should be reported to the state or local health department. Additional information, including precautions and contraindications for immunization, is available from the National Center for Immunization and Respiratory Diseases at http://www.cdc.gov/vaccines or telephone, 800-CDC-INFO (800-232-4636).

DEPARTMENT OF HEALTH AND HUMAN SERVICES • CENTERS FOR DISEASE CONTROL AND PREVENTION

- A two-dose series (Recombivax HB, 10 mcg) is licensed for 11- to 15-year-olds and can be given at 0 and 4 to 6 months later.

Diphtheria and Tetanus Toxoid and Pertussis Vaccine

Diphtheria, tetanus, and pertussis each occur worldwide and are endemic in countries with low immunization levels. Infants and children leaving the United States should be immunized before traveling.

- Optimum protection against diphtheria, tetanus, and pertussis is achieved with at least three but preferably four doses of diphtheria and tetanus toxoids and acellular pertussis vaccine (DTaP).
- Two doses of DTaP received at intervals at least 4 weeks apart can provide some protection; however, a single dose offers little protective benefit.
- Parents should be informed that infants and children who have not received at least three doses of DTaP might not be fully protected against pertussis.

The usual primary series includes four doses given at 2, 4, 6, and 15–18 months of age. A fifth (booster) dose is recommended when the child is 4–6 years of age. The fifth dose is not necessary if the fourth dose in the primary series was given after the child's fourth birthday.

For infants and children <7 years of age, the schedule can be accelerated as soon as the infant is 6 weeks of age, with the second and third doses given 4 weeks after each preceding dose. The fourth dose should not be given before the infant is 12 months of age and should be separated from the third dose by at least 6 months. The fifth (booster) dose should not be given before the child is 4 years of age.

Haemophilus influenzae *Type b Conjugate Vaccine*

Haemophilus influenzae type b (Hib) is an endemic disease worldwide that can cause fatal meningitis, epiglottitis, and other invasive diseases. Infants and children should have optimal protection before traveling.

- Routine Hib vaccination beginning at 2 months of age is recommended for all U.S. children. The first dose may be given when an infant is as young as 6 weeks of age.
- Vaccination before age 6 weeks may induce immune tolerance to subsequent vaccines and should never be done.

A primary series consists of two or three doses (depending on the type of vaccine used) with a minimum interval of 4 weeks between doses.

- A booster dose is recommended when the infant is at least 12 months of age, at least 8 weeks after the previous dose.
- If Hib vaccination is started when the infant or child is 7 months of age or older, fewer doses are required.
- A shortage of Hib vaccine supply in the United States in 2008 may result in deferral of the booster dose at 12–15 months. When the supply is replenished, clinicians may need to review a child's earlier vaccination history with Hib.

Considerations for Travel by Age
- If previously unvaccinated, infants <15 months of age should receive at least two vaccine doses before travel. An interval as short as 4 weeks between these two doses is acceptable.
- Unvaccinated infants and children 15–59 months of age should receive a single dose of Hib vaccine.
- Children >59 months of age, adolescents, and adults do not need to be vaccinated unless a specific condition exists such as functional or anatomic asplenia, immunodeficiency, immunosuppression, or HIV infection.

If different brands of vaccine are administered, a total of three doses of Hib conjugate vaccine completes the primary series. After completion of the primary infant vaccination series, any of the licensed Hib conjugate vaccines may be used for the booster dose when the infant is 12–15 months of age.

A shortage of Hib vaccine supply in the United States in 2008 may result in certain children's being underimmunized. When the supply is replenished, clinicians may need to review a child's earlier vaccination history with Hib.

Polio Vaccine

While polio has been eliminated in the United States, poliovirus continues to circulate in parts of Africa and Asia, including South Asia. In the United States, all infants and children should receive four doses of inactivated poliovirus vaccine (IPV) at 2, 4, 6–18 months, and 4–6 years of age.

- If accelerated protection is needed, the minimum interval between doses is 4 weeks.
- The minimum age for the fourth dose is 18 weeks.
- Infants and children who had initiated the poliovirus vaccination series with one or more doses of oral poliovirus vaccine (OPV) should receive IPV to complete the series.

Rotavirus Vaccine

Rotavirus is the most common cause of severe gastroenteritis in infants and young children worldwide. In developing countries rotavirus gastroenteritis is responsible for approximately 500,000 deaths per year among children <5 years of age. Routine rotavirus vaccination beginning at 2 months of age is recommended for all U.S. infants.

Two different rotavirus vaccines, Rotateq (RV5) and Rotarix (RV1), are licensed for use in U.S. infants. RV5 is to be administered orally in a 3-dose series with doses given at ages 2, 4, and 6 months. RV1 is to be administered orally in a 2-dose series with doses given at ages 2 and 4 months (see Table 7-5). The minimum age for the first dose of rotavirus vaccine is 6 weeks; the maximum age for the first dose is 14 weeks 6 days. Vaccination should not be initiated for infants aged 15 weeks 0 days or older because of insufficient data on safety of the first dose of rotavirus vaccine in older infants. The minimum interval between doses of rotavirus vaccine is 4 weeks. All doses should be administered by age 8 months 0 days.

Measles, Mumps, and Rubella Vaccine

Measles is an endemic disease in areas where measles immunization levels are low, and outbreaks occur even in developed countries. International travelers are at increased risk for measles exposure. Infants and children should be as well protected as possible against measles and one should try to complete the immunization series before traveling. While the risk for serious disease from either mumps or rubella is low, these diseases do circulate in many parts of the world and vaccination is recommended.

Monovalent and Combination Vaccines

In addition to the measles, mumps, and rubella vaccine (MMR), monovalent measles, monovalent mumps, monovalent rubella, and combinations of the components are available from the manufacturer. A combined measles, mumps, rubella, and varicella vaccine (MMRV) is also available for children age 12 months to 12 years. ACIP recommends that MMR or MMRV be administered when any of the individual components is indicated as part of the routine immunization schedule.

Dosing

Two doses of MMR are routinely recommended for all children, usually at age 12 months and again at age 4–6 years.

- The second dose of MMR can be given as soon as 28 days after the first dose. However, if MMRV is used, note that two varicella-containing vaccines should be separated by at least 3 months.

Table 7-5. Schedule for administration of rotavirus vaccine

	RV5 (RotaTeq; Merck)	RV1 (Rotarix; GSK)
Number of doses in series	3	2
Recommended ages for doses	2, 4, and 6 months	2 and 4 months
Minimum age for first dose	6 weeks	
Maximum age for first dose	14 weeks 6 days	
Minimum interval between doses	4 weeks	
Maximum age for last dose	8 months 0 days	

Children age 6–11 months, if they must travel outside the United States, should receive monovalent measles vaccine before departure if it is available, or MMR if monovalent measles vaccine is not available.

- MMR given before age 12 months should not be counted as part of the two-dose series.
- Children who receive MMR before age 12 months will need two more doses of MMR—the first of which should be administered at 12 months of age.

Varicella Vaccine

Varicella (chickenpox) is an endemic disease throughout the world. Two doses of varicella vaccine are recommended for all susceptible children 12 months of age and older. The first dose is recommended at age 12–15 months. The second dose is routinely recommended at age 4–6 years but can be given earlier, provided that at least 3 months have passed since the first dose.

Efforts should be made to ensure varicella immunity before age 13 years, because varicella disease can be more severe among older children and adults. Children 13 years of age and older should receive two doses of varicella vaccine 4–8 weeks apart.

Vaccination is not necessary for children with a history of documented chickenpox. When a prior history of chickenpox is uncertain, the vaccine should be given.

Meningococcal Vaccine

Meningococcal disease, caused by the bacterium *Neisseria meningitidis*, has high morbidity and mortality rates. Epidemics occur in sub-Saharan Africa during the dry season (December through June) (see Map 2-6), and CDC recommends that travelers be vaccinated before traveling to this region. Meningococcal vaccination is a requirement to enter Saudi Arabia when traveling to Mecca during the annual Hajj.

Two vaccines are available in the United States that protect against four serogroups of *N. meningitidis* (A, C, Y, and W-135): the meningococcal conjugate vaccine (MCV4) and the meningococcal polysaccharide vaccine (MPSV4).

- MCV4 is approved for use in persons 2–55 years of age and is recommended by the ACIP for routine vaccination of adolescents at 11–18 years of age. MCV4 is also recommended for persons 2–55 years of age who travel to or reside in areas where *N. meningitidis* is hyperendemic or epidemic.
- MPSV4 can be used when MCV4 is not available.
- Age considerations:
  - The serogroup A polysaccharide in MPSV4 induces an antibody response in some children as young as 3 months. Thus, vaccinating infants traveling to high-risk areas can provide some degree of protection.
  - For children vaccinated at <7 years of age, revaccination in 3 years should be considered if they remain at high risk for infection.
  - For children vaccinated at ≥7 years of age and older, revaccination should be considered in 5 years if they remain at high risk.

Pneumococcal Vaccines

Streptococcus pneumoniae is a leading cause of illness and death worldwide. Two vaccines are available for prevention of pneumococcal disease: the pneumococcal conjugate vaccine (PCV7) is recommended for routine use in children aged ≤5 years and the pneumococcal polysaccharide vaccine (PPSV23) for children aged ≥2 years who have certain underlying medical conditions and adults.

- All infants should be vaccinated with PCV7. Infant vaccination provides the earliest protection, and children aged <2 years have high rates of pneumococcal disease. The primary series for PCV7 includes three doses given at 2, 4, and 6 months of age with a fourth (booster) dose at 12–15 months of age.
- Children 24 months of age and older who are at high risk for pneumococcal disease (e.g., those with sickle cell disease, asplenia, HIV, chronic illness, or

immunocompromising conditions) should receive a dose of PPSV23 at least 2 months following their last dose of PCV7.
- A second dose of PPSV23 is recommended 5 years after the first dose of PPSV23 for persons aged >2 years who are immunocompromised, have sickle cell disease, or functional or anatomic asplenia.

Age-based considerations for children who have not been completely vaccinated:

- Use of PCV7 in children aged 24–59 months:
  - For all healthy children aged 24–59 months who have not completed any recommended schedule for PCV7, administer 1 dose of PCV7.
  - For all children with underlying medical conditions aged 24–59 months who have received three doses, administer one dose of PCV7.
  - For all children with underlying medical conditions aged 24–59 months who have received fewer than three doses, administer two doses of PCV7 at least 8 weeks apart.
- The PCV7 vaccine is not routinely recommended for persons aged >5 years.

Influenza Vaccine

Influenza vaccine can reduce the risk of influenza infection. Influenza circulation occurring predominantly in the winter months in temperate regions (typically November–April in the Northern Hemisphere, April–September in the Southern Hemisphere), but can occur year-round in tropical climates. The vaccine is prepared in two forms: an intramuscular trivalent inactivated vaccine (TIV) approved for persons ≥6 months and a live, attenuated, intranasal vaccine (LAIV) approved for only healthy, nonpregnant persons aged 2–49 years. A history of recurrent wheezing in children 2–4 years is a contraindication to LAIV.

All children 6 months through 18 years of age should receive influenza vaccination annually, as should all children at risk for complicated influenza infection due to chronic medical conditions, including but not limited to asthma, cardiac disease, sickle cell disease, HIV, and diabetes. In addition, all persons who have close contact with healthy children <5 years old (particularly contacts of infants <6 months of age since this group is at high risk for influenza complications but is not eligible for influenza vaccination) or with other persons at increased risk of influenza complications should be vaccinated annually.

- Children receiving TIV should be administered an age-appropriate dose (0.25 mL for those 6–35 months of age and 0.5 mL for those ≥36 months of age).
- One dose of influenza vaccine per season is recommended for most people. Children <9 years of age who are receiving influenza vaccine for the first time or who received only one dose the previous season (if it was their first vaccination season) should receive two doses (separated by a 4-week interval). Only one dose per year is needed in previously vaccinated children and in previously unvaccinated children ≥9 years of age.

Hepatitis A Vaccine or Immune Globulin for Hepatitis A

Hepatitis A virus (HAV) is endemic in most parts of the world, and infants and children traveling to these areas are at increased risk for acquiring HAV infection. Although HAV is often not severe in infants and children <5 years of age, infected children may transmit the infection to older children and adults, who are at higher risk of severe disease.

Hepatitis A Vaccine
Hepatitis A vaccine is now a routine immunization of childhood in the United States. It is recommended for all children at age 1 year (i.e., 12–23 months).

- Vaccination should be ensured for all susceptible children traveling to areas where there is an intermediate or high risk of HAV infection.
- The hepatitis A vaccine is not approved for children <1 year of age.

CHAPTER
7
International Travel with Infants and Children
Vaccine Recommendations for Infants and Children

- The HAV vaccine series consists of two doses at least 6 months apart. One dose of monovalent hepatitis A vaccine administered *at any time before departure* can provide adequate protection for most healthy children. The second dose is necessary for long-term protection.

Immune Globulin

Children <1 year of age who are traveling to high-risk areas can receive immune globulin (IG). For optimal protection, children who are >1 year of age, immunocompromised or have chronic medical conditions, and are planning to depart to an area in <2 weeks should receive the initial dose of vaccine along with IG (0.02 mL/kg) at a separate anatomic injection site.

- IG does not interfere with the response to yellow fever vaccine but can interfere with the response to other live injected vaccines (e.g., measles, mumps, rubella [MMR], and varicella vaccines).
- Administration of MMR should be delayed for at least 3 months and varicella for more than 5 months after administration of IG.
- IG should not be administered for 2 weeks after measles-, mumps-, rubella-, and varicella-containing vaccines. If IG is given during this time, the child should be revaccinated with the live vaccine at least 3 months after administration of IG.
- When travel plans do not allow adequate time for administration of live vaccines and IG before travel, the severity of the diseases and epidemiology of the diseases at destination points will help determine the most appropriate course of preparation.

Other Vaccines

Yellow Fever Vaccine

Yellow fever, a disease transmitted by mosquitoes, is endemic in certain areas of Africa and South America (see Maps 2-3 and 2-4). Proof of yellow fever vaccination is required for entry into some countries (see the Yellow Fever Vaccine Requirements and Recommendations, by Country, section in Chapter 2). Infants and children ≥9 months of age can be vaccinated if they travel to countries within the yellow fever-endemic zone.

Infants are at high risk for developing encephalitis from yellow fever vaccine, a live virus vaccine. Vaccination of infants should be considered on an individual basis. Although the incidence of these adverse events has not been clearly defined, 14 of 18 reported cases of postvaccination encephalitis were in infants <4 months old. One fatal case confirmed by viral isolation was in a 3-year-old child.

Travelers with infants <9 months of age should be advised against traveling to areas within the yellow fever-endemic zone.

- The ACIP recommends that yellow fever vaccine *never* be given to infants <6 months of age.
- Infants 6–8 months of age should be vaccinated only if they must travel to areas of ongoing epidemic yellow fever and a high level of protection against mosquito bites is not possible.
- Physicians considering vaccinating infants <9 months of age should contact the Division of Vector-Borne Infectious Diseases (970-221-6400) or the Division of Global Migration and Quarantine (404-498-1600) at CDC for advice.

Typhoid Vaccine

Typhoid fever is caused by the bacterium *Salmonella enterica* Typhi. Vaccination is recommended for travelers to areas where there is a recognized risk of exposure to *S.* ser. Typhi.

Two typhoid vaccines are available: a Vi capsular polysaccharide vaccine (ViCPS) administered intramuscularly and an oral, live, attenuated vaccine (Ty21a). Both vaccines induce a protective response in 50%–80% of recipients.

- The ViCPS vaccine can be administered to children who are at least 2 years of age, with a booster dose 2 years later if continued protection is needed.

- The Ty21a vaccine, which consists of a series of four capsules (i.e., one ingested every other day) can be administered to children ≥6 years of age. A booster series for Ty21a should be taken every 5 years if indicated.
  - ○ The capsule cannot be opened for administration but must be swallowed whole.
  - ○ All four doses should be ingested at least 1 week before potential exposure.

Japanese Encephalitis Vaccine

Japanese encephalitis (JE) virus is transmitted by mosquitoes and is endemic throughout Asia. The risk can be seasonal in temperate climates, and year-round in more tropical climates. The risk to short-term travelers and those who confine their travel to urban centers is very low. Travelers who plan to take up residence in an endemic area should be vaccinated against JE. The decision to vaccinate a child should follow the recommendations of the Japanese Encephalitis section in Chapter 2.

JE vaccine is administered as a series of three injections on days 0, 7, and 30.

- Children 1–2 years of age receive 0.5 mL of vaccine per dose; those ≥3 years of age receive 1.0 mL of vaccine per dose. No data are available on vaccine efficacy for infants <1 year of age.
- For children who remain at risk, a booster can be given after 3 years.
- JE-VAX carries a risk of hypersensitivity reactions that range from 10 to 180 cases per 100,000 vaccinees. Hypersensitivity reactions can be delayed for 1 to 2 weeks after receipt of the vaccine. Children receiving the vaccine series should be observed for 30 minutes after immunization, and the series should be completed at least 10 days before departure.

The JE vaccine (JE-VAX) currently in use is no longer manufactured. A stockpile of vaccine will be made available until supplies are depleted. A new JE vaccine (IC51, trade name Ixiaro) has been submitted to the FDA for approval, which is anticipated to occur in late 2008 or early 2009. The IC51 vaccine will not initially be approved for use in children <18 years of age. Those children who need JE vaccine will still use the remaining JE-VAX.

Rabies Vaccine

Rabies virus causes an acute viral encephalitis that is virtually 100% fatal. Traveling children may be at increased risk of rabies exposure, mainly from street dogs in developing countries. Bat bites carry a potential risk of rabies throughout the world. There are two strategies for the prevention of rabies in humans.

- Prevention of rabies encephalitis is based on avoiding bite or scratch exposures to potentially infected mammals.
- A child can have a three-shot pre-exposure immunization series, on days 0, 7, and 21 to 28. In the event of a subsequent possible rabies virus exposure, the child will require two more doses of rabies vaccine on days 0 and 3. The decision as to whether to obtain pre-exposure immunization for children should follow the recommendations in the Rabies section of Chapter 2.

For children who have not been pre-immunized and have potentially been exposed to rabies, a weight-based dose of human rabies immune globulin and a series of five rabies vaccine injections are required on days 0, 3, 7, 14, and 28.

Beginning in 2007, there has been a limitation in the supply of rabies vaccine in the United States. Pre-exposure rabies immunization is currently unavailable until the supply of rabies vaccine can be increased. The available doses of vaccine are being prioritized for people undergoing postexposure immunoprophylaxis.

References

1. Mackell SM. Vaccinations for the pediatric traveler. Clin Infect Dis. 2003;37(11):1508–16.

2. CDC. Epidemiology and prevention of vaccine-preventable diseases. Atkinson W,

Hamborsky J, McIntyre L, Wolfe S, editors. 9th ed. Washington, DC: Public Health Foundation; 2006.

3. Broder KR, Cortese MM, Iskander JK, et al.; Advisory Committee on Immunization Practices (ACIP). Preventing tetanus, diphtheria, and pertussis among adolescents: use of tetanus toxoid, reduced diphtheria toxoid and acellular pertussis vaccines. Recommendations of the Advisory Committee on Immunization

Practices (ACIP). MMWR Recomm Rep. 2006;55(RR-3):1–34.

4. Parashar UD, Alexander JP, Glass RI; Advisory Committee on Immunization Practices (ACIP). Prevention of rotavirus gastroenteritis among infants and children. Recommendations of the Advisory Committee on Immunization Practices (ACIP). MMWR Recomm Rep. 2006;55(RR-12):1–13.

TRAVEL AND BREASTFEEDING

Katherine Shealy

Travel need not be a reason to stop breastfeeding. The medical preparation of a breastfeeding traveler (mother or child) differs only slightly from that of other travelers, and depends in part on whether the mother and child will be separated or together during travel. Most travelers should be advised to continue breastfeeding throughout and after travel.

Prior to departure, health-care providers can help breastfeeding mothers find out about available breastfeeding support at their destination. Mothers may wish to have with them a written list of local breastfeeding resources.

- International Board-Certified Lactation Consultants (IBCLCs)—health professionals in approximately 50 countries who specialize in the clinical management of breastfeeding; see www.ilca.org/falc.html.
- La Leche League Leaders (LLLLs)—trained and accredited volunteer mothers in approximately 60 countries who provide mother-to-mother breastfeeding support and help; see www.llli.org.

Mothers who plan to use a breast pump while traveling should have a back-up option available, including written instructions for hand expression.

Immunizations and Medications

In almost all situations, health-care providers can and should select immunizations and medications that are compatible with breastfeeding. It is inappropriate to counsel mothers to wean to be vaccinated, as well as to withhold vaccination due to breastfeeding status.

- Breastfeeding and lactation do not affect dosage guidelines for any immunization or medication (except certain considerations for yellow fever vaccine, see below); regardless of maternal dose, children always require their own immunization or medication.
- In the absence of documented risk to the breastfeeding child of a particular maternal medication, the known risks of stopping breastfeeding outweigh a theoretical risk of exposure via breastfeeding.

Immunizations

- Breastfeeding mothers and children should be vaccinated according to routine, recommended schedules; only preventive vaccinia (smallpox) vaccine is contraindicated for use in breastfeeding mothers.
- Administration of live and inactivated vaccines does not affect lactation, milk supply, or breast milk safety.

Special Consideration: Yellow Fever Vaccination

- When possible, vaccination of breastfeeding mothers should be avoided, due to the possible risk for the transmission of 17D virus to the breastfeeding child.

- Breastfeeding mothers whose travel to high-risk yellow fever-endemic areas cannot be avoided should be vaccinated (see the Yellow Fever section in Chapter 2).

Medications

- The American Academy of Pediatrics (AAP) 2001 Policy Statement: Transfer of Drugs into Human Milk provides an overview of the compatibility or effects on breastfeeding of approximately 250 drugs.
- *Medications and Mothers' Milk* is updated every 2 years and provides a comprehensive review of the compatibility or effects on breastfeeding of approximately 1,000 drugs including generic and trade names, AAP recommendations, risk categories, pharmacologic properties, interactions with other drugs, suitable alternatives, theoretic and relative child dose, pediatric half life, and any other pediatric concerns.

Special Consideration: Antimalarial Medications

- Most experts consider short-term use of doxycycline compatible with breastfeeding.
- Primaquine may be used for breastfeeding mothers and children with normal G6PD levels.
- Breastfeeding mothers should not use atovaquone/proguanil (Malarone) when the breastfeeding infant weighs <5 kg (approximately 11 pounds).

Air Travel

X-rays used in airport screenings have no effect on breastfeeding, breast milk, or the process of lactation. Airlines typically consider breast pumps as personal items to be carried onboard, similar to laptop computers, handbags, and diaper bags.

Prior to departure, mothers who will be traveling by air and expect to have expressed milk with them during travel need to carefully plan how they will transport their milk.

- Airport security regulations for passengers carrying expressed milk vary internationally and are subject to change.
- In the United States, the Transportation Security Administration (TSA) recognizes expressed milk in the category of liquid medications that may be carried on, regardless if the breastfeeding child is traveling, as long as it is declared prior to screening.
  - TSA recommends that travelers carrying expressed milk have with them a printed copy of the TSA website page and URL, www.tsa.gov/travelers/airtravel/children/formula.shtm, to help prevent inadvertent problems at security checkpoints.
- Travelers carrying expressed milk in checked luggage should refer to cooler pack storage guidelines in "Proper Handling and Storage of Human Milk" on CDC's website at www.cdc.gov/breastfeeding/recommendations/handling_breastmilk.htm to protect milk during travel.
- Expressed milk is not considered a biohazard to which Universal Precautions apply. International Air Transport Authority (IATA) regulations for shipping Category B Biological Substances (UN 3373) do not apply to expressed milk; it is considered a food for individual use. Travelers shipping frozen milk should follow guidelines for shipping other frozen foods and liquids.
- Expressed milk does not need to be declared at U.S. Customs upon return to the United States.

Traveling Without a Breastfeeding Child

Travel health-care providers should help mothers determine the best course for breastfeeding based on a variety of factors, including the amount of time she has to prepare for her trip, her flexibility of time while traveling, her options for storing expressed milk while traveling, the duration of her travel, and her destination.

- Mothers should continue feeding at the breast until departure. Feeding from a bottle or a cup is more successful when offered by a caregiver other than the mother.
- Mothers may wish to express and store a supply of milk to be fed to the child during their separation.
- Travel health-care providers should encourage mothers to learn and practice expressing milk by hand prior to departure.
  - Hand expression (i.e., without the use of a breast pump) is the most hygienic and most reliable method of milk expression, especially in environments with uncertain electricity and sanitation options. For more detailed instructions for hand expression, see www.workandpump.com/handexpression.htm.
- Electric breast pumps can also be powered by vehicle lighter adapters and battery pack adapters, which are available from retailers who sell breast pump supplies.
- Expressing milk while separated from the breastfeeding child helps a mother maintain her milk supply during the separation, which makes transitioning back to breastfeeding more likely to be successful, even if expressed milk is not kept to be fed to the child.
- A mother who is interested in resuming breastfeeding after travel should always try first with the child rather than deciding independently that it is not possible. Some children, especially older breastfeeding children, resume breastfeeding regardless of the length of time they are separated from their mother, even if she did not express milk.
- If the mother's milk supply is diminished upon return, she can continue breastfeeding and supplement as needed until her milk supply returns to its prior level.
  - Often a child who is allowed frequent, positive opportunities to breastfeed without time restrictions will bring the milk supply to its prior level.
  - Occasionally a child who is separated from the mother for an extended time has difficulty transitioning back to breastfeeding.

Traveling With a Breastfeeding Child

Breastfeeding provides unique benefits to mothers and children traveling together. Health providers should encourage breastfeeding mothers by explaining clearly the value of continuing breastfeeding during travel.

- *Exclusive breastfeeding*, which is consuming no foods or liquids other than breast milk and consuming breast milk only while at the breast, protects infants from exposure to contamination and pathogens via foods, liquids, or containers (e.g., bottles, cups, utensils).
- Breastfeeding infants require no water supplementation, even in extreme heat environments and in situations where mothers are dehydrated.
- Breastfeeding during air travel protects children from Eustachian tube pain and collapse. Unlike sucking on a bottle or pacifier, suckling at the breast uniquely generates both positive and negative intraoral pressure, which allows children to stabilize and gradually equalize internal and external air pressure.

Health providers should provide information to breastfeeding mothers to support them to be better able to continue breastfeeding during travel.

- Frequent, unrestricted breastfeeding opportunities ensure that the mother's milk supply remains ample and that the child's nutrition and hydration are ideal.

Special Consideration: Travelers' Diarrhea

- *Exclusive breastfeeding* provides infants with unique protection from travelers' diarrhea.
- Breastfeeding is ideal rehydration therapy. Children who are suspected to have travelers' diarrhea should breastfeed more frequently, reduce consumption of other foods and liquids, and should not be offered other fluids to replace breastfeeding.

- Breastfeeding mothers with travelers' diarrhea should continue breastfeeding and increase their own fluid intake.
  - The organisms causing travelers' diarrhea do not pass through breast milk.
  - Breastfeeding mothers should not use bismuth subsalicylate compounds (e.g., Pepto Bismol) due to transfer of salicylate to the child. Compatible alternatives are kaolin-pectin (e.g., Kaopectate) and loperamide (e.g., Imodium). Use of oral rehydration salts (ORS) is fully compatible with breastfeeding.

References

1. Kroger AT, Atkinson WL, Marcuse EK, Pickering LK. General recommendations on immunization: recommendations of the Advisory Committee on Immunization Practices (ACIP). MMWR Recomm Rep. 2006;55(RR-15):1–48.
2. Cetron MS, Marfin AA, Julian KG, et al. Yellow fever vaccine. Recommendations of the Advisory Committee on Immunization Practices (ACIP), 2002. MMWR Recomm Rep. 2002; 51(RR-17):1–11.
3. American Academy of Pediatrics Committee on Drugs. Transfer of drugs and other chemicals into human milk. Pediatrics. 2001;108(3):776–89.
4. Hale TW. Medications and mothers' milk 2008. 13th ed. Amarillo, TX: Pharmasoft Medical Publishing; 2008.
5. Lawrence RA. Breastfeeding: a guide for the medical profession. 4th ed. New York: Mosby-Yearbook; 1994.
6. CDC. Perspectives in disease prevention and health promotion update: universal precautions for prevention of transmission of Human Immunodeficiency Virus, Hepatitis B Virus, and other bloodborne pathogens in health-care settings. MMWR Morbid Mortal Wkly Rep. 1988;37(24):377–88.

INTERNATIONAL ADOPTIONS

Cynthia R. Howard, Chandy C. John

Overview

The number of internationally adopted children arriving annually to the United States has averaged 21,449 children in the past 4 years. These children accounted for 1.85% of all legal immigrants and approximately 10% of all legal pediatric immigrants in 2006 and 2007. The demography of international adoption is in constant flux, and the epidemiology of diseases in this population of children shifts as a consequence.

In 2007, the most common countries of origin for internationally adopted children were China, Guatemala, Russia, Ethiopia, South Korea, Vietnam, Ukraine, and Kazakhstan (Map 7-1). The numbers of children coming from Vietnam and Ethiopia increased 409% and 69%, respectively, during 2006–2007, and in 2007, Vietnam and Ethiopia were represented for the first time in the top six countries of origin. In 2007, 40% of internationally adopted children were <1 year of age, 43% were 1–4 years of age, and 17% were ≥5 years of age. Sixty-one percent were female.

International adoptees are usually underimmunized and are at increased risk for infections such as measles and hepatitis A, due to often-crowded living conditions, malnutrition, lack of clean water, and exposure to endemic diseases that are not common in the United States. The major challenges in health care regarding international adoptees include—

- Absence of a medical history
- Unavailability of biological family history
- Questionable reliability of immunization records
- Variation in pre-adoption living standards
- Different disease epidemiology in countries of origin
- Increased risk for developmental delays

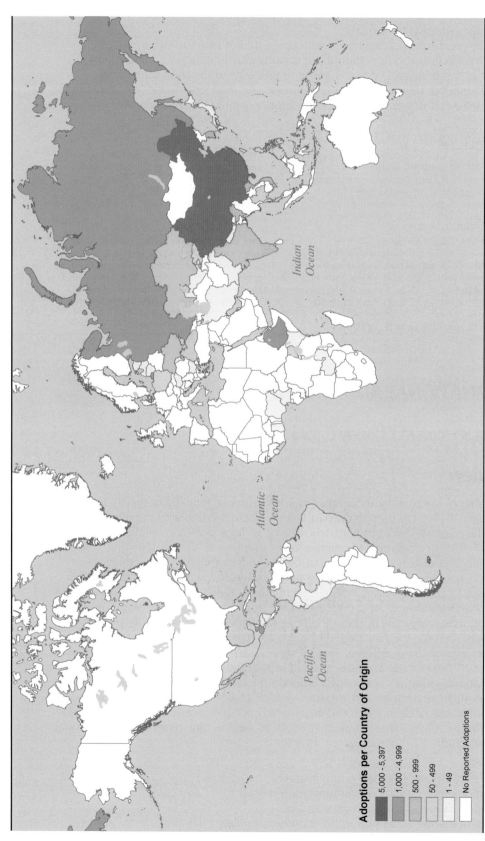

Map 7-1. Countries of origin of adopted children immigrating to the United States, 2007.

(From United States Department of Homeland Security. Yearbook of Immigration Statistics: 2007. Washington, D.C.: U.S. Department of Homeland Security, Office of Immigration Statistics; 2008.)

Adoptions per Country of Origin

5,000 - 5,397
1,000 - 4,999
500 - 999
50 - 499
1 - 49
No Reported Adoptions

Travel Preparation for Adoptive Parents and Their Families

Prospective adoptive parents should be encouraged to consider the following for themselves and other family members:

- A pre-travel visit is strongly recommended for prospective adoptive parents.
- Family members who remain at home, including extended family, and child care providers should also be current on their routine immunizations, as recommended by the Advisory Committee on Immunization Practices (ACIP).
- Protection against measles, hepatitis A, and hepatitis B must be ensured for everyone who will be in the household or providing child care for the adopted child.
- Adults <65 years of age who are due for a tetanus booster should receive the diphtheria, tetanus and acellular pertussis (DTaP) vaccine.
- A one-time inactivated polio booster also is recommended for adults.

Overseas Medical Examination of the Adopted Child

All immigrants, including infants and children adopted internationally by U.S. citizens, and all refugees entering the United States must undergo a medical examination in their country of origin, performed by a panel physician designated by the U.S. Department of State.

- The medical examination is used primarily to detect certain serious contagious diseases that may be the basis for visa ineligibility.
- Prospective adoptive parents should be advised not to rely on this medical examination to detect all possible disabilities and illnesses. Laboratory results from the country of origin may also be unreliable.
- The medical examination consists of a brief physical examination and a medical history, a chest radiograph examination for tuberculosis, and blood tests for syphilis and HIV are required for immigrants ≥15 years of age. Immigration applicants <15 years old are tested only if there is reason to suspect any of these diseases.

The U.S. Department of State website provides additional information about the medical examination at http://adoption.state.gov/about/how/health.html and the vaccination exemption form for internationally adopted children at http://travel.state.gov/pdf/DS-1981.pdf.

Follow-Up Medical Examination after Arrival in the United States

The adopted child should have a medical examination within 2 weeks of arrival in the United States, or earlier if the child has fever, anorexia, diarrhea or vomiting (Table 7-6). Further evaluation will depend on—

- the country of origin,
- the age of the child,
- previous living conditions,
- the number of times a child has been moved from one residence to another (e.g., home, hospital, orphanages, and adoptive families),
- nutritional status,
- developmental status,
- the adoptive family's specific questions, and
- any concerns raised during a pre-adoption medical review.

In one study, >50% of newly arrived adopted children had an undiagnosed medical condition, and of these, >50% were diagnosed as an infectious disease.

Table 7-6. Post-arrival medical examination

Physical

Full exposure, with particular attention to the following:

- Temperature (fever requires further investigation)
- General appearance: alert, interactive, referring to parents, consoled by parents, smiling
- Anthropometric measurements: height/age; weight/age; weight/height; head circumference/age
- Facial features: length of palpebral fissures, philtrum, upper lip (short palpebral fissures, thin upper lip, and indistinct philtrum are characteristic of fetal alcohol syndrome)
- Hair: texture, color
- Eyes: icterus, pallor, strabismus, visual acuity screen
- Ears: hearing screen
- Mouth: palate, teeth
- Neck: thyroid (enlargement secondary to hypothyroidism, iodine deficiency)
- Abdomen: liver or spleen enlargement
- Skin: Mongolian spots, scars, BCG scar
- Lymph nodes: enlargement suggestive of TB

Neurodevelopment

All children should receive a complete developmental examination by a health-care provider with experience in child development.

Screening for Infectious and Noninfectious Diseases

The current panel of tests recommended by the American Academy of Pediatrics (AAP) for screening of infectious diseases is outlined in Table 7-7.

Gastrointestinal Parasites

Gastrointestinal parasites have been found in up to 51% of internationally adopted children. *Giardia intestinalis* is the most common parasite identified. The highest rates of infection have been reported from Russia, Eastern Europe, and China.

Hepatitis A

Serology has proven useful in identifying the young infant or child from a hepatitis A virus-endemic area who may be asymptomatic yet is acutely infected and is shedding virus, with the potential to infect others. In 2007 and early 2008, multiple cases of hepatitis A secondary to exposure to a newly arrived internationally adopted child were reported in the United States.

Hepatitis B

Hepatitis B surface antigen has been reported in 1%–5% of newly arrived adoptees, depending on the country of origin and the year that the study was conducted. The hepatitis B virus (HBV) is highly transmissible within the household. All members of households adopting children who are HBV carriers must be immunized and should have follow-up antibody titers to determine if levels consistent with immunity have been achieved. Children found to be hepatitis B surface antigen-positive should receive additional tests and consultation with a pediatric gastroenterologist.

Hepatitis C

Hepatitis C serologic screening is recommended for children from China, Russia, Eastern Europe, and Southeast Asia. Depending on history of prevalence in the country of origin, receipt of blood products, and maternal drug use, hepatitis C screening of children from other areas may be indicated.

Table 7-7. Screening tests for infectious diseases in internationally adopted children

Hepatitis B virus serologic testing[1]
- Hepatitis B surface antigen (HBsAg)
- Antibody to hepatitis B surface antigen (anti-HBs)
- Antibody to hepatitis B core antigen (anti-HBc)

Hepatitis C virus serologic testing

Syphilis serologic testing
- Nontreponemal test (RPR, VDRL, or ART)
- Treponemal test (MHA-TP or FTA-ABS)

HIV 1 and 2 serologic testing[1]

Complete blood cell count with differential and red blood cell indices

Stool examination for ova and parasites (three specimens)

Stool examination for *Giardia intestinalis* and *Cryptosporidium* antigen (one specimen)

Tuberculin skin test[1]

Note: RPR indicates rapid plasma regain; VDRL, Venereal Disease Research Laboratories; ART, automated reagin test; MHA-TP, microhemagglutination test for *Treponema pallidum*; FTA-ABS, fluorescent treponemal antibody absorption.

1 Repeat at 6 months after initial testing.

From American Academy of Pediatrics. Medical evaluation of internationally adopted children for infectious diseases. In: Pickering LK, Baker CJ, Long SS, McMillan JA, eds. Red book: 2006 Report of the Committee on Infectious Diseases, 27th ed. Elk Grove Village, IL: American Academy of Pediatrics; 2006. p. 184.

HIV

Clinical symptoms of malnutrition, long-term institutionalization, and acquired immunodeficiency may overlap, but positive HIV antibodies in children <18 months of age may reflect maternal antibody, but not infection. Assaying for the virus by HIV DNA with PCR will confirm the diagnosis of HIV in the infant or child. Some experts recommend HIV DNA PCR for any infant <6 months old on arrival. In children >6 months of age, two negative assays for HIV DNA administered 1 month apart are necessary to exclude infection.

Malaria

Smears should be obtained on all children arriving from areas endemic for malaria and for any newly arrived child who has a fever. The child with fever should have three sets of malaria smears at least 12 hours apart before excluding the diagnosis.

Tuberculosis

Internationally adopted children are at four to six times the risk for tuberculosis than their U.S.-born peers.

- The tuberculin skin test (TST) of purified protein derivative is indicated for all children >3 months of age, regardless of their Bacille Calmette–Guérin (BCG) vaccination status. Table 7-8 summarizes interpretation of the TST in internationally adopted children.
- A chest radiograph and complete physical exam to assess for pulmonary and extrapulmonary tuberculosis are indicated for all children with positive TST results.
- Hilar lymphadenopathy is a more sensitive finding for TB in young children than are pulmonary infiltrates or cavitation.
- Some experts recommend a repeat TST 3–6 months after arrival.
- A child who has a positive TST but no evidence of active disease should be treated with isoniazid for 9 months.
- If active disease is found, every effort should be made to isolate the organism and determine sensitivities, particularly if the child is from a region of the world with a high rate of multidrug-resistant TB, such as Russia, Eastern Europe, and Asia.

Table 7-8. Definition of a positive tuberculin skin test (TST) in internationally adopted children

Induration ≥5 mm if—

- evidence of immunosuppression
- history of contact with active tuberculosis
- signs and symptoms of tuberculosis
- abnormal chest radiograph

Induration ≥10 mm in all other internationally adopted children

Eosinophilia

Children with eosinophil counts >450 cells/mm^3 may warrant further evaluation. Evaluation may include testing for parasites that can migrate through tissues and filarial worms such as *Strongloides stercoralis, Toxocara canis, Schistosoma* species, *Ancyclostoma* species, and *Trichinella spiralis.*

Noninfectious Diseases

Screening tests for noninfectious diseases that should be performed in all or selected internationally adopted children are outlined in Table 7-9.

Immunizations

The U.S. Immigration and Nationality Act requires that any person seeking an immigrant visa for permanent residency must show proof of having received the ACIP-recommended vaccines (see Tables 7-2 and 7-3) prior to immigration. This applies to all immigrant infants and children entering the United States, but internationally adopted children <11 years of age have been exempted from the overseas immunization requirements. Adoptive parents are required to sign a waiver indicating their intention to comply with the immunization requirements within 30 days of the infant's or child's arrival in the United States.

Most children throughout the developing world receive BCG, DPT, OPV, and measles vaccine per the original immunization schedule of the United Nations' Expanded Programme of Immunizations (begun in 1974). Upon arrival in the United States, >90% of newly arrived internationally adopted children need catch-up immunizations to meet the ACIP guidelines. Varicella, pneumococcal conjugate, rubella, mumps, and *Haemophilus influenzae* type b vaccines are not usually available in developing countries.

Table 7-9. Screening tests for noninfectious diseases in internationally adopted children

All Internationally Adopted Children

- TST
- TSH
- Iron, iron saturation, IBC
- Lead (Repeat 6 months after initial testing)

Selected Internationally Adopted Children

Test	Indication
Hgb electrophoresis	Any country of origin where sickle cell disease is common (particularly sub-Saharan Africa)
G6PD	Area where G6PD deficiency is common
Metabolic screen	Infant growth +/or developmental delay
Vitamin D screen	Signs consistent with rickets
Calcium	

Note: IBC, iron binding capacity; Hgb, hemoglobin; G6PD, glucose-6-phosphate dehydrogenase.

Table 7-10. Serologic testing available for verifying immunization status

Children >6 Months of Age	Children >12 Months of Age
• Diphtheria antitoxoid antibody • Tetanus antitoxoid antibody • Poliovirus neutralizing antibody for types 1, 2, 3 • Hepatitis B surface antibody	• Diphtheria antitoxoid antibody • Tetanus antitoxoid antibody • Poliovirus neutralizing antibody for types 1, 2, 3[1] • Hepatitis B surface antibody • Rubeola (measles) antibody • Mumps antibody • Rubella antibody • Varicella antibody • Hepatitis A antibody • *H. influenzae* type b IgG • *S. pneumoniae* IgG for serotypes 7–14

Note: IgG, immunoglobulin G.

1 Titer to type 3 polio is often negative after immunization, not an indication to reimmunize.

Reliability of Vaccine Records

- Appears to differ by and even within country.
- Either of two approaches to vaccination can be taken for internationally adopted children: a) reimmunize regardless of immunization record or b) if the child is >6 months of age, test antibody titers (see Table 7-7) to the vaccines potentially administered, and reimmunize only for those to which the child has no protective titers. Serologic testing that can be done in children >6 months and >12 months is outlined in Table 7-10. Antibody titers to pertussis do not correlate with immune status to pertussis.
- If the infant is <6 months old and there is uncertainty regarding immunization status or validity of immunization record, reimmunize according to the ACIP schedule.
- MMR is not given in most of the countries of origin. Measles vaccine is administered as a single antigen. Unless the child has had mumps and rubella, administration of the MMR vaccine is recommended over serologic testing.
- Varicella testing for children coming from tropical countries is not recommended before 12 years of age unless there is a history of disease. In the tropics, varicella is a disease of adolescents and adults.

References

1. United States Department of Homeland Security. Yearbook of Immigration Statistics: 2007. Washington, D.C.: U.S. Department of Homeland Security, Office of Immigration Statistics; 2008. [updated 2008 Apr 2; cited 2008 Nov 30]. Available from: http://www.dhs.gov/xlibrary/assets/statistics/yearbook/2007/ois_2007_yearbook.pdf

2. CDC. Advisory Committee on Immunization Practices (ACIP); recommendations and guidelines. [cited 2008 Nov 26]. Available from: http://www.cdc.gov/vaccines/recs/ACIP/default.htm

3. Lee PJ. Vaccines for travel and international adoption. Pediatr Infect Dis J. 2008;27(4):351–4.

4. Hofstetter MK, Iverson S, Dole K, Johnson D. Unsuspected infectious diseases and other medical diagnoses in the evaluation of internationally adopted children. Pediatrics. 1989;83(4):559–64.

5. American Academy of Pediatrics. Medical evaluation of internationally adopted children for infectious diseases. In: Pickering LK, Baker CJ, Long SS, McMillan JA, eds. Red book: 2006 Report of the Committee on Infectious Diseases, 27th ed. Elk Grove Village, IL: American Academy of Pediatrics; 2006. p.183.

6. Chen LH, Barnett ED, Wilson ME. Preventing infectious diseases during and after international adoption. Ann Intern Med. 2003;139(5):371–8.

7. Miller LC. International adoption: infectious diseases issues. Clin Infect Dis. 2005;40(2):286–93.

8. Stauffer WM, Kamat D, Walker PF. Screening of international immigrants, refugees, and adoptees. Prim Care. 2002;29(4):879–905.

9. Mazzulli T. Laboratory diagnosis of infection due to viruses, *Chlamydia*, Chlamydophila, and mycoplasma. In: Long SS, Pickering LK,

Prober CG, editors. Principles and practice of pediatric infectious diseases, 3rd ed. Orlando: Churchill Livingstone; 2008.

10. Schulte JM, Maloney S, Aronson J, et al. Evaluating acceptability and completeness of overseas immunization records of internationally adopted children. Pediatrics. 2002;109(2);E22.

11. Fuglestad AJ, Lehmann AE, Kroupina MG, et al. Iron deficiency in international adoptees from Eastern Europe. J Pediatr. 2008;153(2):272–7.

12. Mandalakas AM, Kirchner L, Iverson S, et al. Predictors of *Mycobacterium tuberculosis* infection in international adoptees. Pediatrics. 2007;120(3):e610–6.

8

Advising Travelers with Specific Needs

THE IMMUNOCOMPROMISED TRAVELER

Elaine C. Jong, David O. Freedman

Approach to the Immunocompromised Traveler

The pre-travel preparation of travelers with immune suppression due to any medical condition, drug, or treatment, must address several categories of concern:

- Is the traveler's underlying medical condition under stable control? The travel health advisor may need to contact the traveler's primary and specialty care providers (with the patient's permission) to gain a comprehensive medical overview and to verify the drugs and doses composing the usual maintenance regimen.
- Do the conditions, medications, and treatments of the traveler constitute contraindications to or decrease the effectiveness of any of the disease-prevention measures recommended for the proposed trip? Most importantly, these measures include immunizations against vaccine-preventable diseases and drugs used for malaria chemoprophylaxis and management of travelers' diarrhea.
- Do any of the disease-prevention measures recommended for the proposed trip itinerary present a risk for destabilization of the underlying medical condition through direct pathophysiology or drug–drug interactions?
- Are there specific health hazards at the destination that would cause exacerbation of the underlying condition, or an illness of increased severity in the immunocompromised traveler? If so, can specific interventions be recommended to mitigate these risks?

The traveler's immune status is particularly relevant to the administration of travel-related immunizations. Overall considerations for vaccine recommendations, such as destination and the likely risk of exposure to various modes of disease transmission, are the same for immunocompromised travelers as for other travelers, although the consequences of not administering an indicated vaccine may be more severe. In some complex cases when travelers cannot tolerate recommended immunizations and/or malaria chemoprophylaxis drugs, a change of itinerary, an alteration of activities planned during travel, or even deferral of the proposed trip must be considered—depending on the traveler's personal tolerance for risk.

Medical Conditions without Significant Immunologic Compromise

With regard to travel immunizations, travelers whose health status places them in one of the following groups are not considered significantly immunocompromised and should be prepared as any other traveler, although the nature of the previous or underlying disease needs to be kept in mind.

1. Travelers receiving corticosteroid therapy under any of the following circumstances:
   ○ Short- or long-term daily or alternate-day therapy with <20 mg of prednisone or equivalent
   ○ Long-term, alternate-day treatment with short-acting preparations
   ○ Maintenance physiologic doses (replacement therapy)
   ○ Steroid inhalers
   ○ Topical steroids (skin, ears, or eyes)
   ○ Intra-articular, bursal, or tendon injection of steroids
   ○ If >1 month has passed since high-dose steroids (≥20 mg per day of prednisone or equivalent for >2 weeks) have been used. Some experts will wait 2 weeks prior to the administration of measles vaccine following short-term (<2 weeks) of therapy with daily or alternate-day dosing of ≥20 mg of prednisone or equivalent.
2. HIV patients with >500 CD4 lymphocytes.
3. Travelers who received their last chemotherapy treatment at least 3 months previously and whose malignancy is in remission. However, when patients are on immunosuppressive medications (including TNF-blockers) for conditions other than hematologic malignancies and cancer, some clinicians suggest waiting only 1 month since a last dose of such medications before immunization. This recommendation may refer primarily to corticosteroids; it remains unknown exactly what duration off other drugs is optimal for immunization of such patients.
4. Bone marrow transplant recipients who are >2 years post-transplant, not on immunosuppressive drugs, and without graft-versus-host disease.
5. Travelers with autoimmune disease not being treated with immunosuppressive drugs (e.g., systemic lupus erythematosus, inflammatory bowel disease, rheumatoid arthritis, or multiple sclerosis), although definitive data are lacking.
   ○ The ACIP advises the normal use of all live-virus and killed vaccines in multiple sclerosis (MS) patients who are not undergoing a current exacerbation of disease. This advice concurs with that of the National MS Society (www.nationalmssociety.org/), a source well respected by MS patients and their physicians. (In the past, many practicing neurologists have strongly advised their MS patients against the use of live-virus vaccines at any time.)
   ○ If possible, MS patients should not receive any vaccine for 6 weeks after the onset of a disease exacerbation.
   ○ Immunomodulatory agents commonly used in MS patients, such as interferons and glatiramer acetate, are not thought to affect vaccine response or safety, but definitive data are lacking.

Medical Conditions Associated with Immune Suppression

For purposes of clinical assessment and approach to immunizations, immunocompromised travelers fall into one of four groups, based on mechanism and level of immune suppression.

Vaccine use recommendations for different categories of immunocompromised adults are shown in Table 8-1.

Asymptomatic HIV Infection

Asymptomatic HIV-infected persons with CD4 cell counts of 200–500/mm^3 are considered to have limited immune deficits. CD4 counts increased by antiretroviral drugs, rather than nadir counts, should be used in categorizing HIV-infected persons. The exact time at which reconstituted lymphocytes are fully functional is not well defined. To achieve a maximal vaccine response with minimal risk, many clinicians advise a delay of 3 months after reconstitution, if possible, before immunizations are administered. While seroconversion rates and geometric mean titers of antibody in response to vaccines may be less than those measured in healthy controls, seroprotective levels of antibody following immunization with most vaccines studied can be elicited in the majority of HIV-infected patients in this category.

Transient increases in HIV viral load, which return quickly to baseline, have been observed after administration of several different vaccines to HIV-infected persons. The clinical significance of these increases is not known, but they do not preclude the use of any vaccine.

Chronic Conditions Associated with Limited Immune Deficits

Chronic conditions associated with limited immune deficits include asplenia, chronic renal disease, chronic liver disease (including chronic hepatitis C), diabetes mellitus, and complement deficiencies. No information on possible decreased vaccine efficacy or increased adverse events with administration of live attenuated viral or bacterial antigen vaccines is available for this group.

- A blunted response to hepatitis B vaccine has been reported in patients with chronic liver disease; a decreased response to hepatitis B vaccine has also been observed in patients with diabetes. Additional doses of hepatitis B vaccine beyond the primary three-dose series may be necessary.
- Double-dose hepatitis B vaccine preparations are used to promote optimal immunization of persons with chronic renal failure and other patient groups with absent or suboptimal response to standard hepatitis B vaccine doses.
- Adjuvanted hepatitis B candidate vaccines currently undergoing clinical trials look to be more effective for immunization of liver transplant patients and patients with renal insufficiency.
- Persons with asplenia have increased susceptibility to overwhelming sepsis with encapsulated bacterial pathogens. Although response to vaccines may be suboptimal compared with hosts with a functioning spleen, many clinical guidelines recommend immunization with meningococcal vaccine, pneumococcal vaccine, and *Haemophilus influenzae* conjugate vaccine in this patient category, regardless of travel plans. Limited data show that vaccine response in persons who have had a splenectomy was relatively more impaired if splenectomy was performed because of hematologic malignancy rather than for splenic trauma.
- Persons with terminal complement deficiencies appear to have increased susceptibility to meningococcal infections and should be immunized against meningococcal disease.

Severe Immunocompromise (Non-HIV)

Severely immunocompromised persons include those who have active leukemia or lymphoma, generalized malignancy, aplastic anemia, graft-versus-host disease, or congenital immunodeficiency; persons who have received current or recent radiation therapy, solid organ transplant, or bone marrow transplant recipients within 2 years of transplantation; or persons whose transplants occurred >2 years ago but who are still taking immunosuppressive drugs.

Table 8-1. Immunization of immunocompromised adults

	HIV Infection, CD4 cells >200/mm³	Severe Immuno-suppression (HIV/AIDS) CD4 cells <200/mm³	Severe Immuno-suppression (Non-HIV-related)	Asplenia	Renal Failure	Chronic Liver Disease, Diabetes
Live Vaccines						
Bacille Calmette-Guérin (BCG)	X	X	X	U	U	U
Influenza, live attenuated (LAIV)	X	X	X	U	X	X
Measles–mumps–rubella (MMR)[1]	R	W	X	U	U	U
Typhoid, Ty21a	X	X	X	U	U	U
Varicella (adults)[2]	U	X	X	U	U	U
Yellow fever[3]	W	X	X	U	U	U
Inactivated Vaccines						
Haemophilus influenzae (Hib)	C[4]	C[4]	R	R	U	U
Hepatitis A	U[5]	U[5]	U	U[5]	U[5]	U[5]
Hepatitis B	U[5,6]	U[5,6]	U[6]	U[6]	R[7]	U[6]
Influenza (inactivated)	R	R	R	R	R	R
Japanese encephalitis	U	U	U	U	U	U
Meningococcal polysaccharide or conjugate	C	C	U	R	U	U
Pneumococcal polysaccharide	R	R	R	R	R	R
Polio (IPV)	U	U	U	U	U	U
Rabies	U	U	U	U	U	U
Td or Tdap	R	R	R	R	R	R
Typhoid, Vi	U	U	U	U	U	U

C = Consider; R = Recommended for all in this patient category; U = Use as indicated for normal hosts; W = Warning; X = Contraindicated

1 MMR vaccination should be considered for all symptomatic HIV-infected persons with CD4 counts >200/mm³ without evidence of measles immunity. Immune globulin may be administered for short-term protection of those facing high risk of measles and for whom MMR vaccine is contraindicated.
2 Varicella vaccine should not be administered to persons who have cellular immunodeficiencies, but persons with impaired humoral immunity (including congenital or acquired hypo- or dysglobulinemia) may be vaccinated. Immunocompromised hosts should receive two doses of vaccine spaced at 3-month intervals.
3 Yellow fever vaccine. See detail in the text above.
4 Decision should be based on consideration of the individual patient's risk of Hib disease and the effectiveness of the vaccine for that person. In some settings, the incidence of Hib disease may be higher among HIV-infected adults than among non-HIV-infected adults, and the disease can be severe in these patients.
5 Routinely indicated for all men who have sex with men, persons with multiple sexual partners, hemophiliacs, patients with chronic hepatitis, and injection drug users.
6 Test for anti-HBsAg serum titer after vaccination, and revaccinate if initial antibody response is absent or suboptimal (<10 mIU/mL). HIV-infected non-responders may react to a subsequent vaccine course if CD4 cell counts rise to 500/mm³ following institution of highly active antiretroviral therapy. See text for discussion of other immunocompromised groups.
7 Use special double-dose vaccine formulation. Test for anti-HBsAg response after vaccination and revaccinate if initial antibody response is absent or suboptimal (<10 mIU/mL).

- Persons with chronic lymphocytic leukemia have poor humoral immunity even early in the disease course and rarely respond to vaccines.
- Complete revaccination with standard childhood vaccines should begin 12 months after bone marrow transplantation (BMT). However, MMR vaccine should be administered at 24 months after BMT if the recipient is presumed to be immunocompetent. Influenza vaccine should be administered at 6 months after BMT and annually thereafter.
- For solid organ transplants, a higher risk of infection occurs within the first year of transplant than later, so travel to high-risk destinations might best be postponed until after that time.

Vaccine doses received while concurrently receiving immunosuppressive therapy, or during the 2 weeks before starting therapy because of imminent travel, are not considered valid vaccine doses. At least 3 months after therapy is discontinued, these patients should be revaccinated with all vaccines that are still indicated at that time. Persons taking any of the following categories of medications are considered severely immunocompromised:

- High-dose corticosteroids. Most clinicians consider a dose of either >2 mg/kg of body weight or ≥20 mg/day of prednisone or equivalent in persons who weigh >10 kg, when administered for ≥2 weeks, as sufficiently immunosuppressive to raise concern about the safety of vaccination with live-virus vaccines. Furthermore, the immune response to vaccines may be impaired. Vaccine providers should wait at least 1 month after discontinuation of high-dose systemically absorbed corticosteroid therapy before administering a live-virus vaccine.
- Alkylating agents (e.g., cyclophosphamide).
- Antimetabolites (e.g., azathioprine, 6-mercaptopurine).
- Transplant-related immunosuppressive drugs (e.g., cyclosporine, tacrolimus, sirolimus, and mycophenolate mofetil) and mitoxantrone (used in multiple sclerosis).
- Cancer chemotherapeutic agents (excluding tamoxifen). Methotrexate, including low-dose weekly regimens, is classified as severely immunosuppressive, as evidenced by increased rates of opportunistic infections and blunting of responses to certain vaccines among patient groups. Limited studies show that methotrexate monotherapy had no effect on the response to influenza vaccine, but it did impair the response to pneumococcal vaccine.
- Tumor necrosis factor (TNF)-blocking agents such as etanercept, adalimumab, and infliximab are known to blunt the immune response to certain vaccines, such as influenza vaccine. When used in combination regimens with methotrexate for treatment of rheumatoid disease, TNF-blocking agents were associated with an impaired response to pneumococcal vaccine as well. Although the potential benefits of live viral and bacterial vaccines in persons receiving TNF-blocking agents need to be weighed carefully against potential risks, most clinicians would be reluctant to use such vaccines in this situation, as the safety of using live vaccines is unknown for these agents and interleukin-1 receptor antagonist (IL-1ra).

Severe Immunocompromise Due to Symptomatic HIV/AIDS

Knowledge of the HIV-infected traveler's current CD4 lymphocyte count is necessary for pre-travel consultation. HIV-infected persons with CD4 cell counts <200/mm^3, history of an AIDS-defining illness, or clinical manifestations of symptomatic HIV are considered to have severe immunosuppression (see the HIV Infection and Acquired Immunodeficiency Syndrome (AIDS) section in Chapter 5) and should not receive live attenuated viral or bacterial vaccines because of the theoretical risk that the vaccine agent may cause serious systemic disease. The response to inactivated vaccines also will be suboptimal; thus, vaccine doses received by HIV-infected individuals while CD4 cell counts are <200/mm^3 should be ignored, and the individual should be revaccinated at least 3 months after immune reconstitution with antiretroviral therapy.

In newly diagnosed treatment-naïve patients with CD4 cell counts <200/mm^3, travel should be delayed pending reconstitution of CD4 cell counts with antiretroviral therapy.

This delay will minimize risk of infection and avoid immune-reconstitution illness during the travel.

Household Contacts

Household contacts of severely immunocompromised patients may be given live-virus vaccines such as yellow fever, measles–mumps–rubella, or varicella vaccines but should not be given the live attenuated influenza vaccine (LAIV).

Special Considerations for the Immunocompromised Traveler

Yellow Fever Vaccine

Travelers with severe immune compromise should be strongly discouraged from travel to destinations that present a true risk of yellow fever (YF). If travel to a YF-endemic zone (see Maps 2-3 and 2-4) by such individuals is unavoidable and the vaccine is not given, they should be carefully instructed in methods to avoid mosquito bites and should be provided with a vaccination medical waiver (see the Yellow Fever section in Chapter 2).

Patients with limited immune deficits or asymptomatic HIV going to YF-endemic areas may be offered YF vaccine and monitored closely for possible adverse effects. As vaccine response may be suboptimal, such vaccinees are candidates for serologic testing one month after vaccination. (For information about serologic testing, contact the state health department or CDC's Division of Vector-Borne Diseases at 970-221-6400.) Data from clinical and epidemiologic studies are insufficient at this time to evaluate the actual risk of severe adverse effects associated with YF vaccine among recipients with limited immune deficits.

If international travel requirements and not true exposure risk are the only reasons to vaccinate an asymptomatic HIV-infected person or a person with a limited immune deficit, the physician should provide a waiver letter. Travelers should be warned that vaccination waiver documents may not be accepted by some countries; if the waiver is rejected, the option of deportation might be preferable to receipt of YF vaccine at the destination.

Malaria Chemoprophylaxis

When travel destinations are in malaria-endemic areas, immunocompromised travelers should be prescribed appropriate drugs for malaria chemoprophylaxis and receive counseling about avoidance of mosquito bites—the same as for immunocompetent travelers (see the Malaria section in Chapter 2). However, special concerns for immunocompromised travelers include any of the following possibilities:

- Drug–drug interactions between the drugs used for malaria chemoprophylaxis and the drugs in the traveler's maintenance regimen
- The underlying medical condition will predispose the immunocompromised traveler to more serious disease from malaria
- A malaria infection and the drugs used to treat the malaria infection will cause an exacerbation of the underlying disease.

The severity of malaria is increased in HIV-infected individuals. Malaria infection increases HIV viral load and thus may exacerbate disease progression. Table 8-2 gives some examples of potential drug–drug interactions between drugs used for malaria chemoprophylaxis and drugs used in HAART regimens for treatment of HIV infections. Since new drugs and drug combinations for HIV treatment are under continuous development, travel health advisors are encouraged to review the most current information regarding possible drug interactions. An interactive web-based resource for checking on drug–drug interactions involving HAART drugs is found at the University of Liverpool website at www.hiv-druginteractions.org/.

For malaria treatment, the use of quinidine (and by implication quinine) in patients taking nelfinavir or ritonavir is contraindicated because of potential cumulative cardiotoxicity. However, if a patient has severe and complicated malaria, there may be no choice. In these circumstances, as in others, quinidine should be used only with close monitoring. In addition, very careful monitoring should accompany quinidine therapy in those taking amprenivir, delaviridine, or the lopinavir/ritonavir combination. Although the clinical significance, if any, is not known, several protease inhibitors have been shown in laboratory testing to inhibit the growth of malaria parasites.

Some clinical case reports suggest that asplenic individuals may be at greater risk of acquisition and complications of malaria, so asplenic travelers to malaria areas should be counseled to adhere conscientiously to the malaria chemoprophylaxis regimen prescribed for them.

Enteric Infections

Many foodborne and waterborne infections, such as those caused by *Salmonella*, *Campylobacter*, *Giardia*, and *Cryptosporidium*, can be very severe or become chronic in immunocompromised persons. Enteroaggregative *Escherichia coli* is an emerging enteric pathogen causing persistent diarrhea among children, adults, and HIV-infected persons.

Safe food and beverage selection guidelines should be followed by all travelers, but travelers' diarrhea can occur despite strict adherence.

- Selection of antimicrobials to be used for self-treatment of travelers' diarrhea may require special consideration of potential drug–drug interactions among patients already taking medications for chronic medical conditions. Fluoroquinolones and rifaximin are active against several enteric pathogens and do not have significant interactions with HAART drugs. However, macrolide antibiotics may have significant drug–drug interactions with HAART drugs (Table 8-3). Emerging therapies for diarrhea in HIV/AIDS patients may involve probiotics such as *Lactobacillus rhamnosus* GR-1, *L. reuteri* RC-14, and others.
- Waterborne infections might result from swallowing water during recreational activities. To reduce the risk for cryptosporidiosis and giardiasis, patients should avoid swallowing water during swimming and should not swim in water that might be contaminated (e.g., with sewage or animal waste).

Attention to hand hygiene, including frequent and thorough hand washing, is the best prevention against gastroenteritis. Hands should be washed after contact with public surfaces and also after any contact with animals or their living areas.

Table 8-2. Potential interactions between malaria drugs and HIV drugs[1]

Drug	Protease Inhibitors	NRTIs[2]	NNRTI[3]
Mefloquine	Decreased levels of ritonavir Possible decreased levels of atazanavir, lopinavir, and nelfinavir	None known	Decreased levels of mefloquine with efavirenz and nevirapine
Atovaquone/proguanil	Decreased levels of atovaquone with indinavir, lopinavir, and ritonavir Decreased levels of indinavir	None known	No available data
Doxycycline	None known	None known	None known
Chloroquine	Potential interaction with ritonavir	None known	None known
Primaquine	No available data	No available data	No available data

1 Adapted from Table 2 in Bhadelia N, Klotman M, Caplivski D. The HIV-Positive Traveler. Am J Med, 2007;120:574–80.
2 Nucleoside reverse transcriptase inhibitor.
3 Non-nucleoside reverse transcriptase inhibitor.

Table 8-3. Potential interactions between antibiotics against travelers' diarrhea and HIV drugs[1]

Drug	Protease Inhibitors	NRTIs[2]	NNRTI[3]
Fluoroquinolones	No clinically significant interactions	No clinically significant interactions	No clinically significant interactions
Macrolides	Possible increased levels of clarithromycin with ritonavir, atazanavir, and lopinavir	Decreased levels of zidovudine with clarithromycin; no data available for azithromycin	Possible interactions with clarithromycin, efavirenz, and nevirapine
Rifaximin	No available data	No available data	No available data

1 Adapted from Table 2 in Bhadelia N, Klotman M, Caplivski D. The HIV-Positive Traveler. Am J Med, 2007;120:574–80.
2 Nucleoside reverse transcriptase inhibitor.
3 Non-nucleoside reverse transcriptase inhibitor.

Reducing Risk for Other Diseases

Geographically focal infections that pose an increased risk of severe outcome for immunocompromised persons include visceral leishmaniasis (a protozoan infection transmitted by the sandfly) and several fungal infections acquired by inhalation (e.g., *Penicillium marneffei* infection in Southeast Asia and coccidioidomycosis in the Americas). Many developing areas have high rates of tuberculosis (TB), and establishing the TB status of immunocompromised travelers going to such destinations may be helpful in the evaluation of any travel-associated illness that subsequently develops. Depending on the traveler's degree of immune suppression, the baseline TB status may be assessed by obtaining a tuberculin skin test, chest radiograph, or *Mycobacterium tuberculosis* antigen-specific interferon gamma assay.

Patients with advanced HIV and transplant recipients are frequently taking either primary or secondary prophylaxis for one or more opportunistic infections (e.g., pneumocystis, mycobacteria, and toxoplasma). Complete adherence to all indicated regimens should be confirmed before travel (see the HIV Infection and Acquired Immunodeficiency Syndrome (AIDS) section in Chapter 5).

References

1. Recommendations of the Advisory Committee on Immunization Practices (ACIP): use of vaccines and immune globulins for persons with altered immunocompetence. MMWR Recomm Rep. 1993;42(RR-4):1–18.

2. CDC. Epidemiology and prevention of vaccine-preventable diseases (The Pink book). 10th ed. Atkinson W, Hamborsky J, McIntyre L, Wolfe S, editors. Washington D.C.: Public Health Foundation; 2008. Appendix A. Vaccination of persons with primary and secondary immune deficiencies. p. A-18–10. Available from: http://www.cdc.gov/vaccines/pubs/pinkbook/downloads/appendices/A/immuno-table.pdf.

3. Brinkman DM, Jol-van der Zijde CM, ten Dam MM, et al. Resetting the adaptive immune system after autologous stem cell transplantation: lessons from response to vaccines. J Clin Immunol. 2007;27(6):647–58.

4. Kroger, AT, Atkinson, WL, Marcuse, EK, et al. General recommendations on immunization: recommendations of the Advisory Committee on Immunization Practices (ACIP). MMWR Recomm Rep..2006;55(RR-15):1–48.

5. Duchini A, Goss JA, Karpen S, Pockros PJ. Vaccinations for adult solid-organ transplant recipients: current recommendations and protocols. Clin Microbiol Rev. 2003;16(3):357–64.

6. Boerbooms AM, Kerstens PJ, van Loenhout JW, et al. Infections during low-dose methotrexate treatment in rheumatoid arthritis. Semin Arthritis Rhem. 1995;24(6):411–21.

7. Kapetanovic MC, Saxne T, Sjoholm A, et al. Influence of methotrexate, TNF blockers and prednisolone on antibody responses to pneumococcal polysaccharide vaccine in patients with rheumatoid arthritis. Rheumatology (Oxford). 2006;45(1):106–11.

8. Brezinschek HP, Hofstaetter T, Leeb BF, et al. Immunization of patients with rheumatoid arthritis with antitumor necrosis factor alpha therapy and methotrexate. Curr Opin Rheumatol. 2008;20(3):295–9.

9. Furst DE, Breedveld FC, Kalden JR, et al. Updated consensus statement on biological agents, specifically tumour necrosis factor α (TNFα) blocking agents and interleukin-1 receptor antagonist (IL-1ra), for the treatment

of rheumatic diseases, 2005. Ann Rheum Dis. 2005;64(Suppl4):iv2–14.

10. Fomin I, Caspi D, Levy V, et al. Vaccination against influenza in rheumatoid arthritis: the effect of disease modifying drugs, including TNF alpha blockers. Ann Rheum Dis. 2006;65(2):191–4.

11. Bongartz T, Sutton AJ, Sweeting MJ, et al. Anti-TNF antibody therapy in rheumatoid arthritis and the risk of serious infections and malignancies: systematic review and meta-analysis of rare harmful effects in randomized controlled trials. JAMA. 2006;295(19):2275–85.

12. Bhadelia N, Klotman M, Caplivski D. The HIV-positive traveler. Am J Med. 2007;120(7):574–80.

13. Boyle BA, Cohen CJ, DeJesus E, et al. Update on antiretroviral therapy: the 15th CROI. AIDS Reader. 2008;18(5):273–8, C3.

14. Kaplan JE, Masur H, Holmes KK; U.S. Public Health Service; Infectious Disease Society of America. Guidelines for preventing opportunistic infections among HIV-infected persons—2002. MMWR Recomm Rep. 2002;51(RR-8):1–52.

15. Laurence JC. Hepatitis A and B immunizations of individuals infected with human immunodeficieny virus. Am J Med. 2005;118(Suppl 10A):75S–83S.

16. De Sousa dos Santos S, Lopes MH, Simonsen V, Caiaffa Filho HH. *Haemophilus influenzae* type b immunization in adults infected with the human immunodeficiency virus. AIDS Res Hum Retroviruses. 2004;20(5):493–6.

17. Douvin C, Simon D, Charles MA, et al. Hepatitis B vaccination in diabetic patients. Randomized trial comparing recombinant vaccines containing and not containing pre-S2 antigen. Diabetes Care. 1997;20(2):148–51.

18. Nevens F, Zuckerman JN, Burroughs AK, et al. Immunogenicity and safety of an experimental adjuvanted hepatitis B candidate vaccine in liver transplant patients. Liver Transpl. 2006;12(10):1489–95.

19. Beran J. Safety and immunogenicity of a new hepatitis B vaccine for the protection of patients with renal insufficiency including pre-haemodialysis and haemodialysis patients. Expert Opin Biol Ther. 2008;8(2):235–47.

20. Eigenberger K, Sillaber C, Greibauer M, et al. Antibody responses to pneumococcal and haemophilus vaccinations in splenectomized patients with hematological malignancies or trauma. Wien Klin Wochenschr. 2077;119(7–8):228–34.

21. Cohen C, Karstaedt A, Frean J, et al. Increased prevalence of severe malaria in HIV-infected adults in South Africa. Clin Infect Dis. 2005;41(11):1631–7.

22. Kamya MR, Gasasira AF, Yeka A, et al. Effect of HIV-1 infection on antimalarial treatment outcomes in Uganda: a population-based study. J Infect Dis. 2006;193(1):9–15.

23. Khoo S, Back D, Winstanley P. The potential for interactions between antimalarial and antiretroviral drugs. AIDS. 2005;19(10):995–1005.

24. Parikh S, Gut J, Istvan E, et al. Antimalarial activity of human immunodeficiency virus type 1 protease inhibitors. Antimicrob Agents Chemother. 2005;49(7):2983–5.

25. Amenta M, Dalle Nogare ER, Colomba C, et al. Intestinal protozoa in HIV-infected patients: effect of rifaximin in *Cryptosporidium parvum* and *Blastocystis hominis* infections. J Chemother. 1999;11(5):391–5.

26. Huang DB, Mohanty A, DuPont HL, et al. A review of an emerging enteric pathogen: enteroaggregative *Escherichia coli*. J Med Microbiol. 2006;55(pt 10):1303–11.

27. Anukam KC, Oszuwa EO, Osadolor HB, et al. Yogurt containing probiotic *Lactobacillus rhamnosus* GR-1 and *L. reuteri* RC-14 helps resolve moderate diarrhea and increases CD4 count in HIV/AIDS patients. J Clin Gastroenterol. 2008;42(3):239–43.

28. Matulis G, Jüni P, Villiger PM, Gadola SD. Detection of latent tuberculosis in immunosuppressed patients with autoimmune diseases: performance of a *Mycobacterium tuberculosis* antigen-specific interferon gamma assay. Ann Rheum Dis. 2008;67(1):84–90.

TRAVELING WHILE PREGNANT

Christina Dorell, Madeline Sutton

Since as many as 50% of pregnancies are unplanned, women of reproductive age should consider maintaining current immunizations during routine check-ups in case an unplanned pregnancy coincides with a need to travel. Because they decrease risk to the unborn child, preconceptional immunizations are preferred to vaccination during pregnancy. A woman should defer pregnancy for at least 28 days after receiving live vaccines (e.g., MMR, yellow fever), because of theoretical risk of transmission to the fetus. However, small studies of women who received these vaccines unintentionally during pregnancy have not found a definitive link between these vaccines and poor pregnancy outcomes. Therefore, pregnancy termination is not recommended after an inadvertent exposure.

According to the American College of Obstetrics and Gynecology, the safest time for a pregnant woman to travel is during the second trimester (18–24 weeks), when she usually feels best and is in least danger of spontaneous abortion or premature labor. A woman in the third trimester should be advised to defer overseas travel because of concerns about access to medical care in case of problems such as hypertension, phlebitis, or premature labor. Pregnant women should be advised to consult with their health-care providers before making any travel decisions. Collaboration between travel health experts and obstetricians is helpful in weighing benefits and risks based on destination and recommended preventive and treatment measures. Table 8-4 lists relative contraindications to international travel during pregnancy. In general, pregnant women with serious underlying illnesses should be advised not to travel to developing countries.

Preparation for Travel during Pregnancy

Once a pregnant woman has decided to travel, a number of issues need to be considered before her departure.

- An intrauterine pregnancy should be confirmed by a clinician and ectopic pregnancy excluded before beginning any travel.
- General health insurance policies may or may not provide coverage while abroad and during pregnancy. Pregnant travelers should inquire about what their health insurance policies cover, and if needed, obtain a supplemental policy for their trip. Many supplemental travel insurance policies and a prepaid medical evacuation insurance policies do not cover pregnancy-related problems, so this issue should be clarified before obtaining a policy.

Table 8-4. Potential contraindications to international travel during pregnancy

Obstetrical Risk Factors	General Medical Risk Factors	Travel to Potentially Hazardous Destinations
• History of miscarriage	• History of thromboembolic disease	• High altitudes
• Incompetent cervix	• Pulmonary hypertension	• Areas endemic for or with ongoing outbreaks of life-threatening food- or insect-borne infections
• History of ectopic pregnancy (ectopic with current pregnancy should be ruled out before travel)	• Severe asthma or other chronic lung disease	• Areas where chloroquine-resistant *Plasmodium falciparum* malaria is endemic
• History of premature labor or premature rupture of membranes	• Valvular heart disease (if NYHA class III or IV heart failure)	• Areas where live virus vaccines are required or recommended
• History of/or existing placental abnormalities	• Cardiomyopathy	
• Threatened abortion or vaginal bleeding during current pregnancy	• Hypertension	
• Multiple gestation in current pregnancy	• Diabetes	
• Fetal growth abnormalities	• Renal insufficiency	
• History of toxemia, hypertension, or diabetes with any pregnancy	• Severe anemia or hemoglobinopathy	
• Primigravida at 35 years of age and older, or 15 years of age and younger	• Chronic organ system dysfunction requiring frequent medical interventions	

- Check medical facilities at the destination. For a woman in the last trimester, medical facilities should be able to manage complications of pregnancy, toxemia, cesarean sections, and premature or ill neonates.
- Determine beforehand whether prenatal care will be required while abroad and who will provide it. The pregnant traveler should make sure she does not miss prenatal visits requiring specific timing.
- Determine beforehand whether blood is routinely screened for HIV and hepatitis B and hepatitis C at the destination. Pregnant travelers should consider the safety of blood transfusions if needed when making plans for international travel. The pregnant traveler should also be advised to know her blood type, and Rh-negative pregnant women should receive anti-D immune globulin (a plasma-derived product) prophylactically at about 28 weeks' gestation. The immune globulin dose should be repeated after delivery if the infant is Rh positive.
- Determine when influenza season begins and ends in the destination region and administer influenza vaccine accordingly.
- Determine whether the destination region has high prevalence of tuberculosis and whether the planned itinerary will put the traveler at risk for TB. If exposure to TB is determined to be a risk (see the Tuberculosis section in Chapter 5), the pregnant traveler should receive skin testing before and after travel.

General Recommendations for Travel during Pregnancy

A pregnant woman should be advised to travel with at least one companion; she should also be advised that, during her pregnancy, her level of comfort may be adversely affected by traveling. Table 8-5 lists the greatest risks that pregnant women face during international travel.

- Typical problems of pregnant travelers are the same as those experienced by any pregnant woman: fatigue, heartburn, indigestion, constipation, vaginal discharge, leg cramps, increased frequency of urination, and hemorrhoids.
- During travel, pregnant women can take preventive measures, including avoidance of gas-producing food or drinks before scheduled flights (entrapped gases can expand at higher altitudes) and periodic movement of the legs (to decrease venous stasis).
- Pregnant women should always use seatbelts while seated, as air turbulence is not predictable and may cause significant trauma.

Signs and symptoms that indicate the need for immediate medical attention are vaginal bleeding, passing tissue or clots, abdominal pain or cramps, contractions, ruptured membranes, excessive leg swelling or pain, headaches, or visual problems.

Air Travel during Pregnancy

Commercial air travel poses no special risks to a healthy pregnant woman or her fetus. The American College of Obstetricians and Gynecologists (ACOG) states that women with healthy, single pregnancies can fly safely up to 36 weeks' gestation.

Table 8-5. Greatest risks for pregnant travelers

Motor Vehicle Accidents	• Safety belts should be worn whenever possible. • Fasten seatbelts at the pelvic area, not across the lower abdomen. Lap and shoulder restraints are best. • In most accidents, the fetus recovers quickly from the safety belt pressure. However, consult a physician even for mild trauma.
Hepatitis E	• Hepatitis E is not vaccine preventable and is especially dangerous in pregnant women. • Pregnant women should be advised that the best preventive measures are to avoid potentially contaminated water and food, as with other enteric infections.
Scuba Diving	• Scuba diving should be avoided in pregnancy because of the risk of decompression syndrome in the fetus.

- The lowered cabin pressure (kept at the equivalent of 1,524–2,438 m [5,000–8,000 ft]) has minimal effect on fetal oxygenation because of the favorable fetal hemoglobin–oxygen dynamics.
- If supplemental oxygen is going to be required during flight due to pre-existing medical conditions, arrangements for oxygen need to be made in advance.
- Severe anemia, sickle-cell disease or trait, or history of thrombophlebitis are relative contraindications to flying.
- Pregnant women with placental abnormalities or risks for premature labor should avoid air travel.

Airline Policies and Airport Security

Each airline has policies regarding pregnancy and flying; it is always safest to check with the airline when booking reservations, because some will require medical forms to be completed. Domestic travel is usually permitted until the pregnant traveler is in week 36 of gestation, and international travel may be permitted until weeks 32–35, depending on the airline. A pregnant woman should be advised to carry documentation stating the expected day of delivery, contact information for her obstetric provider, and her blood type.

For pregnant flight attendants and pilots, working air travel is restricted by most airlines by 20 weeks' gestation.

Airport security radiation exposure is minimal for pregnant women and has not been linked to an increase in adverse outcomes for unborn children to date. However, because of early reports of a possible association of radiation exposure during pregnancy and subsequent increased risk of childhood leukemia and cancer, a pregnant passenger may request a hand or wand search rather than being exposed to the radiation of the airport security machines.

General Tips

- An aisle seat at the bulkhead will provide the most space and comfort, but a seat over the wing in the midplane region will give the smoothest ride.
- A pregnant woman should be advised to walk every half hour during a smooth flight and flex and extend her ankles frequently to prevent phlebitis.
- Dehydration can lead to decreased placental blood flow and hemoconcentration, increasing risk of thrombosis. Thus, pregnant women should drink plenty of fluids during flights.

Travel to High Altitudes during Pregnancy

There have been no documented reports of adverse pregnancy outcomes related to high-altitude exposure during pregnancy. High-altitude destinations, however, often are remote from medical care in an emergency, and any decision to trek or climb to high altitude while pregnant should take into account the uncertainties of being in a remote environment while pregnant and the unknown possible effects of high altitude on the fetus. Conservative advice for pregnant women is to avoid altitudes above 3,658 m (12,000 ft).

Food and Waterborne Illness during Pregnancy

Pregnant women should be advised of the following:

- Adhere strictly to food and water precautions in developing countries because the consequences may be more severe than diarrhea and may have serious sequelae (e.g., toxoplasmosis, listeriosis).
- Boil suspect drinking water to avoid long-term use of iodine-containing purification systems. Iodine tablets can probably be used for travel up to several weeks, but congenital goiters have been reported in association with administration of iodine-containing drugs during pregnancy.
- Oral rehydration is the mainstay of therapy for travelers' diarrhea (i.e., boiled water, bottled carbonated beverages).

- Bismuth subsalicylate compounds are contraindicated because of the theoretical risks of fetal bleeding from salicylates and teratogenicity from the bismuth.
- The combination of kaolin and pectin may be used, and loperamide should be used only when necessary.
- The antibiotic treatment of travelers' diarrhea during pregnancy can be complicated. Azithromycin or an oral third-generation cephalosporin may be the best options for treatment if an antibiotic is needed.

Malaria during Pregnancy

Advise pregnant women to avoid travel to malaria-endemic areas if possible. Women who do choose to go to malarious areas can reduce their risk of acquiring malaria by taking appropriate malaria chemoprophylaxis and following insect precautions presented in the Malaria section and the Protection Against Mosquitoes, Ticks, and Other Insects and Arthropods section in Chapter 2.

- Use insect repellents as recommended for adults, sparingly, but as needed.
- Pyrethrum-containing house sprays may also be used indoors if insects are a problem.

Antimalarial Medications

For pregnant women who travel to areas with chloroquine-sensitive *Plasmodium falciparum* malaria, chloroquine has been used for malaria chemoprophylaxis for decades with no documented increase in birth defects. For pregnant women who travel to areas with chloroquine-resistant *P. falciparum*, mefloquine should be recommended for chemoprophylaxis. Evidence suggests that mefloquine prophylaxis causes no significant increase in spontaneous abortions or congenital malformations when taken during the first trimester.

Because there is no evidence that chloroquine and mefloquine are associated with congenital defects when used for prophylaxis, CDC does not recommend that women planning pregnancy need to wait a specific period of time after their use before becoming pregnant. However, if women or their health-care providers wish to decrease the amount of antimalarial drug in the body before conception, Table 8-6 provides information on the half-lives of selected antimalarial drugs. After two, four, and six half-lives, approximately 25%, 6%, and 2%, respectively, of the drug remain in the body.

Doxycycline and primaquine are contraindicated for malaria prophylaxis during pregnancy, because both may cause adverse effects on the fetus. Atovoquone/proguanil is currently not recommended for use by pregnant women to prevent malaria because of the lack of safety studies during pregnancy.

Treatment and Management

Malaria must be treated as a medical emergency in any pregnant traveler. A woman who has traveled to an area that has chloroquine-resistant strains of *P. falciparum* should be

Table 8-6. Half-lives of selected antimalarial drugs

Drug	Half Life
Atovaquone	2–3 days
Chloroquine	Can extend from 6 to 60 days
Doxycycline	12–24 hours
Mefloquine	2–3 weeks
Primaquine	4–7 hours
Proguanil	14–21 hours
Pyrimethamine	3–4 days
Sulfadoxine	6–9 days

treated as if she has illness caused by chloroquine-resistant organisms. The management of malaria in a pregnant woman should include frequent blood glucose determinations and careful fluid monitoring (being careful not to give too much intravenous fluid).

Immunizations for Pregnant Travelers

Risk to a developing fetus from vaccination of the mother during pregnancy is primarily theoretical. No evidence exists of risk from vaccinating pregnant women with inactivated virus or bacterial vaccines or toxoids. The benefits of vaccinating pregnant women usually outweigh potential risks when the likelihood of disease exposure is high, when infection would pose a risk to the mother or fetus, and when the vaccine is unlikely to cause harm.

The following table is intended for women who may require immunizations during pregnancy (Table 8-7). Pregnant travelers may visit areas of the world where diseases eliminated by routine vaccination in the United States are still endemic and therefore may require immunizations before travel.

The Travel Health Kit during Pregnancy

Additions and substitutions to the usual travel health kit (see the Travel Health Kits section in Chapter 2) need to be made during pregnancy. Talcum powder, a thermometer, oral rehydration salt packets, prenatal vitamins, a topical antifungal agent for vaginal yeast, acetaminophen, and a sunscreen with a high SPF should be carried. Women in the third trimester may be advised to carry a blood-pressure cuff and urine dipsticks and have their providers train them to use them so they can check for hypertension, proteinuria and glucosuria, any of which would require prompt medical attention. Antimalarial and antidiarrheal self-treatment medications should be evaluated individually, depending on the traveler's itinerary and her health history. Most medications should be avoided, if possible.

Table 8-7. Vaccination during pregnancy

Vaccine/Immunobiologic		Use
Immune globulins, pooled or hyperimmune	Immune globulin or specific globulin preparations	If indicated for pre- or postexposure use. No known risk to fetus
Vaccination of pregnant women is recommended		
Hepatitis B	Recombinant or plasma-derived	Recommended for women at risk of infection
Influenza	Inactivated whole virus or subunit	All women who are pregnant in the second and third trimesters during the flu season (October–March); and women at high risk for pulmonary complications regardless of trimester
Diphtheria–tetanus	Toxoid	If indicated, such as lack of primary series, or no booster within past 10 years
Diphtheria–tetanus–pertussis	Toxoid—acellular	Not contraindicated, but data on safety, immunogenicity and outcomes of pregnancy are not available. ACIP recommends Td when tetanus and diphtheria protection are required but Tdap to add protection against pertussis in some situations. Second or third trimester is preferred.
Hepatitis A	Inactivated virus	Data on safety in pregnancy are not available. Because hepatitis A vaccine is produced from inactivated hepatitis A virus, the theoretical risk of vaccination should be weighed against the risk of disease. Consider immune globulin rather than vaccine.

(Continued)

Table 8-7. Vaccination during pregnancy *(Continued)*

Vaccine/Immunobiologic	Use	
Pregnancy is a precaution, and under normal circumstances vaccination should be deferred; vaccine should only be given when benefits outweigh risks		
Japanese encephalitis	Inactivated virus	Data on safety in pregnancy are not available. Pregnant women who must travel to an area where the risk is high should be vaccinated when the theoretical risks are outweighed by the risk of disease.
Meningococcal meningitis	Polysaccharide	Meningococcal conjugate vaccine (MCV4) is preferred for adults; however, there are no data on safety and immunogenicity in pregnant women. Polyvalent meningococcal meningitis vaccine (MPSV4) can be administered during pregnancy if the woman is entering an epidemic area. Indications for prophylaxis are not altered by pregnancy; vaccine is recommended in unusual outbreak situations.
Pneumococcal	Polysaccharide	The safety of pneumococcal (PPV23) vaccine during the first trimester of pregnancy has not been evaluated, although no adverse events have been reported after inadvertent vaccination during pregnancy. Women with chronic diseases, smokers, and immunosuppressed women should consider vaccination.
Polio, inactivated	Inactivated virus	Indicated for susceptible pregnant women traveling in endemic areas or in other high-risk situations
Rabies	Inactivated virus	Indications for postexposure prophylaxis not altered by pregnancy. If risk of exposure to rabies is substantial, pre-exposure prophylaxis may also be indicated.
Typhoid (ViCPS)	Polysaccharide	If indicated for travel to endemic areas
Typhoid (Ty21a)	Live bacterial	Data on safety in pregnancy are not available; theoretical risk because live-attenuated
Yellow fever	Live attenuated	The safety of yellow fever (YF) vaccination in pregnancy has not been studied in a large prospective trial. Pregnant women who must travel to areas where the risk of YF infection is high should be vaccinated and their infants should be monitored after birth for evidence of congenital infection and other possible adverse effects resulting from YF vaccination. Pregnancy may interfere with the immune response to YF vaccine; therefore, serologic testing to document a protective immune response to the vaccine can be considered (see the Yellow Fever section in Chapter 2 for more details).
Pregnancy is a contraindication to vaccination; vaccine should not be administered to pregnant women		
Tuberculosis (BCG)	Attenuated mycobacterial	Contraindicated due to theoretical risk of disseminated disease. Skin testing for tuberculosis exposure before and after travel is preferable when the risk of possible exposure is high.
Measles–mumps–rubella	Live attenuated virus	Contraindicated; vaccination of susceptible women should be part of postpartum care. Unvaccinated women should delay travel to countries where measles is endemic until after delivery. Unvaccinated pregnant women with a documented exposure to measles should receive IG within 6 days to prevent illness.
Human papillomavirus	Recombinant quadrivalent	Contraindicated. Currently, the vaccine has not been causally associated with adverse outcomes of pregnancy; however, additional information is needed for further recommendations.
Varicella	Live attenuated virus	Contraindicated; vaccination of susceptible women should be considered postpartum. Unvaccinated pregnant women should consider postponing travel until after delivery when the vaccine can be given safely.

References

1. American College of Obstetricians and Gynecologists. ACOG Committee Opinion. Immunization during pregnancy. Obstet Gynecol. 2003;101(1):207–12.

2. ACOG Committee on Obstetric Practice. Committee Opinion No. 264. Air travel during pregnancy. Obstet Gynecol. 2001;98(6):1187–8.

3. Bia FJ. Medical considerations for the pregnant traveler. Infect Dis Clin North Am. 1992;6(2):371–88.

4. CDC. Guidelines for vaccinating pregnant women: from recommendations of the Advisory Committee on Immunization Practices (ACIP). [updated 2007 May; cited 2008 Nov 30]. Available from: http://www.cdc.gov/vaccines/pubs/downloads/b_preg_guide.pdf.

5. Fiore AE, Shay DK, Broder K, et al. Prevention and control of influenza: recommendations of the Advisory Committee on Immunization Practices (ACIP), 2008. MMWR Recomm Rep. 2008;57(RR-07):1–60.

6. Marin M, Güris D, Chaves SS, Schmid S, Seward JF. Prevention of varicella: recommendations of the Advisory Committee on Immunization Practices (ACIP). MMWR Recomm Rep. 2007;56(RR-04):1–40.

7. CDC. Guiding principles for development of ACIP Recommendations for vaccination during pregnancy and breastfeeding. MMWR Morb Mortal Wkly Rep. 2008;57(21):580.

8. Barish RJ. In-flight radiation exposure during pregnancy. Obstet Gynecol. 2004;103(6):1326–30.

9. Boice JD Jr., Miller RW. Childhood and adult cancer after intrauterine exposure to ionizing radiation. Teratology. 1999;59(4):227–33.

10. Physician Desk Reference (PDR) Electronic Library Online [database on the Internet]. Montvale (NJ): Thomson PDR; c2002–2008— [cited 2008 Nov 30]. Malarone tablets (GlaxoSmithKline). Available from: http://elib2.cdc.gov:2111/pdrel/librarian/PFPUI/ 8c1qV3g2Jl2hHF.

11. Mast EE, Margolis HS, Fiore, AE, et al. A comprehensive immunization strategy to eliminate transmission of hepatitis B virus infection in the United States: recommendations of the Advisory Committee on Immunization Practices (ACIP) part 1: immunization of infants, children, and adolescents. MMWR Recomm Rep. 2005;54(RR-16):1–31.

12. Bilukha OO, Rosenstein N, National Center for Infectious Diseases, CDC. Prevention and control of meningococcal disease: recommendations of the Advisory Committee on Immunization Practices (ACIP). MMWR Recomm Rep. 2005;54(RR-7):1–21.

13. Human rabies prevention—United States, 1999. Recommendations of the Advisory Committee on Immunization Practices (ACIP). MMWR Recomm Rep. 1999;48(RR-1):1–21.

14. Typhoid immunization: recommendations of the Advisory Committee on Immunization Practices (ACIP). MMWR Recomm Rep. 1994;43(RR-14):1–7.

15. Cetron MS, Marfin AA, Julian KG, et al. Yellow fever vaccine. Recommendations of the Advisory Committee on Immunization Practices (ACIP), 2002. MMWR Recomm Rep. 2002;51(RR-17):1–11.

16. CDC. Notice to Readers: Revised ACIP recommendation for avoiding pregnancy after receiving a rubella-containing vaccine. MMWR Morb Mortal Wkly Rep. 2001;50(49);1117.

17. Watson JC, Hadler SC, Dykewicz CA, et al. Measles, mumps, and rubella-vaccine use and strategies for elimination of measles, rubella, and congenital rubella syndrome and control of mumps: recommendations of the Advisory Committee on Immunization Practices (ACIP). MMWR Recomm Rep. 1998;47(RR-8):1–57.

TRAVELERS WITH DISABILITIES

Emad Yanni

Any person is defined as a traveler with disabilities whose mobility is reduced because of a physical incapacity (sensory or locomotor), an intellectual deficiency, age, illness, or another cause when using transport and whose situation needs special attention and adaptation of the services made available to all passengers. The medical preparation of a traveler with a stable, ongoing disability does not differ from that of any other traveler.

The keys to safe, accessible travel are to—

- assess each anticipated international itinerary on an individual basis, in consultation with specialized travel agencies or tour operators;
- consult travel health providers for additional recommendations; and
- utilize print and Internet resources.

Air Travel

Regulations and Codes

Carriers may not refuse transportation on the basis of disability. By law, U.S. air carriers must comply with highly detailed regulations that affect people with disabilities. These do not cover foreign carriers serving the United States.

- All U.S. and non-U.S. carriers are required to file annual reports of disability-related complaints with the U.S. Department of Transportation (DOT). The DOT maintains a toll-free hotline (800-778-4838, available 7 am to 11 pm Eastern Standard Time) to provide real-time assistance in facilitating compliance with DOT rules and to suggest customer-service solutions to the airlines.
- The Transportation Security Administration (TSA) has established a program for screening of travelers with disabilities and their equipment, mobility aids, and devices. TSA permits prescriptions, liquid medications, and other liquids needed by persons with disabilities and medical conditions.
- International Air Transport Association (IATA) member airlines voluntarily adhere to codes of practice that are very similar to U.S. legislation based on guidance from the International Civil Aviation Organization. However, smaller airlines overseas may not be IATA members.

Airlines are obliged to accept a declaration by a passenger that he or she is self-reliant. Medical certificates can be required only in specific situations (for example, if a person intends to travel with a possible communicable disease or will require a stretcher or oxygen, or if unusual behavior is anticipated that may affect the operation of the flight).

Assistance and Accommodations

When a disabled person requests assistance, the airline is obliged to provide access to the aircraft door (preferably by a level entry bridge), an aisle wheelchair, and a seat with removable armrests. Aircraft with <30 seats are generally exempt. Airline personnel are not required to transfer passengers from wheelchair to wheelchair, wheelchair to aircraft seat, or wheelchair to lavatory seat. Disabled passengers who cannot transfer themselves should travel with a companion or attendant, but carriers may not without reason require a person with a disability to travel with an attendant.

Only wide-body aircraft with two aisles are required to have fully accessible lavatories, although any aircraft with >60 seats must have an on-board wheelchair and personnel must assist with movement of the wheelchair from the seat to the area outside the lavatory. Wet-acid batteries in electric wheelchairs may require special, separate stowage. Airline personnel are not obliged to assist with feeding, visiting the lavatory, or dispensing medication to travelers.

Airlines may not require advance notice that a person with a disability is traveling; however, they may require up to 48 hours' advance notice and 1-hour advance check-in for certain accommodations that require preparation time, such as the following:

- Medical oxygen for use on board the aircraft, if the service is available on the flight
- Carriage of an incubator, if the service is available on the flight
- Hook-up for a respirator to the aircraft electrical power supply, if the service is available on the flight
- Accommodation for a passenger who must travel in a stretcher, if the service is available on the flight
- Transportation for an electric wheelchair on a flight scheduled to be made with an aircraft with <60 seats
- Provision by the carrier of hazardous material packaging for a battery used in a wheelchair or other assistive devices
- Accommodation for a group of ten or more qualified individuals with disabilities who make reservation and travel as a group

- Provision of an on-board wheelchair on an aircraft that does not have an accessible lavatory

Assessment and Preparation

With high incidence of cardiopulmonary disease and millions of people traveling by air, many people are at risk for significant hypoxia and respiratory symptoms while flying. Generally patients with an oxygen saturation by pulse oximetry above 95% do not require supplemental oxygen and those with a saturation below 92% will require it during air travel. The hypoxia altitude simulation test (HAST) can identify those patients (with an oxygen saturation by pulse oximetry between 92% and 95%) who may benefit from oxygen supplementation during air travel, decreasing their risk for significant cardiopulmonary effects of induced hypoxia at higher altitude.

Internationally standardized codes for classifying disabled passengers and their needs are available in all computerized reservations systems. Disabled passengers should use travel agents experienced in the use of the disability coding; it is critical that appropriate codes and inter-airline messages are sequentially entered for all flights. The delivering carrier is always responsible for a disabled passenger until a subsequent carrier physically accepts responsibility for that passenger.

Service Animals

Service animals are not exempt from compliance with quarantine regulations and so may not be allowed to travel to all international destinations. They are also subject to U.S. Animal Import Regulations on return (see the Taking Animals Across International Borders section in Chapter 6). However, carriers must permit dog guides or other service animals with appropriate identification to accompany an individual with a disability on a flight. Carriers must permit a service animal to accompany a traveler with a disability to any seat in which the person sits, unless the animal obstructs an aisle or other area that must remain clear to facilitate an emergency evacuation, in which case the passenger will be assigned another seat.

Cruise Ships

U.S. companies or entities conducting programs or tours on cruise ships have obligations regarding access for travelers with disabilities, even if the ship itself is of foreign registry (see the Cruise Ship Travel section in Chapter 6). However, all travelers with disabilities should check with individual cruise lines regarding availability of requested or needed items prior to booking. Cruises are available that cater to travelers with special needs, such as dialysis patients.

Useful Links

- MossRehab ResourceNet. Available from www.mossresourcenet.org/travel.htm.
- U.S. Department of Transportation, Aviation Consumer Protection Division:
  - New Horizons Information for the Air Traveler with a Disability. Available from: http://airconsumer.ost.dot.gov/publications/horizons.htm.
  - Nondiscrimination on the Basis of Disability in Air Travel. 14 CFR Part 382 (Federal Rules). Available from: http://airconsumer.ost.dot.gov/rules/rules.htm.
- American Council of the Blind. Lists cruises, books, useful telephone numbers, and links to products for purchase. Available from: www.acb.org/resources/travel.html.
- Access-Able. Resource for mature travelers and those with special needs. Available from: www.access-able.com.
- Transportation Security Administration: travelers with disabilities and medical conditions. Available from: www.tsa.gov/travelers/airtravel/specialneeds.

- Society for Accessible Travel and Hospitality. Available from: www.sath.org.
- Aerospace Medical Association. Medical guidelines for airlines travel. Available from: www.asma.org/publications/medicalguideline.php.
- Mobility International U.S.A. Available from: www.miusa.org.
  - Preparing for Departure. Available from: www.miusa.org/ncde/intlopportunities/survivalsteps/departure/.
  - Equipment and Tools that Make Traveling with a Disability Easy. Available from: www.miusa.org/ncde/tipsheets/tools/.

References

1. Convention on International Civil Aviation. International Civil Aviation Organization. Chapter 8, Annex 9 Attachment 2: ICAO-recommended practices relating to persons with disabilities. [cited 2008 Jul 7]. Available from: http://www.icao.int/icao/en/atb/sgm/disabilities.htm.

2. Bucks, C. A World of Options: A Guide to International Exchange, Community Service and Travel for Persons with Disabilities. 3rd ed. ILR Press;1997.

3. Dine CJ, Kreider ME. Hypoxia altitude simulation test. Chest. 2008;133(4):1002–5.

VFRs: IMMIGRANTS RETURNING HOME TO VISIT FRIENDS AND RELATIVES

Jay S. Keystone

Definition of VFR

A traveler categorized as a VFR is an immigrant, ethnically and racially distinct from the majority population of the country of residence (a higher-income country), who returns to his or her homeland (lower-income country) to visit friends or relatives. Included in the VFR category are family members such as the spouse or children, who were born in the country of residence.

VFRs: An Important Category of Travelers

VFRs are increasing in numbers and importance with regard to travel health, as they represent a group whose morbidity is greater than other travelers.

- Altered migration patterns to North America over the past 30 years have resulted in many immigrants originating from Asia and Latin America instead of Europe.
- Although 12% of the U.S. population is foreign born, in 2007, 38% of those from the United States traveling overseas listed VFR as a reason for travel.
- VFRs experience a higher incidence of travel-related infectious diseases, such as malaria, typhoid fever, tuberculosis, hepatitis A, and sexually transmitted infections than other groups of international travelers.

Disproportionate Infectious Disease Risks in VFRs

There are a number of reasons for an increased risk of infectious diseases in the VFR population:

- Lack of awareness of risk
- 30% or fewer have a pre-travel health-care encounter
- Financial barriers to pre-travel health care

- Clinics are not geographically convenient
- Cultural and language barriers with health-care providers
- Lack of trust in the medical system
- May experience greater last-minute travel plans and longer trips
- Travel to higher-risk destinations, such as staying in homes and living the local lifestyle, which often includes lack of food and water precautions, bed nets, etc.
- Belief that they are "immune." VFR health beliefs likely contribute to lower rates of vaccination against hepatitis A and typhoid and infrequent use of malaria chemoprophylaxis compared with other international travelers.

Malaria

- In 2006, >50% of imported malaria cases in U.S. civilians occurred among VFRs.
- Data from GeoSentinel, the International Society of Travel Medicine and CDC sentinel surveillance network, show VFRs are eight times more likely to acquire malaria than are tourist travelers. Reports from the United Kingdom have shown that VFR travelers to West Africa were 10 times more likely to develop malaria than were tourists.
- Many VFRs assume they are "immune"; however, in most VFRs, especially those who left their countries of origin years previously, immunity has waned and is no longer protective.

Other Infections

- In the United States, >75% of typhoid cases occur in VFRs, mostly from South Asia and Latin America; 90% of paratyphoid A cases are imported from South Asia as well.
- VFR children <15 years of age are at highest risk of hepatitis A, and many are symptomatic. In a British study, most cases were acquired in South Asia.
- Other diseases, such as tuberculosis, hepatitis A and B, cholera, and measles, occur more commonly in VFRs following travel.

Pre-Travel Health Counseling for VFRs

Table 8-8 summarizes VFR health risks and prevention recommendations. It is important to increase awareness among providers and the travelers themselves regarding the unique risks for travel-related infections and the barriers to travel health services. If possible, clinics should try to incorporate culturally sensitive educational materials and language translators, along with providing handouts in multiple languages (see www.tropical.umn.edu/vfr).

Vaccinations

Travel immunization recommendations and requirements for VFRs are the same as those for U.S.-born travelers. It is crucial, however, to first try to establish whether the immigrant traveler has had "routine" immunizations (e.g., measles, tetanus, etc.) or has a history of the diseases. Adult travelers, in the absence of documentation of immunizations, may be considered to be non-immune, and appropriate vaccinations (or serologic studies to check for antibody status) should be provided. There are a few important caveats:

- Immunity to hepatitis A should not be assumed; many young adults and adolescents from developing countries are still susceptible. Pre-travel serologic testing for both hepatitis A and B may be worthwhile.
- Consider varicella immunization for immigrants from South and Southeast Asia and Latin America. These travelers may be more susceptible, because infection occurs at an older age compared with its occurrence in temperate regions. Also, adults with varicella disease have greater morbidity and mortality than do children.

Table 8-8. Specific disease risks, proposed reasons for risk variance, and recommendations to reduce risks specific to travelers visiting friends and relatives

Specific Diseases	Risk of Exposure: VFRs vs. Traditional Travelers	Reason for Risk Variance[1]	Recommendations to Stress with VFR Travelers
Food- and waterborne illness	Increased	Social and cultural pressure (e.g., eat the meal served by hosts)	Frequent handwashing Avoid high-risk foods (e.g., dairy products, undercooked foods) Simplify treatment regimens (e.g., single-antibiotic dose, such as azithromycin, 1,000 mg, or ciprofloxacin, 500 mg) Discuss food preparation (e.g., cleaning vegetables)
Fish-related toxins and infections	Increased	Ingestion of high-risk foods Less pre-travel advice	Avoidance counseling about specific cultural foods (e.g., raw freshwater fish)
Malaria	Increased	Longer stays Higher-risk destinations Less pre-travel advice leading to less use of chemoprophylaxis and fewer personal protection measures Belief that already immune	Education on malaria, mosquito avoidance, and the need for chemoprophylaxis Consider cost in chemoprophylaxis Use of insecticide-treated bed nets
Tuberculosis (particularly multidrug-resistant)	Increased	Increased close contact with local population Increased contact with HIV-coinfected persons	Check PPD 3–6 months after return if history of negative PPD and long stay (>3 months) Educate about tuberculosis signs, symptoms, and avoidance
Bloodborne and sexually transmitted diseases	Increased	More likely to seek substandard, local care (e.g., dental) Cultural practices (e.g., tattoos, female genital mutilation) Longer stays and increased chance of blood transfusion Higher likelihood of sexual encounters with local population	Discuss high-risk behaviors, including tattoos, piercings, dental work, sexual encounters Encourage purchase of condoms prior to travel Consider providing syringes, needles, and intravenous catheters for long-term travel
Schistosomiasis and helminths	Increased	Limited access to piped-in water in rural areas for bathing and washing clothes	Avoid freshwater exposure Use liposomal DEET preparation with freshwater exposures[2] Discourage child from playing in dirt Use ground cover Use protective footwear

(Continued)

Table 8-8. Specific disease risks, proposed reasons for risk variance, and recommendations to reduce risks specific to travelers visiting friends and relatives *(Continued)*

Specific Diseases	Risk of Exposure: VFRs vs. Traditional Travelers	Reason for Risk Variance[1]	Recommendations to Stress with VFR Travelers
Respiratory problems	Increased	Increased close exposure to fires, smoking, or pollution	Prepare for asthma exacerbations by considering stand-by steroids
Zoonotic diseases (e.g., rickettsial, leptopirosis, viral fevers, leishmaniasis, anthrax)	Increased	Rural destinations Stays with family where animals are kept, and increased exposure to insects Increased exposure to mice and rats Sleeping on floors	Avoid animals Wash hands Wear protective clothing Check for ticks daily Avoid thatched roofs, mud walls in Latin America Avoid sleeping at floor level
Envenomations (e.g., snakes, spiders, scorpions)	Increased	Sleeping on floors	Avoid sleeping at floor level Use footwear out-of-doors at night
Toxin ingestion (e.g., medication adverse events, heavy metal ingestion)	Increased	Purchase of local medications Use of traditional therapies Use of contaminated products (e.g., Mexican pottery with lead glaze) Ingestion of contaminated freshwater fish	Anticipate and purchase medications prior to travel Counsel avoidance of known traditional medications (e.g., Hmong bark tea with aspirin) and high-risk items (e.g., large reef fish)
Yellow fever and Japanese encephalitis	Decreased in adults	Unclear, partial immunity due to previous exposure or vaccination	Avoid mosquitoes by taking protective measures and receiving vaccination when appropriate
Dengue fever	Increased (especially risk of DHF and DSS)	DHF and DSS occur on repeat exposure to a second serotype of dengue. VFRs more likely to have had previous exposure	Avoid mosquitoes by taking protective measures

DEET, *N,N*-diethyl-*m*-toluamide; DHF, dengue hemorrhagic fever; DSS, dengue shock syndrome; HIV, human immunodeficiency virus; PPD, purified protein derivative; VFR, visiting friends and relatives.

1 Hypothesis unless reference cited to support assertions.
2 DEET (liposomal preparations) has been demonstrated in animal models to prevent the skin penetration of *Schistosomiasis cercariae*.

Adapted from: Bacaner N, Stauffer B, Boulware DR, Walker PF, Keystone JS. Travel medicine considerations for North American immigrants visiting friends and relatives. JAMA. 2004;291(23):2856–64. Copyright © 2004 American Medical Association.

Malaria Prevention

VFR travelers to endemic areas should not only be encouraged to take prophylactic medications, but also should be reminded of the benefits of barrier methods of prevention, such as bed nets and insect repellents, particularly for children (see the Protection Against Mosquitoes, Ticks, and Other Insects and Arthropods section in Chapter 2). Posters depicting malaria prevention techniques are available on the CDC malaria prevention website at www.cdc.gov/malaria/travel/index.htm.

- VFRs should be advised that drugs such as chloroquine, proguanil, and pyrimethamine are no longer effective in most areas, especially in sub-Saharan Africa. These medications are often readily available and inexpensive in their home countries, but are not efficacious.
- VFRs should also be encouraged to purchase their medications before traveling to ensure good drug quality. Studies in Africa and Southeast Asia show that one third to one half of antimalarial drugs purchased locally were counterfeit or substandard.

References

1. Bacaner N, Stauffer B, Boulware DR, et al. Travel medicine considerations for North American immigrants visiting friends and relatives. JAMA. 2004;291(23):2856–64.
2. Angell SY, Cetron MS. Health disparities among travelers visiting friends and relatives abroad. Ann Intern Med. 2005;142(1):67–72.
3. Leder K, Tong S, Weld L, et al. Illness in travelers visiting friends and relatives: a review of the GeoSentinel Surveillance Network. Clin Infect Dis. 2006;43(9):1185–93.
4. U.S. Department of Homeland Security. Office of Immigration Statistics. Annual Flow Report: U.S. Legal Permanent Residents: 2005 [cited 2006 July 17]. Available from: http://www.uscis.gov/graphics/shared/statistics/publications/2005NatzFlowRpt.pdf.
5. U.S. Census Bureau. The Foreign-Born Population in 2004 [cited 2006 July 17]. Available from: http://www.census.gov/population/pop-profile/dynamic/ForeignBorn.pdf.
6. U.S. Department of Commerce. Office of Travel and Tourism Industries. 2004 profile of U.S. resident travelers visiting overseas destinations reported from: Survey of international air travelers [cited 2006 July 19]. Available from: http://tinet.ita.doc.gov/view/f-2004-101-001/index.html.
7. Skarbinski J, James EM, Causer LM, et al. Malaria surveillance—United States, 2004. MMWR Surveill Summ. 2006;55(4):23–37.
8. CDC. Malaria in multiple family members—Chicago, Illinois, 2006. MMWR Morb Mortal Wkly Rep. 2006;55(23):645–8.
9. Lynch M, Bulens S, Polyak C, et al. Multi-drug resistance among Salmonella Typhi isolates in the United States, 1999–2003. Sixth International Conference on Typhoid Fever and other Salmonelloses; 2005 Nov 12–14; Guilin, China.
10. Steinberg EB, Bishop R, Haber P, et al. Typhoid fever in travelers: who should be targeted for prevention? Clin Infect Dis. 2004;39(2):186–91.
11. Gupta SK, Medalla F, Omondi MW, et al. Laboratory-based surveillance of paratyphoid fever in the United States: travel and antimicrobial resistance. Clin Infect Dis. 2008;46(11):1656–63.
12. Behrens RH, Collins M, Botto B, et al. Risk for British travellers of acquiring hepatitis A. BMJ. 1995;311(6998):193.
13. Scolari C, Tedoldi S, Casalini C, et al. Knowledge, attitudes, and practices on malaria preventive measures of migrants attending a public health clinic in northern Italy. J Travel Med. 2002;9(3):160–2.
14. Schilthuis HJ, Goossens I, Ligthelm RJ, et al. Factors determining use of pre-travel preventive health services by West African immigrants in The Netherlands. Trop Med Int Health. 2007;12(8):990–8.
15. Van Herck K, Van Damme P, Castelli F, et al. Knowledge, attitudes and practices in travel-related infectious diseases: the European airport survey. J Travel Med. 2004;11(1):3–8.
16. dos Santos CC, Anvar A, Keystone JS, et al. Survey of use of malaria prevention measures by Canadians visiting India. CMAJ. 1999;160(2):195–200.
17. Barnett ED, Christiansen D, Figueira M. Seroprevalence of measles, rubella, and varicella in refugees. Clin Infect Dis. 2002;35(4):403–8.
18. Greenaway C, Dongier P, Boivin JF, et al. Susceptibility to measles, mumps, and rubella in newly arrived adult immigrants and refugees. Ann Intern Med. 2007;146(1):20–4.
19. Jacobsen KH, Koopman JS. Declining hepatitis A seroprevalence: a global review and analysis. Epidemiol Infect. 2004;132(6):1005–22.
20. Poovorawan Y, Theamboonlers A, Sinlaparatsamee S, et al. Increasing susceptibility to HAV among members of the young generation in Thailand. Asian Pac J Allergy Immunol. 2000;18(4):249–53.
21. Tufenkeji H. Hepatitis A shifting epidemiology in the Middle East and Africa. Vaccine. 2000;18 Suppl 1:S65–7.
22. Mandal BK, Mukherjee PP, Murphy C, et al. Adult susceptibility to varicella in the tropics is a rural phenomenon due to the lack of previous exposure. J Infect Dis. 1998;178 Suppl 1:S52–4.
23. Lee BW. Review of varicella zoster seroepidemiology in India and Southeast Asia. Trop Med Int Health. 1998;3(11):886–90.
24. Lokeshwar MR, Agrawal A, Subbarao SD, et al. Age related seroprevalence of antibodies to varicella in India. Indian Pediatr. 2000;37(7):714–9.
25. Newton PN, McGready R, Fernandez F, et al. Manslaughter by fake artesunate in Asia—will Africa be next? PLoS Med. 2006;3(6):e197.
26. Bate R, Coticelli P, Tren R, et al. Antimalarial drug quality in the most severely malarious parts of Africa—a six country study. PLoS ONE. 2008;3(5):e2132.

HUMANITARIAN AID WORKERS

Brian D. Gushulak

Through their association with organizations and agencies or their own individual activities, many thousands of people are involved in the delivery of humanitarian aid in diverse locations every year. Following very large-scale events, such as the Asian earthquake and tsunami of 2004, the number of those traveling to provide humanitarian aid and assistance can increase significantly.

In common with other travelers, persons who travel to provide humanitarian aid or disaster relief must first address their personal health and welfare, before, during and after travel. This includes knowledge and preparation for all the usual elements associated with travel to the area. In addition, aid workers can experience specific risks and situations related to the provision of humanitarian care, such as—

- Exposure to the environment that precipitated or sustains a crisis or event, such as a natural disaster or conflict
- Working long hours under adverse or extreme conditions, often in close contact with the affected local population
- Damaged or absent local infrastructure, including availability of food, water, lodging, transportation, and health services
- Reduced levels of security and protection

Accidents and violence are documented risks for humanitarian workers and cause more deaths than disease and natural causes. Thirty percent of these deaths occur during the first 3 months of service. A recent study of deaths among Peace Corps volunteers noted that unintentional injuries were the cause of nearly 70% of deaths, followed by homicide at 17%. Illness was responsible for 14% of the Peace Corps fatalities.

Pre-Travel Considerations

Evaluation and Pre-Travel Medical Care

Giving careful attention to pre-travel evaluation, both medical and psychological, in addition to educating travelers, can help reduce the likelihood of illness and repatriation. Comprehensive medical examinations can prepare travelers by helping to identify previously unrecognized disease and allowing for treatment (e.g., dental work) before travel. Careful evaluation of risk factors (family history, history of alcohol or substance abuse, sexually transmitted diseases, and psychiatric illness) may direct additional evaluation and identify previously unrecognized psychological problems or chronic conditions.

- Identifying alcohol or substance dependence, depression, or other psychiatric illness is important, as these conditions may be exacerbated by stress of the circumstances and can often be a reason for emergency repatriation.
- Those who will be providing medical care as part of their humanitarian activities should be considered in terms of occupational risk and the need for preventive or postexposure interventions.
- Humanitarian workers destined to areas of active conflict or limited policing presence may benefit from specialized security briefings, either provided by the employing agency or private sources.
- Medical facilities may be compromised by the disaster or overwhelmed in responding to the disaster. Therefore, volunteers with underlying conditions or pregnant women should be counseled against travel and encouraged to support the response in other ways.

Regardless of the area of the world in which the aid worker will be deployed, certain basics should be addressed in the pre-travel encounter, including routine vaccinations, malaria prophylaxis (if appropriate), food and water precautions, self-treatment for travelers' diarrhea, risks from insect bites, and injury prevention.

Counseling and Advice

Pre-deployment education and training are essential, as personal illness or injury places a burden on the community the worker has come to support.

- Injuries and accidents are a common risk for travelers anywhere in the world; thus, travelers should be sensitive to their surroundings and carefully select the type of transportation and hour of travel, if possible.
- In disaster and emergency situations, the traveler should also be aware of physical hazards such as debris, unstable structures, downed power lines, environmental hazards, and extremes of temperature.
- Travelers to conflict areas should be aware of landmines and other potential hazards associated with unexploded ordnance.

The amount and detail of health, safety, and security training may increase with the size of sponsoring organizations, but the ultimate responsibility still rests with each individual.

Preparation

Health Items

The traveler should be advised to prepare a travel health kit that is more extensive than the typical kit and should also be familiar with basic first aid to self-treat any injury until medical attention can be obtained. Aid workers may need to disinfect their own water and may want to carry nonperishable food items for emergency use. In addition to a basic travel health kit (see the Travel Health Kits section in Chapter 2), humanitarian aid workers should consider bringing the following items:

Toiletries
- Toothbrush/toothpaste
- Skin moisturizer
- Soap, shampoo
- Lip balm
- If corrective lenses are used:
  - Extra pair of prescription glasses in a protective case, copy of prescription
  - Eyeglasses cleaning supplies and repair kit
  - Extra contact lenses and lens cleaner
- Razor, extra blades[1]
- Nail clippers[1]
- Toilet paper
- Menstrual supplies
- Sewing kit
- Laundry detergent
- Small clothesline/pins

Clothing
- Comfortable, light-weight clothing
- Long pants
- Long-sleeved shirts
- Hat
- Boots
- Shower shoes
- Rain gear
- Bandana/handkerchief
- Towel (highly absorbent travel towel if possible)
- Gloves (leather gloves if physical labor will be performed; rubber gloves if handling blood or body fluids)

Activities of Daily Living
- Sunglasses
- Waterproof watch
- Flashlight
- Spare batteries
- Travel plug adapters for electronics
- Knife, such as a Swiss Army Knife or Leatherman[1]
- If traveling to an area where food and water may be contaminated:
    - Bottled water or water filters/purification system/water purification tablets
    - Nonperishable food items

Safety and Security
- Money belt
- Cash
- Cell phone, equipped to work internationally, or satellite phone (with charger)
- Candles, matches, lighter in a ziplock bag
- Ziplock bags
- Safety goggles

[1]*Note:* Pack these items in checked baggage, since they may be considered sharp objects and confiscated by airport or airline security if packed in carry-on bags.

Personal Items

Because of the loss of life, serious injuries, missing and separated families, and destruction often associated with disasters, relief workers should recognize that situations they encounter may be extremely stressful. Keeping a personal item nearby, such as a family photo, favorite music, or religious material, can often offer comfort in such situations. Checking in with family members and close friends from time to time is another means of support. Satellite phones are now nearly as small as cell phones, can work almost anywhere in the world, and can be rented for less than $10 per day.

Important Documents

In uncertain circumstances extra passport-style photos may be required for certain types of visas or for additional work permits. Travelers should bring photocopies of important documents, such as passports and credit cards, as well as copies of their medical or nursing license, if applicable. Medical information, such as immunization records and blood type, is also helpful to have. The traveler should carry these copies, and also leave a copy with someone back home. In addition, they should carry contact information for whom to notify in an emergency.

Registration with Embassies

Travelers should register before departure with the U.S. Embassy in that country, so that the local consulate is aware of their presence, and they may be accounted for and included in evacuation plans. They should also consider supplemental health insurance to cover medical evacuation should they become ill or injured. See the U.S. Department of State website for additional information: https://travelregistration.state.gov/ibrs/ui/.

Post-Travel Considerations

Returning aid workers should be advised to seek medical care if they sustained injuries during their travel or become ill upon return. To ensure proper evaluation, they should advise their providers of the nature of their recent travel.

Depending upon the length of time away or their activities (i.e., work in health care), returning aid workers may benefit from a complete medical review.

- Homecoming has also been identified as a risk period for difficulties in psychological adjustment, and appropriate treatment or counseling should be sought.

- Individuals who witnessed or have been involved in situations of mass casualties, deaths, or serious injuries of associates or who have been victims of violence (assault, kidnapping, or serious accident) should be considered for referral for critical incident counseling.

Studies have indicated that >30% of aid workers report depression shortly after returning home. The adjustment process can be assisted by a skilled debriefing. Generally, humanitarian workers are able to adapt to the acute and chronic stressors of their work and demonstrate considerable resilience, but they will also benefit from proper rest and support to help them fully adjust back into the home environment.

References

1. Coppola DP. Introduction to international disaster management. Amsterdam: Butterworth-Heinemann; 2006.
2. Peytremann I, Baduraux M, O'Donovan S, et al. Medical evacuations and fatalities of United Nations High Commissioner for Refugees field employees. J Travel Med. 2001;8(3):117–21.
3. Gamble K, Lovell D, Lankester T, et al. Aid workers, expatriates and travel. In: Zuckerman, JN, editor. Principles and practice of travel medicine. Hoboken (NJ): Wiley; 2001. p. 448–66.
4. Sheik M, Gutierrez MI, Bolton P, et al. Deaths among humanitarian workers. BMJ. 2000;321(7254):166–8.
5. Callahan MV, Hamer DH. On the medical edge: preparation of expatriates, refugee and disaster relief workers, and Peace Corps volunteers. Infect Dis Clin North Am. 2005;19(1):85–101.
6. McFarlane CA. Risks associated with the psychological adjustment of humanitarian aid workers. Australas J Disaster Trauma Stud. 2004;1 [cited 2008 Oct 2]. Available from: http://www.massey.ac.nz/%7Etrauma/issues/2004-1/mcfarlane.htm.
7. Campbell S. Responding to international disasters. Nurs Stand. 2005;19(21):33–6.
8. Jung P, Banks RH. Tuberculosis Risk in US Peace Corps Volunteers, 1996 to 2005. J Travel Med. 2008;15(2):87–94.
9. Nurthen NM, Jung P. Fatalities in the Peace Corps: a retrospective study, 1984 to 2003. J Travel Med. 2008;15(2):95–101.
10. Pearn J. Pre-deployment education and training for refugee emergencies: health and safety aspects. J Refug Stud. 1997;10:495–502.
11. CDC Emergency Communication System. Coping with a traumatic event. Atlanta: Centers for Disease Control and Prevention; 2005. [cited 2008 Apr 12]. Available from: http://www.bt.cdc.gov/masscasualties/copingpub.asp.
12. Mitchell AM, Sakraida TJ, Kameg K. Critical incident stress debriefing: implications for best practice. Disaster Manag Response. 2003;1(2):46–51.

ADVICE FOR AIR CREWS

Phyllis E. Kozarsky

Introduction

As airlines expand their reach and as air crews are asked to travel to more exotic destinations, these travelers need to prepare ahead of time for the exposures they may encounter. To some degree, air crews are similar to all travelers to such destinations, but the differences require some modifications of travel health guidance because—

- Layovers within such destinations are very short, often just 24 hours.
- Travel to such destinations is frequent.
- Travel to new destinations may be on very short notice.
- Despite short travel times, air crews may be more adventuresome and thus have greater risk than typical package tourists.

Given these factors, it is worth noting some guidelines for this special group. In general, American carriers traveling to destinations in the developing world try to inform their air crews about health issues they may face. However, airlines do not necessarily have available on their staff occupational health or other providers who are expert in travel medicine, and the airlines may not be aware of special risks at their destinations. Air crews and providers seeing such travelers should therefore encourage airlines to avail themselves of professionals who are knowledgeable in the field and who can help determine recommendations for the various destinations served.

Pilots typically know some of the medications and classes of medications that are not permitted while flying, and providers should always discuss medication options. Those with central nervous system adverse events should not be prescribed, and a trial should be taken in between trips of any medication that could have side effects that may for any reason interfere with flying. Pilots and flights attendants should also be aware that certain foods and beverages containing trace amounts of products could cause a drug screen to turn positive. They should also consider the risks of over-consumption of water (possibly causing hyponatremia) on health and drug tests. If questions arise, an aeromedical examiner (AME) should be consulted. These physicians are responsible for certifying that pilots are fit to fly, examine pilots on a regular basis, and know the medications that are permitted.

General Health Measures

Although pilots are required to have periodic physician visits to ensure they are fit to fly, these may not address some issues that may affect them when they travel internationally, particularly to destinations in the developing world. Flight attendants and others should also consider asking their health-care providers about these recommendations:

- Administering a periodic tuberculin skin test, if traveling frequently to destinations where the prevalence of tuberculosis is much higher than in the United States, where the incidence of antimicrobial resistance is higher, and where the crew member will be in close contact with crowds (www.who.int/tb/challenges/mdr/en/)
- Checking at each visit to make sure that routine immunizations are up to date (see below)
- Immunizing against seasonal influenza every year when the vaccine becomes available

In addition, all medications for chronic conditions should be carried in extra quantities, as they may not be available at some locations, and even if available and less costly, may be counterfeit (see *Perspectives:* Counterfeit Drugs in Chapter 2). The business of the manufacture of counterfeit medications in developing countries is huge and growing; it is impossible to tell from the packaging or from the pills themselves if they are counterfeit. Some counterfeit drugs contain lesser quantities of active ingredient, or none, and others contain toxic contaminants.

Vaccinations

Because of the frequency of travel to international destinations, air crews may have a greater likelihood of exposure to various diseases that are less common in the United States. For example, measles can be a life-threatening illness for adults and is more common in most of the world, including Europe, due to lack of mandatory childhood immunization against the disease in many countries. International flight crews should consider a travel health visit to ensure as complete protection as possible. Some may have very short notice prior to traveling to new destinations; thus, travelers should be asked about this possibility during their visit, so that vaccinations for an upcoming trip—that may not be imminent—may be given, or a series may be started early. The administration of some vaccinations will be determined by education of the traveler about the health risks in the various destinations and the traveler's tolerance for risk.

Routine Vaccinations

All travelers should make sure they are up to date with routine vaccinations (see the separate sections on these vaccine-preventable diseases in Chapter 2):

- **Measles**—If born in the United States prior to 1957, one is assumed to be immune to measles. If born after, it is important to have documentation of having had the disease or having had two vaccine doses against measles. Measles vaccine is typically given as an MMR (measles, mumps, rubella).
- **Varicella**—Strongly recommended for travelers with no history of having had chickenpox.
- **Polio**—A single booster is recommended as an adult. (Although transmission of the polio virus is not a problem in the western hemisphere, it remains a risk in some countries in sub-Saharan Africa and in Asia.)
- **Diphtheria/tetanus/pertussis**—Administered at 10-year intervals for complete protection.
- **Hepatitis B**—Administered to all children and adolescents in the United States, it is advisable for frequent travelers because of unpredictability of exposure.
- **Hepatitis A**—Administered to all children in the United States, it is advisable for all travelers.
- **Others**—Any age-related (e.g., varicella-zoster) or health maintenance-related (e.g., pneumococcal) vaccinations should be considered.

Special Vaccinations for Travel

Although there are no established guidelines or recommendations for the use of travel vaccinations in pilots and air crew, it may be reasonable to offer meningococcal, Japanese encephalitis, yellow fever, and typhoid vaccine to this special population because of their frequent, short-stay, and at times unpredictable travel and destinations.

Malaria Chemoprophylaxis

Crew members are typically informed by their airline which destinations harbor malaria. Some European and Asian air carriers have longer experience in flying to destinations where malaria is endemic, and these airlines have various policies with respect to its prevention. Although there may be malaria transmission in some areas of destination countries, sometimes there is none in the capitals or the larger urban areas to which the major American carriers fly (e.g., China or the Philippines). This is generally not the case in sub-Saharan Africa, where during a short 24-hour layover there can be substantial exposure. Although there may be little risk at the hotels in the destination, risk may be increased at the international airports and during unpredictable delays in transit. There is little published data on the risk of malaria for flight crews with short layovers, but some information suggests that it is less than that for tourists.

Flight crew members should be educated about the risk of malaria at their destinations and have an individual risk assessment for preventive measures. For destinations where there is a high intensity of malaria (e.g., countries in West Africa), crew members should take prophylaxis. For other destinations where crews are thought to be at low risk based on local intensity of transmission, accommodations, and personal behaviors, they may be advised to use insect repellents and no chemoprophylaxis. Flight crews should always—

- Educate themselves as much as possible about malaria.
- Understand the importance of personal protective measures such as repellents, and use them properly.
- Take chemoprophylaxis if recommended by their doctor.
- Know that if fever or chills occur following exposure that it is a medical emergency.
- Know how they can get medical assistance at their destinations or at home in the event of symptoms or signs of malaria.

There are several options for malaria chemoprophylaxis, depending upon the destination city. The combination of country-specific recommendations that can be accessed either in this text (see Malaria Risk Information and Prophylaxis, by Country, section in Chapter 2) or on the CDC Travelers' Health website (www.cdc.gov/travel) should help with this decision, along with the individual assessment.

Chemoprophylaxis Options for Pilots and Air Crew

- **Mefloquine:** The current US FDA-approved product label for mefloquine contains a caution against using mefloquine for malaria prophylaxis in pilots.
- **Chloroquine:** There are no contraindications for use of chloroquine in pilots or air crew. Chloroquine may not be the preferred option for many because of the need to continue taking the drug for 4 weeks after the last exposure, thus requiring over 4 weeks of drug administration for even a single night of exposure.
- **Atovaquone–proguanil:** There are no contraindications for use of atovaquone–proguanil in pilots or air crew members. In addition, because of the short-stay nature of their travel, use of atovaquone–progunil as chemoprophylaxis may be preferred because of the need to take the drug for only 7 days after leaving an area of exposure risk.
- **Doxycycline:** There are no contraindications for use of doxycycline in pilots or air crew. Doxycycline may not be the preferred option for many because of the need to continue taking the drug for 28 days after the last exposure, thus requiring over 4 weeks of drug administration for even a single night of exposure.
- **Primaquine:** There are no contraindications for use of primaquine in pilots or air crew. Like atovaquone–proguanil, use of primaquine as chemoprophylaxis may be attractive because of the need to take the drug for only 7 days after leaving an area of exposure risk.

Food and Water Precautions and Travelers' Diarrhea

Pilots and air crew members should follow the same safe food and water guidelines and prevention and management of travelers' diarrhea as other travelers (see the Travelers' Diarrhea section in Chapter 2). Pilots and air crew should be well versed in the recognition and self-treatment of travelers' diarrhea to avoid unnecessary morbidity that would impact their job performance.

Blood-Borne Infections and Sexually Transmitted Diseases (STDs)

Although these risks and preventions are addressed in greater detail in other sections, it is worth reiterating that frequent travelers have a greater likelihood of engaging in casual and unprotected sex. It is common to think that others from western countries would have the same risk of HIV and STDs; however, travelers have far higher rates of such infections. Dental procedures and activities such as acupuncture, tattooing, and piercing also are ill advised during travel to developing countries.

References

1. Bagshaw M, Nicolls DS. Aircraft cabin environment. In: Keystone JS, Kozarsky PE, Freedman DO, Nothdurft HD, Connor BA, editors. Travel medicine. 2nd ed. Philadelphia: Mosby; 2008. p. 447–61.
2. Byrne NJ, Behrens RH. Airline crews' risk for malaria on layovers in urban sub-Saharan Africa: risk assessment and appropriate prevention policy. J Travel Med. 2004;11(6):359–63.
3. Byrne N. Urban malaria risk in sub-Saharan Africa: where is the evidence? Travel Med Infect Dis. 2007;5(2):135–7.

LONG-TERM TRAVELERS AND EXPATRIATES

Anne E. McCarthy

Unique Considerations for Long-Term Travel

A prolonged stay of 6 months or more in low- and middle-income countries, whether for tourism or employment purposes, leads to an increase in the risk of travel and non-travel-related illness. The risk includes both infectious diseases and trauma, due in part to the cumulative risk over months to years of potential exposure. Any illness may necessitate interaction with the local health-care system, which may have limited resources.

The most commonly reported health problems in long-term travelers include diarrheal diseases, respiratory illness, and skin conditions. Infectious diseases, although important causes of morbidity, are not common causes of travel-related mortality, even in long-term travelers. A Canadian study of international travel-related death documented the rare occurrence due to vaccine-preventable or exotic disease. Similarly, a U.S. study found that those residing abroad were more likely to sustain fatal injuries, particularly due to motor vehicle crashes and drowning, suggesting that time should be spent educating these travelers about road and water safety.

Those spending prolonged periods abroad are likely to eventually relax preventive measures, resulting in increased risk of acquiring vector-, food-, and water-borne diseases. This risk will in turn lead to an increased chance of requiring local medical care, which may have limited resources (personnel and therapeutic) and may have suboptimal therapy (such as counterfeit or poor-quality medications). Approximately 3% of >4,000 UK diplomats living overseas required medical evacuation, most (70%) of which were due to unsuitable medical facilities.

Pre-Travel Care

Providing pre-travel care for these special-needs travelers includes prevention strategies, as well as therapy for illness that may be inevitable with time.

- Prior to departure, all long-term travelers should undergo an extensive medical and dental examination to exclude underlying disease.
- The pre-travel consultation for long-term and expatriate travelers should include consideration of vaccine-preventable and other diseases, discussion about acquiring medical care while abroad, and appropriate medical care and evacuation insurance.
  - With prolonged travel, there may be more than just the immediate destination to consider, since over time there may be travel to surrounding regions and possibly repeated short-term exposures that translate into significant cumulative risk.
  - Expatriates often live in areas or cities with low or negligible infectious risks but take frequent recreational or business trips to regional destinations with increased risk.

Vaccine-Preventable Infectious Diseases

Routine vaccines, including influenza vaccination, should be updated. As well, a number of travel-related vaccines warrant consideration.

- **Hepatitis A** and **typhoid** vaccines are appropriate given the cumulative risk, although the traveler should be aware that the latter does not provide full protection.
- **Hepatitis B** vaccine is increasingly provided in the United States; however, many adults may not have protection. They may be at substantial risk, as demonstrated by a survey of mostly short-term travelers, where 15% of 400 travelers had potential blood and body fluid exposure.
- **Meningococcal disease** is more likely in travelers with prolonged exposure to local populations in endemic or epidemic areas; quadravalent vaccine should be considered for those at risk.
- **Japanese encephalitis** vaccine is costly and is usually recommended for travelers with prolonged rural exposure; however, the potential for travel outside the primary destination must be considered in light of the possible cumulative risk.
- **Rabies** prevention is of increased importance with prolonged residence in endemic countries. Foreign residents in Nepal reported an exposure risk of 5.7/1,000 persons/year, compared with 1.9 per 1,000 persons/year for tourists. Rabies

prevention strategies are complicated by the cost and availability of pre-exposure vaccine and by the potential lack of availability of safe or effective postexposure prophylaxis in some countries. In one survey, only 38% of 293 missionary personnel stationed abroad had received pre-exposure prophylaxis. More concerning was that just 8% of the 38 potential exposures received appropriate postexposure care.

Non-Vaccine-Preventable Infectious Diseases

Malaria

Standard strategies appropriate for malaria prevention in short-term travel may need to be modified and adapted for those with long-term malaria risk. These travelers or expatriates often do not optimize personal protection measures for bite avoidance (insect repellents and insecticide-treated nets and clothing) on a daily basis and adhere poorly to continuous prophylaxis regimens or do not wish to take medications long term. A retrospective cohort analysis study conducted by reviewing pharmacy records and by interviews in person of chemoprophylaxis adherence in 183 expatriate households in coastal Nigeria showed that only 127 (69%) collected their prophylaxis regularly, and overall only 39% of households were compliant. Many cited concerns about the real and perceived risks for adverse drug reactions, particularly with long-term use.

There are no consensus guidelines on the prevention of malaria in long-term travelers. Many different malaria prevention strategies have been recommended, such as initial prophylaxis followed by discontinuation or intermittent use at times of higher risk (seasonal chemoprophylaxis) If the long term traveler chooses not to take chemoprophylaxis, they should have good access to medical care and seek medical attention when sick for the best quality diagnosis and treatment (see the Malaria section in Chapter 2).

Long-term travelers—

- Must be aware of their risk.
- Should optimize bite prevention with the use of window screens and bed nets.
- Should be educated on malaria symptoms and the need to seek early medical attention for a febrile illness.

Other Diseases

Diarrhea and gastrointestinal diseases are common in long-term travelers residing in the tropics, and these individuals should be educated about the management of acute diarrhea, including rehydration, the use of antimotility agents, and empiric antimicrobial therapy. Prolonged diarrhea is more suggestive of a protozoal etiology.

HIV and sexually transmitted infection risks have increased in travelers and expatriates. Furthermore, the consistent use of condoms in expatriates is low (around 20%). Long-term travelers should be educated about the risk of HIV and STDs in their destination. The potential for occupational exposure to HIV is important to consider in health-care workers; postexposure prophylaxis with highly active antiretroviral therapy and risk avoidance should be included in the pre-travel consultation (see the Occupational Exposure to HIV section in Chapter 2).

Transfusion is an important risk for hepatitis C infection in expatriates. The risk of hepatitis E, spread by the fecal–oral route, is highest in Asia, although it has been transmitted in many different tropical locations. Pregnant women are at highest risk of fulminant disease. Other infections vary with location and include schistosomiasis, which may be prevented by not swimming or wading in fresh water. Tuberculosis risk eventually equates to that of the local population, increasing with length of stay and contact with the local population.

Summary

Long-term travelers and expatriates require realistic and individualized pre-travel counsel on the prevention and management of infectious and noninfectious illnesses. The need for eventual medical care should be anticipated, and strategies to reduce the risk of counterfeit or ineffective medication should be discussed.

References

1. Banta JE, Jungblut E. Health problems encountered by the Peace Corps overseas. Am J Public Health Nations Health. 1966;56(12):2121–5.

2. Leutscher PD, Bagley SW. Health-related challenges in United States Peace Corps Volunteers serving for two years in Madagascar. J Travel Med. 2003;10(5):263–7

3. MacPherson DW, Gushulak BD, Sandhu J. Death and international travel—the Canadian experience: 1996 to 2004. J Travel Med. 2007;14(2):77–84.

4. Guse CE, Cortés LM, Hargarten SW, et al. Fatal injuries of US citizens abroad. J Travel Med. 2007;14(5):279–87.

5. Hillel O, Potasman I. Correlation between adherence to precautions issued by the WHO and diarrhea among long-term travelers to India. J Travel Med. 2005;12(5):243–7.

6. Cockburn R, Newton PN, Agyarko EK, et al. The global threat of counterfeit drugs: why industry and governments must communicate the dangers. PLoS Med. 2005;2(4):e100.

7. Patel D, Easmon CJ, Dow C, et al. Medical repatriation of British diplomats resident overseas. J Travel Med. 2000;7(2):64–9.

8. Correia JD, Shafer RT, Patel V, et al. Blood and body fluid exposure as a health risk for international travelers. J Travel Med. 2001;8(5):263–6.

9. Pandey P, Shlim DR, Cave W, et al. Risk of possible exposure to rabies among tourists and foreign residents in Nepal. J Travel Med. 2002;9(3):127–31.

10. Arguin PM, Krebs JW, Mandel E, et al. Survey of rabies preexposure and postexposure prophylaxis among missionary personnel stationed outside the United States. J Travel Med. 2000;7(1):10–4.

11. Berg J, Visser LG. Expatriate chemopophylaxis use and compliance: past, present and future from an occupational health perspective. J Travel Med. 2007;14(5):357–8.

12. Chen LH, Wilson ME, Schlagenhauf P. Prevention of malaria in long-term travelers. JAMA. 2006;296(18):2234–44.

13. Toovey S, Moerman F, van Gompel A. Special infectious disease risks of expatriates and long-term travelers in tropical countries. Part I: malaria. J Travel Med. 2007;14(1):42–9.

14. Toovey S, Moerman F, van Gompel A. Special infectious disease risks of expatriates and long-term travelers in tropical countries. Part II: infections other than malaria. J Travel Med. 2007;14(1):50–60.

15. Cobelens FG, van Deutekom H, Draayer-Jansen IW, et al. Risk of infection with Mycobacterium tuberculosis in travellers to areas of high tuberculosis endemicity. Lancet. 2000;356(9228):461–5.

TRAVELING WITH CHRONIC MEDICAL ILLNESSES

Deborah Nicolls Barbeau

General Preparation: Practical Considerations

Although traveling abroad can be relaxing and rewarding, the physical demands of travel (e.g., maneuvering through a crowded terminal, rushing to catch a flight) can be stressful, particularly for travelers with underlying chronic medical illnesses. With adequate preparation, however, those with chronic medical illnesses can have safe and enjoyable trips.

The following is a list of recommendations for travel advisors to help those with chronic medical illnesses:

- **Ensure that any chronic illnesses are stable.** Persons with underlying medical illness should see their physicians to ensure that the management of their illness is optimized.
- **Recommend seeking pre-travel consultation early, at least 4–6 weeks prior to departure.** This is to ensure that there is adequate time to respond to immunizations and, in some circumstances, to try medications prior to travel.
- **Provide a physician's letter.** The letter should be on office letterhead stationery, outlining existing medical conditions, medications prescribed (including generic names), and any equipment required to manage the condition.

- **Advise travelers to pack medications in carry-on luggage in their original containers.** Ensure sufficient quantities of medications for the entire trip, plus extra in case of unexpected delays. When crossing time zones, medications should be taken based on elapsed time, not time of day.
- **Educate regarding important drug interactions.** Medications used to treat chronic medical illnesses may interact with medications prescribed for self-treatment of travelers' diarrhea or malaria chemoprophylaxis. Discuss all medications used, either daily or on an as-needed basis.
- **Recommend consideration of supplemental insurance.** Consideration should be given for three types of insurance policies: 1) trip cancellation in the event of illness prior to travel; 2) supplemental insurance so that money paid for health care abroad may be reimbursed, since most medical insurance policies do not cover health care in other countries; and 3) medical evacuation insurance (see the Travel Insurance and Evacuation Insurance section in Chapter 2).
- **Help devise a health plan.** This plan should give instructions for managing minor problems or exacerbations of underlying illnesses and should include information about medical facilities available in the destination country (see the Obtaining Health Care Abroad for the Ill Traveler section in Chapter 2).
- **Recommend that the traveler wear a medical alert bracelet.**
- **Always advise the traveler about packing a health kit** (see Travel Health Kits section in Chapter 2).

Specific Chronic Medical Illnesses

Issues related to specific chronic medical illnesses are addressed in Table 8-9. These recommendations should be used in conjunction with the other recommendations given throughout this book. Additional resources for information include—

- American Heart Association: www.americanheart.org
- American Lung Association: www.lungusa.org
- American Diabetes Association: www.diabetes.org
- National Kidney Foundation: www.kidney.org
- Global Dialysis: www.globaldialysis.com
- Crohn's and Colitis Foundation of America: www.ccfa.org
- U.S. Department of State: www.state.gov

Also, many international health-care facilities are accredited by Joint Commission International, an affiliate of the Joint Commission, which is the largest accreditor of U.S.-based health-care organizations. A list of accredited international facilities is available at their website, www.jointcommissioninternational.org (see the Obtaining Health Care Abroad for the Ill Traveler section in Chapter 2).

If travelers or their health-care providers have concerns about fitness for air travel, the medical unit affiliated with the airline is also a valuable source for information.

References

1. Aerospace Medical Association; Medical Guidelines Task Force. Medical guidelines for airline travel, 2nd ed. Aviat Space Environ Med. 2003;74(5 Suppl):A1–19.
2. McCarthy AE. Travelers with pre-existing disease. In: Keystone JS, Kozarsky PE, Freedman DO, Nothdurft HD, Connor BA, editors. Travel medicine. 2nd ed. Philadelphia: Mosby; 2008. p. 249–55.
3. Chandran M, Edelman SV. Have insulin, will fly: diabetes management during air travel and time zone adjustment strategies. Clinical Diabetes 2003;21:82–5.
4. Simons FER. 9. Anaphylaxis. J Allergy Clin Immunol 2008;121(2 Suppl):S402.

Table 8-9. Special considerations for travelers with chronic medical illnesses

Condition	Absolute and relative contraindications to airline travel	Pre-travel considerations	Immunizations	Miscellaneous
Cardiovascular diseases	• Uncomplicated MI within 2–3 weeks • Complicated MI within 6 weeks • Unstable angina • CHF, severe, decompensated • Uncontrolled hypertension • CABG within 10–14 days • CVA within 2 weeks • Uncontrolled arrhythmia • Eisenmenger syndrome • Severe symptomatic valvular HD	• Supplemental oxygen • Plan for self-management of dehydration and volume overload, may include adjusting medications • Bring copy of recent EKG • Bring pacemaker or AICD card • DVT precautions	• Influenza • Pneumococcal • Consider hepatitis B	• Have sublingual nitroglycerine available in carry-on bag • Mefloquine not recommended for persons with cardiac conduction abnormalities, particularly for those with ventricular arrhythmias
Pulmonary diseases	• Severe, labile asthma • Recent hospitalization for asthma • Active respiratory infection • Pneumothorax within 2–3 weeks • Pleural effusion within 14 days • High supplemental oxygen requirements at baseline • Major chest surgery within 10–14 days	• Supplemental oxygen • Discuss with airline need for other equipment on plane (e.g., nebulizer) • Plan for self-management of exacerbations (including COPD, asthma) • DVT precautions	• Influenza • Pneumococcal • Consider hepatitis B	• Consideration for carrying short course of antibiotics or steroids for exacerbations • Consider advising an inhaler available in carry-on bag, even if not routinely used
Gastrointestinal diseases	• Surgery, including laparoscopic, within 10–14 days • Gastrointestinal bleed within 24 hrs • Colonoscopy within 24 hrs • Partial bowel obstruction	• Emphasize food and water precautions • Consider prescribing prophylactic antibiotic for TD • Recommend avoiding undercooked seafood if cirrhosis or heavy alcohol use (*Vibrio vulnificus*)	• Influenza • Pneumococcal • Hepatitis A • Hepatitis B	• May experience increased colostomy output during air travel • H_2-blockers and PPIs increase susceptibility to TD • Use mefloquine with caution in any chronic liver disease
Renal failure and chronic renal insufficiency	• None	• Emphasize food and water precautions • Plan for self-management of dehydration, which can worsen renal function • Arrange dialysis abroad if needed • Adjust medications for CrCl	• Influenza • Pneumococcal • Hepatitis B	• Know HIV, hepatitis C, and hepatitis B status • Atovaquone/proguanil (Malarone) contraindicated when CrCl <30 mL/min

(Continued)

Table 8-9. Special considerations for travelers with chronic medical illnesses *(Continued)*

Condition	Absolute and relative contraindications to airline travel	Pre-travel considerations	Immunizations	Miscellaneous
Renal failure and chronic renal insufficiency *(Continued)*				• Kidney Foundation and Global Dialysis websites can help with finding dialysis centers, check for JCI accreditation
Diabetes mellitus	• None	• Plan for self-management of dehydration, diabetic foot and pressure sores • Insulin adjustments • Should check FSBG at 4- to 6-hour intervals during air travel • Discuss changes in insulin regimen or oral agent with diabetes specialist • Provide physician's letter stating need for all equipment, including syringes, glucose meter, and supplies	• Influenza • Pneumococcal • Consider hepatitis B	• Keep insulin and all glucose meter supplies in carry-on bag • Bring food and supplies needed to manage hypoglycemia during travel • Check feet daily for pressure sores
Severe allergic reactions	• None	• Plan for managing allergic reaction while traveling, and consider bringing short course of steroids for possible allergic reactions • Should carry injectable epinephrine and antihistamines (H_1 and H_2-blockers)—always have on person		• Many airlines already have policies in place for dealing with peanut allergies • Make sure to carry injectable epinephrine in case of severe reaction while in flight

AICD = automatic implantable cardioverter defibrillators, CABG = coronary artery bypass graft, CHF = congestive heart failure, COPD = chronic obstructive pulmonary disease, CrCl = creatinine clearance, CVA = cerebrovascular accident, DVT = deep vein thrombosis, EKG = electrocardiogram, FSBG = fingerstick blood glucose, HD = heart disease, JCI = Joint Commission International, MI = myocardial infarction, PPIs = proton-pump inhibitors, TD = travelers' diarrhea.

9

Health Considerations for Newly Arrived Immigrants and Refugees

INTRODUCTION

According to the U.S. Department of Homeland Security, approximately 60 million non-U.S. citizens enter the United States annually (Figure 9-1). These 60 million foreign persons (not citizens or nationals of the United States) are from countries around the world and include immigrants, refugees, migrants adjusting their visa status, persons with nonimmigrant visas, and persons in short-term transit status. On average, approximately 500,000 legal immigrants and refugees arrive in the United States annually; immigrants make up approximately 90% and refugees close to 10% of these arrivals.

A medical examination is mandatory for these immigrants and refugees. Individuals who are currently in the United States who apply for adjustment of their immigration

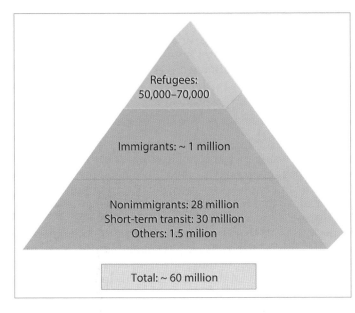

Refugees:
50,000–70,000

Immigrants: ~ 1 million

Nonimmigrants: 28 million
Short-term transit: 30 million
Others: 1.5 milion

Total: ~ 60 million

Figure 9.1. Annual estimate of migrants entering the United States. (Modified from U.S. Department of Homeland Security. Refugee admissions in 2007: 48,217.)

status to that of permanent resident are also required to have a medical assessment. CDC's Division of Global Migration and Quarantine (DGMQ) provides the U.S. Department of State and the U.S. Citizenship and Immigration Services with technical instructions for conducting medical examinations.

BEFORE ARRIVAL IN THE UNITED STATES: PANEL PHYSICIANS AND THE OVERSEAS MEDICAL EXAMINATION

Maria V. Cano, Mary P. Naughton, Luis S. Ortega

Panel Physicians

A panel physician is a medically trained, licensed and experienced doctor practicing overseas, who is appointed by the local U.S. Embassy or Consulate. Over 670 panel physicians selected by U.S. Department of State (DOS) consular officials perform pre-departure medical examinations as required by CDC (www.cdc.gov/MigrationHealth) and the U.S. Citizenship and Immigration Services (USCIS) (www.uscis.gov).

The Immigration and Nationality Act (INA), which, along with other immigration laws, treaties, and conventions of the United States, relates to the immigration, temporary admission, naturalization, and removal of foreigners, mandates that all immigrants and refugees migrating to the United States are required to undergo an overseas medical screening examination performed by panel physicians.

On October 6, 2008, CDC amended the regulations that govern the required overseas medical examination for immigrants and refugees. In addition to the communicable diseases specified in the INA, the following disease categories were added: (1) quarantinable diseases designated by Presidential Executive Order, and (2) diseases that meet the criteria of public health emergency of international concern which require notification to the World Health Organization under the revised International Health Regulations of 2005. CDC also amended the provisions that describe the scope of the medical examination by incorporating a more flexible, risk-based approach based on medical and epidemiologic factors. This approach will determine which diseases are included in the medical screening and testing of immigrants and refugees in areas of the world that are experiencing outbreaks of specific diseases. In addition, CDC updated the screening requirement for tuberculosis (TB) to be consistent with current medical knowledge and practice. These changes will reduce the health security threat to the United States from emerging diseases without imposing undue burden on either the immigrants and refugees or the health-care system in the United States.

Physical Exam

The mandated medical examination focuses primarily on detecting diseases determined to be inadmissible conditions for the purposes of visa eligibility and on preventing the importation of diseases of public health importance. These medical conditions include infectious diseases such as tuberculosis and HIV infection, mental disorders associated with harmful behavior, and substance abuse or addiction (see www.cdc.gov/yellowbook/MedicalExam). In addition, the visit to the panel physician provides opportunities for providing preventive medicine interventions, such as updating vaccines and administering presumptive therapy for parasitic or other infectious diseases that may be affecting a specific refugee population at the time of migration, including nematode infections, malaria, and specific vaccine-preventable diseases.

Classification of Applicants

For the purposes of determining the inadmissibility of an applicant, medical conditions are categorized as Class A or B. Class A conditions are defined as those which preclude an immigrant or refugee from entering the United States. Class B conditions are defined as physical or mental abnormalities, diseases, or disabilities serious enough or permanent in nature, as to amount to a substantial departure from normal well-being. Follow-up evaluation soon after U.S. arrival is recommended for immigrants or refugees with Class B TB conditions. If an immigrant or refugee is found to have an inadmissible condition that may make him or her ineligible for a visa, a visa may still be issued after the illness has been adequately treated or after a waiver of the visa ineligibility has been approved by USCIS (see www.cdc.gov/yellowbook/VisaMedicalWaiver).

Proof of Vaccination

In 1996, a subsection was added to the INA requiring that persons seeking immigrant visas for permanent residency show proof of receipt of at least the first dose of all vaccination series recommended by the Advisory Committee on Immunization Practices (ACIP) (see www.cdc.gov/vaccines/recs/acip). Although these regulations apply to all adult immigrants and most immigrant children, internationally adopted children who are <10 years of age have been exempted from the immunization requirements. Refugees are not required to meet the INA immunization requirements at the time of entry into the United States but must show proof of vaccination at the time they are eligible to apply for permanent U.S. residence, typically after one year of arrival. Updated instructions regarding vaccination requirements are provided to panel physicians and are available on the CDC website (see the 2007 Technical Instructions for Vaccination for Panel Physicians at www.cdc.gov/yellowbook/PanelVaccination).

Technical Instructions

DGMQ is responsible for providing technical instructions to the panel physicians in performing the overseas medical screening examination. The testing modalities recommended for the medical examination include a medical history, a physical examination, and diagnostic tests (see Table 9-1). DGMQ also monitors the quality of the overseas medical examination process through its Quality Assessment Program. There are over 670 panel physician sites (i.e., health-care staff, radiology facilities, laboratories) worldwide.

Table 9-1. Testing for required overseas medical screening examination

Health Condition	Testing
Tuberculosis (TB)	Chest radiograph, followed by AFB smear and sputum culture if chest radiograph suggests TB
HIV	Serology
Syphilis	Serology
Other sexually transmitted diseases	Physical examination
Hansen's disease	Physical examination
Mental disorders with associated harmful behavior	History
Drug abuse or addiction	History, physical exam
Vaccinations	History and vaccination records Serology

Additionally, DGMQ is responsible for notifying state or local health departments of all arriving refugees, immigrants with Class A conditions (with waiver), and immigrants with Class B TB conditions who are resettling in their jurisdiction and need follow-up evaluation and possible treatment. DOS forms, known as DS forms, which summarize the results of the overseas medical examination and include classification of health conditions, are collected at U.S. ports of entry at the time of arrival. This information is transmitted to state or local health departments electronically through CDC's Electronic Disease Notification System.

State and local health departments are asked to report to DGMQ the results of these U.S. follow-up evaluations and any significant public health conditions among recently arrived immigrants and refugees, as a way to better understand epidemiologic patterns of disease in recently arrived immigrants and refugees and to monitor the quality of overseas medical examination.

References

1. Office of Immigration Statistics (OIS), U.S. Department of Homeland Security. Yearbook of immigration statistics: 2007. Washington, D.C.: U.S. Department of Homeland Security; 2008.

2. U.S. Citizenship and Immigration Services. U.S. Department of Homeland Security. Immigration and Nationality Act. Washington D.C.: U.S. Department of Homeland Security; 2008. [cited 2008 Nov 19]. Available from: http://uscis.gov.

3. Scope of the Examination, 42 C.F.R. Sect 34.3. 2007. [cited 2008 Jun 2]. Available from

http://frwebgate.access.gpo.gov/cgi-bin/get-cfr.cgi.

4. Maloney S, Ortega L, Cetron M. Overseas medical screening for immigrants and refugees. In: Walker PF, Barnett ED, editors. Immigrant medicine. Philadelphia: Saunders; 2007.

5. CDC. Technical instructions for panel physicians. Atlanta: Centers for Disease Control and Prevention; 1991–2008 [updated 2008 Oct 29; cited 2008 Nov 19]. Available from: www.cdc.gov/yellowbook/PanelInstructions.

AFTER ARRIVAL IN THE UNITED STATES: RECOMMENDATIONS FOR SCREENING AND IMMUNIZATIONS OF NEW IMMIGRANTS AND REFUGEES

Patricia F. Walker, William M. Stauffer, Elizabeth D. Barnett

Notification of Refugee Arrival

State health departments are notified about refugee new arrivals. A secure electronic system, the Electronic Disease Notification System (EDN), alerts states of refugee arrivals who have Class A and B conditions.

Newly arrived refugees receive stateside evaluation and treatment, usually conducted at state or local health departments, within 3 months of U.S. arrival. However, there is no standardized nationwide protocol for the postarrival health assessment; therefore, the content of postarrival refugee health evaluations varies from state to state. There is no formal mechanism or funding for evaluation of nonrefugee immigrants, and funding sources are often inadequate to provide comprehensive services. Further, both refugees and immigrants often have other daily demands to achieve integration into their new living environment, which may compete with their need for health evaluations and treatment. To address the special health challenges of refugees, the Office of Refugee Resettlement in the U.S. Department of Health and Human Services, provides guidance, resources, and oversight for refugee medical assistance, initial medical screening, and refugee health/mental health technical assistance and consultation (see www.acf.hhs.gov/programs/orr).

Medical Screening for New Arrivals

Medical examinations are performed by approximately 3,000 physicians known as civil surgeons who have received specific training. Civil surgeons are designated by district directors of the USCIS.

After their arrival in the United States, it is recommended, but not required, that all refugees and immigrants receive new arrival medical screening. In addition to medical screening, this visit provides an opportunity for preventive services such as immunizations and initiation of treatment for latent tuberculosis and individual counseling (e.g., nutritional health, mental health), as well as the opportune moment for establishment of ongoing primary care. Recommendations for this initial medical evaluation, ideally, should be tailored to the specific population and based on such factors as receipt of predeparture presumptive therapy (i.e., malaria and intestinal parasites), ethnicity, and epidemiologic risks for the country of origin, as well as the country, or countries, of first asylum.

Domestic Health Assessment

Many refugees and immigrants originate from countries with a high prevalence of tropical and other infectious diseases, which may present a threat to public health or to the health of the individual. In addition, untreated chronic health conditions are common. Infectious diseases with long latency periods can be particularly challenging, including tuberculosis, hepatitis B, and certain intestinal nematodes such as *Schistosoma* species and *Strongyloides stercoralis*.

All migrants who are medically screened should have a detailed history and physical examination. New arrival medical screening should also include the following (see Box 9-1):

- Basic laboratory screening
- Testing for tuberculosis
- Immunizations, as needed
- Dental, hearing, and vision evaluation
- Screening for mental health issues

Many refugees and immigrants will not have had age-appropriate cancer screening, such as pap smears, mammography, and colon cancer screening, and these needs should be addressed at early follow-up visits. Clinicians should be aware of cancers with a higher prevalence in many immigrant populations, such as cervical, liver, stomach, and nasopharyngeal cancer.

CDC is developing postarrival domestic medical screening guidelines for refugees. These refugee health guidelines are available from www.cdc.gov/yellowbook/RefugeeGuidelines. Other published resources are available to the clinician to obtain expert opinion of appropriate medical screening in refugees. The reference section includes a list of clinical resources for providers and organizations.

Box 9-1. Recommended components of domestic health assessment

- Review all available records, chest radiograph
- Complete history and physical examination
- Vision and hearing screening
- Dental evaluation
- Mental health assessment
- Tuberculosis[1]
- Laboratory testing (hepatitis B, hematologic testing,[1] urinalysis,[1] lead,[1] and HIV testing, when clinically appropriate)
- Presumptive treatment of malaria[1]
- Evaluation for intestinal parasites[1]
- Evaluation and update of immunizations as needed

---

[1]Formal refugee health guidelines are available from www.cdc.gov/yellowbook/RefugeeGuidelines.

References

1. Seybolt L, Barnett ED, Stauffer W. U.S. Medical screening for immigrants and refugees: clinical issues. In: Walker P, Barnett E, editors. Immigrant medicine. Philadelphia: Saunders; 2007. p. 135–50.

2. Barnett ED. Infectious disease screening for refugees resettled in the United States. Clin Infect Dis. 2004;39(6):833–41.

3. Stauffer WM, Maroushek S, Kamat D. Medical screening of immigrant children. Clin Pediatr. 2003;42(9):763–73.

4. Ivey SL, Faust S. Immigrant women's health: screening and immunization. West J Med. 2001;175(1):62–5.

5. Avery R. Immigrant women's health. Infectious diseases—Part 1. Clinical assessment, tuberculosis, hepatitis, and malaria. West J Med. 2001;175(3):208–11.

6. Barnett ED. Immunizations and infectious disease screening for internationally adopted children. Pediatr Clin North Am. 2005;52(5):1287–309.

7. Miller LC. International adoption: infectious disease issues. Clin Infect Dis. 2005;40(2):286–93.

8. Chen LH, Barnett ED, Wilson ME. Preventing infectious diseases during and after international adoption. Ann Intern Med. 2003;139(5 Pt 1):371–8.

9. Stauffer WM, Kamat D, Walker PF. Screening of international immigrants, refugees, and adoptees. Prim Care. 2002;29(4):879–905.

MIGRANT HEALTH RESOURCES

William M. Stauffer

Although the Yellow Book has generally addressed pre-travel health issues for persons visiting countries outside the United States, a large group of "travelers" does not fit this traditional definition. These "travelers" are generally individuals who originate in other countries and migrate to the United States, either temporarily or permanently. Recognized migrants to the United States include immigrants (documented and undocumented), refugees, asylees, and adoptees. In addition, students and corporate workers are frequent visitors to the United States. Many clinics serving the traditional travel population also function as contact points with the U.S. medical system for these populations, particularly for immigrants and refugees. This section provides resources to assist clinicians and organizations that serve these populations to access up-to-date patient-care guidelines, education materials online, and print resources.

Clinical References

Organizational Guidelines

- **Centers for Disease Control and Prevention**—Predeparture and post-arrival presumptive treatment and medical screening guidelines for refugees relocating to the United States available at www.cdc.gov/yellowbook/RefugeeGuidelines
- **American Academy of Pediatrics**—Online Red Book guidance on medical screening and vaccination issues in adoptees, refugees and immigrants at http://aapredbook.aappublications.org/
- **Canadian Collaboration for Immigrant and Refugee Health (CCIRH)**—Clinical preventive guidelines for newly arriving immigrants and refugees for primary care at www.ccirh.uottawa.ca

Websites

- **Centers for Disease Control and Prevention**
  - ○ Division of Global Migration and Quarantine—Information on immigrants and refugee who are resettling to the United States, plus resources at www.cdc.gov/MigrationHealth

- o Division of Parasitic Diseases—Clinical and public policy information on parasitic diseases at www.cdc.gov/ncidod/dpd
  - o Travelers' Health at www.cdc.gov/travel/
  - o International Emergency and Refugee Health Branch—Health information pertaining to complex humanitarian emergencies at www.cdc.gov/nceh/ierh/
- **Minnesota Department of Health**
  - o Refugee Health Provider Resources—Multiple resources for clinicians in refugee health at www.health.state.mn.us/divs/idepc/refugee/hcp/index.html
- **Healthy Roads Media**
  - o Health education materials, including video, in a variety of languages at http://healthyroadsmedia.org
- **University of Michigan Program for Multicultural Health**
  - o Cultural competency and language resources at www.med.umich.edu/multicultural/ccp/Language.htm
- **The EthnoMed Site**
  - o Information about cultural beliefs, medical issues, and other related issues pertinent to the health care of recent immigrants at http://ethnomed.org/ethnomed/
- **The 24 Languages Project**
  - o Over 200 health education brochures in 24 languages at http://library.med.utah.edu/24languages/
- **Medical Leadership Council on Cultural Proficiency**
  - o Database of patient information resources in a variety of languages and organizations providing services in languages other than English at http://medicalleadership.org/resource_interpreter.aspx
- **Refugee Health Information Network**
  - o Multilingual information for health providers, refugees and asylees in print, audio, and video formats at www.rhin.org/health_info.aspx
- **U.S. Committee for Refugees and Immigrants**
  - o Toolkits on multiple health issues for health-care providers, immigrants, and communities in multiple languages at www.refugees.org/article.aspx?id=1851
- **U.S. Citizenship and Immigration Services**
  - o Information regarding adjustment of status at www.uscis.gov

Reference Books

Textbooks with a Focus on Migrant Health

- **Immigrant Medicine.** Walker PF, Barnett ED, editors. Philadelphia: Saunders; 2007.
- **Migration Medicine and Health: Principles and Practice.** Gushulak BD, MacPherson D, editors. Hamilton (ON): BC Decker; 2006.
- **Travel Medicine and Migrant Health.** Lockie C, Walker E, Calvert L, Cossar J, Knill-Jones R, Raeside F, editors. Edinburgh: Churchill Livingstone; 2000.
- **Refugee and Immigrant Health. A Handbook for Health Professionals.** Kemp C, Rasbridge LA, editors. New York: Cambridge University Press; 2004.

Textbooks with a Focus on Tropical Diseases

- **Manson's Tropical Diseases.** 21st ed. Cook GC, Zumla AI, editors. Saunders Ltd; 2002.
- **Hunter's Tropical Medicine and Emerging Infectious Diseases.** 8th ed. Hunter GW, Strickland GT, Magill AJ, editors. Philadelphia: W.B. Saunders Company; 2000.
- **Tropical Infectious Diseases.** 2nd ed. Guerrant RL, Walker DH, Weller PF, editors. Philadelphia: Churchill Livingstone; 2006.
- **Douglas and Bennett's Principles & Practice of Infectious Diseases.** 5th ed. Mandell GL, Bennett JE, Dolin R, editors. Philadelphia: Churchill Livingstone; 2000.
- **Atlas of Tropical Medicine and Parasitology.** 6th ed. Peters W, Pasvol G, editors. Mosby; 2006.

General Resources

Reading Lists

- **Global Health Education Consortium's Global Health Bibliography**
  - Bibliography of selected citations for use by students and faculty in global health at http://globalhealthedu.org/resources/Pages/GlobalHealthBibliography.aspx
- **University of Minnesota reading list on refugee and immigrant health**
  - Comprehensive reading list for persons interested in refugee and immigrant health at www.globalhealth.umn.edu/globalhlth/pathway/reading.html

Educational Opportunities

- **University of Minnesota/CDC ASTMH-accredited course in Global Health** (focus on immigrant and refugee health)
  - ASTMH-accredited tropical medicine course that has a special focus on immigrant and refugee health at www.globalhealth.umn.edu/globalhlth/course.html
- **ASTMH-accredited courses in Tropical and Travel Medicine**
  - List of ASTMH accredited tropical and travel medicine courses at www.astmh.org in the "Approved Diploma Courses" section of the "Education & Training" drop-down menu.

Non-CDC Organizations

- **U.S. Department of Health and Human Services—**
  - Office of Refugee Resettlement: www.acf.hhs.gov/programs/orr/
  - Office of Global Health Affairs: www.globalhealth.gov/
  - Substance Abuse and Mental Health Services Administration, Points of Wellness: www.refugeewellbeing.samhsa.gov/linksAcademic.aspx
- **United Nations High Commissioner on Refugees—**www.unhcr.org/cgi-bin/texis/vtx/home
- **World Health Organization Refugee page—**www.who.int/topics/refugees/en/
- **American Society of Tropical Medicine and Hygiene—**www.astmh.org/
- **International Organization for Migration—**www.iom.int
- **International Society of Travel Medicine Health of Migrants and Refugees Committee—**www.istm.org
- **Global Health Education Consortium (GHEC)—**www.globalhealth-ec.org/

Other Resources

- **Pre-Travel Handouts for non-English speaking patients** (multiple topics in over 15 languages)—www.tropical.umn.edu/VFR

Appendices

APPENDIX A: PROMOTION OF QUALITY IN THE PRACTICE OF TRAVEL MEDICINE

Stephen M. Ostroff

Travel medicine is a relatively young area of medical practice. Although it encompasses a growing body of scientific information and requires specific areas of expertise, there is currently no recognized specialty or subspecialty of travel medicine in the United States or elsewhere in the world. Health-care providers offering travel medicine-related services are not "board-certified" in travel medicine. Instead, travel medicine physicians are credentialed in other disciplines, usually infectious diseases, internal medicine, family practice, or general practice. The same applies to nurses and other allied health professionals. Clinics in the United States that offer travel medicine services are also not specifically credentialed for this purpose.

Given these circumstances, how can travelers maximize the likelihood their provider will deliver quality medical care and that the advice, preventive measures, and treatment services they are given fall within accepted standards? Similarly, how can providers assure patients they have sufficient knowledge of the subject matter relevant to travel medicine?

Although research into the quality of travel medicine-related care is limited, several studies do suggest that travelers who access a provider with training in travel medicine are more likely to receive appropriate pre- and post-travel advice and care. Similarly, 2006 guidelines on travel medicine published by the Infectious Diseases Society of America (see below) recommend that pre- and post-travel care be obtained from a practitioner with expertise in travel medicine. This is especially relevant for those going to exotic destinations or with special needs or medical problems.

Below is a partial list of resources for travel medicine providers wishing to enhance their expertise in travel medicine. Individuals seeking travel-related medical services may want to inquire about whether their provider or clinic participates in these organizations or activities.

International Society Of Travel Medicine (ISTM)

Founded in 1991, ISTM (www.istm.org) is the pre-eminent organization dealing exclusively with travel medicine. Although less than 20 years old, it has more than 2,300 members worldwide, with the largest proportion in the United States.

Among the activities sponsored by the ISTM are—

- The Journal of Travel Medicine
- An active listserv where members share information and can ask questions
- A biennial travel medicine meeting and annual regional submeetings
- A directory of domestic and international travel clinics affiliated with ISTM members
- An annual examination leading to a Certificate of Knowledge in Travel Medicine available to physicians, nurses, and other professionals offering travel advice

The Certificate of Knowledge in Travel Medicine has been administered by ISTM since 2003. The Body of Knowledge, which is the scope of the specialty of travel medicine and is the basis for examination questions, was last updated in 2006 and is published on the ISTM website. Content areas within the Body of Knowledge include—

- Travel medicine-related epidemiology
- Immunology and vaccinology (including travel-related vaccines)
- Pre-travel consultation and management
  - Patient evaluation
  - Travelers with special needs
  - Special itineraries
  - Prevention and self-treatment
  - Precautions
- Diseases contracted during travel
  - Vector-borne diseases
  - Person-to-person transmitted diseases
  - Foodborne and waterborne diseases
  - Diseases related to bites and stings
  - Diseases due to environmental hazards
- Other conditions associated with travel
  - Conditions occurring during travel
  - Conditions due to environmental factors
  - Threats to personal safety and security
  - Psychocultural issues
  - Post-travel management
- General travel medicine issues
  - Medical care abroad
  - Travel clinic management
  - Travel medicine information resources

Since it was introduced, the Certificate of Knowledge in Travel Medicine examination has been taken by more than 1,200 practitioners in 53 countries. The society hosts exam preparation meetings periodically. Practitioners interested in travel medicine should strongly consider membership in the ISTM.

American Society of Tropical Medicine and Hygiene (ASTMH)

Formed in 1951, ASTMH (www.astmh.org) has a subsection that deals exclusively with tropical and travel medicine, known as the American Committee on Clinical Tropical Medicine and Travelers' Health (ACCTMTH).

ASTMH's activities include—

- The American Journal of Tropical Medicine and Hygiene
- An annual meeting
- A listserv
- A clinical tropical medicine clinic directory
- A biennial examination leading to a Certificate of Knowledge in Clinical Tropical Medicine and Travelers' Health available to those who have passed an ASTMH-approved tropical medicine course or have tropical medicine practice experience

The content areas of the ASTMH Certificate of Knowledge in Clinical Tropic Medicine and Travelers' Health are as follows:

- Basic science and fundamentals
- Infectious and tropical diseases (including parasites, bacteria, fungi, and viruses)
- Other diseases and conditions
- Diagnostic and therapeutic approach to clinical syndromes
- Travelers' health
- Public health in the tropics
- Epidemiology and control of disease
- Laboratory diagnosis

More than 800 persons have passed the ASTMH examination. The society offers a periodic Intensive Update Course in Clinical Tropical Medicine and Travelers' Health, which is in part designed to prepare those planning to take the Certificate of Knowledge examination.

Wilderness Medical Society

Organized in 1983, this society (www.wms.org) focuses on adventure travel, including wilderness travel and diving medicine. Its activities include—

- The journal Wilderness and Environmental Medicine
- An annual meeting and subspecialty meetings
- Courses leading to certification in Advanced Wilderness Life Support (AWLS)
- A wilderness medical curriculum that, when successfully completed, qualifies members for Fellowship in the Academy of Wilderness Medicine (FAWM)

Infectious Diseases Society of America (IDSA)

IDSA (www.idsociety.org) is the largest organization representing infectious diseases clinicians in the United States. Although IDSA does not deal exclusively with travel medicine, it maintains a strong interest in this topic. In 2006, IDSA published extensive evidence-based guidelines on the practice of travel medicine in the United States (Box A-1). It also publishes travel-related research in its two journals.

- Journal of Infectious Diseases and Clinical Infectious Diseases
- The Practice of Travel Medicine: Guidelines by the Infectious Diseases Society of America. Clin Infect Dis. 2006;43(12):1499–1539, available at www.journals.uchicago.edu/doi/pdf/10.1086/508782.

Aerospace Medical Association

This organization (www.asma.org) represents professionals in the fields of aviation, space, and environmental medicine who deal with air and space travelers. Its activities include—

- The journal Aviation, Space, and Environmental Medicine
- An annual meeting
- Continuing medical education in topics related to aerospace medicine

While Traveling Outside the United States

Both the ISTM and ASTMH websites contain the names of non-U.S.-based clinics and health-care providers affiliated with members of these organizations. Travelers are advised to review these lists before departure to identify health-care resources at their travel destination. A number of countries have websites related to travel medicine that also provide access to health-care providers, including—

- Canada (Health Canada) (www.hc-sc.gc.ca/hl-vs/travel-voyage/index_e.html)
- Great Britain (National Travel Health Network and Centre) (www.nathnac.org)
- South Africa (South African Society of Travel Medicine) (www.sastm.org.za)
- Australia (Travel Medicine Alliance) (www.travelmedicine.com.au)

Emergency travel-related medical care and medical evacuation may be accessed through a number of private companies. One example is International SOS, which operates throughout the world. Provider locations and details may be found at www.internationalsos.com.

References

1. Hill DR, Ericsson CD, Pearson RD, et al. The practice of travel medicine: guidelines by the Infectious Diseases Society of America. Clin Infect Dis. 2006;43(12):1499–539.
2. Kozarsky P. The Body of Knowledge for the practice of travel medicine—2006. J Travel Med. 2006;13(5):251–4.
3. Spira A. Setting the standard. J Travel Med. 2003;10(1):1–3.

APPENDIX B: ESSENTIAL ELECTRONIC RESOURCES FOR THE TRAVEL MEDICINE PRACTITIONER

David O. Freedman

Selected Electronic Resources in Travel Medicine

The table below provides URLs for selected websites that have information of generally high quality that are of use to those with a primary focus on pre-travel medical preparation of the international traveler. Checking more than one authoritative website on a specific issue is always recommended. Authoritative recommendations may still contain some element of opinion, and also some sites are timelier in updating than others. Fortunately, most sites now put an indicator at the bottom of each page stating when the last update was done.

Electronic Discussion Forums and Listeservs

"Listservs" are electronic distribution lists that function by using e-mail with or without a browser-based interface. Anyone who has joined a particular listserv group can e-mail a posting to a central server. The posting is then disseminated to all members who have subscribed to the same list. Moderated listservs will have each posting reviewed and accepted by a moderator or editor; on unmoderated listservs each posting will be instantly disseminated to all other subscribers. To join one of these listservs, an e-mail message must be sent to the server, or in some cases a form can be filled out on a website that automatically generates the required e-mail. Once a person is accepted as a list member, the computer will generate, by e-mail, a list of instructions on how to participate in the discussion for that group.

- TravelMed is an unmoderated discussion of issues related to the practice of travel medicine (see www.istm.org/listserv.aspx for further information).
- TropMed is a moderated discussion of issues related to the practice of tropical medicine, with some discussion of pre-travel issues as well (see www.astmh.org/AM/Template.cfm?Section=Clinicians#CED).

Some listservs are set up to provide information only and do not allow interactive discussion. For example, with MMWR-TOC subscribers receive an e-mail each Thursday evening with the table of contents of that week's Morbidity and Mortality Weekly Report. Subscribers can then decide whether to download the whole issue from the CDC server. Similar arrangements are in place for the Emerging Infectious Diseases Journal (EID), for Eurosurveillance, and for the WHO Weekly Epidemiological Record (WER). The travel advisories listserv automatically e-mails the membership whenever a U.S. Department of State Consular Information sheet is updated or changed, or when a travel advisory or warning is issued.

The CDC website has an e-mail notification system called GovDelivery. Subscribers select topics for which to receive e-mail updates from content developers when new information about that topic is added to the CDC website. Although GovDelivery is available for many health topics, the Travelers' Health website has two topics available for subscription: 1) Homepage, News, and Announcements (Travel) and 2) Notices and Outbreaks (Travel). When new items are posted on the CDC Travelers' Health website, subscribers can receive an e-mail informing them about what items were recently added. Users can set up a profile with details such as adding a password; deleting, adding, or modifying subscription topics; and specifying how frequently e-mails are sent. For more information or to subscribe, see www.cdc.gov/emailupdates/index.html.

CDC also has RSS (Really Simple Syndication) feeds, which is another form of electronic notification of website updates. Since this system is external to e-mail accounts, to receive RSS feeds, users must have an RSS reader. Readers are available for download from commercial organizations; some are free to download and others are available for purchase. CDC Travelers' Health has two topics for feeds: 1) Travel Notices and 2) Updates to the Yellow Book. For more information, see wwwn.cdc.gov/travel/contentRss.aspx.

Table B-1. Selected websites for the travel medicine practitioner

Authoritative Travel Medicine Recommendations

CDC Travelers' Health Homepage	http://www.cdc.gov/travel
CDC Travelers' Health Yellow Book Homepage	http://www.cdc.gov/yellowbook
U.S. Department of State Country-Specific Consular Information	http://travel.state.gov/travel/cis_pa_tw/cis/cis_1765.html
World Health Organization International Travel Health Homepage	http://www.who.int/ith/en
The Practice of Travel Medicine: Guidelines by the Infectious Diseases Society of America	http://www.journals.uchicago.edu/doi/pdf/10.1086/508782

Emerging Diseases and Outbreaks

WHO Epidemic and Pandemic Alert and Response Homepage	http://www.who.int/csr/en
WHO Epidemic and Pandemic Alert and Response Disease Outbreak News	http://www.who.int/csr/don/en/

(Continued)

Table B-1. Selected websites for the travel medicine practitioner *(Continued)*

Emerging Diseases and Outbreaks *(Continued)*

WHO Epidemic and Pandemic Alert and Response Homepage Disease Links Page	http://www.who.int/csr/disease/en/
CDC Health Alert Network Message Archive	http://www2a.cdc.gov/HAN/ArchiveSys/
GeoSentinel-Surveillance Network of the International Society of Travel Medicine and CDC	http://www.geosentinel.org
ProMED-Program for Monitoring Emerging Diseases	http://www.promedmail.org/
HealthMap-Global Disease Alert Map	http://www.healthmap.org/en

Surveillance and Epidemiologic Bulletins

CDC MMWR Weekly, Recommendations and Reports, and Surveillance Summaries	http://www.cdc.gov/mmwr
WHO Weekly Epidemiological Record	http://www.who.int/wer/
Eurosurveillance	http://www.eurosurveillance.org/
PAHO Links to National Bulletins in the Americas	http://www.paho.org/English/DD/AIS/vigilancia-en.htm
US Department of Defense Global Emerging Infections System	http://www.geis.fhp.osd.mil/

Vaccine Resources

US Advisory Committee on Immunization Practices Statements on Individual Vaccines	http://www.cdc.gov/vaccines/pubs/ACIP-list.htm
Vaccine Information Statements for Patients Download Site	http://www.cdc.gov/vaccines/pubs/vis/default.htm
CDC Information on Vaccination Shortages	http://www.cdc.gov/vaccines/vac-gen/shortages/default.htm
American Academy of Pediatrics Table on Approval Status and Recommendations for New Vaccines	http://aapredbook.aappublications.org/news/vaccstatus.shtml
CDC Pink Book: Epidemiology and Prevention of Vaccine-Preventable Diseases	http://www.cdc.gov/vaccines/pubs/pinkbook/default.htm
CDC Pink Book: Appendices	http://www.cdc.gov/vaccines/pubs/pinkbook/pink-appendx.htm
Vaccines Used in U.S. and Foreign Markets	http://www.immunize.org/izpractices/p5120.pdf
Translation of Foreign Vaccine-Related Terms into English	http://www.immunize.org/izpractices/p5121.pdf
Vaccine-Preventable Disease Terms in Multiple Languages	http://www.immunize.org/izpractices/p5122.pdf
WHO Country by Country Routine Immunization Schedules	http://www.who.int/vaccines/GlobalSummary/Immunization/ScheduleSelect.cfm
U.S. Vaccine Package Inserts from the Vaccine Safety Institute	http://www.vaccinesafety.edu/package_inserts.htm
PATH Vaccine Resource Library	http://www.path.org/vaccineresources/

Consumer-Oriented Travel Health Information and Products

High Altitude	http://www.high-altitude-medicine.com/
Travel Health ONLINE	http://www.tripprep.com/
MDTravelHealth.com	http://www.mdtravelhealth.com
Chinook Medical Gear, Inc.	http://www.chinookmed.com
Magellan's, Inc.	http://www.magellans.com
Travel Medicine, Inc.	http://www.travmed.com/

(Continued)

Table B-1. Selected websites for the travel medicine practitioner *(Continued)*

Overseas Medical and Safety Assistance

U.S. Department of State Guidelines	http://travel.state.gov/travel/abroad_health.html
Overseas Security Advisory Council Reports	http://www.osac.gov/
FAA Data on Air Safety Standards in Foreign Countries	http://www.faa.gov/avr/iasa/
International Association for Medical Assistance to Travellers	http://www.iamat.org/
International SOS Assistance	http://www.intsos.com/
MedEx Insurance Worldwide Travel Assistance and International Medical Insurance	http://www.medexassist.com/

Disability Resources

MossRehab ResourceNet	http://www.mossresourcenet.org/travel.htm
Aviation Consumer Protection Divsion	http://airconsumer.ost.dot.gov/publications/horizons.htm
Society for Accessible Travel and Hospitality	http://www.sath.org/
Mobility International USA	http://www.miusa.org/

Maps and Country Information

Perry Castañeda Library Map Collection	http://www.lib.utexas.edu/Libs/PCL/Map_collection/map_sites/map_sites.html
CIA—The World Factbook	https://www.cia.gov/library/publications/the-world-factbook/
U.S. Department of State Background Notes	http://www.state.gov/r/pa/ei/bgn/
United Nations Maps	http://www.un.org/Depts/Cartographic/english/htmain.htm
Falling Rain Global Gazetteer and Place Name Altitude Finder	http://www.fallingrain.com/world/

Professional Medical Societies with a Major Focus on Travelers' Health

International Society of Travel Medicine	http://www.istm.org/
American Society of Tropical Medicine and Hygiene	http://www.astmh.org/
Divers Alert Network	http://www.diversalertnetwork.org/
Wilderness Medical Society	http://www.wms.org/
Undersea and Hyperbaric Medical Society	http://www.uhms.org/
American Travel Health Nurses Association	http://www.athna.org
Christian Medical and Dental Associations	http://www.cmdahome.org/

Disease Pages

WHO Global Health Atlas	http://www.who.int/GlobalAtlas/
CDC Diseases and Conditions A-Z List	http://www.cdc.gov/DiseasesConditions/
Oxford Malaria Atlas Project	http://www.map.ox.ac.uk/MAP_overview.html
CDC Influenza Home Page	http://www.cdc.gov/flu/
Global Polio Eradication Initiative	http://www.polioeradication.org/
PAHO Malaria	http://www.paho.org/english/ad/dpc/cd/malaria.htm
PAHO Dengue	http://www.paho.org/english/ad/dpc/cd/dengue.htm

General Travel Aids

Embassies in the United States	http://www.state.gov/s/cpr/rls/
Embassies in the United States Web Links	http://www.embassy.org/embassies/index.html
Times around the World	http://www.timeanddate.com/worldclock/
Tourism Offices Worldwide	http://www.towd.com/

(Continued)

Table B-1. Selected websites for the travel medicine practitioner *(Continued)*

General Travel Aids *(Continued)*

Visa Plus-ATM Locator	http://visa.via.infonow.net/locator/global/jsp/SearchPage.jsp
Mastercard Cirrus ATM Locator	http://www.mastercard.com/cardholderservices/atm/

U.S. Organizations Offering Training in Travel Medicine

International Society of Travel Medicine	http://www.istm.org/
American Society of Tropical Medicine and Hygiene	http://www.astmh.org/
Gorgas Memorial Institute	http://www.gorgas.org
Tulane Department of Tropical Medicine	http://www.sph.tulane.edu/tropmed/
University of Washington School of Medicine	http://depts.washington.edu/cme/home/

References

1. Freedman DO. Sources of travel medicine information. In: Keystone JS, Kozarsky PE, Freedman DO, Nothdurft HD, Connor BA, editors. Travel medicine. 2nd ed. Philadelphia: Mosby; 2008. p. 29–34.

2. Keystone JS, Kozarsky PE, Freedman DO. Internet and computer-based resources for travel medicine practitioners. Clin Infect Dis. 2001;32(5):757–65.

APPENDIX C: TRAVEL VACCINE SUMMARY TABLE

David R. Shlim

Table C-1 is a quick reference for administering or prescribing travel-related vaccines. Before administering, please review detailed instructions, precautions, and side effects under the specific vaccines discussed in this book or in the manufacturer's package insert.

Table C-1. Travel vaccine summary

Vaccine	Dose	Route	Schedule	Booster	Age
Hepatitis A (HAVRIX)	1.0 mL (1440 ELISA units)	IM	0 and 6–12 months	None	Ages 19 years or older
Hepatitis A (HAVRIX) pediatric	0.5 mL (720 ELISA units)	IM	0 and 6–12 months	None	Ages 1–18 years
Hepatitis A (VAQTA)	1.0 mL (50 units)	IM	0 and 6–18 months	None	Ages 19 years or older
Hepatitis A (VAQTA) pediatric	0.5 mL (25 units)	IM	0 and 6–18 months	None	Ages 1–18 years
Combined hepatitis A and hepatitis B (TWINRIX)	1.0 mL (20 µg of hepatitis B antigen and 720 ELISA units of hepatitis A antigen)	IM	0, 1 month, and 6 months	None	Ages 18 years or older
Combined hepatitis A and hepatitis B (TWINRIX), accelerated schedule	1.0 mL (20 µg of hepatitis B antigen and 720 ELISA units of hepatitis A antigen)	IM	Days 0, 7, and 21, with a fourth dose at 12 months	None	Ages 18 years or older

(Continued)

Table C-1. Travel vaccine summary *(Continued)*

Vaccine	Dose	Route	Schedule	Booster	Age
Japanese encephalitis (JE-VAX)[1]	0.5 mL for ages 1–2 years; 1.0 mL for ages 3 years or older	SQ	Days 0, 7, and 30	3 years[2]	Ages 1 year or older
Meningococcal conjugate (Menactra)	0.5 mL	IM	1 dose	>5 years[3]	Ages 2–55 years
Meningococcal polysaccharide (Menomune)	0.5 mL	SQ	1 dose	3 years, if vaccinated before 4 years of age; 5 years, if vaccinated at >4 years of age	Ages 2 years or older
Inactivated polio (Adult)	0.5 mL	SQ or IM	One dose at >18 years of age, if patient has already had an acceptable polio vaccine series	None	Age 18 years or older[4]
Rabies (IMOVAX)	1.0 mL	IM	Pre-exposure series: Days 0, 7, and 28	See the Rabies section in Chapter 2	No age restrictions
Rabies (RabAvert)	1.0 mL	IM	Pre-exposure series: Days 0, 7, and 28	See the Rabies section in Chapter 2	No age restrictions
Typhoid capsular polysaccharide (Typhim Vi)	0.5 mL	IM	1 dose	Every 2 years	Ages 2 years or older
Typhoid oral (Vivotif)	1 pill	Orally	1 pill every other day for 4 doses	Every 5 years	Ages 6 years or older
Yellow fever (YF-VAX)	0.5 mL	SQ	1 dose	Every 10 years	Never give to infants <6 months of age. Give only under special circumstances for ages 6–8 months. Ages 9 months or older, same dose for children and adults[5]

ELISA, Enzyme-Linked ImmunoSorbent Assay; IM, intramuscular; SQ, subcutaneous.

1 This vaccine is no longer manufactured, and current supplies are limited. A new JE vaccine (IC-51, trade name Ixiaro) may be approved and available by 2009. However, the new vaccine will not initially be approved for children aged <18, and JE-VAX will still be the vaccine of choice for this age group as long as it remains available.

2 Booster recommendations beyond the first booster have not been established. Most authorities recommend every 3 years if the traveler remains at risk.

3 Booster recommendations have not been established.

4 For catch-up immunization in pediatric population, see Table 7-4.

5 Special considerations apply in deciding whether to administer yellow fever vaccine. Please review the Yellow Fever section in Chapter 2 before administration.

Index

Note: Page numbers followed by the letter b refer to boxes; those followed by the letter f refer to figures; those followed by the letter m refer to maps; and those followed by the letter t refer to tables.

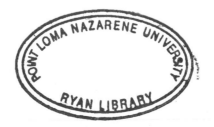